A Textbook of Veterinary Special Pathology

Infectious Diseases of Livestock and Poultry

J.L. Vegad

Former Professor & Head,
Department of Pathology,
College of Veterinary Science & Animal Husbandry,
Jabalpur - 482 001

A.K. Katiyar

Associate Professor & Head,
Department of Pathology,
College of Veterinary Science & Animal Husbandry,
Jabalpur - 482 001

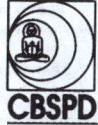

CBSPD

CBS Publishers & Distributors Pvt Ltd

New Delhi • Bengaluru • Chennai • Kochi • Kolkata • Lucknow • Mumbai
Hyderabad • Jharkhand • Nagpur • Patna • Pune • Uttarakhand

Disclaimer

Science and technology are constantly changing fields. New research and experience broaden the scope of information and knowledge. The authors have tried their best in giving information available to them while preparing the material for this book. Although all efforts have been made to ensure optimum accuracy of the material, yet it is quite possible some errors might have been left uncorrected. The publisher, the printer and the authors will not be held responsible for any inadvertent errors, omissions or inaccuracies.

A Textbook of Veterinary Special Pathology

ISBN: 978-81-239-2788-6

Copyright © Publisher

First CBS Reprint: 2015
Reprint: 2016, 2017, 2018, 2019, 2021, 2023, **2025**

Published by **Satish Kumar Jain** and produced by **Varun Jain** for

CBS Publishers & Distributors Pvt Ltd

4819/XI Prahlad Street, 24 Ansari Road, Daryaganj, New Delhi 110 002, India.
Ph: 011-23266838, 23289259   Website: www.cbspd.com
e-mail: delhi@cbspd.com

Corporate Office: 204 FIE, Industrial Area, Patparganj, Delhi 110 092
Ph: 011-4934 4934   Fax: 011-4934 4935
e-mail: publishing@cbspd.com; publicity@cbspd.com

Branches

- **Bengaluru:** Seema House 2975, 17th Cross, KR Road, Banasankari 2nd Stage, Bengaluru 560 070, Karnataka, India
  Ph: +91-80-26771678/79   Fax: +91-80-26771680   e-mail: bangalore@cbspd.com
- **Chennai:** 18/8B, Subbarayan Street, Shenoy Nagar, Chennai 600 030, Tamil Nadu, India
  Ph: +91-44-42032115, 26681266   e-mail: chennai@cbspd.com
- **Kochi:** 42/1325, 1326, Power House Road, Opp KSEB, Power House, Ernakulum Kochi 682 018, Kerala, India
  Ph: +91-484-4059061-65,67   Fax: +91-484-4059065   e-mail: kochi@cbspd.com
- **Kolkata:** 147, Hind Ceramics Compound, 1st Floor, Nilgunj Road, Belghoria, Kolkata-700056, West Bengal, India
  Ph: +033-25633055, 033-25633056   e-mail: kolkata@cbspd.com
- **Lucknow:** Basement, Khushnuma Complex, 7 Meerabai Marg (Behind Jawahar Bhawan), Lucknow-226001, UP, India
  Ph: +0522-4000032   e-mail: tiwari.lucknow@cbspd.com
- **Mumbai:** PWD Shed, Gala no 25/26, Ramchandra Bhatt Marg, Next to JJ Hospital Gate no. 2, Opp. Union Bank of India, Noorbaug, Mumbai-400009, Maharashtra, India
  Ph: 022-66661880/89   e-mail: mumbai@cbspd.com

Representatives

• Hyderabad	0-9885175004	• Jharkhand	0-9811541605	• Nagpur	0-8692091830
• Patna	0-9334159340	• Pune	0-9664372571	• Uttarakhand	0-9716462459

Printed at Neekunj Print Process, Sonipat, Haryana, India

About the Authors

DR. J.L. VEGAD was Professor and Head, Department of Veterinary Pathology at Jawaharlal Nehru Krishi Vishwa Vidyalaya, Jabalpur, for 25 years, and taught pathology for 37 years. He then also worked as Professor Emeritus of the ICAR for two years. He obtained Ph.D. from New Zealand (1968) under a Commonwealth Scholarship. His contributions to the study of acute inflammatory response in the Sheep and the Chicken are pioneering. He has published more than 150 research papers, 60 of them in British, American and New Zealand journals. Three of his Ph.D. students received the 'Jawaharlal Nehru Award' of the ICAR. In 1988-89, he was a Visiting Professor at the University of California, Davis, U.S.A. He is on the editorial Board of 'Comparative Haematology International' for the past ten years; and has recently contributed a chapter on 'buffalo haematology' in the 5th edition (2000) of Schalm's Veterinary Hematology. He has the distinction of receiving the 'Rafi Ahmed Kidwai Memorial Award' of the ICAR, New Delhi. Dr. Vegad is the author of 'A Textbook of Veterinary General Pathology' and 'A Textbook of Veterinary Systemic Pathology'; and is also President of the Indian Association of Veterinary Pathologists.

DR. A.K. KATIYAR is Associate Professor and Head, Department of Veterinary Pathology, Jawaharlal Nehru Krishi Vishwa Vidyalaya, Jabalpur. For the past 33 years, he has been teaching pathology to undergraduate and postgraduate students. He obtained M.V.Sc. (Gold Medalist) from Mhow and Ph.D. (Honours) from Jabalpur. His main research contributions are to the study of inflammatory and reparative responses in the chicken; and is currently engaged in the study of inflammation in the buffalo. He has contributed 65 research papers, 16 of them in British journals, including one review article in the 'Veterinary Bulletin'. Dr. Katiyar is also co-author of 'A Textbook of Veterinary Systemic Pathology.

PREFACE

This book is a continuation of our earlier two works: "**A Textbook of Veterinary G eneral Pathology by J. L. Vegad**" and "**A Textbook o f Veterinary Systemic Pathology by J. L. Vegad and A. K. Katiyar**". Greatly encouraged b y the r esponse o f t hese two p ublications, from s tudents and teachers alike, w e embarked on the daunting task of writing this third book with a triple objective. Firstly, to complete the unfinished portion of infectious diseases, thereby covering the entire subject of veterinary pathology. Secondly, to put d iseases of d omestic animals a nd poultry t ogether at o ne place. W e believe that this combined information would be most helpful to the students, and would also save them from the burden of buying books on poultry diseases. Thirdly, to offer a book that caters for the requirements of our students - one that is easy to follow, also deals with diseases under Indian conditions, and is of a n a ffordable p rice. Foreign books being too expensive are beyond t he reach of most students.

In recent years there has been a tremendous upsurge in our understanding of the p athogenesis of i nfectious diseases. A n emphasis h as therefore b een given on the molecular mechanisms involved. The diseases have been discussed in a pattern that includes introduction, cause, spread, pathogenesis, c linical signs, gross a nd microscopic c hanges, zoonotic i mportance, and d iagnosis. Infections caused b y all c lasses o f p athogen have been covered, including those of prion. For an easy comprehension, all chapters include a brief review of general considerations, elements in the production of an infectious disease, evasion of t he immune r esponse by t he pathogen, a nd the host reaction. A special feature o f the b ook is t hat important p ortions in e ach chapter h ave been put in bold letters for a better grasp of the subject. Emphasis has been given on clarity of writing, as lucidity enhances understanding and facilitates learning. S incere e fforts have b een made t o achieve as much b revity as i s compatible w ith the t horoughness a nd sufficient d iscussion to permit e asy understanding. The abbreviations used are 'L' for Latin and 'G' for Greek.

We hope the information provided proves very useful to both undergraduate and postgraduate students, the teaching c ommunity, and also the f ield veterinarians, p articularly those w orking in the field o f disease diagnosis. Discussion on poultry diseases would be especially helpful to the poultry diagnosticians and even to the enlightened poultry farmers. The book also refers to the diseases of wildlife. Besides, wherever considered appropriate, comparative a spects of human diseases h ave been n arrated side b y side, highlighting the zoonotic implications. As such the book may also serve as a good reference for the medical personnel.

We are grateful to Shri Suneel Gomber, Manager, International Book Distributing Co., Lucknow, for the publication of this book. We like to extend our sincere thanks to Dr. Madhu Swamy for going through the manuscript. We are, especially grateful to Dr. A. S. Panisup, Senior Scientist, In charge Pathology Laboratory, National Research Centre on Equines, Hisar (Haryana) for providing valuable information on equine diseases. Dr. A. B. Shrivastava was helpful in furnishing information pertaining to wildlife. Shri Phillip Francis did an excellent job of typing. Shri Sharad Vegad, Shri Anand Parmar and Shri Vijay Parmar of Jabalpur Graphics, Dr. N. K. Jain, Dr. S. Suresh of Phoenix Group, Ku. Neeti Katiyar, and Shri Amit Vegad were most generous in extending help relating to computer and other work. Finally, it is indeed a great pleasure to express our profound appreciation to members of our families, especially to Smt. Nita Vegad and Smt. Indra Katiyar for their tolerance and understanding.

J. L. Vegad

A. K. Katiyar

CONTENTS

CONTENTS

Viral Diseases

Viruses are submicroscopic infectious agents. That is, they are too small to be seen in an ordinary light microscope. They are among the smallest and simplest of all life forms. Other micro-organisms, such as bacteria, **Mycoplasma**, **Chlamydia** and **Rickettsia** species, and protozoa contain DNA, ribosomes and cytoplasmic organelles. They all multiply by binary fission. **Viruses, in contrast, are not cells**. They are little more than bundles of genes - strands of DNA or RNA - the molecules that carry the blueprints (detailed schemes) for all life. In other words, **they contain only one type of nucleic acid, DNA or RNA**, double-stranded or single-stranded. They have no ribosomes, or cytoplasmic organelles, and do not multiply by binary fission.

Until a virus enters a cell, it is more dead than alive. Alone, a virus cannot reproduce. It is as lifeless as a speck of dust. Viruses are obligate intracellular parasites. That is, they depend on host-cell machinery for protein synthesis and replication (multiplication). They are essentially nucleoprotein entities, or genetic elements surrounded by a protective coat. They are capable of passing these genetic elements from one cell to another. In other words, at its core (centre), a virus is pure information, encoded in the molecules of DNA or RNA.

The interaction between virus and host cell determines whether the relationship is going to be harmful (pathogenic) or not. Most viral infections are subclinical. That is, infection does not lead to overt (open) disease. **Viruses, however, are responsible for most important and often fatal infections of domestic animals and poultry,** such as rinderpest, swine fever, canine distemper, Ranikhet disease, and infectious bursal disease, as well as certain neoplastic conditions. The result of infection depends on many factors. These include the nature of the specific virus and its cell tropism, genetic resistance of the species or breed affected, and immune response, age, nutritional status, and hormone levels of the individual animal/bird affected.

Classification and Nomenclature of Viruses

The biochemical, ultrastructural, and molecular characteristics of viruses form the basis of their classification. Many classification systems for viruses have been employed; and schemes for their classification are still evolving.

The **tropism (affinity)** of viruses for specific tissues is one of the characteristics that has been used in grouping similar viruses. This led to their classification as **neurotropic, epitheliotropic, pneumotropic,** and **other designations**. This feature, however, is variable, because many viruses infect numerous types of tissue. Tropism may also vary depending on the species affected, age of the animal, and other circumstances.

The **two principal characteristics used in the current classification are virion morphology and nucleic acid type**. These are supplemented with other characteristics, such as mode of replication, cell tropism, means of transmission, antigenicity, susceptibility to physical and chemical agents, and clinical and pathological effects. Using these parameters, viruses are grouped into families, sub-families, genera, and species. Families are designated by adding suffix **"-viridae"**, sub-families by **"-virinae"**, and genera by **"-virus"**. Virus families, grouped on the basis of main characteristics, are presented in **Table 1.**

Table 1. Classification of viruses according to genetic characteristics

Characteristics	Family	Example
Single-stranded RNA (ss RNA)		
Enveloped		
No DNA in replication	Coronaviridae	Transmissible gastroenteritis virus
Positive-sense genome		
	Togaviridae	Swine fever virus
Negative-sense genome	Bunyaviridae	Rift Valley fever virus
	Orthomyxoviridae	Influenza virus
	Paramyxoviridae	Canine distemper virus
	Rhabdoviridae	Rabies virus
DNA step in replication	Retroviridae	Feline leukaemia virus
Non-enveloped	Caliciviridae	Vesicular exanthema virus
	Picornaviridae	Foot-and-mouth disease virus
Double-stranded RNA (ds RNA)		
Enveloped	Nil	
Non-enveloped	Birnaviridae	Gumboro disease virus
	Reoviridae	Bluetongue disease virus
Single-stranded DNA (ss DNA)		
Enveloped	Nil	
Non-enveloped	Circoviridae	Chicken anaemia virus
	Parvoviridae	Feline panleukopaenia virus
Double-stranded DNA (ds DNA)		
Enveloped	Herpesviridae	Pseudorabies, infectious bovine rhinotracheitis virus
	Poxviridae	Cowpox, swinepox viruses
Non-enveloped	Adenoviridae	Bovine adenovirus
	Iridoviridae	African swine fever virus
	Papovaviridae	Shope papilloma virus

Structure

Each 'virus-particle' (virion) has a central core of DNA (deoxyribonucleic acid) or RNA (ribonucleic acid), surrounded by a protein coat called the **capsid** (Fig. 1). The capsid is composed of a large number of units, called **capsomeres**. The nucleic acid core and its capsid, together, are referred to as **nucleocapsid**. The nucleocapsid may be surrounded by a lipoprotein **envelope (peplos)**, or may lack this envelope ('**naked**'). The envelope is derived from nuclear or cytoplasmic membranes of the cell in which the virion is produced. Basically, the envelope is a phospholipid bilayer in which are embedded specific proteins. The phospholipids are similar to those of the host cell. Radially arranged (i.e., arranged like rays) structures (**peplomers**) may project from the outer surface of the envelope (**Fig. 1**). The **envelope** is, therefore, made up of an **inner lipid layer**, a **protein coat**, and **peplomers** as the **outermost layer**. Some virions may have more than one envelope.

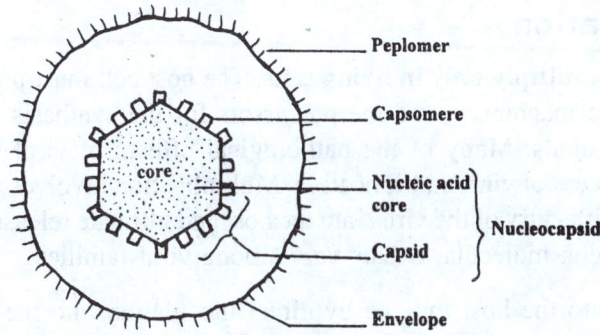

Fig. 1. Schematic diagram showing the structure of a complete virus particle (the virion).

The nucleocapsid of the virion contains the **genome** (genetic material) of the virus. The envelope contains the specific material which determines the **viral antigenicity**, and interacts with receptor sites on the cell membrane of the host cell to initiate infection.

Virions (virus-particles) range in size from the large poxvirus, measuring **300 nm** by 250 nm by 100 nm, to the parvoviruses, which are only 20 nm in diameter (**Table 2**). The shape of the virion is determined by the organization of the capsid and its relationship to the central core of nucleic acid. **Two basic groups** of structures or **symmetries** are recognized: (1) **icosahedral** or **cubic symmetry** in which condensed nucleic acid is surrounded by a capsid in the form of a 20-faceted (faced) icosahedron [G. icosa = twenty + hedron]. Thus, icosahedron is a polyhedron having 20 faces. [A hedron is a geometrical figure having a specified number of surfaces/faces]. Each facet (face) is composed of a specific number of capsomeres, depending on the virus group. (2) **helical, spiral**, or **screw symmetry** in which the nucleic acid and capsomeres are bound together forming filamentous or rod-like particles.

Table 2. Various classes of pathogens and their size

Taxonomic class	Size
Viruses	18 - 450 nm*
Mycoplasmas	300 - 800 nm
Chlamydiae	200 - 1500 nm
Rickettsiae	490 - 2700 nm
Bacteria, spirochaetes, mycobacteria	0.8 - 30 μm**
Fungi	5 - 300 μm
Protozoa	1 - 50 μm
Helminths	3 mm - 10 m

* One nanometre = One billionth of a metre
**One micrometre = One millionth of a metre

Multiplication

Viruses multiply only in living cells. The host cell must provide the energy and synthetic machinery, and the precursors for the synthesis of viral proteins and nucleic acids. Many of the pathological effects of viral infections result from the process of viral multiplication. Multiplication involves a series of events beginning with entry of the virus into the host and ultimate release of new **virions**. The in-between molecular events vary among viral families.

Entry into the host may be by direct inoculation into the bloodstream, as occurs with arthropod-borne viruses (e.g., **Togaviridae**). However, most viruses enter by penetrating the skin, or mucosal barrier of the respiratory or gastrointestinal tract. If the portal (route) of entry is the target organ, further transport is not necessary. However, many viruses must be transported to their final site of replication and disease production. This may involve primary replication in cells at the portal of entry, and then spread through the lymphatics or the bloodstream (e.g., with certain herpesviruses), direct spread through lymphatics or bloodstream (e.g., with reoviruses), spread through infected lymphocytes (e.g., with cytomegaloviruses), or spread through neuronal axons (e.g., with rhabdoviruses, which cause rabies). Vertical transmission provides another mechanism of entry. Viruses may cross the placenta to the foetus (e.g., with cytomegalovirus), or be carried as part of the germplasm (e.g., with certain retroviruses).

General steps in a virus replication cycle include:

Attachment

The first step in virus infection is interaction of a **virus particle** (virion) with a specific **receptor** site on the surface of a cell. That is, attachment to cells involves specific binding of virus to the cell surface. **The presence or absence of specific** receptors accounts for the susceptibility of a given cell type or types, or the tissue tropism of the virus. Entry of a virus does not mean infection. This is because certain species (i.e., animals/birds) lack appropriate receptors for specific viruses.

Penetration

After binding, the virus particle is taken up inside the cell. This step is referred to as **penetration, engulfment,** or **viropexis.** Penetration occurs immediately following attachment. With enveloped viruses, the virion envelope fuses with the plasma membrane allowing entry of the nucleocapsid. Non-enveloped viruses enter by receptor-mediated endocytosis (pinocytosis) of the virion, or by translocation (change of location) of the virion across the plasma membrane.

Uncoating

After penetration, the virion is **uncoated.** That is, the RNA or DNA of the virus particle is exposed by removal of the capsid (protein coat). The infectivity of the virus is lost at this point. The process is mostly dependent on cellular enzymes. Uncoating is followed by the **"eclipse phase"**, when no virions are seen. Infection of a cell (attachment and penetration), does not necessarily lead to viral multiplication and cell damage. For a productive infection, the cell must be **permissive. That is, it should have appropriate receptors and be capable of supporting replication.** Entry does not necessarily mean permissiveness. **Non-productive infection** may also occur from infection by defective viruses. **A defective virus** is one that is functionally defective in some aspect of replication. That is, viruses may enter a cell and their RNA or DNA may persist in the cell without a productive infection. The RNA or DNA may or may not get incorporated into the cell genome, but it continues to persist. Such persistent infections may, under appropriate circumstances, get activated to **productive infection,** or lead to **cell transformation.**

Multiplication

The most essential step in virus replication is that specific messenger RNAs (mRNAs) must be transcribed from the viral nucleic acid for successful expression and duplication of genetic information. **Transcription** is the mechanism by which specific information encoded in a nucleic acid chain is transferred to the mRNA. (The enzyme which brings about transcription is known as **transcriptase**). In other words, viral multiplication involves expression of viral genes, leading to replication of the viral genome **and production of new virions.** Once transcription is achieved, viruses use cell components to translate the mRNA. **Translation** is the mechanism by which a particular base sequence in mRNA results in production of a specific amino acid sequence in a protein.

The process of transcription varies with the type of viral nucleic acid, enzymes carried within the virion, and the intracellular location of the virus. **That is, various**

classes of viruses use different pathways to synthesize the mRNA, depending upon the structure of the viral nucleic acid. With the exception of single-stranded **positive-sense** RNA viruses, **in which viral RNA can serve directly as messenger RNA,** all viral nucleic acid must be transcribed to mRNA. DNA viruses that replicate in the nucleus use host RNA polymerase (i.e., transcriptase) for transcription to mRNA, **whereas all other viruses depend on transcriptases carried within the virion.** Some viruses, such as orthomyxo-, paramyxo- and rhabdoviruses, which are single-stranded RNA viruses, carry RNA polymerases (transcriptases) to synthesize mRNAs. RNA viruses of this type are called **negative-sense (negative-strand)** viruses, since their single-strand RNA genome is complementary to mRNA, which is designated **positive-sense (positive-strand).** With this background, multiplication of various classes of viruses will be discussed, briefly.

Multiplication of Single-Stranded RNA (ss RNA) Viruses

Multiplication of single-stranded RNA viruses may occur in one of the following three ways:

1. **Positive (+) strand viruses: Togaviruses** and **picornaviruses are positive (+) strand viruses.** Positive (+) strand viruses are those viruses **in which viral RNA can serve directly as mRNA.** In other words, nucleotide sequences of RNA are directly translated. After infecting a cell, viral RNA links to ribosomes and is directly translated to proteins. The viral RNA gives rise to a polymerase which allows direct synthesis of a complementary negative (-) strand RNA from the parental (+) strand. The (-) strand then serves as a template for synthesis of additional (+) strands, which in turn can repeat the process and ultimately form viral progeny. Since replication does not depend on any enzyme carried by the virion, RNA extracted from (+) strand RNA viruses is **infectious.**

2. **Negative (-) strand viruses: Arenaviruses, bunyaviruses, orthomyxoviruses, paramyxoviruses** and **rhabdoviruses are negative (-) strand viruses.** The first step in their multiplication requires that viral RNA be transcribed into a (+) mRNA. This step depends on **a transcriptase carried within the virion.** Translation products of the mRNA then serve to allow transcription of (-) strand virion RNA into a complementary (+) strand, which serves as a template for synthesis of (-) strand virion RNA for assembly into progeny. In contrast to (+) strand RNA viruses, RNA extracted from (-) strand RNA viruses is **not infectious, since replication depends on virion transcriptase.**

3. **Retroviruses: These viruses have a DNA step in replication.** Their viral RNA serves as a template for the synthesis of viral DNA. This step depends on the enzyme **reverse transcriptase** (RNA-dependent DNA-polymerase) **carried within the virion.** Viral RNA is then digested by a RNA nuclease, also carried by the virion, and a complementary copy of viral DNA is made. This results in the formation of **double-stranded DNA, which is integrated into cellular DNA.** Viral multiplication results from transcription (by host cell transcriptase)

of integrated viral DNA into complementary viral RNA. Positive (+) mRNA, which codes for the necessary protein to be packaged along with the viral RNA into viral progeny, is also produced.

Multiplication of Double-Stranded RNA (ds RNA) Viruses

This is represented by **reoviruses** which are double-stranded RNA viruses. Their RNA is transcribed by **virion polymerase**. The (-) strand of the genome is transcribed into (+) strand mRNA, which is translated into viral proteins and enzymes. The same (+) strands serve as templates for transcription into complementary negative (-) strands, yielding double-stranded RNA for assembly into virions.

DNA viruses also have **several methods of multiplication**. These are:

Multiplication of Single-Stranded DNA (ss DNA) Viruses

Single-stranded (DNA) parvoviruses replicate in the nucleus. They depend on host cell enzymes for synthesis of complementary DNA to form double-stranded DNA. This, in turn, is transcribed into mRNA and genomic DNA.

Multiplication of Double-Stranded DNA (ds DNA) Viruses

The double-stranded DNA of **papovavirus, adenovirus**, and **herpesvirus** is transported in the virion to the **nucleus**, in which cellular enzymes are used for production of mRNA. Replication of DNA uses host-cell polymerase in the case of papovaviruses, whereas' herpesviruses and adenoviruses use virally coded polymerase. A large number of virally coded proteins, which are made in the cytoplasm, are involved in the multiplication and assembly process. **Poxvirus multiplication occurs in the cytoplasm**. The virion is uncoated by both cellular enzymes and enzyme products of an early transcribed mRNA. Cytoplasmic DNA replication is under the control of enzymes carried within the virion and translation products of early and late mRNA.

Release of New Virions

Non-enveloped viruses mature within the host cell, either in nucleus or cytoplasm, **and depend on cell lysis for their release. Enveloped viruses** obtain their surrounding membranes by budding. Budding may result in the **release of virus without causing cell lysis**. All negative-strand RNA viruses, togaviruses and retroviruses are released through **budding**. That is, the virion is extruded through the cell membrane, which along with some viral proteins becomes the virion envelope. Retroviruses and arenaviruses bud without causing cell damage. That is, they are **non-cytolytic**. Other budding viruses, such as togaviruses, paramyxoviruses, and rhabdoviruses, however, are cytolytic.

Poxviruses are released by both mechanisms. Intracellular virions develop a membrane and acquire an envelope from Golgi apparatus, which fuses with the plasma membrane releasing virions with a double-layered envelope. Most poxvirus virions, however, are released without an envelope on disruption of the cell. **Both**

types of particles are infectious. However, those released by budding more readily attach to host cells. Herpesviruses, in contrast to all other enveloped viruses, acquire their envelope from the inner lamella of the nuclear membrane. These enveloped v irions pass within cisternae, without contact with the cytoplasm, to the cell surface and are released. This allows viral release without cell disruption. However, productive herpesvirus infection is always cytolytic.

Cellular Injury

Once a virus has entered a susceptible and **permissive cell** (i.e., a cell with appropriate receptors and one which can support replication), **the effect on the cell varies with the nature of the interaction between virus and cell**. Basically, there are **three types of interaction**: 1) cytocidal, 2) infection without apparent pathological effect, and 3) cell transformation.

1) **Cytocidal viruses cause cell lysis or necrosis**, a feature of many herpesviruses, picornaviruses, parvoviruses, adenoviruses and flaviviruses. All the mechanisms that lead to cell death are not fully understood, but they are related to alterations in host-cell metabolism. **Viruses do not generate toxins like bacteria**. However, protein products coded for and produced by the virus, such as **capsid proteins, are often toxic**. Moreover, **the coding of viral proteins results in a shutdown (stoppage) of host protein synthesis, and ultimately of host DNA and RNA synthesis, which is incompatible with cell survival**.

2) **Non-cytocidal viruses cause infection without apparent cytopathic effect (CPE)**. This may take two forms : 1) **Persistent infection**, and 2) **latent infection. In persistent infection**, viral replication and release take place **without killing the cell**. This occurs in infection with arenaviruses and retroviruses. Virions are released by budding without cellular damage. Another form of persistent infection is called **chronic infection**. After recovery from acute disease, in which cell lysis may be an important outcome of the host cell-virion interaction, virus is not eliminated from the host, but remains within selected populations of cells and continues to be reproduced at low levels. **These chronic infections may result in:** 1) infectious carriers as is the case with foot-and-mouth disease, 2) chronic disease, as seen in African swine fever, or 3) in disease appearing several years after the initial infection, a s s een in canine d istemper encephalitis (old dog encephalitis).

Latent viral infection differs from persistent infection in that the virion genome resides in the cell but there is no replication of the virus. A ll herpesviruses (alpha, beta, gamma) establish latent infections following initial exposure. **The alpha or neurotropic herpesviruses,** such as infectious bovine rhinotracheitis virus and herpesvirus simplex, enter neurons in cranial or spinal ganglia through axons, **in which they reside as episomal DNA, probably for**

the life of the host. Under appropriate circumstances, the latent virus can be **reactivated**, in which case virions move down to axons and enter a productive cycle in epithelial cells. This results in shedding of virus, and in some cases, overt (visible) lesions and disease. **Beta herpesviruses** (cytomegaloviruses) establish latent infection in epithelial cells of secretory glands, the kidneys and lymphoreticular cells. **Gamma herpesviruses** (lymphotropic herpesviruses) usually establish latent infections in lymphoid cells.

Slow virus infection represents a special form of persistent infection. It is restricted to viral infections with very long incubation periods that result in slowly progressive fatal disease. Examples include lentiviruses (e.g., maedi/visna virus, human immunodeficiency virus - HIV) and the "viruses" causing scrapie, mink encephalopathy, and chronic wasting disease of mule deer and elk. **Lentiviruses are retroviruses**.

Cell lysis also occurs following an immune response to virus-infected cells. Most viruses, both cytocidal and non-cytocidal, impart new antigens to the surface of infected cells, that are recognized by host as foreign. **A cell-mediated immune response** brought about by specifically sensitive **cytotoxic T lymphocytes** leads to destruction of virus infected cells. **This is one of the most important defence mechanisms in viral disease**. The destruction of infected cells limits the release and spread of new virions. **Natural killer (NK) cells** may also play a role in lysis of virus-infected cells, as may antibody and complement. The importance of these mechanisms in resistance to and recovery from viral infections is exemplified by the seriousness of viral disease in immunodeficiencies, particularly those affecting T cell functions.

A cytopathic effect (CPE) of great diagnostic importance is the formation of **inclusion bodies**. Although not a feature of all viral infections, they are characteristic of many. **Inclusion bodies consist of aggregates of virions and viral proteins**. In most replicating cycles, surplus of viral proteins do not assemble into virions. **Inclusion bodies may be intranuclear, intracytoplasmic, basophilic, or eosionphilic**. They are **intranuclear** in herpesvirus, adenovirus, and parvovirus infections; and **intracytoplasmic** in poxvirus, paramyxovirus, reovirus, and rhabdovirus infections. Certain viruses induce **both intranuclear and cytoplasmic inclusion bodies**, such as the viruses causing canine distemper and measles, and often, cytomegaloviruses. The relative proportions of virions and proteins vary between viral infections. Adenovirus inclusion bodies are aggregates of **virions (basophilic)**, or of **viral proteins (eosinophilic)**. Herpesvirus inclusion bodies contain a mixture of virions and viral protein.

Syncytial cell formation, such as multinucleated cells, polykaryocytes, is another **cytopathic effect** of certain viral infections. Syncytial cells are a regular and often diagnostically important feature of herpesvirus and paramyxovirus lesions.

3) **Cell transformation:** Certain viruses have the ability to transform *in vitro* normal cells to cells with characteristics of cancer cells, or to induce tumours in animals either naturally or experimentally. They are referred to as **oncogenic viruses** and include both DNA and RNA viruses. DNA viruses capable of inducing tumours include polyomaviruses, papillomaviruses, adenoviruses, herpesviruses, and hepatitis B-like viruses. Cell transformation by DNA viruses is non-productive, as viral progeny are not produced. Under appropriate settings, however, oncogenic herpesviruses, polyomaviruses, and adenoviruses may induce productive infection, causing cell death. In transformed cells, the DNA of polyomaviruses, adenoviruses, and hepatitis virus is integrated into cellular DNA. The RNA tumour viruses are members of the retrovirus family and are collectively known as **oncornaviruses.** In contrast to DNA tumour viruses, oncornaviruses simultaneously transform cells during a productive, but non-cytocidal, infection. The viral genome becomes integrated into host-cell DNA as a DNA copy of viral RNA.

After this general consideration, a discussion of various viral diseases will now follow. **The diseases will be taken up in the same order as listed in Table 1.** That is, **first,** diseases caused by the families of **single-stranded RNA viruses** will be presented, **followed by double-stranded RNA virus families, single-stranded DNA virus families, and double-stranded DNA virus families.**

Diseases caused by Single-Stranded RNA (ss RNA) Families

Coronaviridae

The viruses of this family consist of one molecule of **single-stranded, enveloped, positive-sense RNA.** The family is so named because unique club-shaped peplomers, which project from the outer surface of the envelope, give the appearance of a **c**rown in negatively stained electron micrographs (L. **corona = c**rown). The virions (virus particles) are pleomorphic, averaging about 100 nm in diameter.

Virion (viral) RNA acts as mRNA, first producing a RNA polymerase, which forms a minus strand template that serves to make new positive-sense virion RNA. **Replication occurs in the cytoplasm.** The envelope is acquired by budding through internal cytoplasmic membranes of endoplasmic reticulum and the Golgi apparatus. The virions are then transported in vesicles to the cell membrane for release.

Coronavirus

Important diseases caused by coronaviruses include :

Transmissible gastroenteritis of swine

Porcine coronaviral encephalomyelitis
Feline infectious peritonitis
Calf neonatal diarrhoea
Canine coronavirus infection
Avian infectious bronchitis
Turkey bluecomb disease

Transmissible Gastroenteritis of Swine

First described in 1946, transmissible gastroenteritis of **pigs** (TGE) is a highly contagious viral disease, e specially in **young pigs**. Clinically, the disease i s characterized by vomiting, diarrhoea, dehydration and a high mortality rate, **often 100% in piglets under 2 weeks of age.**

Cause

The causative agent is a **coronavirus**. This virus is different from another porcine coronavirus, the haemagglutinating encephalomyelitis virus of piglets, which agglutinates *in vitro* the red blood cells of chicks and rats. **The TGE virus lacks this property**. The virus of TGE is antigenically related to feline infectious peritonitis virus and canine coronavirus.

Spread

The exact mode of transmission of TGE is uncertain. The **carrier pig** is probably the major source of infection and transmission of the disease. Once infection has gained access to the herd, transmission probably occurs **by both oral and respiratory routes**. Virus can be spread by aerosol. Respiratory transmission appears significant in adults. Replication in the respiratory tract is followed by excretion of the virus in nasal secretions and milk within one day of infection and also in faeces. Excretion in milk results in rapid transmission to suckling piglets, which, in turn, may excrete large quantities of virus within 2 days of infection. Immunity to clinical disease in newborn piglets is dependent on the level of secretory IgA antibody in the colostrum of the sow.

Pathogenesis

The virus infects the upper respiratory tract and the intestine, but the major clinical signs are associated with the intestinal infection. The virus infects mature differentiated columnar epithelial cells of the intestinal villi, but not the undifferentiated cells of the crypts. Replication occurs within 4-5 hours with sloughing of the infected cells and release of virus. After several replication cycles, there is a marked reduction in villous size with villous atrophy. The loss of epithelial cells results in increased migration of undifferentiated cells from the crypts to line the shortened villi. With virulent virus, epithelial cells at all levels of the small intestine are infected with major lesions occurring at the proximal jejunum, and to a lesser extent the ileum.

Signs

In piglets less than 10 days of age, the disease is characterized by acute diarrhoea, vomiting, excessive thirst, weight loss, and dehydration. These lead to death in 2-5 days. Morbidity and mortality rates may approach 100%. **In older piglets and adults**, clinical signs may not be seen, or there may be profuse diarrhoea, vomiting, depression, and failure to gain or maintain weight. The morbidity rate in older pigs may also approach 100%, but the mortality rate is low.

Lesions

In pigs dying of TGE, few gross lesions are seen. The carcass is dehydrated, and curdled milk is usually present in the stomach. The mucosa of the stomach and small intestine is congested and often shows petechiae. **Microscopically, there is marked shortening and fusion of villi in the small intestine**. Villous length is reduced several times, and villi are lined with flattened to cuboidal epithelial cells **rather than with the normal columnar cells**. The brush border of the epithelium is absent, the cytoplasm vacuolated, and the nuclei small and pyknotic. **Ultrastructurally**, microvilli are shortened and irregular. There is swelling and disruption of mitochondria and vacuolation of the endoplasmic reticulum. The lamina propria is infiltrated with mononuclear cells and neutrophils, but inflammatory exudation is not a striking feature. **Villous atrophy** results from the combined effect of virus induced villous cell destruction and improper maturation of cells as they advance from the crypts to the villi.

Diagnosis

Presumptive diagnosis can be made from the clinical signs, and supported by finding the histopathological lesions in the small intestine. The virus can be detected in fresh tissue and faeces by an ELISA test, specific immunofluorescence or immunoperoxidase test, or by neutralization in tissue culture systems. It can be differentiated from the haemagglutinating encephalomyelitis virus by its lack of haemagglutination of erythrocytes *in vitro*.

Porcine Coronaviral Encephalomyelitis

Two clinical entities in newborn piglets, **both caused by coronaviruses**, have been described. **The first**, manifested by encephalomyelitis, was reported in 1959 from Canada. The causal agent was called "haemagglutinating encephalomyelitis virus", and the disease as a **"haemagglutinating encephalomyelitis virus disease of pigs"**. **The second**, reported from England in 1969, was named after its clinical features as **"vomiting and wasting disease of piglets"**. The causative agent of this disease proved to be a virus identical to the haemagglutinating encephalomyelitis virus. Thus, it appears that similar viruses may produce different clinical pictures under differing conditions. The virus can also be recovered from clinically normal pigs.

Spread

The virus gains entry through the respiratory tract, and spreads to the brain by way of peripheral nerves. **The pathogenesis is uncertain.**

Signs

Baby pigs usually show the signs of the disease 4-7 days after birth, which include anorexia, lethargy, vomiting, and constipation. These are soon followed by signs of central nervous system involvement, which include hyperaesthesia (unusual sensitivity to stimuli, such as making a shrill cry and paddling movements in response to a sudden noise), stiff gait, and progressive posterior paralysis. In advanced stages, the pigs lie prostrate (i.e., lying with body extended), show dyspnoea (difficult breathing), become blind, and are in coma (i.e., in a state of deep unconsciousness). **The vomiting and wasting disease** also starts within a few days after birth. Signs include vomiting and retching (trying to vomit), inappetence (loss of appetite, anorexia), excessive thirst (polydipsia) but impaired ability to drink. They fail to gain weight, become emaciated, and usually die within a week or two.

Lesions

Lesions first appear in sensory nuclei of brain. Non-suppurative encephalomyelitis follows, with neuronal necrosis, glial nodules, diffuse gliosis, and perivascular aggregations of lymphocytes.

In vomiting and wasting disease, vomiting is thought to be due to the natural tendency of the coronaviruses to infect the gastrointestinal tract, and wasting due to the involvement of nerves and peripheral ganglia.

Diagnosis

Presumptive diagnosis can be made by clinical signs and lesions, but must be confirmed by identification of the virus. Also, the virus must be differentiated from other coronaviruses, and also from the Teschen disease group of enteroviruses.

Feline Infectious Peritonitis (FIP)

A disease of **cats**, FIP is caused by a **coronavirus. Cats of all ages are susceptible**. The disease is of worldwide distribution. Although the disease occurs only sporadically, serological surveys suggest an infection rate up to 90% in many populations. This may be because many infections are subclinical. Their progression to clinical disease may be facilitated by immunosuppression from concurrent infections with feline leukaemia virus, or feline immunodeficiency virus (FIV).

Signs

FIV is a slowly progessive fatal disease with a course of one to several months. Signs vary with the distribution of lesions and the extent of peritoneal or pleural effusion (accumulation of fluid). If effusion is extensive, the disease is called as the **"effusive"** or **"wet"** form. When effusion is not extensive, the disease is called **"non-effusive"** or **"dry"**. Affected cats are febrile, and there is chronic weight loss, anorexia, and depression. There may also be gradual abdominal enlargement, dyspnoea, vomiting and diarrhoea. In some cats neurological signs develop. These include ataxia (muscular incoordination), paresis (partial paralysis), seizures (convulsions), and blindness.

Lesions

The abdominal cavity contains excessive fluid, often as much as one litre. The fluid is yellow, viscid (thick and sticky), and transparent, though it contains flakes of fibrin. A grey-white granular exudate is present over all serosal surfaces, and is especially thick over the liver and spleen (**fibrinous peritonitis**). A similar inflammatory lesion and exudate affects the pleural cavity and pericardium. Multiple granulomatous nodules are present in the liver, pancreas, kidney, lungs and other organs. In prolonged cases, organization of fibrinous exudate can result in severe distortion of abdominal viscera. **Microscopically**, the peritonitis or pleuritis is a classical **fibrinous inflammation** consisting of a layer of fibrin of varied thickness. The fibrin layer contains neutrophils, lymphocytes, and macrophages. Fibroplasia (fibrosis) and proliferation of capillaries may occur in prolonged cases.

In other organs, such as the liver, pancreas, kidney, lymph nodes, muscular layers of the gastrointestinal tract, meninges, and eye, the **microscopic lesions** consist of multiple foci of necrosis, or granulomatous inflammation, usually in a blood vessel. The cellular infiltrate includes macrophages, lymphocytes, plasma cells and neutrophils. The lesion appears to be a primary vasculitis, mediated through immune mechanisms. Circulating immune complexes have been demonstrated in affected cats, and also in renal glomeruli and the granulomatous lesions.

Diagnosis

The clinical signs are usually sufficient for diagnosis. The characteristic gross and microscopic changes are not seen in other forms of peritonitis. Specific immunofluorescence can be demonstrated in tissues of cats infected with the virus.

Coronaviral Calf Diarrhoea

Many organisms, namely, bacteria, fungi, mycoplasma, chlamydia, or viruses, are involved in diseases of **young calves** characterized by **diarrhoea**. **Rotaviruses are the most important cause of calf diarrhoea.** However, **coronaviruses** are also recognized as a cause of acute diarrhoea in calves. Usually coronavirus diarrhoea affects calves less than three weeks of age. The onset is acute and diarrhoea lasts 4-5 days. **Although less severe than rotavirus diarrhoea, dehydration and electrolyte imbalance can lead to death**. Coronavirus has also been associated with diarrhoea in adult cattle.

Lesions

The virus has an affinity for the epithelial cells of the villi of the small intestine. Replication of the virus in these cells results in loss of epithelium and blunting and fusion of villi. In the colon, surface and crypt epithelial cells are attacked, with loss of surface cells and cystic dilation and accumulation of cellular debris in underlying crypts.

Diagnosis

The virus can be demonstrated by immunofluorescent techniques in affected cells in the small and large intestine, and in the affected mesenteric lymph nodes. Virus can also be demonstrated in intestinal epithelial cells shed into the intestinal lumen. Diagnosis depends on confirmed identification of the aetiological agent

Canine Coronavirus Infection

A coronavirus, first reported in 1971, is now recognized as a cause of **diarrhoea in dogs**. It is related to those of transmissible gastroenteritis of pigs and feline infectious peritonitis. Infection is most **severe in young dogs**. Signs include diarrhoea, vomiting and dehydration lasting about a week. Most animals recover. The intestinal lesions resemble other enteric coronavirus infections, with marked shortening and fusion of intestinal villi.

Infectious Bronchitis (Avian Infectious Bronchitis)

Infectious bronchitis (IB) was first reported in 1931, from USA. **It is a highly infectious and contagious respiratory disease of chickens**. Infection of chickens with the virus is widespread. Besides causing disease of the respiratory tract, the virus may also affect the **oviduct, and some strains have a tendency for the kidneys** and other tissues. The infection is of great economic importance due to its **adverse effect on egg production and egg quality in layers, and on production in broilers**. Infection of IB virus along with other pathogens, such as mycoplasma or certain strains of *Escherichia coli* is common, and increases the severity and duration of the resulting disease.

Causal Agent

The causal organism, IB virus, is a **coronavirus. Many antigenically different serotypes** are recognized by virus neutralization and haemagglutination inhibition tests, **but all possess a common group antigen** that can be demonstrated by ELISA and agar gel precipitation, or immunofluorescence tests. Some serotypes show an affinity for the **respiratory tract** (Massachusetts and Connecticut serotypes), while others are mainly **nephrotoxic** (T, Gray and Holte serotypes). It is now thought that new serotypes appear from time to time. **Concurrent infection of chickens with more than one serotype occurs.** Variation in virulence occurs among isolates of the virus. The virus is rapidly killed by common disinfectants.

Host

Only the chicken is naturally infected. The **respiratory form** is more severe in **young chicks,** whereas the **nephritic form** is mainly seen **in birds under 10 weeks of age**. Intercurrent infections with other pathogens predispose to more severe and prolonged respiratory disease. These include viruses of Ranikhet disease and infectious laryngotracheitis, and bacteria such as *Escherichia coli, Haemophilus paragallinarum, Mycoplasma gallisepticum* and *M. synoviae.* Immunosuppressive agents such as infection with Gumboro disease virus may reduce the protective immune response.

Spread

Direct airborne transmission of virus from the respiratory tract of one bird to another, and one flock to another, **is the most common method of spread**. However, transmission through **infected faeces** may also be important. Spread by fomites can occur, **but transmission through the egg is exceptional**. Infection can persist in individual birds in a flock for many months and also may cycle from bird to bird. The greatest source of infection are those birds in which virus is rapidly replicating and is being excreted. These include susceptible chickens which have recently been infected and also those in which virus replication is stimulated by such factors as the **onset of laying**.

Pathogenicity

Infectious bronchitis virus (IBV) readily infects the respiratory tract and produces **characteristic lesions in the trachea**. The virus can replicate in tissues of the respiratory tract, intestinal tract, kidneys and the **oviduct. The virus replicates in the cytoplasm**. New virus starts to appear 3-4 hours after infection, with maximum output per cell being reached within 12 hours. However, one nephropathogenic IBV strain (Australian T strain) elicits little inflammatory response in the respiratory tract.

In many cases, recovery occurs unless the chickens are very young, or airsacculitis (inflammation of airsac) develops from secondary bacterial infection, or kidney disease follows the respiratory phase. Virulent strains of IBV, however, induce severe respiratory disease with mortality. Virulence for the reproductive tract differs among IBV strains. Different IBV strains can produce a range of effects in susceptible layers **varying from changes in shell pigment with no production drop to production drops of 10-50%**.

Signs

Infection may be asymptomatic,, or may result in signs of the respiratory or reproductive system disease. Besides, there may be general malaise and retarded growth. **The respiratory syndrome is the most common in birds of all ages**. Signs include rales, gasping and sneezing, watery nasal discharge, lachrymation, and facial swelling. Signs may be seen within a few days in almost all birds, since **the infection spreads rapidly**, and the period of incubation is 1-3 days. Mortality is negligible in uncomplicated cases. **Mortality, up to 30%, may occur in the renal form in broilers**.

Two syndromes reflect disease **of the reproductive tract**. The most common is due to **damage to the functional oviduct**. This results in **reduced egg production and quality**. Reduced egg production may sometimes be in excess of 50%. Return to full laying may take 4-6 weeks, but the expected potential production is never attained. Respiratory signs may or may not accompany the fall in egg production.

Resumption of production may be accompanied by **deterioration in egg quality**. Eggs may be smaller than normal, misshapen, lacking symmetry, or show corrugations in outline. The shells may be depigmented, have calcareous deposits, are thinner than normal, or the shell may be absent entirely. Internally, the albumen loses its viscosity (thickness and stickiness) ("**watery whites**"), and the chalazae are often broken so that the yolk floats free.

The less common form of the reproductive tract disease is associated with abnormal development of the oviduct following infection of very young susceptible chicks with certain strains of virus. There may be partial or complete failure of the oviduct to develop, or at maturity the ova are taken up by the malformed oviduct, and are shed into the body cavity. Such birds fail to lay ("**blind layers**").

In the **nephritic form**, usually affecting young growing birds, there is marked depression, often with respiratory signs, and mortality as high as 30% in the severe form. In the milder form, there may be little or no mortality.

In **yet another form** of disease reported recently, there are either very mild respiratory signs or none at all. There is a fall in egg production of 5-10%, and reduction in pigment of shells, some becoming completely white. Production may return to normal in 2-3 weeks.

Lesions

Grossly, there may be serous, catarrhal, or caseous exudate in the trachea, nasal passages, and sinuses. Airsacs may appear cloudy, or contain a yellow caseous exudate. A **caseous plug** may be formed in the lower trachea or bronchi of chicks that die. Small areas of pneumonia may be seen around the large bronchi. Nephropathic infections produce **swollen and pale kidneys with the tubules**

and ureters distended with urates. In the intestinal infection, there are no gross lesions of the intestinal tract.

Microscopically, the mucosa of the trachea is oedematous. Trachea and bronchi show loss of cilia, rounding and sloughing of epithelial cells, and slight infiltration of heterophils and lymphocytes within 18 hours of infection. Regeneration of the epithelium starts within 48 hours. Hyperplasia is followed by massive infiltration of the lamina propria by lymphoid cells and a large number of germinal centres, which may be present after 7 days. If airsac involvement occurs, there is oedema, epithelial cell desquamation, and some fibrinous exudate within 24 hours. The kidney lesions are mainly those of an interstitial nephritis. The virus causes granular degeneration, vacuolation and desquamation of the tubular epithelium, and massive infiltration of heterophils in the interstitium in acute stages of the disease. The lesions in tubules are most prominent in medulla. Focal areas of necrosis may be seen. During recovery, the inflammatory cell population changes to lymphocytes and plasma cells. In **urolithiasis, the ureters are distended with urates** and often contain large calculi composed mainly of urates. Disease of the functional oviduct results in decreased height and loss of cilia from epithelial cells, dilation of the tubular glands, infiltration of subepithelial tissues with mononuclear cells (monocytes, lymphocytes, plasma cells) and proliferation of lymphoid follicles, and later oedema and fibroplasia.

Diagnosis

The clinical features, gross and microscopic lesions, may be suggestive **but are not diagnostic of IB**. The respiratory form may resemble other acute respiratory diseases such as Ranikhet disease (RD), infectious laryngotracheitis (ILT), and infectious coryza (IC). RD is generally more severe than IB. Nervous signs may be observed with virulent strains of RD, **and in laying flocks drop in production may be greater than with IB**. ILT tends to spread more slowly in a flock, but respiratory signs may be more severe than with IB. Infectious coryza can be differentiated **on the basis of facial swelling which occurs only rarely in IB. Production decreases and shell quality problems in flocks infected with the egg drop syndrome (EDS) adenovirus are similar to those seen with IB, except that internal egg quality is not affected in the case of EDS.**

Diagnosis of IB can be confirmed by isolation and identification of the causative agent. The trachea being a primary target for IBV, is the best sampling site. It is easiest to demonstrate the IB virus in the trachea in the early stages of infection when it is replicating most rapidly. About 7-10 days after infection the virus is difficult to find. In the later stages, **caecal tonsils** may be used because the virus here is cleared later than in the trachea. Samples from the lungs, kidneys, and oviduct should be considered depending on the clinical history of the disease. Samples for virus isolation are inoculated into embryonated chicken eggs, or tracheal organ culture (TOC). Another method for the demonstration of the virus is to examine sections or scrapings of the tracheal mucosa by **immunofluorescence, or immunoperoxidase assays**. This is a simple and satisfactory method when virus is plentiful, i.e., the first 7 days after infection. For the detection of antibodies to IB virus, the method that can be used include virus neutralization (VN), immunodiffusion (ID), haemagglutination inhibition (HI), immunofluorescence (IF) and ELISA. **The ELISA is more sensitive than other tests, but greater cross-reactivity is observed between strains.** More recently, confirmation of IBV is done by nucleic acid-based method. IBV RNA has been detected in infected tissues using the reverse-transcriptase/polymerase chain reaction (RT/PCR) method.

Turkey Bluecomb Disease

Also known as "**coronaviral enteritis of turkeys**", bluecomb disease is **an acute, highly infectious disease caused by a coronavirus. It affects turkeys of all ages**. The disease is characterized by loss of appetite, constant chirping (i.e., making a short, high-pitched sound), weight loss, depression and watery droppings. The sick birds show darkening of the head and skin. Infection occurs through the oral route, and the disease spreads rapidly through a flock and from flock to flock on the same farm. The disease is spread from farm to farm by personnel, equipment, and vehicles. **There is no evidence that the disease is egg transmitted.**

Gross lesions are seen mainly in the intestinal tract. Contents of the duodenum, jejunum, and caeca are watery and gaseous. The duodenum may be swollen, pale and flaccid. Caeca are distended and filled with watery, yellow-brown contents having a foetid odour. **Microscopically**, intraluminal mononuclear cell exudate is present in the duodeno-jejunal area.

Diagnosis

In turkey of any age, typical signs with characteristic **gross and micro-**scopic lesions are suggestive of bluecomb disease, **but not diagnostic.** ELISA test has been found useful in detecting coronaviruses in intestinal contents from turkey poults with diarrhoea.

Togaviridae

The Family **Togaviridae** is made up of a large number of viruses. The family is so named because of the presence of a cloak (toga = cloak, gown), kind of an outer garment surrounding the virus. **This refers to the envelope possessed by all members of the family**. The family incorporates those viruses previously classified as **arboviruses** (ar = arthropod, bo = borne) as well as a number of related viruses which do not involve arthropod transmission cycle (**Table 3**). There is still some confusion about these classifications, but each member of this family is a spherical **single-stranded, enveloped, positive-sense RNA virus**, 40-70 nm in diameter.

The **family has four genera** which contain animal pathogens. These are: **alphavirus, arterivirus, flavivirus,** and **pestivirus.**

Table 3. Diseases caused by Togaviridae*

Genus: Alphavirus
(Group A arboviruses)
Equine encephalomyelitis
Western
Eastern
Venezuelan
Genus: Arterivirus
Equine viral arteritis
Porcine reproductive and respiratory syndrome
Genus: Flavivirus
(Group B arboviruses)
Japanese B encephalitis
Louping-ill
Genus: Pestivirus
Swine fever
Bovine viral diarrhoea-mucosal disease
Border disease

*The genera **'flavivirus'** *and* **'pestivirus'** *are also classified as a separate family, the* **Flaviviridae**.

The genus **'alphavirus'** is made up of those viruses previously known as **'group A arboviruses'**. It includes some 26 serologically related viruses, **all of which are arthropod-borne**. Three of these are pathogens for **horses**, as well as humans, **namely**, Western equine encephalomyelitis, Eastern equine encephalomyelitis, and Venezuelan equine encephalomyelitis. The genus **'flavivirus'** (L. flavi = yellow) is made up of some 60 antigenically related viruses. It includes those viruses previously called **'group B arboviruses'**. Some schemes identify this group as a separate family, **Flaviviridae. All flaviviruses of medical importance are arthropod-borne.**

With rare exception, alphaviruses and flaviviruses are transmitted by the bites of arthropods, usually **mosquitoes** and **ticks**. For each virus, there are specific arthropods (insects) for perpetuation of the transmission cycle. This factor restricts the geographical distribution of the disease. **Arthropods become infected on biting a viraemic vertebrate host**. The virus multiplies first in the insect's gut, and ultimately passes through the haemolymph to other tissues, including the salivary gland, from where it can be passed to another vertebrate host through bites. **The insect remains infected throughout life,** and although there is continuous virus multiplication no harm is done to the insect. In some virus insect relationships, the virus can be transmitted from generation to generation. Certain diseases seen in domestic animals represent spillover from an arthropod-wild animal cycle. **Such is the case with Eastern** and **Western equine encephalomyelitis** and yellow fever (an acute destructive viral disease of humans). In these situations, the wild vertebrate hosts (often birds) do not develop disease, but do develop an adequate viraemia to allow perpetuation of the cycle. In contrast, h orses develop disease, but t ypically there is not significant viraemia. Thus, usually they are **dead-end hosts**. The virus probably gains access to the nervous system through centripetal spread by w ay of p eripheral and cranial nerves. M ost **alphavirus and flavivirus infections are inapparent.**

The remaining two genera, **arterivirus and pestivirus, are not dependent on an arthropod transmission cycle**. The genus 'arterivirus' is made up of only two members, equine arteritis virus, and the recently recognized virus of the porcine reproductive and respiratory syndrome. The 'pestivirus' genus includes swine fever virus, bovine viral diarrhoea virus (mucosal disease) and Border disease of sheep. Some classifications place the genus **pestivirus** along with the flavivirus in the family **Flaviviridae**.

Diseases caused by Alphaviruses (Group A Arboviruses)

Equine Encephalomyelitis

A **disease of the central nervous system of horses** was recognized in the United States, as early as 1912. The disease was the cause of serious losses, particularly in the central part of the country. In 1930, equine encephalomyelitis virus was isolated. This discovery proved very important in the understanding and control of viral encephalitis in many species, **including humans**. The virus isolated is now known as the "**Western**" s train of equine encephalomyelitis virus, to distinguish it from an antigenically different virus isolated from horses in the eastern part of the United States, the "**Eastern**" strain. A third strain of virus which produces similar signs and lesions was isolated in Venezuela, and is known as the "**Venezuelan**" strain.

The demonstration, in 1933, that **mosquitoes** may serve as vectors of the virus of equine encephalomyelitis, provided an explanation for many of its epidemiological features. Soon it was discovered that the equine encephalomyelitis viruses are **infective to a large number of animals, including humans**. However, in other species (dogs, pigs, goats, calves, domestic fowl) the infection is usually inapparent.

Spread

The enzootic (peculiar to a locality) cycles of these three encephalomyelitis viruses involve mosquitoes, birds, reptiles, and rodents, with occasional epizootic spillover into horses and humans. **The cycles are still not completely understood**. The Western strain infects a variety of birds, and is transmitted by **Culex** mosquitoes, which also f eed on mammals. The Eastern strain also infects a variety of birds, but uses a different mosquito that rarely feeds on mammals. With amplification of the mosquito-bird cycle, other species of mosquitoes, such as **Aedes**, become infected and transmit the virus to horses. Reptiles and amphibians may also be infected and may play a role in perpetuation of the Western and Eastern strains. The infection in most avian species is asymptomatic. The Venezuelan strain involves an enzootic cycle between rodents, birds, and **Culex** mosquitoes. Other species of mosquitoes, including **Aedes**, can transmit the virus among horses, and due to high levels of viraemia, even mechanical insect transmission is believed possible. **As a result of mosquito transmission, the diseases are seasonal**.

Even though equine encephalomyelitis is an important disease **in horses** and **humans, infection of these species is incidental** because generally viraemia is not adequate to infect mosquitoes, **except in Venezuelan strain, where viraemia levels can be high**.

Since the signs and lesions caused by the three strains of virus are basically the same, they are considered together.

Signs

The signs of derangement of the central nervous system usually appear suddenly after an incubation period of 1-3 weeks. Affected horses lose awareness of their surroundings and wander aimlessly, walk continuously in circles, are unresponsive to commands, and may strike violently against objects or crash through fences. High fever often occurs at the outset, but may return to normal by the time nervous symptoms appear. As the disease advances, stupor (unconsciousness) appears, and paralysis of various groups of muscles sets in. This flaccid paralysis (i.e., having defective or no muscular tone) increases rapidly. The animal lies down, is unable to stand, and soon succumbs. About 50% of horses infected with the Western strain of virus die. In the Eastern strain, this figure reaches 90%, and in Venezuelan strain, between 50% to 80%.

Lesions

No gross lesions are characteristic of this disease. The viruses of equine encephalomyelitis **attack neurons**. Hence, the damage is to these cells (**microscopic lesions**). Affected neurons undergo various degenerative changes, ending in **necrosis**. The changes are characterized by dissolution and loss of tigroid substance (**tigrolysis**) and chromatin (**chromatolysis**), fragmentation of the neuron, and its removal by phagocytes (**neuronophagia**). The process attracts leukocytes and glial cells, which form **small nodules** around the injured neurons. Such nodules persist even after the neuron has completely disappeared. The grey matter around the neurons may become oedematous and diffusely infiltrated with lymphocytes, neutrophils, and a few erythrocytes. Lymphocytes which escape from nearby arterioles are often trapped in the Virchow-Robin space, to form a wide collar of densely packed cells around the blood vessels. This **"perivascular cuffing"** may extend into the white matter, where it is the only significant change. Although perivascular cuffing is a striking microscopic finding, it is not specific for equine encephalomyelitis. It occurs in numerous inflammatory lesions of the central nervous system.

The distribution of the lesions varies, depending somewhat on the strain of virus. **With Eastern strain**, the grey matter is diffusely involved, the lesions are numerous, and neutrophils are often a prominent component of the exudate. Neutrophils appear to result from severity of the infection and the short fatal course of the disease. Thus they are not absolutely diagnostic of the **Eastern type**. Infection with any strain of the virus results in lesions in the grey matter of the cerebral or cerebellar cortex, but they are most numerous in the olfactory bulbs, thalamus, hypothalamus, brain stem, and in both dorsal and ventral grey columns of the spinal cord.

Zoonotic Implications

The susceptibility of humans to the causative virus gives the disease **great public health importance. Humans can become infected with all three types**. The first human cases were reported in 1933, in the United States, when **an outbreak in children followed an epidemic in horses**. Human infections generally follow equine infections in about 2 weeks. The infection in humans is a mild, influenza-like illness in which recovery occurs spontaneously. When clinical encephalitis does occur, it is usually in very young or older people. There is a strong relationship between the mosquito population and the incidence of the disease in horses and humans. There are usually widespread mortalities in horses before the disease occurs in humans. Western equine encephalomyelitis infections have occurred **among laboratory workers** as a result of aerosol infections from laboratory accidents and from handling of infected laboratory animals.

Diagnosis

A presumptive diagnosis can be made on finding the microscopic lesions diffusely distributed through the grey matter of the central nervous system. A confirmed diagnosis can be made only on the basis of isolation and identification of the virus.

Diseases caused by Arteriviruses

Equine Viral Arteritis

Equine viral arteritis (EVA) is manifested clinically **as an acute systemic disease**, and by **abortion in mares**. There are specific lesions in the walls of the small arteries. The causative virus is generally classified as a togavirus, but recently it has been shown to be related to the **coronavirus group**. First reported from the United States in 1957, the disease is now present in most countries, **including India**. Serological surveys conducted in the United States indicate that infection with EVA virus is widespread, but clinical disease is not common, suggesting that most infections are subclinical. **The infection is rarely fatal, but up to 80% of pregnant mares may abort** during or shortly after clinical disease.

This is the main cause of its economic importance. **In India**, the disease was first reported in 1990. Following this, a serological survey has been carried out by the National Research Centre on Equines, Hisar, employing *Escherichia coli* expressed antigen in an enzyme-linked immunosorbent assay (ELISA) to detect EVA specific antibody in horses. Out of a total of 264 samples tested from 9 states, 15 samples, 5 from Uttar Pradesh and 10 from Haryana, were found positive. All the seropositive samples were from aborted mares belonging to army establishments.

Spread

Horses of all age groups are susceptible. Infection occurs primarily **through the respiratory route by inhalation** of droplets derived from the nasal exudate of infected horses which remain infective for 8-10 days. Infection also occurs by ingestion of contaminated material and from **venereal transmission** by carrier stallions. The virus is also shed in **urine** and in **semen**. Infected stallions can be long-term carriers and continue to **shed virus for up to 2 years**. This may be the major method of spread on stud farms. The tissues and fluids of infected aborted foetuses contain large quantities of the virus.

Pathogenesis

Following infection, there is **viraemia** causing **severe vascular damage**, especially in the small arteries, intestinal tract, visceral lymph nodes, and the adrenals. A haemorrhagic enteritis results and causes diarrhoea and abdominal pain. Pulmonary oedema and pleural effusion are manifested by severe dyspnoea. Petechiation of the mucosae and the conjunctiva, and oedema of the limbs, also occur. Death, when it occurs, is due to a combination of dehydration and anoxia. The abortion is caused by a severe necrotizing myometritis. The foetus is unaffected but contains virus.

Signs

An incubation period of 1-6 days is followed by the appearance of fever (102°-106° F), a purulent nasal discharge, conjunctivitis, and excessive lachrymation. Respiratory signs are secondary in importance. Cough and dyspnoea develop. The appetite is reduced or absent, and in severe cases there may be abdominal pain, diarrhoea, and jaundice. Oedema of the limbs is common. **In stallions**, oedema of the belly wall may extend to involve the prepuce and scrotum. The disease is acute and severe, and deaths may occur without secondary bacterial invasion. The course in non-fatal cases is usually between 3-8 days. Secondary bacterial invasion is manifested by catarrhal rhinitis and infection of the respiratory tract. Abortion occurs within a few days of the onset of clinical illness, in contrast to the much later abortions which occur in equine viral rhinopneumonitis. There is a pronounced leukopaenia due to reduction of the lymphocytes, usually 1-3 days after the onset of fever. The virus is present in the blood during the febrile period.

Lesions

The **gross lesions** consist of congestion, oedema, and petechiae in the conjunctiva, nasal mucosa, pharynx, larynx, and guttural pouches; oedema of the subcutis of the legs; hydrothorax and petechiae in the pleura; oedema in the mediastinum, base of the heart, and the interlobular pulmonary septa; oedema and enlargement of the mediastinal lymph nodes; petechiae on the endocardium and epicardium; and distension of the pericardial sac with fluid. In addition, the peritoneal cavity often contains an excessive amount of fluid, **sometimes as much as 8-10 litres**. Petechiae are commonly found on the visceral and parietal peritoneum; the mesenteric lymph nodes are large and oedematous, and wall of the small intestine, caecum and colon is often oedematous. Haemorrhages into the adrenal cortex are frequently found.

The **microscopic lesions** confirm the presence of widespread oedema, vascular dilation, and to a smaller extent, haemorrhages. Generally, the veins are distended with blood and the lymphatics with lymph. Otherwise they are not affected. On the other hand, small arteries throughout the body show severe changes, especially in those tissues which exhibit gross lesions. **The most severe arterial changes are seen in the submucosa of the caecum and colon.** The earliest change is replacement of small parts of the arterial media by a **homogeneous eosinophilic material**. This displaces the nuclei and cytoplasm of the muscular coat of the artery, and is accompanied by oedema and some cellular infiltration in the adventitia. In more advanced lesions, areas of necrosis appear in the media, either as small foci, or as more extensive zones of necrosis. This is accompanied by leukocytic infiltration. Scattered bits of nuclear chromatin are also seen in these areas.

Ultrastructurally, vascular lesions are mainly endothelial cell damage characterized by dilation of endoplasmic reticulum, and the presence of viral particles 58 nm in diameter within cytoplasmic vacuoles. Swelling of endothelial cells and platelet thrombi obliterate capillary lumina. Oedema appears to be the direct result of injury to capillaries. Degeneration of smooth muscle cells appears to be secondary lesion not associated with direct viral injury.

No specific lesions are present in aborted foetuses. The abortion results from generalized vascular disease in the mare, or from necrotizing myometritis which may occur independently of generalized vascular disease.

Diagnosis

EVA is much more severe than equine viral rhinopneumonitis and equine influenza. The microscopic lesions of EVA are characteristic enough to differentiate from equine viral rhinopneumonitis, in which the characteristic lesions include foci of necrosis in lungs, liver, and lymph nodes with **intranuclear inclusion bodies**. The microscopic lesions of arteries also serve to differentiate it from equine infectious anaemia, which is also accompanied by petechiation of the mucosa and jaundice in acute cases. Leptospirosis may present a rather similar clinical picture to EVA, but can be distinguished serologically. Complement fixation, serum neutralization, and ELISA tests are available for serological diagnosis.

Porcine Reproductive and Respiratory Syndrome (PRRS)

PRRS is a newly recognized disease of **pigs** characterized by reproductive failure in sows, pneumonia in young pigs, and pre-weaning mortality. It was recognized first in the United States in 1987. The agent is classified as an **arterivirus**.

Air-borne spread is suspected. The syndrome is still not well-defined. The **clinical signs** and severity of the infection vary. The main manifestation is late-term abortion, stillbirths, premature farrowings, and the births of weak piglets. Other signs in sows and boars include fever, inappetence, lethargy and laboured breathing. Mortality in adults is low. Clinical signs, particularly respiratory distress, are much more severe in young piglets. **Mortality in piglets may approach 100%.**

The exact basis for abortion is not clear. No specific **lesions** have been noted in the placenta, or in foetuses. The consistent **microscopic feature** is an **interstitial pneumonia** characterized by extensive thickening of the alveolar septa with presence of mononuclear cells and interlobular oedema. Infiltration of lymphocytes, histiocytes, and plasma cells into alveoli has been described. There may be necrosis and squamous metaplasia of airway epithelium with mononuclear infiltration from the nasal passages through the lung. Secondary infections are common in young piglets and may contribute to mortality.

Diseases caused by Flaviviruses (Group B Arboviruses)

Japanese B Encephalitis

Japanese B encephalitis is primarily a disease of humans, who provide the source of infection for animals (horses, pigs and cattle). The disease is most prevalent in Japan, China, and other parts of Asia. **In India, serological evidence of Japanese B encephalitis in horses has been reported.** It is **arthropod-borne** with an enzootic cycle involving **Culex** mosquitoes, pigs, and birds, mainly ducks.

Infection is most important in humans when the virus causes encephalitis. Horses and other equines may also develop encephalitis. However, infection in cattle is almost always asymptomatic. In **pigs**, the virus is an important cause of abortion and neonatal mortality.

Lesions

In fatal infections in humans neuronophagic nodules are observed in all parts of the grey matter. In the spinal cord, the lesions tend to become confluent, whereas in the cerebral cortex and cerebellum, the lesions are generally discrete (separate).

The neuronophagic nodules indicate involvement of neurons. In animals, including aborted and stillborn pigs, **similar lesions are seen**, particularly in the grey matter of the cerebral cortex and basal ganglia.

Diagnosis

Although the presence of typical lesions may suggest Japanese B encephalitis, these lesions cannot with certainty be differentiated from those of louping ill, Teschen disease, or even equine encephalomyelitis. To make a definitive diagnosis, it is necessary to isolate the causative virus, or demonstrate specific neutralizing antibody production after infection.

Ovine Encephalomyelitis (Louping-Ill)

Louping-ill is a tick-borne encephalitis, mainly of sheep, which occurs in Britain and Ireland. **Humans are susceptible, but infection is usually mild.** Encephalitis can also occur in **horses**, and sporadic cases have been described in **cattle**. The disease is of main importance, however, in sheep. Affected animals, usually **lambs**, exhibit a peculiar **"louping" gait** (leaping, jumping gait), which gives the disease its common name. The tick, *Ixodes ricinus* transmits louping ill to sheep under natural conditions, which accounts for seasonal occurrence of the disease.

Pathogenesis

After tick-borne infection the virus proliferates in the regional lymph node to produce a **viraemia** which peaks at 2-4 days. Invasion of the central nervous system occurs in the early viraemic stage. The occurrence of clinical disease is associated with replication of the virus in the brain, severe inflammation throughout the central nervous system, and necrosis of brainstem and ventral horn neurons.

Signs

In most sheep infection is inapparent. There is an incubation period of 2-4 days followed by a sudden onset of high fever (up to 107° F) for 2-3 days, followed by a return to normal. In animals which develop neurological disease, there is **a second febrile phase** during which nervous signs appear. Affected animals stand apart, and there is marked tremor of muscle groups **and** rigidity of the musculature, particularly in the neck and limbs. This causes jerky, stiff movements and a bounding gait (i.e., characterized by jumping movement), which gives rise to the name **"louping-ill"** (to loup = to jump). Incoordination is most marked in the hind limbs. The sheep walks into objects and may stand with the head pressed against them. Hypersensitivity to noise and touch (hyperaesthesia) may be seen. With time, the increased muscle tone is followed by recumbency, convulsions and paralysis, and death occurs within 1-2 days. **Young lambs may die suddenly with no specific nervous signs.**

The **clinical picture in cattle** is very similar to that observed in sheep with hyperaesthesia, blinking of the eyelids and rolling of the eyes. Convulsions are more likely to occur in cattle. **Horses** also show a similar clinical picture as sheep.

Lesions

Louping-ill virus causes destruction of neurons diffusely throughout the grey matter. However, they are most concentrated in the cerebellum, where loss of Purkinje cells and focal glial or inflammatory nodules are also observed. In the ventral horn of the spinal cord and medulla, motor neurons are often affected. The lesions are similar in intensity and distribution to those of Teschen disease (porcine encephalomyelitis).

Zoonotic Importance

In humans, an influenza-like disease followed by meningo-encephalitis occurs after an incubation period of 6-18 days. While recovery is common, the disease is fatal and residual nervous deficiencies can occur.

Diagnosis

A presumptive diagnosis can be made on the basis of microscopic lesions in the brain and spinal cord, but definitive diagnosis depends on isolation and identification of the virus.

Diseases caused by Pestiviruses

Swine Fever (Hog Cholera, Swine Plague)

Swine fever, also known as hog cholera, is **an acute, febrile, highly contagious and often fatal disease of pigs**, caused by a **pestivirus**. Chronic or inapparent infection also occurs, including persistent congenital infection in newborn pigs, infected during foetal life. First recognized in 1885 in the United States, its viral aetiology was established in 1903. The disease is now worldwide in distribution, **including India**. There is only one antigenic type of the virus, but there are a number of strains of variable virulence and antigenicity. The virus of swine fever has an antigenic relationship to that causing bovine virus diarrhoea.

Spread

The pig is the only domestic animal which is naturally infected by the virus. The source of virus is always an infected pig and its products. **The infection is usually acquired by ingestion, but inhalation** is also a possible route. In case of infection with a virulent virus, all excretions, secretions and body tissues of affected pigs contain the virus, and it is excreted in the urine for some days before clinical illness appears, and for 2-3 days after clinical recovery. The resistance and high infectivity of the virus make spread of the disease by inert materials, especially uncooked meat, a problem. **The virus probably survives for considerable periods** as it is quite resistant to chemical and physical influences. Birds and humans may also act as physical carriers of the virus. Farmers, veterinarians and v accination t eams c an transmit t he virus by c ontaminated i nstruments and d rugs.

Pathogenesis

The tonsil is the primary site of virus invasion following oral exposure. Primary multiplication of the virus occurs in the tonsils within a few hours after infection. The virus is then transported through lymphatics, and enters blood capillaries resulting in an **initial viraemia** by about 24 hours. At this time, the virus can be found in the spleen and other sites, such as peripheral and visceral lymph nodes, bone marrow, and Peyer's patches. The virus exerts its pathogenic effect on endothelial cells, lymphoreticular cells, macrophages, and epithelial cells. **Most of the lesions are produced by hydropic degeneration and proliferation of vascular endothelium which result in the occlusion of blood vessels**. This effect on the vascular system results in the characteristic lesions of congestion, haemorrhage and infarction from changes in arterioles, venules, and capillaries. **Thrombosis of small and medium-sized arteries** is another feature. Leukopaenia is common in the early stages, followed by a leukocytosis, anaemia, a nd thrombocytopaenia. **Leukopaenia** in t he early stages is pronounced, the total c ount falling from a n ormal range of 14,000-24,000/µl to 4000-9000/µl. This can be of value in differentiation from bacterial septicaemias.

Signs

After an incubation period of about 7 days, depression and a **high fever** (106° F) are first seen. These signs are accompanied by **severe leukopaenia** in which the total leukocyte count may be less than 4000/µl. The disease spreads rapidly to all susceptible animals in contact with the infected animals. Besides weakness and inappetence, nervous s ymptoms are u sually observed. These include lethargy (lack of energy or dullness), occasional convulsions, grinding of the teeth, and difficulty in locomotion. In pigs with light skin, erythematous lesions a ppear, particularly o n the s kin of the abdomen, a xillae, and i nner surface of the legs. **Most animals die within 10 days after the onset of signs**. A few that live longer, show intestinal and pulmonary involvement. **In natural outbreaks, nearly 100% of the susceptible animals in a herd may be expected to die**. The disease in nature is limited to domestic and wild pigs.

Infection with a virus of reduced virulence can result in a longer course, which has been called "**chronic**" **swine fever**. Following an apparent remission (lessening of severity), there is an aggravation of the disease, resulting in death as late as 40-70 days after the initial signs of infection. **Pigs with chronic disease play an important role in the dissemination of swine fever, because they excrete virus intermittently throughout the entire course of the infection**. Pigs vaccinated with live attenuated virus may also excrete virulent virus, and serve as a source of infection to non-immune pigs.

A variety of **foetal and neonatal abnormalities** have been attributed to exposure to the virus during pregnancy. The most critical period of exposure appears to be after 20 days of gestation. Abnormalities include mummification, anasarca, ascites, stillbirth, cerebellar hypoplasia, and neonatal death. Virus crosses the placenta and invades foetal tissues, and can be demonstrated or isolated from piglets. Infection *in utero* can also lead to lesions resembling swine fever in adult pigs, or to the birth of persistently infected pigs which shed the virus.

Lesions

The virus of swine fever exerts a direct effect on the vascular system, and the signs and lesions result from changes in the capillaries. For this reason, the **gross lesions** appear as areas of congestion, haemorrhage, or infarction. In acute cases and in pigs which die early in the disease, gross lesions may be difficult to detect. But in cases of longer duration, they are found in a variety of organs. **Lesions are seen in this order of frequency:** kidney, lymph nodes, urinary bladder, skin (in white-skinned pigs), spleen, larynx, lungs, and large intestine. With less frequency, lesions occur in the heart, liver, small intestine, and stomach.

In the vascular system, the specific action of the virus is manifested by **petechiae** and **ecchymoses**. The earliest and most pronounced **microscopic lesions** are found in the capillaries and pre-capillaries. The most constant change is **swelling and proliferation of endothelial cells,** accompanied by decrease in staining intensity. **Ultrastructurally,** mitochondria are swollen and lose their cristae. The endothelial nuclei are enlarged, increased in number, pale-staining, and may pile up to occlude the lumen, or are desquamated and lost. The capillary basement membrane is pale, eosinophilic, hyaline, and homogeneous. These changes may extend to the collagen and reticular fibres which surround the vessel. **The capillary wall may become completely hyalinized, resulting in partial or complete occlusion.** Fat droplets may be seen in the capillary walls. Thrombosis is rare in arterioles or smaller vessels. In small and medium-sized arteries, the lesions are similar to those in capillaries, but are less frequent. The media and adventitia may be hyalinized, and occasionally show necrosis. Thrombosis sometimes occurs. Similar lesions may be seen in veins, but are rare in lymphatics.

In the central nervous system, the lesions are related to the vasculature. Apart from congestion of vessels, **gross changes are not seen in the brain. The most striking microscopic lesion** occurs from accumulation of lymphocytes in the perivascular (Virchow-Robin) spaces around arteries and veins. This **perivascular cuffing** comprises lymphocytes, mononuclear cells, plasma cells, and occasionally, eosinophils. **Neutrophils are not a part of the inflammatory exudate.** Thrombi, emboli, or patches of softening are conspicuously absent. Small nodules of proliferated microglia are present in both white and grey matter.

Changes in the neurons are much less significant; they are neither specific, nor common. There is no demyelination. **Inclusion bodies are found in a few cases, but are not considered specific**. These inclusions are **intranuclear**, round, homogeneous, eosinophilic (acidophilic) or sometimes basophilic, and several may be found in a single neuron.

In the spleen, infarction due to lesions in the arteries occurs **in about 50% of cases**. **Grossly**, the infarcts are sharply outlined, red, irregular in shape, and elevated. Some are definitely wedge-shaped. **Microscopically**, degenerative changes in the wall of follicular or trabecular arteries are characterized by proliferation of endothelium, hyalinization, and necrosis in the media and adventitia with resultant thrombosis. Haemorrhagic infarction is seen as sharply demarcated areas of necrosis.

Gross lesions are seen in **lymph nodes** in more than 80% of animals which die of swine fever. Lesions vary from swelling and hyperaemia with bright red subcapsular haemorrhages to dense dark-coloured haemorrhages obscuring the entire nodal architecture. Pronounced changes are observed in the capillaries, arterioles, and venules. Swelling and proliferation of endothelial nuclei are striking, and are accompanied by occlusion of the lumen. In the skin, erythematous areas resulting from cyanosis are the most common gross lesions. They usually appear as areas of purplish discoloration, 1-15 cm in diameter, on the ventral surface of the abdomen and thorax, the medial surface of the thigh and leg, ears, skin of the perineum, and the snout. The cyanotic changes can be readily detected in white-skinned pigs, and rarely in the black breeds. The typical changes in the vascular system are also responsible for these cutaneous lesions.

In the kidneys, sharply demarcated petechiae, 1-5 mm in diameter are visible grossly just beneath the capsule, and deep in the renal cortex. These petechiae give the kidney a characteristic appearance, known as "**turkey egg kidney**". **Microscopically**, haemorrhages are found in the interstitial stroma and in Bowman's spaces. These haemorrhages are due to the typical lesions in the vessels. **The digestive system** is usually **affected in pigs dying after a more prolonged course**. The characteristic lesion is a spherical ulcer in the mucosa, particularly in the colon. These ulcers are sharply circumscribed, single or multiple. They originate as small congested areas and develop into encrusted button-shaped foci ("**button ulcers**") a few millimetres in diameter. Cut sections reveal a sharply demarcated zone of necrosis in the underlying mucosa and submucosa. This lesion develops after occlusion of a small artery by swelling and hydropic changes in its endothelium. **Thus, the "button ulcer" is the result of infarction.**

Diagnosis

The diagnosis can usually be made on the basis of clinical signs, and gross and microscopic lesions. The presence of the virus can be demonstrated by the application of fluorescent antibody staining to infected cell cultures. This test has proved reliable. Fluorsescent antibody staining can also be applied directly to tissue sections. The agar gel precipitation test (AGPT) detects antigen in tissues by means of a precipitin formed with immune sera. Usually pancreas is tested. The enzyme-linked immunosorbent assay test (ELISA) is useful for large-scale testing of sera in eradication programmes.

In differential diagnosis, swine fever has to be differentiated from salmonellosis, acute erysipelas, and acute pasteurellosis. Salmonellosis is usually accompanied by enteritis and dyspnoea; and in acute erysipelas and acute pasteurellosis subserous haemorrhages a re ecchymotic rather than petechial.

Bovine Virus Diarrhoea (BVD) and Mucosal Disease (MD)

A contagious disease of cattle in New York State was first described in 1946. Its viral aetiology was demonstrated and the infection was termed "**virus diarrhoea**". The disease was characterized by high morbidity but low mortality. In the same year, a disease of cattle w as also described in Canada that was similar to virus diarrhoea, but was more severe and had a high mortality. The disease was termed "**mucosal disease**". Virus diarrhoea and mucosal disease have since been described in other countries, **including India**.

It is now established that **each of these diseases is caused by antigenically related pestiviruses**, and that the different clinical picture of morbidity and mortality is determined by the **viral strain variations** and mode of infection. **Bovine viral diarrhoea virus (BVDV) occurs in two bio-types: cytopathogenic** and **non-cytopathogenic** on the basis of their effects in tissue culture cells. Virus diarrhoea occurs sporadically in cattle between 6 months and 2 years of age as a transient, highly contagious acute infection with a high morbidity rate, but is usually a mild disease with cytopathogenic BVDV. However, new strains of BVDV have caused outbreaks with high mortality.

On the other hand, **mucosal disease** develops in cattle which become infected *in utero* with non-cytopathogenic BVDV. These animals develop a persistent infection to which they are immunotolerant. Mucosal disease develops in these animals when the persistent non-cytopathogenic BVDV undergoes a transformation to cytopathogenic BVDV through a process of RNA recombination. **The disease generally appears in cattle between 6 months and 2 years of age, and results in death**.

Border disease of sheep (discussed next) **is caused by the same virus**, or a basically indistinguishable variant. The virus of swine fever is also related. Pigs can be infected with BVDV, but the virus ordinarily does not cause clinical disease. In pregnant sows, it may cause foetal death and resorption.

Spread

The v irus is transmitted **by direct c ontact between animals**, and by **transplacental transmission** to the foetus. The virus is present in nasal discharge, saliva, faeces, urine, tears, milk and semen, each of which would allow wide dissemination of the virus. Discharges from the reproductive tract of an infected cow, including aborted foetuses can be potent source of virus. Nose-to-nose contact is an effective method of spreading the virus from persistently infected animals to susceptible animals. Persistently infected bulls may also introduce the virus into artificial breeding units. The **foetus** can be infected by transplacental transmission of the virus in the infected dam. **Persistently viraemic female can remain clinically normal for several years, and may introduce infection into a herd.**

Pathogenesis

The pathogenesis of disease due to infection with the bovine viral diarrhoea virus is governed by several features of the infection. These include the occurrence of viraemia, the ability of the virus to compromise (damage) the immune system, the age of the animal, the previous vaccination status of the animal, the occurrence of transplacental infection, the induction of immune tolerance, and the emergence of foetal immune competence at about 180 days of gestation. Apart from those infected with the virus *in utero* most cattle are immuno-competent to the virus, and will successfully control a natural infection, develop antibodies, and eliminate the virus so that latency and shedding do not occur. **However, the pathogenesis of the lesions remains obscure.**

Signs

The clinical signs include **high fever** (105°-108 ° F), anorexia, depression, and diarrhoea accompanied by excessive salivation, with stringy mucus hanging from the muzzle to the ground. Severe leukopaenia is observed in the early stages. Ulcers develop in the mouth, nose, and muzzle of severely affected animals. Other signs include mucous or mucopurulent nasal discharges and cough. The nasal and oral mucosa, and the conjunctiva are congested. Disturbances in distribution of body heat may be observed by touching. The ears, muzzle, and extremities may be cold, while other parts of the body may be very warm. Dehydration and suspension of milk secretion and rumination occur in severe infections. Abortions, stillbirths, and mummified foetuses are common after acute attacks. Septic metritis after abortion may result in death. Calves born alive may be persistently infected and later succumb to mucosal disease. Congenital cerebellar hypoplasia, cataracts, retinal atrophy, microphthalmia, and optic neuritis have been noted **in calves born to infected dams**.

Lesions

The main gross lesions are found in the gastrointestinal tract. Sharply defined, irregularly-shaped **ulcers or erosions of the mucosa** are found on the dental pad, palate, lateral surfaces of the tongue, and inside of the cheeks. Ulcers may also occur on the muzzle and at the external nares. On the mucosa of the **pharynx**, irregularly-shaped ulcers of varying size may be covered by a tenacious grey exudate. Necrotic lesions may be confined to the pharynx, or may extend to the larynx. Some animals develop pneumonia.

In the **oesophagus**, the entire mucous membrane may contain **shallow erosions or ulcers** with sharply defined, irregular margins and a red base. These ulcers may coalesce to form elongated ulcers or erosions, with necrotic material adhering. The **abomasal mucosa** may be diffusely reddened, or may contain petechiae and a few ulcers. Haemorrhages may be present in the omasum. The mucosa of the **small intestine, caecum,** and **colon** is hyperaemic and may show small haemorrhages and ulcers, particularly over Peyer's patches, where necrosis of intestinal glands and lymphoid tissue, reminding lesions of **rinderpest**, is often seen. There also may be necrosis in **lymph nodes** and the **spleen,** which may contribute to immunosuppression. Necrotizing enteritis, probably immune-mediated, develops in many organs and tissues, including the gastrointestinal tract. **In the foetus,** lesions similar to those of the adult may be seen in the gastrointestinal tract.

In cattle with chronic mucosal disease, there is chronic ulceration of the oral cavity as well as the skin. Lameness and deformed hooves are a clinical feature.

Diagnosis

The similarity of the lesions of virus diarrhoea to the gastrointestinal lesions of rinderpest, and the oral lesions of malignant catarrhal fever, complicates the differential diagnosis. Cross-immunity and cross-serum neutralization tests can be used to differentiate rinderpest from virus diarrhoea. Malignant catarrh can be differentiated by its slower spread and the characteristic ocular, nasal and brain lesions. **Virus isolation and identification provide the only precise means of diagnosis.** Two recently described ELISA tests are of high serological sensitivity. A single dilution ELISA test has been developed which has a high level of correlation with the virus neutralization test. An ELISA test has also been used to detect BVDV antibodies using recombinant antigen and monoclonal antibodies.

Border Disease of Sheep

Also known as "**hairy-shaker lamb**", "**fuzzy lamb**" and "**hypomyelinosis congenita**", the disease was first recognized as **a sporadic disease of lambs** in 1959 in the Welsh Border Country between England and Wales. Hence the name "**Border disease**". It is characterized by birth of lambs with a hairy coat, severe tremors within a month of birth, and poor growth and viability. The disease is caused by a **pestivirus**, which is serologically related to bovine virus diarrhoea virus and to swine fever virus. The latter two viruses have been shown capable of infecting sheep, and causing a border disease-like syndrome. Border disease is now known to occur worldwide. Goats are also susceptible. **In India** studies carried out, based on SFV antigen by agar-gel immunodiffusion (AGID) test in **sheep and**

goats, gave a positive reaction, indicating the possibility of the presence of border disease infection. However, this needs to be confirmed.

Spread

Lambs which are infected *in utero*, that is, prior to the development of immunological competence, may survive the infection but are born persistently infected with border disease virus. These sheep excrete virus in nasal secretions, saliva, urine and faeces, **and provide the major source of infection to healthy sheep. Thus, border disease is a congenital disease of sheep.** Infection can be introduced into a flock with the purchase of a persistently infected sheep. Transmission is by sheep-to-sheep contact. Experimental transmission has been achieved with both oral and conjunctival challenge.

Pathogenesis and Signs

Infection in adult sheep is subclinical and the virus is eventually eliminated. However, **in pregnant ewes,** the virus crosses the placenta and infects the foetus leading to several possible results. Early *in utero* infection may result in immune tolerance and birth of lambs that are permanent carriers and shedders of the virus. These serve as the main source of infection to other sheep. Early infection may also lead to **embryonic death** and **abortion.** Foetuses infected before 90 days gestation, which survive and do not develop immune tolerance, **develop typical border disease.** Affected lambs are born with an abnormally coarse, long, and straight (free from curves and bends) birthcoat (external growth of hair at birth), described as "**hairy**". This is most noticeable in fine-fleeced and medium-fleeced breeds. Neurological signs include continuous tremors, tonic-clonic contraction of skeletal muscles, and uncoordinated movements. The combination of abnormal fleece and neurological signs has given the affected lambs name "**hairy shakers**". In lambs which survive, neurological signs and fleece abnormalities gradually disappear in the first few months of life. These lambs eliminate the virus and do not become shedders.

Lesions

Grossly, there may be hydranencephaly, an undersized cerebral cortex, and the presence of cysts or cavities in the brain and spinal cord. Cerebral arteries and arterioles show periarteritis, with an infiltration of lymphocytes and macrophages. Decreased levels of circulating thyroid hormones have been noted, which may contribute to the retardation of growth.

Microscopically, the fleece changes result from an atypical growth and differentiation of primary hair follicles. Primary follicles are enlarged and contain enlarged primary fibres, of which a high proportion is more heavily medullated than normal. There are fewer secondary follicles. The main lesion in the central nervous system is **hypomyelinogenesis** in all parts of the brain and spinal cord. There is also an increase in the number of glial cells in the cerebral white matter.

Glial nuclei are increased in number and, in myelin stains, nerve fibres are twisted, distorted, and swollen, giving them a beaded appearance.

Diagnosis

Diagnosis is based on clinical, epidemiological and histopathological evidence along with serology and virus isolation.

Bunyaviridae

This family of viruses derives its name from **Bunyamwera**, a place in Uganda where the type species **"Bunyamwera virus"** was isolated. The family contains over 200 viruses divided into five genera. **But only a few are important pathogens of animals.** Most of the viruses are arthropod borne, with mosquitoes, ticks, sandflies or **Culicoides** species serving as vectors. Transovarian transmission is known in some of them.

The **virions** of this family are spherical and enveloped, 90-100 nm in diameter. The envelope contains at least one virus specified glycoprotein. The genome consists of a **negative-sense, single-stranded RNA** in three pieces. **The virions develop in the cytoplasm of host cells,** and mature by budding into smooth-surfaced membranes in or adjacent to the Golgi region.

The three most important diseases of animals caused by members of the **Bunyaviridae are "Rift Valley fever, Akabane disease,** and **Nairobi sheep disease**. **Cache Valley virus** has emerged as a cause of arthrogryposis-hydranencephaly complex in sheep.

Rift Valley Fever

Rift Valley fever is an acute viral disease, which principally **affects mainly sheep** and **cattle, causing heavy mortality in young lambs and calves, and abortion in pregnant ewes and cows.** The disease was first reported as an acute highly fatal infection of lambs in 1912 from Kenya, where the disease occurred on farms in the Rift Valley. Like many other newly reported diseases of unknown aetiology, this one was named after the location where it was first observed. Rift Valley fever has a wide distribution in Africa, but has not been recognized in domestic animals outside that continent.

Spread

The disease is usually transmitted by arthropod vectors, particularly **culicine mosquitoes.**

Signs

After an incubation period of 20-70 hours, the course in **young lambs** is short. They are disinclined to move, refuse to eat, exhibit some form of abdominal pain, and soon thereafter become recumbent, and are unable to rise. **Death may occur**

within 24 hours. The lambs may die even before symptoms are observed. In **adult sheep** also, the infected animal is found dead without showing any sign of illness. Vomiting may be observed as the only symptom. However, pregnant ewes usually abort. **In cattle**, the disease may appear as a storm of abortions. The symptoms include a brief febrile period with inappetence, profuse salivation, diarrhoea, abdominal pain, roughened hair coat, and cessation of lactation. The mortality rate in cattle is not high. However, erosions of the buccal mucosae, necrosis of the skin of the udder or scrotum, laminitis, and coronitis may occur.

Lesions

The most constant and characteristic lesions are found in the **liver. In the sheep**, the organ is grossly enlarged, its surface is mottled grey to red and shows numerous grey to white subcapsular opaque foci. **Microscopically**, these foci are seen as areas of necrosis involving parenchymal cells near the central veins. The affected cells have swollen, eosinophilic, hyaline cytoplasm, and pyknotic or fragmented nuclei. **Intranuclear inclusions** have been described, but their specificity is in doubt, since replication occurs in the cytoplasm of affected cells. The gallbladder wall may be thickened by oedema and contain subserosal haemorrhages.

Haemorrhages may occur in the subcutis of the axillae, and the medial and lower aspects of the limbs. Haemorrhages may also be seen in the peritoneum of the gastrointestinal tract and diaphragm, as well as under the pleura, pericardium, and endocardium, and in the myocardium. Similar haemorrhages may occur in the submucosa and muscular layer of the gastrointestinal tract, and in the pancreas, kidney, adrenal, lung, thymus, and lymph nodes. The lymph nodes are enlarged and appear moist and red. Ulceration of the intestinal mucosa may be seen in the ileum, caecum, and colon. The lungs are always hyperaemic and oedematous, often with subpleural and diffuse haemorrhages. Consolidation may be fibrinous in character. Kidneys are usually enlarged, bear haemorrhages, and show microscopic evidence of necrosis. That is, swelling and loss of cell outline in tubular epithelium, albuminous casts in tubules, haemosiderin in tubular epithelium and congestion. The spleen is usually enlarged and exhibits subcapsular petechiae.

Zoonotic Importance

Humans may contract the infection during the course of an epizootic among domestic animals, or by handling the virus in the laboratory. **Humans are particularly susceptible and can easily become infected**. The initial symptoms, after an incubation period of 4-6 days, are malaise, nausea, hyperthermia, epigastric pain, and a sensation of fullness over the region of the liver. There is usually complete anorexia, followed by rigors, severe headache, photophobia (intolerance to light), characteristic flushing of the face, pain in the back and joints, vertigo, and sometimes epistaxis. The disease in human is rarely fatal, and immunity follows recovery. However, serious sequelae, such as thrombophlebitis, retinopathy, and retinal detachment, have been reported.

Diagnosis

Rift Valley fever should be suspected in outbreaks of **a highly fatal disease affecting both lambs and calves**, especially if persons who are associated with the sick animals, or who handle infective materials, show mild febrile symptoms. Sometimes human cases of an influenza type may provide the first indication of the existence of an epizootic of Rift Valley fever. Also, the occurrence of abortion in adult animals and the presence of the gross and microscopic lesions, particularly those of the liver, permit a presumptive diagnosis. Neutralization of infective blood by immune serum using mice as test animals, confirms the diagnosis. A serum neutralization test with mice can also be employed.

Akabane Disease (of Cattle)

Also known as "**congenital arthrogryposis hydranencephaly syndrome**", Akabane disease caused by **a bunyavirus** termed **Akabane virus** is an **arbovirus infection of cattle**, which leads to **disease of the foetus without systemic lesions in the pregnant cow**. No disease occurs in bulls. Natural disease also has been recently described in **sheep** and **goats**. The disease in newly born calves, lambs, and kids is characterized by congenital arthrogryposis (fixed joints) causing deformities of the limbs and vertebral column, or by hydranencephaly (formation of a big space or cavity in the cerebrum).

Spread

The virus is transmitted by **mosquitoes** (**Culex** and **Aedes** species), and the midges (small mosquito-like insects). The disease has occurred in Japan, Australia, Israel, and the Middle East.

Pathogenesis

A viraemia occurs in the dam for 3-4 days. The virus passes from the dam, which is unaffected, to the foetus, and causes arrest of differentiation in its growing neural tube. Which part of the tube is most affected depends on the stage of its development, and therefore on the age of the foetus. Usually, **three forms** of the disease are observed. The **first ones** to appear are calves with arthrogryposis (infected at 105-174 days of pregnancy). They are therefore at an older foetal age when infected than others. The **next group** is those with arthrogryposis accompanied by hydranencephaly. The **third group** is those with hydranencephaly only (infected between days 76 and 104 of pregnancy).

Signs

The **cow is unaffected**. The two syndromes, **arthrogryposis** and **hydranencephaly**, occur separately. Arthrogryposis occurs in the early stages of the outbreak and hydranencephaly at the end. Calves with both defects occur in the middle of the outbreak. In some outbreaks, only one of the manifestations of the disease is seen.

Calves with arthrogryposis (fixed joints) are unable to rise, stand, or walk. One or more limbs are fixed at the joints. There is a congenital articular rigidity. The muscles of affected limbs are severely wasted. Severe deformity of the vertebral column, such as **kyphosis** (abnormal dorsal curvature of the spine) or **scoliosis** (lateral curvature of the spine), or **lordosis** (abnormal ventral curvature of the spine), is common. These abnormalities are believed to be of neurogenic origin. Calves with hydranencephaly have no difficulty in rising or walking. **The major defects are blindness and a lack of intelligence**. They will suck if put onto the teat, but if this is not done, they stand and bleat (utter a mournful cry). They have no dam-seeking reflex.

Apart from skeletal and neurological defects, cases of abortion, stillbirth, and premature birth are also regarded as being caused by **Akabane virus** infection in cows. They are usually observed at the beginning of the outbreak before neurological defects occur.

Lesions

In the foetus, the virus invades the brain and skeletal muscle, producing encephalomyelitis and polymyositis (simultaneous inflammation of many muscles), **Encephalitis** occurs regardless of the age of the foetus when affected. However, **myositis** occurs only when the foetus is infected during the first half of gestation. The foetus may die and abort, be stillborn, or be born with deformities, such as **arthrogryposis in all four legs**. The non-suppurative encephalomyelitis is characterized by extensive necrosis and endothelial proliferation, leading to formation of cysts, **porencephaly** (occurrence of cavities in brain), and **hydranencephaly** (formation of cavities in cerebral hemispheres due to lack of proper development. The cavities are filled with cerebrospinal fluid). **Hydrocephalus** is a common manifestation. There is loss of neurons in the ventral horn of the spinal cord. Myositis is accompanied by swelling, necrosis and fragmentation of muscle fibres (myofibres). At birth, muscles are smaller than normal and replaced by adipose tissue, giving rise to the names "**runt-muscle disease**" and "**runt-muscle fibre**". **Microscopically**, there is thinning and loss of myofibres. Many lack transverse striations.

In **differential diagnosis**, Akabane disease must be differentiated from other forms of congenital arthrogryposis.

Nairobi Sheep Disease

This is a **bunyavirus infection of sheep and goats**, which occurs in East Africa, mainly in Kenya. The virus is **transmitted** by the **tick Rhipicephalus**, in which transovarian infection occurs. The virus does not affect cattle, but it can cause **a mild febrile disease in humans**.

Clinical disease occurs when susceptible animals are moved from the Nairobi area into enzootic areas for marketing purposes, or when there are breakdowns in tick control measures. **Clinical signs** include sudden onset of fever, anorexia, nasal discharge, dyspnoea, and severe diarrhoea, sometimes with dysentery and abortion in pregnant ewes. Adult animals are more severely affected, and death usually occurs in 3-9 days. The affected sheep develop an acute haemorrhagic gastroenteritis. **The disease is severe, and is regarded as the most pathogenic virus infection of sheep and goats in eastern Africa.** The mortality rate may be as high as 90 per cent.

Diseases that can be confused with Nairobi sheep disease are peste-des-petits-ruminants (PPR), rinderpest, parasitic gastroenteritis, and salmonellosis.

Cache Valley Virus Infection

This viral infection is widespread throughout North America. It infects a variety of species, including domestic and wild ruminants, horses, pigs and **humans.** Mostly these infections are **asymptomatic.** The virus, however has been associated with arthrogryposis, hydranencephaly, and other foetal abnormalities in **sheep** in Texas, USA. Experimental *in utero* inoculation of pregnant sheep between 27 and 54 days of gestation has confirmed that Cache Valley virus infection can lead to arthrogryposis and hydranencephaly, as well as foetal mummification, resorption, and oligohydramnios (abnormally small amount of amniotic fluid).

Orthomyxoviridae

The Family **Orthomyxoviridae** (G. ortho = correct, **true**; myxo = mucus) is composed of the true influenza viruses. They are currently classified in **one genus, "influenzavirus".** Based on antigenic differences between their nucleoprotein (NP) and matrix (M) proteins (antigens), influenza viruses are divided into **three types: A, B and C. All the three types occur in humans, but in animals only type A viruses are of concern as causes of natural disease. They cause equine, swine, and avian influenza.**

The three A type viruses are about 120 nm in diameter and irregularly spherical. They are often filamentous on initial isolation. The virion **envelope** is covered with a layer of **two kinds of glycoprotein spikes (peplomers)** (Fig. 2), which contain strain-specific antigens, either **haemagglutinin (HA)** or **neuraminidase (NA).** The **genome** is **negative-sense, single-stranded RNA,** divided into **eight separate segments** (seven in type C). The virion contains a transcriptase, and **multiplication occurs in the nucleus and cytoplasm of infected cells.** Virions mature by budding from the plasma membrane.

Influenza viruses are spread by aerosols (suspended particles in air), and establish infection in the respiratory tract, where they attach and replicate in respiratory epithelium from the nares to bronchioles. There has been a great concern as to the potential of influenza viruses as **teratogenic** (producing abnormal structures in the foetus) **agents**. Experimentally, a variety of foetal abnormalities have been induced, but their role in natural disease, is uncertain.

Equine Influenza

Equine influenza is an infectious respiratory disease of horses caused by an influenzavirus (type A). The disease is characterized by mild fever, and a severe, persistent cough. Equine influenza virus was first isolated and identified in 1958 in Czechoslovakia (**A/Equi 1 serotype**). A second serotype (**A/Equi 2**) was isolated in 1963 in Miami, USA. **Thus, the virus is of two serotypes, based on antigenic differences in their haemagglutinin**. Both serotypes are of worldwide distribution, **including India**, and cause similar syndromes. **Equine influenza is highly infectious and spreads rapidly**.

The disease was first recorded in India in 1987, and has since been reported from Haryana, Punjab, Himachal Pradesh, and Delhi. It causes 80-100% morbidity and 0-1% mortality, with an average fatality rate of 0.5%. It was **A/Equi-2** which was found to be responsible for the major outbreak. A/Equi-1 has also been suspected on the basis of serological evidence.

Spread

The transmission of the virus occurs by **droplet inhalation**, but spread through infected fomites (substances which absorb and transmit the virus) may also occur. All age groups of horses, including newborn foals, are susceptible. The greatest risk appears to be between thre age of 2-6 months. This is because serum levels of possibly acquired antibodies are lost by foals at 2 months of age. Most cases occur in 2 year old or younger horses, probably because horses of 3 years of age, or older, are immune.

Pathogenesis

The disease is principally an inflammation of the upper respiratory tract. The virus is inhaled, multiplies in the epithelial cells of the respiratory mucosa, especially in the upper part of the tract, and causes erythema, oedema, and focal erosions. Viraemia, if it occurs, is mild and brief. Because of the way in which virus disrupts, or completely removes the epithelial cilia from the airways, secondary bacterial infection may occur, and complicate the disease in both adult and young animals.

Signs

The disease begins with a fever (101°-106° F) after an incubation period of 2-3 days. The main sign is cough, which is dry in the beginning and moist later. It begins soon after the temperature rise, and lasts for 1-3 weeks. Nasal discharge is not a prominent sign, and if it occurs, is watery only. There is no marked swelling of the submaxillary lymph nodes, but they may be painful on palpation in the early stages. Depression, reluctance to move, and anorexia are inconstant findings. **The disease is rarely fatal in adult horses, but deaths have been**

reported in young foals from a viral pneumonitis or secondary pneumonia.

Lesions

Erosions have been observed in the mucosa of nose, pharynx, larynx, and trachea. In the lungs, lesions have been described as peribronchitis, bronchitis with hyaline membranes in the alveoli, periarteritis, and bronchopneumonia.

Diagnosis

The serological tests available include complement fixation, haemagglutination inhibition, serum neutralization and ELISA tests. **Positive diagnosis depends on**: 1) demonstration of serum-neutralizing antibodies, 2) isolation and identification of the virus, or 3) demonstration of viral antigens with immunological staining techniques. Equine influenza must be differentiated from equine rhinopneumonitis and equine viral arteritis. Equine rhinopneumonitis may resemble influenza, but as a respiratory disease it is mainly an infection of young horses. Differentiating features of equine viral arteritis include oedema of the limbs, colic, diarrhoea, conjunctivitis, and photophobia. Viral arteritis is also associated with abortion.

Swine Influenza

Swine influenza is a specific, **highly contagious disease of pigs** characterized clinically by fever, and signs of respiratory involvement. It is caused by **type A influenza virus** of the orthomyxovirus group. The virus acts in combination with a Gram-negative bacterium, *Haemophilus influenzae suis*. **The swine influenza virus is closely related to the virus of human influenza type A**. Swine influenza first appeared in the United States immediately following the 1918 pandemic of human influenza, and it was generally believed that it was caused by adaptation of human influenza virus to pigs. This view has been reinforced by the **recent appearance of swine influenza A in the human population**, not in pandemic form. Molecular microbiology has now revealed the antigenic diversity of the virus. Several different H and N antigens have been identified, and grouped on the basis of serological tests. The H3 N2 strain, similar to H3 N2 strain found in the human population, has been isolated from an outbreak in England. The H1 N1 strain of the virus can be found in pig tissues at slaughter.

Spread

The influenza viruses may be transmissible between humans and pigs. Pigs may become infected with related type A human influenza strains during epidemics of human influenza, but show no clinical signs of infection. **The human strains have been isolated from pigs in Hong Kong, and pigs may serve as a reservoir for pandemics in humans as well as a source of genetic information for recombination between human and porcine strains.**

Swine lungworms can act as intermediate host and reservoir for the swine influenza virus during inter-enzootic periods. The virus is introduced into susceptible pigs by lungworm larvae. Infection is provoked by the presence of *H. influenzae suis*. The disease can then spread to other pigs in the herd by direct contact.

Pathogenesis

Swine influenza is primarily a disease of the upper respiratory tract, the trachea and bronchi being particularly involved. However, secondary lesions may develop in the lung because of the drainage of copious exudate from the bronchi. These lesions disappear rapidly, leaving no residual damage. This is in contrast to the lesions of enzootic pneumonia in pigs, which persist for very long periods. Secondary pneumonia, usually due to infection with *Pasteurella multocida*, occurs in some cases and is the cause of most fatalities.

Signs

The disease affects mainly **young pigs**. After an incubation period of 24-48 hours, animals exhibit fever, rhinitis, cough and inappetence. These symptoms usually subside after 3-5 days, but in some cases, transitory (brief) fever may recur within 3 weeks. Dyspnoea associated with severe pulmonary involvement is observed in some cases, and death occurs after severe pneumonia. The mortality rate is usually not high (about 1%), but in some outbreaks may assume serious proportions. The morbidity rate may approach 100%.

Lesions

The specific lesions of swine influenza are restricted to the trachea, bronchi, bronchioles, alveolar ducts, and alveoli. The **gross changes** in part consist of mucopurulent exudate, which lies over the tracheal and bronchial mucosa and fills smaller branches of the bronchi. Plugging of these bronchi and bronchioles results in sharply demarcated areas of atelectasis. Consolidation of lung parenchyma occurs around the bronchi.

. **Microscopically**, the virus produces necrosis of the lining cells of alveoli and bronchi, and to a smaller extent, those of the lower part of the trachea. Because of the loss of nuclei and hyalinization of cytoplasm of the epithelial cells, this necrosis process often appears as a hyaline membrane. Proliferation of the epithelial cells accompanies these necrotic changes. In the bronchi and bronchioles, the growth of epithelium progresses to such a degree that it fills the adjacent alveoli. The pneumonia is characterized by necrosis of alveolar walls with formation of hyaline membranes lining the alveolar sacs. It is accompanied by congestion, focal haemorrhages, severe perivascular and intralobular oedema, and infiltration with leukocytes, mainly mononuclear cells. Areas of collapsed lung parenchyma appear as a result of obstruction of bronchi by pus, mucus, and desquamated cells. Peribronchiolar alveoli are often consolidated as a result of infiltration of mononuclear cells, or the ingrowth of respiratory epithelium. Consolidated alveoli are restored to a functional state by phagocytic removal of the consolidated areas by mononuclear cells.

Diagnosis

The symptoms and gross and microscopic lesions provide a basis for the presumptive diagnosis of swine influenza. **Definitive diagnosis depends on:** 1) demonstration of a significant elevation of virus-neutralizing, or anti-haemagglutinin antibodies in the sera of pigs during the course of an infection, 2) isolation and identification of the swine influenza virus type A, or 3) demonstration of viral antigens with immunological staining techniques.

Avian Influenza

A disease causing extremely high mortality in fowls was first described in 1878, in Italy, and was called **"fowl plague"**. (**'Plague'** is a Latin word for 'blow'. Therefore, any epidemic disease which caused high mortality was called 'plague'. Thus, rinderpest was first called **'cattle plague'**, swine fever as **'swine plague'**, and peste-des-petits-ruminants as **'goat plague'**). In 1901, the causative organism of fowl plague was shown to be a virus. However, it was not until 1955, that its relationship to mammalian influenza A virus was demonstrated. It then became clear **that "fowl plague' virus was actually type A influenza virus**. Soon it was established that influenza A viruses capable of causing the **avian influenza were of two subtypes**: 1) viruses of **low virulence**, and 2) viruses of **high virulence**, capable of causing severe disease in poultry and **inflicting up to 100% mortality**. The term **"highly pathogenic avian influenza (HPAI)"** has been used for these viruses. Thus, fowl plague was caused by highly pathogenic strains of avian influenza viruses. The viruses of low virulence could be antigenically indistinguishable from those of high virulence.

In view of the recent outbreak of a highly pathogenic **avian influenza in Hong Kong, in December 1997**, necessitating slaughter of the entire chicken population of more than 1.5 million, and even threatening a human pandemic, the disease is discussed at some length.

Cause

Avian influenza virus is **an enveloped RNA virus**. The viral genome is composed of eight segments of single-stranded RNA (Fig. 2) of a negative-sense (i.e., the virus RNA is complementary to the messenger RNA). Proteins are associated with the RNA genome to form the **"nucleoprotein-RNA-polymerase complex"**. Virions are roughly spherical or filamentous particles 80-120 nm in diameter. The matrix surrounding the genome complex is enveloped in a lipid membrane. The surface of this lipid membrane of the virion, that is **envelope**, is covered by two different surface **"projections"** or **"spikes"** 10-12 nm in length (**Fig. 2**).

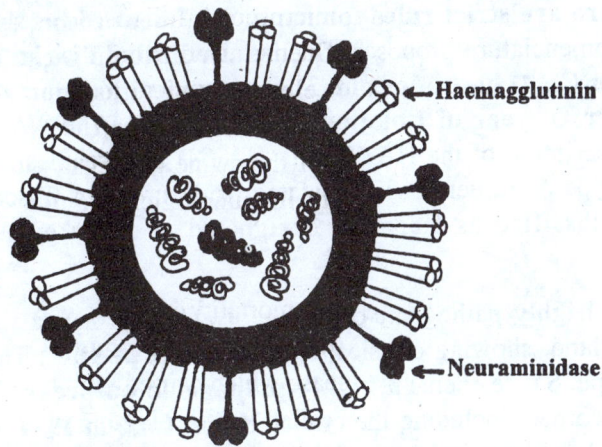

Haemagglutinin

Neuraminidase

Fig. 2. Diagram of (avian) influenza A virus. The "**spikes**" are about 10-12 nm in length. Inside the membrane and matrix shell are eight segments of single-stranded RNA.

These surface spikes are glycoprotein, and have haemagglutination and neuraminidase activity. **The surface spikes** (i.e., surface antigens) **are of two different shapes:** 1) **haemagglutinin (HA),** and 2) **neuraminidase (NA). HA is a rod-shaped trimer** (i.e. m ade of t hree structural s ubunits), and **NA a mushroom-shaped tetramer** (made of four subunits) (**Fig. 2**). **So far, only type A influenza viruses have been isolated from the birds.** Influenza A viruses are subtyped on the basis of HA and NA surface antigens. It is these antigens t hat are i mportant in **p rotective immunity,** a nd show t he g reatest variation. Since these antigens play a crucial role in the pathogenesis of the disease, they are discussed further.

The haemagglutinin is responsible for the attachment of the virion to cell surface receptors (sialyl-oligosaccharides), a nd i s responsible for the haemagglutinating activity of the v irus. Antibodies a gainst the HA are v ery important in n eutralization of t he virus, **a nd protection against infection. Neuraminidase enzyme** activity is **responsible for the release of new virus from the cell,** by its action on the neuraminic acid in the receptors. Antibodies to NA are also important **in protection, by restricting the spread of virus from infected cells.**

Classification based on Haemagglutinin and Neuraminidase

Type A avian influenza viruses are divided into subtypes, according to the antigenic nature of the HA and NA. The typing is done using a group of antisera specific f or the d ifferent subtypes. A t present there are **15 distinct** (separate) **HAs** and **nine distinct NAs.** Each virus possesses one HA and NA subtype, and most of the possible combinations have been isolated from avian species. **There are strict rules for naming influenza isolates.** The standard system of nomenclature proposes that the name **should include:** 1) **antigenic type** (A, B or C), 2) **host of origin**, 3) **geographical location**, 4) **strain reference number**, 5) **year of isolation**, and 6) **the HA and NA subtypes**, i.e., antigenic description of the HA (H) and NA (N) in parenthesis (brackets). For example, a type A influenza virus isolated from turkey in Wisconsin (USA) in 1968, and classified as H8N4, is designated as A/turkey/Wisconsin/1/68 (H8N4).

The first highly pathogenic outbreak of avian influenza was recorded in 1959 in Scotland, showing classical signs of "fowl plague". The virus was of H5N1 subtype. Since then **13 highly pathogenic outbreaks** of the disease have been recorded, including the **one of Hong Kong in 1997.** Of the remaining 12, three have occurred in England, 4 in Australia, 1 in Ireland, 1 in USA, 1 in Canada, 1 in Mexico and 1 in Pakistan (in 1995). To stamp out the disease, in the Ireland outbreak in 1983, some 2,70,000 ducks were slaughtered; in the USA outbreak (Pennsylvania) in 1983-84 over 1,7000,000 birds in 448 flocks were destroyed; and recently in 1997 in Hong Kong outbreak 1,500,000 chickens were mercilessly slaughtered. **It is important to note that all the outbreaks have been of either H5 or H7 subtype.**

Hosts

Avian influenza viruses are distributed throughout the world in many domestic birds, including chickens, turkeys, ducks, geese, guinea-fowl, pheasants, and quails, and also in the feral bird population, i.e., in wild birds. However, the number and frequency of isolations from other species have been overshadowed by the presence of these viruses in waterfowl, particularly **ducks. Ducks have yielded more viruses than any other group.** Moreover, **though the ducks may be infected, they do not suffer from the clinical disease** because of the marked resistance these birds show even **to strains that are highly virulent for chickens and turkeys.** Ducks therefore act as reservoirs and carriers of avian influenza and spread the virus to **chickens and turkeys,** which **suffer the disease clinically.**

Spread

Avian influenza A viruses are **enveloped** viruses, and are therefore **relatively sensitive to inactivation.** They are inactivated by heat, extremes of pH, formalin, and dryness. On the other hand, in the field situation, influenza viruses are often released in nasal secretions and faeces of infected birds, and therefore the **viruses are protected by the presence of organic material. This greatly increases their resistance to inactivation.**

Infected birds excrete virus from the respiratory tract, conjunctiva, and faeces. Therefore likely modes of transmission include both **direct con-**

tact between infected and susceptible birds, and **indirect contact** including **aerosol (droplets),** or exposure to virus-contaminated **fomites.** Since infected birds can excrete high levels of the virus in their **faeces,** spread readily occurs by anything contaminated with **faecal material,** e.g., feed, water, equipment, supplies, c ages, delivery v ehicles, i nsects, and e ven shoes, c lothes e tc. o f humans that come in contact with infected birds or premises. In view of the relatively slow and inefficient spread observed in natural infections, **the fae-cal/oral route appears to be the main route of spread.** A lthough there i s ample evidence for **horizontal spread, there is no evidence to indicate that the viruses can be transmitted vertically.**

Although waterfowl, mainly ducks, appear to be responsible for most in-fluenza i ntroductions to d omestic poultry, o ther possibilities s hould not b e ruled out. For example, **H1 N1 viruses pass readily between pigs, humans, and turkeys,** and the introduction of viruses of this subtype to turkey flocks by infected pigs has b een well documented.

Pathogenesis

Although avian influenza v iruses of t he H5 a nd H7 subtypes have b een associated with severe disease in c hickens, there are many examples of H5 and H7 virus isolates that are n ot pathogenic. **This suggests that antigenic configuration alone does not determine pathogenicity.** A remarkable insight has been gained in recent years i n our understanding of t he mechanisms of virulence of the virus and pathogenesis of the disease.

The avian influenza virus adsorbs to glycoprotein receptors containing sialic acid on the cell surface. The virus then enters the cell by **receptor-medi-ated endocytosis.** As with any virus, pathogenicity is a property of the interaction of the host and virus. The tissue tropism of a virus is involved in its pathogenicity. For example, viruses restricted to the respiratory or intestinal tract will produce quite a different disease problem than a virus which becomes systemic and reaches vital organs. **The basis for tissue tropism is receptor specificity.** Receptor recognition by the virus is an important factor in both tissue tropism and pathogenicity. Since so far no cellular receptor has been identified for influenza viruses, the role of virus-receptor interactions in disease is unclear.

However, there has been a major breakthrough in our understanding of the mechanism of virulence and molecular basis for pathogenicity. Recent studies at a molecular level reveal that infectivity depends **on post-translational cleavage of the haemagglutinin molecule.** That is, on a split or division (cleavage) of the haemagglutinin molecule after it has been formed/synthesized (post-translational). This cleavage is brought about by **host proteases,** and takes place at the **cleavage site.** It was further revealed that the susceptibility of the haemagglutinin molecule to cleavage by host proteases **depends on the number of basic amino acids at the cleavage site. Trypsin-like enzymes can cleave if only a single amino acid** arginine is present at the cleavage site, whereas other host proteases require multiple basic amino acids. This remarkable finding has a direct bearing on the virulence of the virus, as explained below.

The ability of proteases in the host cell to achieve cleavage of haemagglutinin molecules is important in deciding the extent of virus replication, and in the production of infective virus particles. **The HAs of low to moderately virulent influenza viruses have only a single basic amino acid arginine at the cleavage site.** These viruses are therefore cleaved in tissues where trypsin-like enzymes are found, i.e., the respiratory and digestive tract. Since they cannot be cleaved elsewhere, no infective virus is produced at other places. As a result, **their growth and pathogenicity are limited to the respiratory and digestive tracts.** On the other hand, **the highly pathogenic viruses possess HAs with multiple basic amino acids at the cleavage site.** Therefore, their HAs can be cleaved by proteases found throughout the body. **These viruses therefore invade and replicate in many tissues and organs, resulting in the production of infective virus throughout the body, generalized disease, and death.** It appears that multiple basic amino acids are involved in protease recognition and cleavage of the HA of highly pathogenic viruses. It is interesting to note that the mechanism involved in the pathogenicity of avian influenza virus has similarities to that of the Ranikhet disease virus (Newcastle disease virus) (see pathogenesis of Ranikhet disease).

In addition to the cleavability of the haemagglutinin molecule, **other factors may also influence virulence.** For example, the less pathogenic virus isolates may possess a **glycosylation site** (a carbohydrate chain) in the cleavage region. Its presence may block efficient cleavage. **A single mutation removing this glycosylation site has resulted in a highly pathogenic strain.** Also, concurrent bacterial infections play a major role in aggravating the effect of less pathogenic viruses. This could occur because **bacteria provide proteases capable of cleaving the haemagglutinin of these low or moderately virulent viruses in the absence of multiple basic amino acids.** This enables them to replicate and spread widely in the host.

Although it is not yet clear how influenza virus actually kills host cells, recent studies have shown that tissue culture cells infected with influenza virus undergo **apoptosis (programmed cell death).** The *in vivo* significance of apoptosis in influenza remains to be determined.

Signs

The signs of disease are extremely variable and depend on the species affected, age, sex, concurrent infections, type of the virus, environmental factors etc. The disease caused by different viruses varies in severity from high mortality with sudden deaths, to a very mild form, or even inapparent infection. Often the first sign of highly **pathogenic avian influenza** in chickens or turkeys is the sudden onset of **high mortality, which may approach 100% within a few days**. Other clinical signs include cessation of egg laying, respiratory signs including coughing, sneezing, rales, excessive lachrymation; pronounced depression and decreased activity; decreased feed consumption and emaciation; oedema of head and face; cyanosis of unfeathered skin; nervous disorder; and diarrhoea. Any of these signs may occur singly or in various combinations. Outbreaks of highly virulent avian influenza tend to be self-limiting **because few birds survive the disease to act as carriers.**

The **less virulent viruses** may cause drop in egg production or complete cessation, respiratory disease, anorexia, depression, sinusitis, and low mortality. Ducks and other waterfowl tend to be refractory (resistant), even to the viruses that are highly pathogenic for chickens. However, they may be carriers. For waterfowl, **a faecal-water-cloacal route of transmission is believed to be important** in addition to the faecal-water-oral route.

Lesions

The **gross lesions** vary greatly in their location and severity, depending on the species of the bird and pathogenicity of the infecting virus. They are therefore unhelpful in diagnosis. **With less pathogenic viruses**, mild lesions are observed in the sinuses, characterized by catarrhal, fibrinous, serofibrinous, mucopurulent, or caseous inflammation. Other lesions include oedema of the tracheal mucosa with serous or caseous exudate, thickened airsacs with fibrinous or caseous exudate, and catarrhal to fibrinous enteritis. **In the case of highly pathogenic viruses**, there may be no prominent lesions because the birds die very quickly, before gross lesions can develop. However, a variety of congestive, haemorrhagic, transudative, and necrotic changes have been observed. **Initial changes** include oedema of the head with swollen sinuses, and cyanotic, haemorrhagic wattles and combs. **As the disease progresses**, lesions comprise necrotic foci in the liver, spleen, kidneys, and lungs. Besides necrotic foci visceral organs may also show oedema, hyperaemia and haemorrhage. Not all the highly pathogenic strains produce the same gross lesions. Moreover, influenza virus infection may be accompanied by bacterial involvement. Therefore, lesions may reflect the effect of both virus and bacteria.

Microscopically, changes include oedema, hyperaemia, haemorrhages, and foci of perivascular lymphoid cuffing, mainly in the myocardium, spleen, lungs, brain, wattles, liver and kidney. Parenchymal degeneration and necrosis occur in spleen, liver, and kidney. Brain lesions include foci of necrosis, perivascular lymphoid cuffing, glial foci, vascular proliferation, and neuronal changes, i.e., lesions of mild to severe diffuse, non-suppurative encephalitis. **However, none of the lesions are pathognomonic for the disease.**

Zoonotic Implications

A growing body of evidence suggests that pandemic strains of human influenza often arise as a result of recombination between human and animal strains. Genetic reassortment between human and avian viruses is suggested as the mechanism by which "new" human pandemic strains arise. The frequency of variation among influenza viruses is high, and occurs in two ways: **drift** and **shift**. **Antigenic drift** involves **minor antigenic changes** in the haemagglutinin and/or neuraminidase, whereas **antigenic shift** involves **major antigenic changes** in the HA and/or NA.

Influenza viruses are readily recovered from migratory waterfowl, particularly **ducks**, throughout the world. **Infected ducks can shed virus for prolonged period without showing clinical sign.** This reservoir can serve as a source of viruses for other species, including humans, animals, and birds. It appears that ducks may act as the "**melting pot**" where various strains of influenza virus can come together and undergo genetic reassortment, **resulting in "new" strains of influenza.** This new virus could possess surface antigens very different from those previously experienced by the human population. The result could be an influenza pandemic as the new strain rapidly spreads through a susceptible population. In the past, three antigenic shifts have taken place among human influenza viruses leading to pandemics in the human population. Each of these shifts had its origin traced to China. Moreover, China is known to contain a large reservoir of different influenza A viruses among wild and domestic species, **particularly ducks**. The mass production of ducks and the closeness of human habitations to duck farms in China have been implicated as an ideal situation for establishing new antigenic strains and introducing these viruses to the human population. There is enough antigenic and genetic evidence to suggest that the haemagglutinin gene in the virus responsible for the 1968 pandemic in humans **originated from a virus circulating in ducks**. Furthermore, H1N1 viruses present in pigs, turkeys and ducks may be involved in inter-species transmission, so a **swine-avian-human connection** could have a **public health significance**. The agent responsible for the great human pandemic of 1918 was either very similar, or identical, to the agent producing swine influenza. Recent polymerase chain reaction (PCR) analysis of influenza virus **from the lungs of a soldier who died in the 1918 influenza pandemic** that killed 20 million people worldwide identified a swine influenza virus belonging to the same family of influenza viruses causing illness today.

Direct transmission of viruses between birds and humans does not occur. Until now, there were no reports of avian viruses producing disease outbreaks in human populations. Therefore, the potential public health concern was based primarily on circumstantial evidence, not actual events. However, the recent events in Hong Kong (during the second half of 1997) have confirmed this potential danger, and dispelled all doubts. **A strain of influenza type A virus (H5N1), previously known to infect only birds, was for the first time found associated with infection and illness in humans affecting 16 people and causing several deaths**. Surveillance among poultry in Hong Kong indicated continued circulation of type A (H5N1) viruses since March 1997. The human c ases, m ostly i n **children**, w ere c haracterized by a cute o nset, accompanied by fever, cough, sore throat, and running nose. Some adult cases developed viral pneumonia, respiratory distress syndrome, and renal failure. As mentioned, influenza A (H5N1) virus was known previously to infect birds only, **and these were the first cases in which humans were affected**. Infected humans had been in contact with sick poultry afflicted with avian influenza. Although no human influenza A (H5N1) infections have been identified outside Hong Kong, w orldwide surveillance f or influenza is critical t o monitor the circulation of v arious i nfluenza s trains. The c oncern among p ublic health experts is that this **H5 influenza virus** could be the cause of the next worldwide epidemic (pandemic) of human influenza. The previous two introductions of **new "H" subtypes** into humans occurred in Asia. The **"Asian flu"** was caused by an "**H2 virus**", and occurred in 1957. In 1968, an "**H3 virus**" caused "**Hong Kong flu**" epidemic, and variations of that H3 virus have been the major cause of concern for human influenza since that time. **When a different "H" subtype emerges** as the cause of human influenza, severe disease and death losses can occur, **because no one then has residual immunity to the"new H" strain** (H5 in recent Hong Kong case) **from vaccination or past infections.**

Diagnosis

Since clinical symptoms can vary greatly, clinical diagnosis is considered only presumptive. A confirmed diagnosis is based on isolation and identification of the virus. Samples for isolation should include faeces, or intestinal contents and trachea. V irus characterization i nvolves subtype i dentification by the use of specific antisera. Detection of antibodies to the virus is a very useful indirect diagnostic tool. The most commonly used tests are the haemagglutination inhibition test and double immunodiffusion to detect antibodies to the NP. Other serological tests to detect antibodies include virus neutralization, single radial haemolysis, and the more recently developed ELISA assays. Complement fixation test is generally unsatisfactory for avian serum. The other d isease that m ust be considered in t he differential d iagnosis is Ranikhet d isease.

Paramyxoviridae

Viruses classified in the Family **Paramyxoviridae** (G. para = alongside; myxo = mucus) are pleomorphic, **enveloped** viruses, with **RNA** occurring **as a single negative-sense molecule**. (The family was so named because whereas **Orthomyxoviridae** family contained 'true' (G. artho = true) influenza viruses, this family a lso alongside (G. p ara) c ontained i nfluenza viruses known as "**parainfluenza viruses**".) The virions of this family may be spherical or filamentous, 100-500 nm in diameter. The family **now** has **four genera**: **paramyxovirus, morbillivirus, rubulavirus,** and **pneumovirus.** The principal members of this family are listed in **Table 4.** The viruses grouped in the genus "**paramyxovirus**" contain neuraminidase, whereas viruses in the other genera do not. Those in the genus "**morbillivirus**" are antigenically related and induce similar diseases.

Table 4. Diseases caused by Paramyxoviridae

Paramyxoviruses
    Mumps
    Parainfluenza - 1 (human, swine)
    Parainfluenza - 2 (human, canine)
    Parainfluenza - 3 (human, bovine, ovine)
    Parainfluenza - 4 (human)
Morbilliviruses
    Measles
    Canine distemper
    Rinderpest
    Peste-des-petits-ruminants (PPR)
    Equine morbillivirus
Rubulaviruses
    Newcastle disease (Ranikhet disease)
    (Avian paramyxovirus - 1)
    Avian paramyxoviruses (type 2-9)
Pneumoviruses
    Respiratory syncytial virus (human)
    Respiratory syncytial virus (bovine)
    Avian pneumovirus
    (Turkey rhinotracheitis, TRT)
    Swollen head syndrome (SHS) of chickens

Diseases caused by Paramyxoviruses

Mumps

Mumps virus is also a member of the paramyxovirus genus, but is not pathogenic for domestic animals.

Parainfluenza

The parainfluenza viruses **are important respiratory pathogens, of both animals and humans,** especially the young. The numerous isolates are divided into four types or groups, which contain related viruses of varying virulence.

Parainfluenza - 1

These viruses have been recovered from humans, **pigs,** rats and mice. **In children,** the three viruses, parainfluenza 1, 2 and 3, are a major cause of upper respiratory disease (**croup**) and pneumonia. **In pigs,** the infection is usually subclinical and of no c onsequence.

Parainfluenza - 2

These viruses h ave been r ecovered from h umans, **dogs** and monkeys. The prototype (first model) of this group was recovered from a monkey, and is called **Simian** (L. simia = monkey) **virus 5 (SV 5)**. Canine parainfluenza 2 virus causes upper respiratory disease of dogs, especially in k ennels, and i s considered one of the main causes of "**kennel cough syndrome**". Infection is manifested by coughing associated w ith rhinitis, t racheitis, bronchitis, and less often, conjunctivitis, and b ronchopneumonia.

Parainfluenza - 3

This virus infection has been demonstrated in humans, cattle, sheep, pigs, cats, monkeys, and apes. **Infection in cattle and sheep is common. Clinical signs** include a short course of fever, rhinitis with nasal discharge, lachrymation, coughing and d yspnoea. Interstitial p neumonia with p roliferation of septal cells and bronchiolar and alveolar epithelium, and also form ation of multinucleated cells with both **intranuclear and cytoplasmic inclusions** may occur. The importance of bovine and ovine parainfluenza - 3 infection is that **it predisposes to other respiratory pathogens**, particularly to *P asteurella haemolytica* which causes shipping fever.

Diseases caused by Morbilliviruses

The **morbillivirus genus** contains several v ery important p athogens t o humans and animals (Table 4). **Measles, canine distemper, and rinderpest are the three classical members of this group.** The viruses are morphologically indistinguishable a nd **antigenically closely related**. T he main d ifference among canine distemper, rinderpest and measles viruses **is in their natural hosts**.

Measles

Measles is a highly infectious exanthematous disease of humans, mainly **children**, caused by a **morbillivirus**. The virus and its pathogenic effects are closely related to canine distemper and rinderpest. Measles is also known to be infectious for several species of **monkeys**, including rhesus. Although measles is rare in their native habitats (the natural environment), few rhesus monkeys escape infection once they are brought into captivity. Clinical disease is rarely recorded. However, monkeys may exhibit conjunctivitis, and an exanthematous rash, which lasts for 3-14 days.

Canine Distemper

Canine distemper is **a highly contagious**, common, **serious systemic disease** of dogs, caused by **a morbillivirus**. The disease is worldwide in distribution, and is characterized by a **diphasic (biphasic) fever**, leukopaenia, gastrointestinal and respiratory catarrh, and usually pneumonic and neurological complications. The often changing clinical symptoms can confuse canine distemper with such diseases as canine hepatitis, herpesvirus, parainfluenza, and leptospirosis. Besides dogs, canine distemper also occurs in wolf and fox.

Spread

The main route of infection is **through inhalation of aerosol droplet secretions from infected animals**. Some infected dogs may shed virus for several months. The virus is sensitive to most disinfectants, and is unstable outside the host.

Pathogenesis

Infection occurs through the respiratory route with initial viral replication in respiratory epithelium and alveolar macrophages. Soon virus spreads to the **tonsils** and **bronchial lymph nodes**. Before clinical signs appear, cell-associated virus (mostly associated with lymphocytes) circulates through the bloodstream to other organs, including the brain. Free virus (viraemia) has also been demonstrated in the bloodstream. However, it is not clear whether the central nervous system is invaded as a result of viraemia, or by the cell-associated virus. **Viral replication and consequent direct damage to neurons and astrocytes occur**. Indirect damage to oligodendroglial cells result in **demyelination**. There is no evidence of direct damage to oligodendrocytes. However, occurrence of the demyelinating encephalitis is due to the development of a local immune response, similar to that of experimental allergic encephalomyelitis. The mechanism by which **"old dog encephalitis (ODE)"** develops is not clear. ODE is a rare condition characterized by ataxia (muscular incoordination), compulsive (irresistible) movements, such as head pressing, and hypermetria (unusual movements). It may occur in the adult dog without a prior history of canine distemper virus related clinical signs. It is believed that the distemper virus remains suppressed in the central nervous system, and following some unknown stimulus, causes defective replication without development of complete viral particles. However, the **"defective virus"** spreads from cell to cell. It is suggested that the suppressed virus does not express antigens on the surface of infected cells. **This allows its persistence and escape from the immune system.**

In distemper encephalitis **extensive demyelination of neurons** occurs. This demyelination seen in chronic distemper is a result of the local antiviral response. Macrophages, which are very numerous in these brain lesions, ingest immune complexes and infected cells. As a result, they release free radicals and other toxic products. It is these toxic products that damage nearby cells, especially oligodendroglia, and thus cause demyelination. It has been suggested that some of the demyelinating encephalitis results from autoimmune attack. Thus, most animals suffering from this syndrome make antibodies against myelin proteins, and it has been suggested that these cause tissue destruction.

Recent studies have shown that dogs with **rheumatoid arthritis** have much higher levels of antibodies against canine distemper in their synovial fluids, than normal dogs. This suggests that in dogs canine distemper virus may be present in rheumatoid joints and that it may play a role in the pathogenesis of the disease.

Signs

Exposure of susceptible dogs to the virus results in **an acute fever**, which appears after 7-8 days of incubation. Within 96 hours, body temperature usually drops rapidly to about normal levels. It remains normal up to the 11th or 12th day, when it climbs to **a second peak. This diphasic (biphasic) fever curve is a characteristic feature of the disease.** Coryza, purulent conjunctivitis, and bronchitis occur in varying degrees. Bronchopneumonia may occur. Usually, vesiculo-pustular lesions appear on the abdomen. In some cases, there is hyperkeratosis of the digital pads (**"hard pad disease"**). Usually, leukopaenia and thrombocytopaenia also develop. In many cases, diarrhoea results in severe dehydration and emaciation. Signs of meningo-encephalitis occur in about 50% of affected dogs. However, lesions are present in a much higher percentage. Nervous signs may develop during the acute phase of the disease, and continue even after disappearance of other signs. Nervous signs include chewing movements, excessive salivation, incoordination, circling, neuro-muscular tics (spasmodic muscular contractions involving face, head, neck, or shoulder muscles), nystagmus (involuntary movement of the eyeball), torticollis (twisted neck), and convulsions. Blindness and paralysis are less common. Although the disease may occur in a mild, non-fatal form, most animals with severe nervous, respiratory, and enteric signs die from the infection. In a small number of dogs, which recover, the virus remains latent in the brain and causes **"old dog encephalitis"** years later.

Lesions

In the **respiratory system**, purulent or catarrhal exudate is found on the nasal and pharyngeal mucosa. **Microscopically, characteristic cytoplasmic and intranuclear inclusion bodies** are often seen in cells associated with the exudate. These inclusions are **eosinophilic** when stained by H. & E. In the cytoplasm, they are round or ovoid and vary from 5-20 μm in diameter. They are usually homogeneous and sharply demarcated. The intranuclear inclusions, which are similar to the cytoplasmic in appearance, cause only slight enlargement of the nucleus and little margination of the chromatin. The immunofluorescence techniques can be used to demonstrate that these inclusions contain viral antigen.

Principal lesion in the **lung** is a purulent **bronchopneumonia**, in which bronchi and adjacent alveoli are filled with neutrophils, mucin, and tissue debris. In some cases, **multinucleated giant cells** form in the bronchial lining, alveolar septa, and freely in the alveoli. This form of **giant-cell pneumonia** is similar to that associated with measles in humans and monkeys. Cytoplasmic, and less often intranuclear inclusions, are found in the giant cells, and in cells of the bronchiolar and bronchial epithelium. **In the skin**, particularly of the abdomen, a vesicular and pustular dermatitis may occur. The vesicles and pustules are confined to the Malpighian layer of the epidermis. There is usually some congestion of the underlying dermis, and occasionally lymphocytic infiltration. Nuclear or cytoplasmic inclusion bodies may be present within epithelial cells of sebaceous glands. On the foot pads, extensive proliferation of the keratin layer of the epidermis results in a clinically recognized lesion, which is called "**hard-pad disease**". However, this lesion can develop in other diseases (e.g., toxoplasmosis), **and is therefore not specific for canine distemper.**

The **urinary epithelium**, particularly of the renal pelvis and bladder, contain congested vessels, and microscopically, **cytoplasmic or intranuclear inclusion bodies**. The **stomach** and **intestines** contain large numbers of cytoplasmic and some intranuclear inclusions in the lining epithelium. Apart from these inclusions, few lesions are observed. There is necrosis of both T cell and B cell areas in lymph nodes and the spleen. No significant lesions occur in the liver. However, inclusions may be present in the biliary epithelium.

In the central nervous system, the virus has an affinity for the myelinated portions of the brain and spinal cord. Thus, in contrast to such infections as equine encephalomyelitis, Teschen disease (porcine encephalomyelitis), and poliomyelitis (of humans), **the neurons are not primarily affected.** The distribution and nature of the lesions in canine distemper, therefore, differ from those in most viral encephalitides. The lesions at one time were thought to be caused by some other agent, and were referred to as "**McIntyre's encephalitis**". The structures most constantly affected are the cerebellar peduncles, the myelinated tracts of the cerebellum, and the white columns of the spinal cord. The lesions are characterized by sharply delimited areas of destruction, particularly in the myelinated tracts of the areas mentioned. Under low-power microscopy, sharply defined holes (vacuoles) of irregular size give the affected tracts a "**spongy**" **appearance (status spongiosa).** Often, collections of lymphocytes in the Virchow-Robin spaces around nereby vessels are present. Sometimes, "**gitter**" **cells** gather around areas of necrosis in the white matter. Gemistocytic astrocytes ("**gemistocytes**") are prominent in the exudate, and contain **intranuclear inclusions, which is a characteristic feature of this lesion.** In the **cerebrum**, the most prominent lesion is an increase in the number of capillaries, probably from proliferation, or from their distension and congestion. Apart from the changes in the myelinated tracts, degenerative changes also develop in neurons. There is pyknosis, chromatolysis, gliosis, and neuronophagia. Rarely, cytoplasmic or nuclear inclusion bodies can be found in neurons. Neuronal necrosis may be present in the cerebral and cerebellar cortex, medullary nuclei, and spinal cord.

In the retina, there is congestion, oedema, perivascular cuffing with lymphocytes, and gliosis. Neuritis of the optic nerve with demyelination and gliosis may also be present. Intranuclear inclusions are present in glia of the retina and optic nerve. The lesions lead to retinal atrophy of all layers. The so called "**old dog encephalitis**", the most striking lesion in the central nervous system, is characterized by perivascular cuffing with almost pure populations of lymphocytes. Intranuclear inclusion bodies may be found in glial cells and neurons.

Of particular interest in clinical diagnosis of distemper is the finding that **cytoplasmic inclusions** appear **in some circulating neutrophils** of affected dogs. Less often, similar inclusions are found in circulating lymphocytes. In some cases, inclusion bodies can be demonstrated in the conjunctival epithelium.

Diagnosis

Distemper should be considered in the diagnosis of any febrile condition in puppies. Diagnosis can be made on the basis of a history of the typical clinical disease, and the demonstration of characteristic lesions and cytoplasmic and intranuclear inclusion bodies. Immunological staining techniques, or viral isolation and identification confirm the diagnosis.

Clinical diagnosis can be confirmed by finding typical inclusion bodies in smears of cells of the respiratory epithelium, or peripheral blood. Unfortunately, the inclusions are not present in all cases. Therefore, their absence does not rule out the diagnosis of distemper. In dogs, toxoplasmosis often occurs in association with canine distemper. Lesions of both diseases should be searched if evidence of either infection is present.

Rinderpest (Cattle Plague)

Rinderpest is **an acute, highly contagious disease of cattle** caused by a **morbillivirus**. The disease has been the foremost cause of death in cattle in most African and Asian countries, **including India**. In fact, the need to fight the disease was instrumental in the establishment of the first veterinary college in 1762 in Lyon, France. Mortality varies from 25%-90%, depending on the strains of virus and the resistance of the animals. **Clinically**, the disease is characterized by high fever, necrotic stomatitis, diarrhoea, and high mortality. Buffaloes, sheep, pigs, goats, and camels are also susceptible. **In wildlife**, rinderpest has been reported in deer, antelope, wild buffaloes, wild boars, bushbuck, warthogs and giraffe. The rinderpest virus is antigenically closely related to the viruses of canine distemper, peste-des-petits-ruminants (PPR) of sheep and goats, and measles of humans. Many strains of rinderpest virus occur, but all are immunologically identical. Therefore, the immunity which develops after infection, or vaccination with one strain, **protects against all other strains. Rinderpest has not been reported since June 1995 in our country.**

Spread

Rinderpest virus is quite fragile. Therefore, close contact between infected and non-infected animals is necessary for spread of the disease, because the virus does not survive for long outside the host. The virus is excreted by infected animals in urine, faeces, nasal discharges, and sweat. Transmission occurs through contaminated feed, or by **inhalation** of aerosol (infected droplets). **Ingestion** of food contaminated by the discharges of clinical cases, or animals in the incubation stage, may also be important modes of infection, especially in pigs.

Pathogenesis

The virus is inhaled in infected droplets. It penetrates through the epithelium of the upper respiratory tract and multiplies in the **tonsils** and **regional lymph nodes.** From here it enters the blood in mononuclear cells, which disseminate the virus to other lymphoid organs, the lungs, and epithelial cells of mucous membranes. **The virus has a high degree of affinity for lymphoid tissue and alimentary mucosa. There is a pronounced destruction of lymphocytes in tissues.** This is the cause of **marked leukopaenia.** The virus is intimately associated with leukocytes, only a small proportion being free in plasma. The focal, necrotic stomatitis and enteritis are the direct result of the viral infection and replication in the epithelial cells in the alimentary tract. However, since the virus induces a strong antibody response shortly after infection, there is a rapid decrease and elimination of virus from the body as the clinical signs and lesions become visible. **Death is usually from severe dehydration,** but in less acute cases, death may be from activated latent parasitic or bacterial infections. These aggravate because the animal is immunosuppressed as a result of the destruction of lymphoid organs by the virus.

Signs

The onset of illness is indicated by a sharp rise in body temperature (104° 105° F), accompanied by restlessness, dryness of the muzzle, and constipation. Other signs include photophobia (intolerance to light), excessive thirst, starry (shining) coat, retarded rumination, anorexia, and excessive salivation. A maculo-papular rash may develop on parts of the body, where hairs are fine. The fever usually reaches its peak on the 3rd or 5th day, but **drops abruptly with the onset of diarrhoea,** even though other symptoms get intensified. Lesions in the oral mucosa may appear by the 2nd or 3rd day of fever, but become clearly visible only after the onset of diarrhoea. As the diarrhoea increases in intensity, it is accompanied by abdominal pain, increased respiration, severe dehydration, and emaciation. This is followed by prostration, subnormal temperature, and death, usually after a course of 6-12 days.

A marked leukopaenia occurs at the height of infection. The total count usually falls to below 4000/μl, and is due to **an abrupt drop in lymphocytes**. Immunity after a natural infection is long and persists for life. The protection is associated with the induction of humoral antibodies, first IgM, and later IgG and IgA.

Lesions

As already mentioned, **the rinderpest virus has a particular affinity for epithelial tissues of the gastrointestinal tract**, where it produces severe characteristic changes. **In lymphoid tissue, the virus causes necrosis of lymphocytes.** This is striking in microscopic sections of lymph nodes, spleen, and Peyer's patches. The destruction of lymphocytes is first seen as a fragmentation of nuclei in the germinal centres, and in a short time, most of the mature lymphocytes disappear. **Multinucleated giant cells containing eosinophilic cytoplasmic inclusion bodies** are often present. Rarely, intranuclear inclusions are also seen. Oedema and congestion of capillaries are seen microscopically. The destruction of lymphoid cells leaves a fibrillar, eosinophilic, acellular matrix at sites of the lymphoid follicles. **Grossly**, changes are most marked in the **Peyer's patches**, which may be darkened with haemorrhages and slough out, leaving **deep craters (ulcers)** in the intestinal wall.

In the digestive system of cattle, rinderpest virus produces typical lesions. The virus is carried to the oral mucosa by the bloodstream. In the squamous epithelium of the oral cavity, the first change is necrosis of a few epithelial cells in deep layers of the stratum malpighii. These cells have pyknotic and fragmented nuclei and eosinophilic cytoplasm. They are shrunken and separated from the adjoining space by a clear space. As these necrotic areas increase in size and extend towards the surface, the cornified layer above them becomes elevated. This causes them to appear grossly as tiny, greyish-white, slightly raised puncta (points). Multinucleated giant cells form in the stratum spinosum. **Eosinophilic cytoplasmic inclusion bodies** form in the mucosal epithelial cells and giant cells. Intranuclear inclusion bodies are rare. **Vesicles are not formed in this disease**. With time, the foci of necrosis coalesce to form large areas of **erosions**. Since the basal layer of the squamous epithelium is rarely penetrated, ulcers seldom form. The erosions are shallow, with a red raw floor, and a sharply demarcated margin. **The lesions in the oral mucosa have a selective distribution: inside the lower lip, the adjacent gum, the cheeks near commissures, and the ventral surface of the free portion of the**

tongue. In severe cases, lesions extend to the hard palate and pharynx, and in fulminant cases, to all the mucous surfaces of the tongue. The oesophageal lesions are similar to those in the mouth, but are less severe. The rumen, reticulum, and omasum rarely exhibit any lesions.

The **abomasum** is one of the most common sites of the lesions of rinderpest. They are most severe in the **pyloric region**, where necrotic foci of microscopic size in the epithelium are accompanied by congestion and haemorrhage in the underlying lamina propria. **Grossly**, this results in irregular superficial bright red to dark brown streaks. These streaks follow the edges of the broad plicae and extend into the fundus, but become more numerous and diffuse in the pylorus. Oedema may be extensive in the submucosa of plicae, making it to appear thickened. As necrosis of the epithelium progresses, the epithelium sloughs away, leaving sharply outlined irregular erosions with a red raw floor oozing blood. In the **small intestine**, severe lesions are less common than in the mouth, abomasum, or large intestine. However, Peyer's patches are exceptionally vulnerable. The lymphoid tissue may become so necrotic that patches slough out, **leaving deep raw craters in the intestinal wall**.

The large intestine, as a rule, is more seriously damaged than the small intestine, with prominent lesions in the ileo-caecal valve, caeco-colic junction, and the rectum. The crest of the folds of mucous membrane throughout the caecum is bright red because of numerous petechiae, which appear more like diffuse haemorrhages. **Microscopically**, the petechiae (haemorrhages) are markedly distended capillaries, packed with erythrocytes, in the lamina propria. **Streaks of congestion along the folds of mucosa produce a characteristic "Zebra-striped" (Zebra markings), or "barred" appearance**. As the disease progresses and the mucosa becomes eroded, diffuse congestion and bleeding from the raw surfaces may occur over large areas. When opened, the mucosa is diffusely red, and the lumen contains partially clotted blood.

Lesions at the **caeco-colic junction** include congestion, erosion, and increased thickness of the wall, partly the result of oedema in the submucosa and muscularis. The changes in the **colon** and **rectum** vary from a few longitudinal streaks of congestion along the crest of the folds of the mucosa to erosions of the mucosal epithelium. The characteristic streaks of cogestion and haemorrhage are more common and striking **in the rectum than in the colon**. The **liver** is affected only secondarily in rinderpest, with chronic passive congestion resulting from cardiac and pulmonary complications. Lesions in the **gallbladder** vary from scattered petechiae to diffuse blotches of haemorrhage.

In the **respiratory system**, the epithelium is susceptible to the virus. Petechiae occur on the turbinates and larynx. **In the trachea, streaks of haemorrhages in the mucosa are almost always found**. Most common are longitudinal streaks of rusty haemorrhage in the anterior third of the trachea. The **lungs** appear to be involved only secondarily. In acute cases, lungs usually appear grossly normal. In long-standing cases, lesions include both interlobular and alveolar emphysema and small areas of consolidation. The lesions of the **heart** also appear to be secondary and include subendocardial haemorrhages over the papillary muscles of the left ventricle. The right ventricle is seldom involved. In the **urinary system**, lesions comprise oedema around the renal pelvis and desquamation of pelvic epithelium. In the **urinary bladder**, the epithelium may be desquamated and the underlying stroma infiltrated with erythrocytes. The infiltrates are grossly seen as thin red blotches. Lesions in the skin, though not common, may be seen as a maculo-papular rash over thinly haired portions of the body, the vulva, and prepuce. **Microscopically**, they resemble those of the oral mucosa.

A virus very closely related to rinderpest, and causing an acute, highly fatal disease of sheep and goats is called "**peste-des-petits-ruminants (PPR)**" (discussed next). It does not naturally affect cattle, nor does experimental infection lead to disease in cattle. **It does, however, confer immunity to rinderpest virus.**

Diagnosis

The clinical, gross, and microscopic features of the disease are adequate for a presumptive diagnosis. This should, however, be confirmed by immunological methods w hich include a gar gel i mmunodiffusion (AGID), c omplement fixation, c ounter-immunoelectrophoresis (CIEP), i mmunofluorescence, and immuno-peroxidase tests, an ELISA which is accurate and easy to perform, and a rapid dot-enzyme immunoassay test suitable for field use. **Using specific cDNA probes, isolates o f rinderpest and PPR viruses can now be differentiated.** A test employing the **polymerase chain reaction (PCR)** has been developed that can detect viral RNA in tissues otherwise unsuitable for standard techniques. Isolation of the virus and its identification are now possible in tissue culture to confirm the diagnosis.

Peste-Des-Petits-Ruminants (PPR, Goat Plague)

"**Peste-des-petits-ruminants (PPR)**" is a French name and means "**plague of small ruminants**", i.e., **goats** and **sheep**. The disease was called "**plague**" because it inflicted h eavy mortality. '**Plague**' is a Latin word f or '**blow**'. Therefore, in p ast, a ny epidemic disease which caused h igh m ortality w as called '**plague**'. Thus, rinderpest was first called "**cattle plague**"; swine fever as "**swine plague**", and avian influenza as "**avian plague**". PPR is thus commonly known as "**goat plague**". Other synonyms include **erosive stomatitis** and **enteritis of goats**, and **stomatitis-pneumoenteritis complex.** **The disease in goats is clinically and pathologically indistinguishable from rinderpest.**

PPR is an acute, highly contagious disease of goats and sheep, caused by a **morbillivirus** (ssRNA). The disease was first recognized in 1942 in Ivory Coast, in French West Africa. **In India**, it was first reported in 1989 in native sheep flocks in Villupuram district of Tamil Nadu, and is now widely spread in the country. **Each year it inflicts heavy losses in goats and sheep.** In recent past, several outbreaks have been reported from Tamil Nadu, Andhra Pradesh, Uttar Pradesh, Rajasthan, Karnataka, Jammu and Kashmir, Bihar, West Bengal and Himachal Pradesh. PPR is characterized by fever, anorexia, lymphopaenia, erosive st omatitis, diarrhoea, oculo-nasal purulent d ischage, and r espiratory distress. **It is a rinderpest-like disease, and is highly fatal in goats, less so in sheep.** PPR is antigenically closely related to the viruses of rinderpest, canine distemper, and measles (of humans). All these are also morbilliviruses. In particular, PPR and rinderpest (RP) viruses cross-immunize and cross-protect, so much so that **tissue culture rinderpest vaccine has been found to be an effective prophylactic against PPR.** Morbidity and mortality rates in sheep and goats in enzootic areas are generally high (above 50%), and can be up to 90% of the flock during outbreaks. **The disease is more severe in goats than in sheep, and is rapidly fatal in young animals.** There is a belief that rinderpest became prevalent in sheep and goats in Africa and Asia only after the introduction of goat-adopted rinderpest vaccine from which the virus of PPR probably evolved through mutation.

Spread

As in rinderpest, close contact with an infected a nimal, or contaminated fomite, is required for the disease to spread. Large amounts of the virus are present in all body excretions and secretions, especially in diarrhoeic faeces. **Infection is mainly by inhalation**, but could also occur through the conjunctiva and oral mucosa. **The disease is particularly fulminating in goats, and is usually fatal.**

Pathogenesis

The v irus penetrates the retro-pharyngeal m ucosa, sets u p a v iraemia, and specifically damages the alimentary, respiratory, and lymphoid systems. Infected cells undergo necrosis, but in the respiratory mucosa and lungs, there is a lso proliferation of cells. Some virulent st rains cause d eath from severe diarrhoea and d ehydration, p articularly i n **young goats** before r espiratory lesions become severe. In others, death may occur f rom concurrent diseases such as pneumonic pasteurellosis and coccidiosis. Entero-toxigenic *Escherichia coli* may also aggravate the diarrhoea. Lymphoid necrosis is not as marked in this disease as in rinderpest. Most sheep and some adult goats recover and they carry **antibodies that confer life-long immunity.**

Signs

The disease can be **acute** or **subacute. The acute form is seen mainly in**

goats, and is similar to rinderpest in cattle. Signs generally appear 3-6 days after being in contact with an infected animal. A **high fever** (above 104° F) is accompanied by dullness, sneezing, and serous discharges from the eyes and nostrils. A leukopaenia occurs from destructive effect of the virus on lymphocytes, but this is not as marked as in rinderpest. Within a day or two, distinct necrotic lesions develop in the mouth and extend over the entire oral mucosa, forming diphtheritic plaques. There is profound halitosis (offensive breath) and the animal is unable to eat because of the sore mouth and swollen lips. Nasal and ocular discharges become mucopurulent and the exudate dries up, matting (gluing) the eyelids and partially occluding the external nares (nostrils). **Diarrhoea develops 3-4 days after the onset of fever**. It is profuse and the faeces may be mucoid and blood-tinged. Dyspnoea and coughing occur later, and the respiratory signs are aggravated when there is secondary bacterial pneumonia. Superficial erosions may occur in the mucosa of the vulva and prepuce. **Death usually occurs within a week of the onset of illness**. Pregnant animals may abort. **Subacute reactions** are more common in sheep, and are manifested by catarrh, low-grade fever, and intermittent diarrhoea. Most recover after a course of 10-14 days. **Animals recovering from the disease (both goats and sheep) have a lasting immunity, as in rinderpest.**

Lesions

Grossly, discrete (separate) or extensive areas of erosion, necrosis, and ulceration, present in the oral mucosa, pharynx and upper oesophagus, may extend to the abomasum and distant small intestine. Haemorrhagic ulceration is marked in the ileo-caecal region, colon, and rectum, where they produce typical **"Zebra stripes"**. Retropharyngeal and mesenteric lymph nodes are enlarged. Spleen may also be enlarged. Severe lesions are often present throughout the respiratory tract. A mucopurulent exudate extends from the nasal opening to the larynx. The trachea and bronchi may be hyperaemic, and contain froth due to pulmonary congestion and oedema. An interstitial pneumonia is usually present. **Grossly**, the pneumonia is characterized by areas of red consolidation and atelectasis. These usually involve the antero-ventral lobes, particularly the right lobe. With bacterial complications (mostly **Pasteurella**), there may be purulent or fibrinous bronchopneumonia and pleuritis.

Microscopic lesions in the **alimentary tract** are similar to those in rinderpest, **but are often more severe**. Syncytial cells (**multinucleated giant cells**) are present in the early stages of the lesion in the stratified squamous epithelium of the upper respiratory tract. **Intracytoplasmic inclusion bodies** may be abundant in necrotic glands of the small and large intestines. **In the respiratory tract**, there is proliferative rhino-tracheitis, bronchitis and bronchiolitis, and within the alveoli **proliferation of type II pneumocytes and formation of huge syncytial giant cells. Intracytoplasmic and**

intranuclear eosinophilic inclusion bodies are common in the epithelial cells of the airways and in the type II pneumocytes and syncytial cells. The inclusion b odies can be shown to contain viral antigens by immuno-histochemical st ains.

Diagnosis

Presumptive diagnosis can be made from the clinical signs and postmortem findings. **Pneumonia is usually a feature of PPR, but not rinderpest**. Confirmation can be achieved by isolation of the virus and its identification. Blood at the height of the fever is the best source of the virus. Virus has been successfully isolated in primary l amb or k idney cultures. F or provisional diagnosis antigen in lymph nodes can be detected by agar gel immunodiffusion (AGID) or by counter-immunoelectrophoresis technique (CIEP). Unlike rinderpest, cases of PPR usually contain high levels of antigen at death. Since PPR and rinderpest in goats are indistinguishable both clinically and pathologically, it is important to confirm by other means that it is PPR virus and n ot r inderpest virus t hat c aused the d isease. For this, i mmunocapture sandwich ELISA has been developed which employs specific PPRV and RPV detector MABs (monoclonal antibodies). Also, specific cDNA probes for selected segments of N genes of the two viruses are useful in differentiating PPR and RP, on postmortem materials. **Differential diagnosis** is also possible by complement fixation and virus neutralization tests. More recently, a **reverse transcriptase-polymerase chain reaction (RT-PCR)** has been found valuable in confirmatory diagnosis in tissues otherwise unsuitable for standard techniques, and also in differentiating PPR from RP.

Morbillivirus Pneumonia of Horses

In 1994, an outbreak of respiratory disease occurred in a stable of horses in Queensland, Australia, in which **many sick horses died**. A trainer and a stable se rvant also b ecame ill, and the trainer later died. The disease in the horses and the trainer was characterized by **interstitial pneumonia**, with marked pulmonary oedema. Syncytial cells with **cytoplasmic inclusion bodies** were prominent in the walls and endothelium of pulmonary capillaries and arterioles, as w ell as i n lymph n odes, spleen, s tomach, heart, k idneys, and b rain. A morbillivirus was r ecovered, which appears to be a newly recognized virus. Its origin is not known. No further occurrence of the disease has been reported.

Diseases caused by Rubulavirus

The genus **Rubulavirus** includes Newcastle disease virus (Ranikhet d isease virus), and the other avian paramyxoviruses. **Nine serogroups (serotypes) of avian paramyxoviruses have been recognized**: PMV-1 to PMV-9. **Of these, Newcastle disease virus (PMV-1) remains the most important pathogen for poultry**, but PMV-2 and PMV-3 can also be responsible for serious disease.

The method of nomenclature used for influenza A isolates has been adopted for avian paramyxoviruses, **so that an isolate is named by**: 1) serotype, 2) species or type of bird from which it was isolated, 3) geographical location of isolation, 4) reference number or name, and 5) year of isolation (see avian influenza).

Newcastle Disease (Ranikhet Disease)
(Paramyxovirus type -1)

Also known as **"avian pneumo-encephalitis"** and in India as **"Ranikhet disease"**, Newcastle disease is **an acute, rapidly spreading disease of domestic poultry** and other birds, **caused by paramyxovirus type 1 (PMV - 1)**. The disease is characterized by rapid onset, respiratory signs, and nervous manifestations; and variable mortality. The first outbreaks of Newcastle disease were recorded in 1926, in Java, Indonesia; and in 1927 by Doyle in Newcastle-upon-Tyne, England. **In India**, the disease was first recorded at **Ranikhet**, in Kumaon hills (District Nainital, U.P.), by Edward in 1927; hence the name **"Ranikhet disease"**. The name **"Newcastle disease"** was coined by Doyle. It later became clear that other less severe diseases were caused by viruses indistinguishable from Newcastle disease virus (NDV). In the United States, a relatively mild respiratory disease, often with nervous signs, was first described in the 1930s, and termed **"avian pneumo-encephalitis"**. It was caused by a virus indistinguishable from NDV in serological tests. Soon numerous NDV isolations that produced extremely mild, or no disease in chickens, were made around the world. Today, the disease is almost world-wide in distribution, except in the Scandinavian countries. **In India, it is the most important viral disease of poultry.**

Cause

Newcastle disease is caused by **a group of closely related viruses, which form the avian paramyxovirus type 1 (PMV-1) serotype**. Paramyxoviruses are RNA viruses showing helical capsid symmetry with a single-stranded genome of negative polarity. They are **enveloped**. The envelope is formed from modified cell membrane as the virus is budded from the cell surface after capsid assembly in the cytoplasm. Although virus particles are very pleomorphic, usually they are rounded and 100-500 nm in diameter. The surface of the virus particle is covered with **projections** about 8 nm in length.

For many years, NDV strains and isolates were considered to form a serologically homogeneous group. However, recently developed more precise serological techiques, mostly the use of mouse monoclonal antibodies, have shown that **considerable antigenic variation exists between different strains of NDV**. (The term **"strain"** is generally used to mean a well-charac-terized isolate of the virus). A striking feature of NDV strains and isolates is their ability to cause quite distinct signs and severity of disease, even in the same host species. Based on the disease produced in chickens, NDVs have been placed in five pathotypes:

1. **Viscerotropic velogenic**: The NDVs cause a **highly virulent form of the disease**. Haemorrhagic lesions are characteristically present in the intestinal tract.

2. **Neurotropic velogenic**: These NDVs cause **high mortality** following respiratory and nervous signs.

3. **Mesogenic**: These NDVs cause **low mortality** following respiratory and sometimes nervous signs.

4. **Lentogenic**: These respiratory NDVs cause **mild or inapparent respiratory infection.**

5. **Asymptomatic**: The enteric NDVs cause **inapparent enteric infection**.

However, such groups should be regarded only as a guide as there is always some degree of overlap and some viruses cannot easily be placed in a specific pathotype.

Surface Projections (Spikes)

As these have an important bearing on the molecular basis of pathogenicity, they are discussed at some length. As already mentioned, the ND virus particles have typical **projections** or "spikes" covering the surface. These are inserted into the envelope. They are of two types: 1) **The longest** (about 8 nm) **consists** of single glycoprotein (HN) with which both haemagglutination and neuraminidase activities are associated. 2) **The smaller spikes** are formed by the F (fusion) glycoprotein. These are associated with the ability of the virus envelope to fuse with cell membranes, allowing insertion of virus genetic material into the host cell, and to cause fusion of infected cells, resulting in the characteristic cytopathic effect of syncytial formation.

Spread

Over 200 species of birds have been reported to be susceptible to natural infection of NDV. The spread from bird to bird depends on the organs in which the virus multiplies. Birds showing respiratory disease shed the virus in aerosols (droplets) of mucus, which may be inhaled by susceptible birds. Viruses which are restricted to intestinal replication may be spread by ingestion of contaminated faeces, either directly or in contaminated food or water, or by inhalation of small infective particles produced from dried faeces. Viruses transmitted by the respiratory route may spread extremely rapidly, whereas viruses excreted in the faeces and transmitted by the oral/faecal route may spread extremely slowly.

Humans seem to play the central role in the spread of NDV, usually by the movement of live birds, contaminated vehicles, fomites, and poultry products (such as unfumigated eggs, dead birds and faeces for fertilizer), from affected premises to susceptible birds. A key to the successful spread of the **virus is its ability to survive in the dead host or excretions.** In infected carcasses virus may survive for several weeks at cool ambient (surrounding) temperatures, or several years if held frozen. Faeces in which virus may be present in high titres, is also an excellent medium for the survival of the virus, and even at 37° C infectivity has been retained for over a month. The virus has been found to survive for several days on the mucous membrane of the **human respiratory tract** and has been isolated from sputum.

Pathogenesis

The initial step is attachment of the virus to cell receptors. This is mediated by the **HN glycoprotein**. Attachment at the replication site is followed by fusion of the virus membrane with the cell membrane. **Fusion of the viral and cell membranes is brought about by action of the fusion (F) glycoprotein.** Thus, the **nucleocapsid complex** enters the cell. **Intracellular virus replication takes place entirely within the cytoplasm.** The F glycoprotein is synthesized as a non-functional precursor, **FO**, which requires cleavage (a split, division) to F1 and F2 by host proteases **for the production of infective viral particles.** The HN of some strains of NDV may also require **post-translational cleavage** (i.e., after the HN molecule has been formed). This cleavage plays a crucial role in the molecular basis of its pathogenicity, as discussed below.

Cleavage Site

During the replication of virus, it is necessary for the precursor glycoprotein FO to be cleaved to F1 and F2, **for the progeny virus particles to be infective.**

This **post-translation cleavage** (i.e., split after the **FO molecule** has been formed) is mediated by **host cell proteases.** The cleavage takes place at the **cleavage site. If cleavage fails to take place, non-infectious virus particles are produced.** **Trypsin** is capable of cleaving FO for all strains of NDV. In fact, *in vivo* treatment of non-infectious virus by trypsin restores infectivity.

The **importance of FO cleavage** was easily demonstrated in *in vitro* experiments. Viruses normally unable to replicate or produce plaques in cell culture systems, were able to do both **if trypsin was added to the culture medium.** The viruses pathogenic for chickens could replicate *in vitro* in a wide range of cell types **with or without trypsin, whereas strains of low virulence could replicate only when trypsin was added.** This indicated that FO molecules of virulent viruses can be cleaved by host proteases found in a wide range of cells and tissues, but **FO molecules** in viruses of low virulence were restricted in their sensitivity, **and these viruses could grow only in cer-**

tain types of host cells. Results obtained from nucleotide sequencing have revealed some fundamental differences in the amino acid sequences at the cleavage site between viruses of low virulence (lentogenic) and virulent viruses (velogenic or mesogenic). It was found that viruses of low virulence have only a single basic amino acid arginine at the cleavage site, whereas virulent viruses contain multiple (additional) basic amino acids at the site of cleavage. It was further revealed that the susceptibility of the FO molecule by host proteases depends on the number of basic amino acids at the cleavage site. Trypsin-like enzymes can cleave if only a single amino acid is present at the cleavage site, whereas other host proteases require multiple (additional) basic amino acids.

Thus, it is interesting that the mechanism controlling the pathogenicity of Newcastle disease virus resembles that described for the avian influenza virus (see avian influenza). The presence of additional basic amino acids in virulent strains means that cleavage can be brought about by proteases present in a wide range of host tissues and organs, but in lentogenic viruses (i.e., in viruses of low virulence), cleavage can be caused by only those proteases that recognize the single amino acid arginine, i.e., by trypsin-like enzymes, such as are present in the respiratory and intestinal tracts. Since they cannot be cleaved elsewhere, no infective virus is produced at other places. Therefore, their growth and pathogenicity are limited to the respiratory and digestive tracts. On the other hand, the virulent viruses, because they possess additional amino acids at the cleavage sites in the FO molecule, can be cleaved by proteases found throughout the body. The virulent viruses thus invade and replicate in many tissues and organs, resulting in the production of infective virus throughout the body, generalized disease, and death.

Signs

The clinical signs vary considerably with the pathotype of the infecting virus. In addition, the species of bird, the immune status, age, and conditions under which they are reared also greatly affect the clinical signs, while the presence of other organisms may greatly aggravate even the mildest forms of disease. As such, no signs can be regarded as pathognomonic of the disease.

The highly virulent (velogenic) viruses may produce peracute infections, where the first indication of disease is sudden death. Typically, signs such as depression, prostration (lying down), diarrhoea, oedema of the head (facial oedema) and nervous signs may occur, with mortality reaching 100%. The appearance of shell-less or soft-shelled eggs, followed by complete cessation of egg laying, may be an early sign in adult fowl. The moderately virulent (mesogenic) viruses usually cause severe respiratory disease. This is followed by nervous signs, with mortality up to 50% or more. In laying hens, there may be a marked drop in egg production which may last for several weeks. The viruses of low virulence (lentogenic) may cause no disease, or mild respiratory distress for a short time. However, the presence of other organisms, such as avian pneumovirus, infectious bronchitis, and vaccine strains of NDV, or poor management may cause disease similar to that seen with more virulent virus.

Lesions

Gross Lesions

As with clinical signs, the gross lesions and the organs affected depend on the strain and pathotype of the virus. There are no pathognomonic lesions for any form of the disease. Viruses producing clinically inapparent infections cause **no gross lesions**. The presence of **haemorrhagic lesions in the intestine** has been used to distinguish v iscerotropic velogenic (VVND) viruses from neurotropic velogenic (NVND) viruses. These lesions are usually prominent in the proventriculus, caeca, and small intestine. They are markedly haemorrhagic and result from necrosis of the intestinal wall, or lymphoid foci such as caecal tonsils. These lesions include **haemorrhage in the mucosa of the proventriculus, enlarged and necrotic caecal tonsils, necrosis and haemorrhage in intestinal lymphoid aggregates, and splenic necrosis on the capsular surface**. Usually, gross lesions are not observed in the central nervous system, regardless of the pathotype. **Gross changes are not always present in the respiratory tract**. Viruses causing respiratory disease may induce **haemorrhagic lesions and marked congestion of trachea. Airsacculitis** (airsacs being cloudy and congested) may be present even after infection with relatively mild strains, and thickening of the airsacs with catarrhal or caseous exudates is often observed. Laying hens infected with velogenic viruses usually reveal egg yolk in the abdominal cavity. The **ovarian follicles** are often flaccid (lacking firmness) and degenerate, and may even show haemorrhagic stigmata (i.e., spots). Haemorrhage and discoloration of the other reproductive organs may occur.

Microscopic Lesions

Microscopic lesions are as varied as the clinical signs and gross lesions. They are, therefore, of no value in the diagnosis. Lesions in the **central nervous system** are those of non-purulent encephalomyelitis with neuronal degeneration, foci of glial cells, perivascular infiltration of lymphocytes, and proliferation of endothelial cells. Lesions usually occur in the cerebellum, medulla, mid brain, brain stem and spinal cord, **but rarely in the cerebrum**. Lesions in the **vascular system** include hyperaemia, oedema, and haemorrhage in many organs. Regressive changes in the **lymphopoietic system** consist of disappearance of lymphoid tissue. **Necrotic lesions are found throughout the spleen**. Marked degeneration of the medullary region is seen in the bursa. The haemorrhagic-necrotic lesions in the **intestinal tract** develop in lymphoid aggregates. Lesions in the **upper respiratory tract** may be severe and related to the degree of respiratory distress. Lesions may extend throughout the length of the trachea. Cilia may be lost within 2 days of infection. In the mucosa, congestion, oedema, and dense cellular infiltration of lymphocytes and macrophages may be seen. Oedema, cell infiltration, and increased thickness and density of the airsacs may occur.

Zoonotic Significance

Although Newcastle disease virus can produce a transitory (of brief duration) **conjunctivitis in man**, the condition has been limited mainly to **laboratory workers and vaccination teams** exposed to large quantities of virus. And, before vaccination was practised, it was seen in **persons eviscerating poultry in processing plants**. The disease has not been reported in individuals who rear poultry, or consume poultry products.

Diagnosis

None of the clinical signs or lesions can be regarded as specific/pathognomonic. At best, they can only be suggestive of the disease. The presence of specific antibodies in the serum gives little information on the infecting strain of the ND virus, and therefore, has limited diagnostic value. Nevertheless, in certain circumstances the demonstration that infection has taken place is sufficient for diagnostic purpose. The **various serological tests** include single radial immunodiffusion, agar gel precipitin, virus neutralization (VN) in chick embryos, and plaque neutralization. ELISA has become popular, especially as part of flock screening procedure. Currently, the haemagglutination inhibition test (HI test) is most widely used. Good correlation has been reported between ELISA and HI tests.

At present the only sure method of diagnosis, which allows identification of the strain, **is isolation of the virus and its characterization**. Sampling from live birds should consist of both cloacal swabs (or faeces) and tracheal swabs, regardless of the clinical signs. From dead birds, intestines, intestinal contents and tracheas should be taken, together with affected organs and tissues. Isolation can be carried on various cell systems and also eggs. NDV may be confirmed by HI test using specific NDV antiserum. However, mere isolation and identification of the virus is not adequate, the characterization of the pathotype, which relates to virulence, is necessary. This can be done by using a group of **monoclonal antibodies** to find out whether the isolate has the ability to react or not against them. This enables differentiation and grouping of NDV isolates. However, the usefulness of this technique may not be as an alternative to pathogenicity tests for primary isolates of ND virus, but as rapid confirmation of the isolations during outbreaks.

Avian Paramyxovirus Type 2 (PMV - 2)

PMV - 2 viruses have been reported to infect both **chickens and turkeys**. Little is known about their spread, but mechanisms appear very similar to NDV. However, reports indicate relatively slow spread through a flock, and that closely situated flocks do not always become infected.

Clinically, PMV - 2 viruses may cause **mild respiratory disease and reduced egg production**. However, in the presence of secondary bacterial infections, or environmental stress, the clinical picture may be far more serious, with severe respiratory disease, cessation of egg production, and even high mortality. **No signs or postmortem lesions are specific for the disease**. Definitive diagnosis can be made by demonstration of antibodies to PMV - 2 viruses by HI tests, and by virus isolation and identification. Virus isolation procedures in embryonated eggs are similar to those for Newcastle disease virus.

Avian Paramyxovirus Type 3 (PMV - 3)

PMV - 3 viruses have been obtained from **only turkeys**. There are no reports of PMV - 3 viruses infecting chickens. **Clinically**, in turkeys, these viruses produce mild respiratory disease, and a reduction in number and quality of eggs. Procedures for the isolation of the viruses in embryonated eggs are similar to those used for ND virus.

Diseases caused by Pneumoviruses

The genus **Pneumovirus** contains **three important viruses**: human respiratory syncytial virus (HRSV), bovine respiratory syncytial virus (BRSV), and avian pneumoviruses. The two respiratory mammalian syncytial viruses are related antigenically to each other.

Human Respiratory Syncytial Virus (HRSV)

Human RSV is the most important cause of lower respiratory tract infection in **infants and children**. The virus was first recovered from chimpanzees with upper respiratory disease. Many species of non-human primates (monkeys) can be infected with HRSV, but clinical disease is usually absent except in chimpanzees.

Bovine Respiratory Syncytial Virus (BRSV)

Bovine RSV occurs worldwide, and affects **cattle** and **sheep**, particularly the young. The incidence of infection is high, and the virus is one of the major causes of respiratory disease in cattle. The disease may be mild or severe, with a high morbidity but a low mortality rate. **Clinically**, there is fever, coughing, hyperpnoea (an increased respiratory rate), serous oculo-nasal discharge, and lethargy. The virus causes an interstitial pneumonia with necrosis of bronchial, bronchiolar, and alveolar epithelium. **Inclusion-bearing multinucleated giant cells form at these sites**. Infection with BRSV predisposes the respiratory tract to other viruses, such as parainfluenza-3, and bacterial pathogens, such as *Pasteurella haemolytica*, causing significantly more severe pneumonia. The lesions of BRSV closely resemble those caused by parainfluenza-3 virus, from which they must be differentiated.

Avian Pneumoviruses

There are **two important diseases of poultry** produced by the avian pneumovirus: 1) **turkey rhinotracheitis (TRT)**, and 2) **swollen head syndrome (SHS) of chickens.**

Turkey Rhinotracheitis (TRT)

Also known as **"turkey coryza"**, turkey rhinotracheitis (TRT) **is an acute disease of the upper respiratory tract of turkeys**, caused by an **avian pneumovirus**. The condition usually affects flocks between 3 and 10 weeks of age. The syndrome is characterized by rapid onset, with high flock morbidity which frequently approaches 100%. **Clinical signs** may include depression, change of voice, gasping, moist tracheal rales, snicking (making slight sharp sound), coughing, submandibular oedema, foamy ocular discharge, and excess mucus noticeable at the external nares. Recovery is rapid, and may be complete in 7-14 days with low or no mortality. However, in complicated cases, high mortality rates, often exceeding 50%, have been reported. These are associated with secondary bacterial infection, particularly *Escherichia coli*.

Swollen Head Syndrome (SHS)

Swollen head syndrome (SHS) is a condition which affects chickens of all types, but **mainly broilers and broiler parents. A pneumovirus** is believed to be the primary cause, but bacteria may be involved as secondary pathogens. SHS was first described in Britain at about the same time when turkey rhinotracheitis (TRT) was first seen there. However, despite some early confusion, it is now established that there is no association between TRT and SHS, **and that both diseases are separate.**

Signs

In Broiler Parents

Affected broiler breeders sit with the neck arched so that the head rests on the back **(opisthotonus)**. If birds are picked up, this sets off a fit of incoordination causing them to roll over, and they experience a difficulty in regaining a normal posture. Their heads continue to shake for some time after returning to a normal sitting position. There is usually **swelling around the eyes, and over the top of the head**. Affected birds usually have a green, foul-smelling diarrhoea which causes soiling around the vent. Morbidity is usually low (1%), but birds showing clinical symptoms **usually die**. In general **only females are affected**, but sometimes a small number of males show similar symptoms. The disease usually occurs around peak of lay (30 weeks). In most cases, it lasts 2-3 weeks, but in some outbreaks, birds continue to die throughout the life of the flock. There is usually **a drop in egg production** (of no more than 5%) which lasts as long as the other clinical signs persist.

In Broilers

The clinical signs consist of **head swelling** which **is more severe than in breeders, giving the face a puffy appearance** caused by subcutaneous oedema around the eyes and over the head, and down into the inter-mandibular tissue and wattles. Respiratory signs include coughing and sneezing, and many birds have a severe tracheitis and often die from secondary septicaemia caused by *Escherichia coli*.

Lesions

In broiler breeders, the most important lesion is an **extensive peritonitis**. This appears as a moist inflammatory lesion in the ovarian region containing released yolk free in the peritoneum. Puffiness of the skin is seen over the head. Gelatinous fluid and inspissated pus are observed subcutaneously. There are no other significant lesions except at times a mild tracheitis. The lesions in **broilers** consist of fine petechiation of the turbinate mucosa. Removal of the skin over the head reveals yellow, oedematous subcutaneous tissue.

Rhabdoviridae

The Family **Rhabdoviridae** (G. rhabdo = rod, figuratively **bullet-shaped**) contains a large number **of enveloped, single-stranded, negative-sense RNA viruses**. They are bullet-shaped, about 70 nm wide and 180 nm long. The lipoprotein envelope contains prominent peplomers that contain glycoprotein, **which mediates attachment to the host-cell receptor**. The virion contains a transcriptase essential to initiate replication. Both positive-strand and negative-strand viral RNA is replicated, **but only the negative strand is packaged into virions.**

The family contains a large number of different viruses infectious for humans, domestic animals, fish, invertebrates, and plants. Many are transmitted by arthropods. There are **two genera: Vesiculovirus** and **Lyssavirus**. In addition, there are a large number of rhabdoviruses which have yet to be classified. The **three most important diseases of animals** caused by rhabdoviruses are: 1) **vesicular stomatitis** from the genus "**Vesiculovirus**"; 2) **rabies** from the genus "Lyssavirus"; and 3) **bovine ephemeral fever** from the "**unclassified**" rhabdoviruses.

Disease caused by Vesiculovirus

Vesicular Stomatitis

Vesicular stomatitis is **an infectious disease** caused by a **vesiculovirus**, and characterized clinically by the development of **vesicles on the mouth and feet**. Thus, it has close similarities to foot-and-mouth disease and vesicular exanthema. While primarily a disease of **horses**, it has come to assume major importance as a disease of **cattle** and **pigs**. Goats and sheep are resistant.

Insects are believed to be the principal vectors of transmission. Mosquitoes, black flies, sand flies, gnats, and midges have been identified as possible vectors. **The disease is limited to the western hemisphere**.

As in foot-and-mouth disease, there is a primary viraemia with subsequent localization of the virus in the mucous membrane of the mouth, and the skin around the mouth and coronets. **Clinical signs in cattle** include mild fever, and the development of vesicles on the dorsum of the tongue, dental pad, lips and the buccal mucosa. The vesicles rupture, and the resulting irritation causes profuse salivation and anorexia. In some outbreaks, vesicles have been almost completely absent. Vesicles are usually found on the cheeks and tongue. At other sites there is an abrasive, necrotic lesion. Recovery is rapid, affected animals being clinically normal in 3-4 days. **In horses**, the signs are more or less similar but usually the lesions are limited to the dorsum of the tongue or the lips. **In pigs**, vesicles develop on or behind the snout or on the feet, and lameness is more common than in other animals.

Lesions are most common on the **tongue** and **oral mucosa**, but may also occur on the teats and the coronary band. Since infection occurs through the bites of insects, lesions develop at the site. Viraemic spread to other sites does not play a role. **Microscopically**, there is intercellular oedema in the stratum spinosum. This leads to cell dissociation and necrosis. Neutrophils and macrophages infiltrate the necrotic tissue, which sloughs, leaving erosions that are subject to secondary infection. The intra-epithelial oedema may become abundant enough to result in a **vesicle**. Healing usually occurs in 7-10 days.

Zoonotic Importance

Occasional human infections give the disease **some public health significance**, but the disease is mild, resembling influenza.

Diagnosis

The lesions of vesicular stomatitis are basically similar in distribution, location and microscopic appearance to those of foot-and-mouth disease and vesicular exanthema. The lesions of these three diseases cannot be finally distinguished on morphological grounds, in spite of less prominent vesicle formation in vesicular stomatitis. Vesicular stomatitis, unlike foot-and-mouth disease, rarely causes myocarditis and is never fatal. To confirm diagnosis virus may be isolated for identification in tissue culture systems, or be seen in ultramicroscopic sections.

Disease caused by Lyssavirus

Rabies (Hydrophobia, Lyssa, Rage)

Rabies is **an acute, viral encephalomyelitis** (inflammation of both brain and spinal cord), which **affects all warm-blooded animals, including humans. It is a highly fatal disease, mortality rate being close to 100%.** The disease is transmitted by the bites of affected animals. Although rabies occurs throughout the world, a few countries are free of the disease by virtue of their island status, or due to successful eradication programmes, or because of strict quarantine regulations. New Zealand and Australia never had the disease. Britain, Hawaii, Japan and Scandinavia are currently free of the disease. In the United States, Canada, and Western Europe, where rabies in dogs has been effectively controlled through vaccination, **the disease is endemic in wildlife,** particularly foxes, skunks, raccoons, and bats. Cats are the most often affected domestic animals in the United States. In Asia, Africa, Latin America, and the Middle East, rabies is endemic in **dogs** and **wildlife,** and **numerous cases occur each year in humans.** In Europe, fox rabies predominates.

Cause

Lyssavirus of rabies is truly neurotropic and causes lesions only in nervous tissue. It is one of the larger viruses (180 nm long and 80 nm wide), **and is relatively fragile.** It is susceptible to most disinfectants, and **dies in dried saliva in a few hours.** The virus can be propagated in tissue culture, and chick embryos. Strains of rabies virus isolated from naturally occurring cases are referred to as "**street virus**", and attenuated laboratory strains are referred to as "**fixed virus**".

Spread

The source of infection is always an infected animal, and the method of spread is almost always by the bite of a rabid animal, although contamination of skin wounds by fresh saliva may result in infection. **Saliva is rich in virus.** Rarely, virus may be introduced through **intact or abraded mucous membrane.** Virus may be present in the saliva, and be transmitted by an infected animal some days before the onset of clinical signs. **Rarely,** transmission has been recorded by non-salivary routes. These include aerosol transmission to man in the laboratory. Rare cases of rabies have occurred in humans from breathing the air in a cave where thousands of bats were living.

Traditionally, the **dog,** and to a minor extent the **cat,** have been considered to be the principal source of infection. However, native fauna (animal life), including **foxes, wolves,** skunks, blood-sucking vampire bats, insectivorous and frugivorous (fruit-eating) bats, racoons, **mongoose,** and **squirrels** may provide the major source of infection in countries where domestic carnivora are well controlled. Vampire bats are important in the spread of the disease, particularly to cattle in Mexico, Central and South America, and parts of the Caribbean. **As a rule, rabies in humans results from the bite of a rabid dog, cat, fox, or wolf.** These animals also transmit the disease to **cattle, horses, and sheep,** which seldom spread it further. Bats are the important species in which symptomless carriers are known to occur. That is, they harbour and transmit the virus, often without showing clinical signs of the disease. Multiplication of the virus without **invasion of the nervous system** is known to occur in fatty tissues in bats, and may be the basis of the **'reservoir' mechanism** known to occur in this species.

Not all bites from rabid animals result in infection, because the virus is not always present in the saliva. Also, it may not gain entrance to the wound if the saliva is wiped from the teeth by clothing, or the coat of the animal. The virus may appear in the **milk** of affected animals, but spread by this means is unlikely **as infection through ingestion is not known to occur**. Domestic animals are rarely a source of infection although chance transmission to humans may occur if the mouth of a rabid animal is manipulated during treatment, or examination. The virus may be present in the saliva for periods up to 5 days before signs are seen. **In humans**, most bites of a rabid animal do not lead to infection. **However, once disease is established, it is nearly always fatal**. **Bites to the head are much more likely to lead to rabies**, than those of the extremities. Contrary to what was once thought, all animals that become infected do not succumb to the disease. This is true in bats, as already mentioned. Although the diseae is usually fatal once clinical signs appear, recovery has been recorded in several animals, including dog, and also in man. **Inapparent infection can also occur in dogs**, leaving them immune to challenge.

Pathogenesis

After entry of the virus, following bite of rabid animals, there is **a variable incubation period of 1 week to 1 year**, with a mean of 1-2 months. Several factors, including the virulence of the strain, quantity of infectious virus in the saliva, and the susceptibilty of the species, play a role in establishing rabies in the recipient animal. The length of the incubation period after viral exposure varies greatly and depends on the anatomical distance between the bite site and the central nervous system, the severity of the bite, and the amount of infectious virus in the saliva.

Virus first replicates in the myocytes (muscle cells) at the site and is shed into extracellular spaces. **The virus then enters the nervous system at motor end plates**, and binds to the receptor for acetylcholine, a neurotransmitter. Following entry into the peripheral or cranial nerves, **the virus spreads within the axons of nerve cells to the ventral horn cells of the spinal cord at a rate of 3-4 mm/hour**. The form of virus during its axoplasmic flow is unclear. Intact virions have not been demonstrated in axons during this phase of the infection. Virus replication occurs first in the spinal cord cells, and then it spreads to the brain, from where virus is disseminated throughout the central nervous system. **There is no evidence that a viraemia is present for the dissemination of rabies virus to the central nervous system**. Direct trans-neuronal transfer of virus from neuronal perikarya (the cell bodies of neurons) and dendrites to adjacent axon terminals is a mechanism of dissemination of rabies in the central nervous system. Brain stem, cerebral cortex, and hippocampus are particularly susceptible to rabies infection, **and the**

destruction of neurons in these regions gives rise to clinical symptoms of rabies.

There is eventual **centrifugal spread** (i.e., away from the centre, towards periphery) **via nerves** throughout the body to other tissues, including the salivary glands. Rabies virus can spread from the CNS to salivary glands, cornea, and tonsils, **via their nerve supply. Viral replication in salivary gland occurs rapidly and infected saliva is the major source of infection.**

The only lesions produced are in the central nervous system, and spread from the site of infection occurs **only by way of the peripheral nerves**. This method of spread accounts for the **extremely variable incubation period** which varies to a large extent with the site of the bite. Bites on the head usually result in a shorter incubation period than bites on the extremities. The severity and the sites of lesions govern to a large extent, whether the clinical picture will be one of "**furious form**" or "**paralytic (dumb) form**". When irritation phenomena (induced by the virus in the nerve cells) occur, they are followed by paralysis as the stimulated nerve cells are subsequently destroyed. However, this is not always the case. Destruction of spinal neurons results in paralysis and in the "**paralytic (dumb) form**" of the disease. But when the virus invades the brain, irritation of higher centres produces manias (madness), excitement, and convulsions. **Death is usually due to respiratory paralysis.**

Signs

After the bite of a rabid animal, or penetration of the virus through the skin by some other means, the incubation period varies from a few days to several months. Rabid animals of all species exhibit typical signs of CNS disturbance. **In any animal, the first sign is a change in behaviour**. Animals usually stop eating and drinking. The disease progresses rapidly after the onset of paralysis, **and death is virtually certain within 10 days of the first signs**. The clinical symptoms usually appear in one of two forms: 1) the "**dumb or paralytic form**" and 2) "**furious form**".

In the "**dumb or paralytic form**" of rabies, the animal falls into a stupor (unconsciousness), and has a peculiar staring expression. This form is characterized by early paralysis of the throat and muscles of mastication, usually with **profuse salivation and inability to swallow**. Dropping of the lower jaw is common in dogs. These animals are not vicious, and rarely attempt to bite. The paralysis progresses rapidly to all parts of the body, and coma and death follow in a few hours. **In the "furious form"**, the animal becomes irrational and viciously aggressive. This form is the classical "**mad-dog syndrome**". The animal goes into rages (violent anger), biting and slashing at any moving object or even inanimate objects, such as sticks and trees. The furious champing of the jaws (i.e., chewing noisely) is accompanied by excessive salivation. The saliva flows from the mouth or is churned into foam, which may adhere to the lips and face. A basic change in temperament occurs. Wild animals which normally avoid humans go into the open and attack humans. The rabid dog, fox, or wolf tends particularly to attack a moving person or animal. As the disease progresses, muscular incoordination and seizures become common. Paralysis may follow either the **"furious"** or **"dumb" stage** of the disease. **Death occurs within 10 days of the first symptoms.**

Rabies in cattle follows the same general pattern. Those with the furious form are dangerous, attacking and pursuing man and other animals. Lactation stops abruptly in dairy cattle. A most typical clinical sign in cattle is a **characteristic bellowing** (making a deep loud cry). This may continue intermittently until shortly before death. **Horses and mules** show extreme agitation evidenced by rolling as with colic. They may bite or strike viciously, and because of size and strength, become unmanageable in a few hours.

Lesions

There are no gross lesions. **The lesions of rabies are microscopic, limited to the central nervous system, and extremely variable in extent.** They may not be easily recognizable except for early necrosis of neurons with **specific cytoplasmic inclusion bodies in the affected nerve cells.** In some cases, there is **diffuse encephalitis** characterized by perivascular cuffing, neuronophagic nodules and other changes of destruction of neurons throughout the brain. These changes are particularly prominent in the **brain stem, hippocampus and the gasserian ganglia.** (Gasserian ganglion lies on the sensory root of the trigeminal nerve, and from it originate the three branches - ophthalmic, maxillary, mandibular). **Lesions in the gasserian ganglia are specific,** develop earlier and are more constant than elsewhere. The main lesion consists of the collections of proliferating glial cells encroaching on the neurons and replacing them. **These collections** of proliferating glial cells are known as **"Babes' nodules".**

In 1903, spherical cytoplasmic inclusion bodies with specific tinctorial (staining) characteristics were described by Negri in neurons of dogs, cats, and rabbits which were experimentally infected with rabies virus. These inclusion bodies have been called **"Negri bodies"**, and are accepted as specific indications of infection with rabies virus. **Electron microscopic studies** indicate that Negri bodies represent well-defined electron-dense masses, which may or may not contain, or be associated with rabies virions. The nature of the matrix is not understood, but may represent a necessary component for viral replication, or a reaction on the part of the infected neuron. **Negri bodies are not always present in rabies.** Certain strains of rabies virus do not produce inclusion bodies, indicating that Negri bodies are not necessary for viral replication. **Negri bodies are always intracytoplasmic.** In the **dog**, they are found mostly in the **hippocampus**, but in **cattle** they are more numerous in the **Purkinje cells of the cerebellum**. It is possible for all neurons, even those of the ganglia, to contain these inclusions. **Negri bodies have a distinct limiting membrane,** and may be encircled by a narrow, clear halo. In tissue sections, they usually measure from 2-8 µm in diameter. One or several may be present in the affected nerve cell. These inclusions may be completely within the cell body, or they may occur in dendrites, where they are likely to be elongated, conforming to the shape of these processes. A granular, slightly basophilic internal structure can be seen in preparations with Mann's stain.

The staining characteristics of the Negri body are of great interest. **The haematoxylin and eosin method does not differentiate Negri bodies well**. The Schleifstein modification of Wilhite stain is particularly successful with tissue fixed in Zenker's solution. When stained by this method, Negri bodies are bright magenta (deep purplish-red), contrasting with the purplish cytoplasm of the neuron. **In impression smears, Seller's stain is effective**. The inclusion body is bright red or magenta against the pale blue background of the neuronal cytoplasm. Mann's and Giemsa's stains are also useful, particularly in impression smears. No matter which stain is used, it is important that the person who examines the material to confirm the diagnosis, be thoroughly familiar with the characteristics of the stain and the appearance of Negri bodies. The final identification of Negri bodies should not be left to the beginner.

When the virus centrifugally invades the salivary gland, degenerative changes leading to necrosis may be seen in the acinar epithelium, mainly affecting mucogenic cells of the mandibular salivary gland. Virus can readily be demonstrated within these cells by fluorescent antibody techniques, and electron microscopy. A moderate infiltration of lymphocytes and plasma cells accompanies the degenerative changes.

Zoonotic Implications

The prime importance of rabies is its transmissibility to humans with **veterinarians being at special risk**. By far the greatest proportion of humans requiring pre-treatment for rabies in our country have been exposed to a rabid dog. Human rabies is extremely rare in countries where rabies in dogs has been controlled by regular vaccination. According to a survey conducted by the World Health Organization in 1987, dogs were responsible for 91% of all human rabies cases; cats 2%; other domestic animals 3%; bat 2%; foxes 1%; and all other wild animals, less than 1%. **The disease is a major occupational hazard for veterinarians who should receive pre-exposure prophylaxis**.

Diagnosis

The diagnosis of rabies can be based on the **symptoms** if they are typical, but should be confirmed by laboratory examination. Dogs or other species, suspected of rabies because of abnormal behaviour, should be kept in isolation where they cannot bite others, **for 10 days. If the animal is rabid, it will die and the diagnosis can then be confirmed by laboratory examination**. The animal can be classified non-rabid if it is alive at the end of 10 days. Still it will be desirable to carry out a postmortem examination. The laboratory examination includes the following four tests. It is essential that **at least two of them be used on all specimens**.

1. A fluorescent antibody test (FAT) on impression smears from the brain, preferably hippocampus, medulla o blongata, c erebellum o r gasserian g anglion. The test can be completed in about 2 hours and is **highly accurate**. The reliability of the fluorescent antibody test confirmed by the mouse inoculation test is over 99%.

2. A histological search of Negri bodies in tissue sections with r esults available in 4 8 hours. H owever, the l imitation of t his technique i s that t he brains of as many as 30% of infected animals may not contain demonstrable Negri b odies.

3. T hose specimens w hich are n egative on F AT, and h ad contacts w ith humans, are **inoculated into experimental mice**. Mice of all ages are susceptible to rabies virus, **but newborn mice less than 3 days of age are most sensitive**. Following intracerebral inoculation, newborn mice usually die within 14 days, but should be examined daily for at least 4 weeks before the test is considered negative. The virus is demonstrated in the brains of mice that die by: 1) finding Negri bodies, 2) by a neutralization test in other mice, or preferably, 3) by the fluorescent antibody identification of the virus. Rabies virus may also be isolated by injecting suspected brain suspensions into tissue culture. Positive results can be obtained in 24 h ours, and the virus identified by the fluorescent antibody m ethod.

4. Recently, a newer **peroxidase-antiperoxidase staining technique** has been used. It can be performed on paraffin-embedded tissue, and has largely replaced reliance on the presence of Negri bodies, or mouse inoculation.

In dogs, in which rabies is suspected but cannot be demonstrated, an attempt should be made to determine the cause of death, or cause of encephalitis. Diseases to consider are canine hepatitis, toxoplasmosis, and canine distemper. Differentiation between canine hepatitis and canine distemper is very important, **since inclusion bodies may occur in both of these diseases**. Both are much more common in dogs than is rabies. However, in canine distemper involving the brain **intranuclear inclusion bodies are found in endothelial cells** in association with rupture of capillary w alls and microscopic haemorrhages. I nclusion bodies in canine d istemper are e asily seen i n glial cells, particularly in the nuclei of gemistocytic astrocytes a nd microglia. F luorescent antibody t echniques s how that d istemper inclusions o ccur in n eurons, but they are less readily demonstrable with other methods, **Cytoplasmic inclusions are less common in the brain in canine distemper.**

Groups of tiny spherical bodies **without a limiting membrane** are seen in the cytoplasm of neurons **in non-rabid animals**. Since at one time they were thought t o be associated with rabies, they were called "**Lyssa bodies**". **It is now clear that they are not specific for rabies**. They have been described in the dog, cat, fox, a nd laboratory w hite mouse. A lthough they can be easily confused w ith Negri b odies, **they lack an internal structure, are more acidophilic, and are highly refractile. In the brains of normal cats**, there are also other cytoplasmic inclusions with staining characteristics similar to those of Negri bodies. These **feline inclusions** cannot be differentiated morphologi-cally from Negri bodies. Therefore, it may be necessary to carry out animal inoculation, o r fluorescent a ntibody techniques w hen rabies i s suspected i n **the cats**.

Disease caused by Unclassified Rhabdovirus

Bovine Ephemeral Fever

Also known as "**three-day sickness**", "**bovine epizootic fever**", and "**stiff sickness**", ephemeral fever is **an infectious disease of cattle** characterized by transitory fever, muscular shivering, stiffness, lameness, and enlargement of the peripheral lymph nodes.The disease is caused by an unclassified, insect-borne **rhabdovirus**.

Spread

The virus is probably transmitted by **biting insects**. Experiments indicate that stable flies and mosquitoes are probably not responsible for transmission of this virus. **Culicoides** species (**sand flies**) are suspected to be the vectors, along with **mosquitoes**, but confirming evidence is lacking.

Pathogenesis

After an incubation period of 2-10 days, a viraemia develops with localization and inflammation in mesodermal tissues, particularly joints, lymph nodes, and muscles. The virus is thought to grow mainly in the reticulo-endothelial cells in the lungs, spleen, and lymph nodes, and not in vascular endothelium or lymphoid cells.

Signs

Calves are least affected, and those less than 6 months of age show no clinical sign. **Fat cows and bulls are worst affected**. In most cases the disease is acute, and c haracterized by t ransitory (of b rief duration) f ever, inappetence (ano-rexia), hyperpnoea (increased breathing) or dyspnoea (difficult breathing) of short d uration, mucous o r purulent n asal discharge, shivering, and s hifting lameness. In some cases, rumination may cease for a few d ays and ruminal stasis, diarrhoea, or constipation m ay occur. O ccasional posterior p aralysis has been described. **Many animals become ill, but few die from the disease.**

Lesions

Gross lesions include general vascular e ngorgement, oedematous lymph nodes, congestion of abomasal mucosa, hydropericardium, hydrothorax, rhinitis, tracheitis, and pulmonary oedema. Tendovaginitis (inflammation of a tendon and its sheath), fasciculitis (inflammation of a bundle of muscle fibres), and cellulitis (inflammation of connective tissue) and focal necrosis of muscle have also been described. **Microscopically**, lesions are limited to venules and capillaries, particularly in muscles, tendon sheaths, synovial membranes, fascia, and skin. Endothelial cells m ay be h yperplastic, and the vessels surrounded by oedema and leukocytic infiltration.

Diagnosis

The diagnosis is not difficult on the basis of its transient (brief) nature, and its rapidity of spread. Diagnosis may be confirmed by isolation and identification of the virus, or by identifying viral antigens in tissues of affected animals by s pecific immunofluorescent techniques.

Retroviridae

The Family Retroviridae contains a diverse group of RNA viruses. Retroviruses constitute the only family of RNA tumour viruses. The family is divided into **three sub-families: 1) oncoviruses or oncornaviruses** (L. oncos = tumour) **or RNA tumour viruses, or RNA oncogenic viruses, 2) lentiviruses** (L. lenti = slow), and 3) **foamy viruses or spumaviruses** (L. spuma = foam). Important members of each group are listed in **Table 5**.

Table 5. Diseases caused by Retroviridae

Oncoviruses (RNA tumour viruses)
(Sub-family: Oncovirinae)

    Type C Oncovirus Group (most are exogenous)
    Feline leukaemia virus
    Feline sa rcoma virus
    Bovine leukaemia virus
    Ovine leukaemia virus
    Porcine leukaemia virus
    Human T cell leukaemia virus
    Avian t ype C o ncoviruses
        Avian leukosis/sarcoma viruses (ALSV)
        Reticuloendotheliosis virus
        Lymphoproliferative disease of turkey virus

    Type B Oncovirus group (endogenous)
    Mouse mammary tumour virus (endogenous)
    (mammary-tumour milk virus)

Type D Oncovirus group (exogenous)
Jaagsiekte virus
(pulmonary adenocarcinoma virus of sheep)

Lentiviruses (exogenous)
(Sub-family: Lentivirinae)
    Visna/maedi virus
    Caprine arthritis-encephalitis virus
    Human immunodeficiency v irus (HIV-1, HIV-2)
        Simian immunodeficiency virus
        Feline immunodeficiency virus
        Bovine immunodeficiency virus
        Equine infectious anaemia virus

Spumaviruses (foamy viruses, inapparent infections)
(Sub-family: Spumavirinae)
    Bovine syncytial virus
    Feline s yncytial virus

The Family **Retroviridae** is so named because these viruses contain the enzyme **reverse transcriptase**, an RNA-dependent DNA-polymerase (L. retro = reverse), which is c arried in t he virion of all r etroviruses.The genome of these viruses consists of **two single-stranded positive-sense molecules of RNA** (i.e., diploid ssRNA). **In contrast to other RNA viruses, the information stored in the virion nucleic acid is not directly translated. Instead, a double-stranded DNA replica of viral RNA i s generated through reverse transcriptase**. This multistep process depends on and is catalyzed by virally encoded reverse transcriptase. The v irally generated DNA is **synthesized in the cytoplasm** but afterwards may be integrated into host-cell DNA, and i s termed "**provirus integrated DNA**". Expression of provirus DNA can occur whether or not the viral DNA is integrated. However, perpetuation of the virus is most efficient if integration occurs. The proviral DNA of certain retroviruses is integrated in germ cells and transmitted vertically ("**genetic transmission**") with e very cell t hus containing p roviral DNA. T hese viruses a re known a s "**endogenous**", a nd usually remain quiescent (quiet, inactive). T hat is, t hey are not expressed, and are of low or no pathogenicity. **Vertical transmission** can also occur by viri on passage across the placenta ("**congenital transmission**"). Viruses t ransmitted by t he **horizontal route are termed** "**exogenous**", and are the most important retroviruses as causes of disease.

Retroviruses typically cause a chronic cellular infection that does not lead to early cell lysis. In fact, with the **oncoviruses**, infection leads to **uncontrolled cellular proliferation**. This is in contrast to most other RNA viruses, in which infection and replication lead to **cell death**.

All retroviruses contain three or four genes in common. Each b ears genes for reverse transcriptase referred to as "**pol genes**" (polymerase), a gene for core proteins called the "**gag gene**" (group specific antigens), and a gene encoding for virion peplomer p roteins called the "**env gene**" (envelope). Members of the oncovirus sub-family may contain a fourth gene responsible for cellular transformation. This is called the "**viral oncogene**" (**V-onc**).

All retroviruses share a similar morphology. They consist of an inner core of RNA, surrounded by a capsid, which in turn is surrounded by a lipid-containing envelope bearing glycoprotein projections. Virions are 80-130 nm in diameter. **Replication of oncoviruses occurs only in dividing cells, whereas lentiviruses can replicate in non-dividing cells**.

Diseases caused by Oncoviruses

In 1908, Ellermann and Bang demonstrated the cell-free transmission of avian leukosis, and afterwards demonstrated avian leukosis viruses. After this discovery, the search for oncogenic viral causes of leukaemia in humans and animals was intensified. A specific RNA virus was first discovered in mice by Ludwig Gross in 1951. Now, several viruses of laboratory and domestic animals, and also humans, have been found to be associated with lymphoma and leukaemia. Most of these are **oncoviruses**.

Although s ub-family O ncovirinae has t he largest g roup o f retroviruses and a number of them are oncogenic, **not all members have been shown to be oncogenic**. O n the basis of morphology and the se quence in which t hey were originally described, **retrovirus particles are classified into four types: A, B, C and D**.

A-type particles were originally identified as the **immature nucleocapsids of mouse mammary tumour virus**, the **mature** enveloped virions of which became the prototype (original model) **B-type particles**. A-type particles appear as intracytoplasmic, hollow, 60-90 nm spherical structures with a double-contoured w all.

B-type retrovirus particles are represented by the **mature** extracellular enveloped virions of **mouse mammary tumour virus. These particles originate from intracytoplasmic A-type particles**.

C-type particles comprise most of the avian and mammalian leukaemia viruses. They do not develop from preformed, cytoplasmic A-type particles. Instead, their nucleocapsid formation occurs simultaneously with development of t he viral e nvelope from t he cell m embrane. The i nitial s tage o f nucleocapsid a ssembly appears i n the cytoplasm as a crescent-shaped (i.e., shaped like the new moon, semilunar) object just beneath the cell membrane which becomes the viral envelope. Since the developing nucleocapsid is 'crescent' or 'C-shaped', these retrovirus particles are called 'C-type particles'.

D-type r etrovirus particles c omprise several simian (of monkey) retroviruses, and the retrovirus associated with **jaagsiekte in sheep**. Type D particles, like B particles, develop from intracytoplasmic A-type nucleocapsids which bud through the cell membrane to acquire their envelope.

Diseases caused by Type C Oncoviruses

Feline Leukaemia

Also known as 'feline lymphoma' and 'feline lymphosarcoma', the disease is caused by "feline leukaemia virus (FeLV)". The virus is associated with a variety of disorders, and collectively are the most important cause of **deaths in cats**. FeLV occurs worldwide, with an incidence of up to 50% in densely populated areas. **The virus is transmitted horizontally**, primarily through salivary and nasal secretions of the affected cats. **Two main results** occur following infection: 1) **A self-limiting infection** (or **"regressive infection"**): In this, the initial virus replication in lymphoid tissue is either totally eliminated by the immune system or may remain as provirus, which is contained (prevented from spreading) through immune mechanisms. About 60% of infected cats fall into this category and do not develop any FeLV-associated disease. Provirus can, however, become activated if there is immune dysfunction. In such an event, infected cats may become viraemic and develop FeLV disease. 2) **The second outcome is progressive infection with persistent viraemia**. The initial viral replication in lymphoid tissues, usually in the oropharynx, is not contained and is followed by viraemia and generalized viral infection of lymphocytes, macrophages, intestines, salivary glands, pancreas and urinary bladder. **These cats are infectious because virus is excreted through these sites.**

Persistent infection and **viraemia** are ultimately followed by several disease processes, which lead to death. This usually requires months or years following infection. However, some infections may cause illness or death within a few weeks. Most viraemic cats die within 3 years of infection. The disorders caused by FeLV are grouped into **"cytoproliferative diseases"** and **"cytosuppressive diseases"**. The particular outcome depends on the viral subtype and the age of cat at the time of infection, as well as immune status and genetic make up of the cat. Infection early in life is likely to be followed by viraemia. **The main disorders resulting from FeLV infection are:**

1. **Malignant lymphoma** with or without leukaemia is the **most common** malignancy in cats. **It results from viral activation of cellular proto-oncogenes**. On the basis of anatomical distribution, several forms are recognized: 1) **Thymic lymphoma** occurs mainly in young cats. It is characterized by large tumour masses originating in and replacing the thymus gland and filling the mediastinum; 2) **Alimentary lymphoma** is seen more in older cats. It is characterized by solid tumours which infiltrate the gastrointestinal tract, abdominal lymph nodes, liver, spleen, and kidney; 3) **Multicentric lymphoma** is seen usually in mature cats.

It is characterized by generalized lymphoma, affecting many organs and tissues; and 4) **unclassified lymphoma**. This usually presents as isolated tumour masses in non-lymphoid tissues, such as the eye, or central nervous system. Most cases of malignant lymphoma, with the exception of the alimentary form, are of T cell origin.

2. **Lymphocytic leukaemia**. This may occur in connection with malignant lymphoma.

3. **Erythroid and myeloid leukaemias** (myeloproliferative disorders). **These are the most common leukaemias in cats**, which may occur together. Myelofibrosis is another outcome.

4. **Fibrosarcoma** occurs from infection with **feline sarcoma virus**. This virus is a defective mutant of FeLV. It lacks part of the viral genome and is unable to replicate. However, in the presence of FeLV virus replication occurs. This is because FeLV serves as a **helper virus**, providing the missing genes.

5. **Myelosuppression syndrome**. This is characterized by **anaemia** and/or **leukopaenia** (lymphopaenia and neutropaenia). It is a frequent outcome of FeLV infection. It results from suppression of erythropoiesis and myelopoiesis. The anaemia may become very severe.

6. **Immunosuppression** is seen at some stage in most cats infected with FeLV. It is characterized by progressive loss of function, and a decrease in numbers of both T and B lymphocytes as well as neutrophils.

7. **Enteropathy** is characterized by chronic diarrhoea and wasting. It results from FeLV infection of crypt cells of the intestinal epithelium.

8. **Infertility** results from foetal death and resorption due to FeLV infection of the placenta and foetus.

9. **Neurological disease** has been observed in FeLV-infected cats, but has not been studied in detail.

Diagnosis

The presence of the virus may be demonstrated by electron-microscopic photographs of replicating C-type particles. A fluorescent antibody test is used to detect antigen in leukocytes in blood smears. A third method is to isolate the virus in feline cell cultures from plasma, or oral swabs of cats.

Bovine Leukaemia

Also known as "**bovine lymphoma**", "**malignant lymphoma of cattle**", and "**enzootic bovine lymphoma**", bovine leukaemia is caused by a C-type oncovirus called "**bovine leukaemia virus (BLV)**", first isolated in 1969. **The virus affects**

B lymphocytes, leading to either persistent lymphocytosis, or generalized lymphoma. Infection is spread horizontally.

Enzootic bovine lymphoma, a B-cell lymphoma of adult cattle caused by bovine leukaemia virus, usually involves the lymph nodes. Often lymphoma is restricted to mesenteric lymph nodes, pelvic nodes, and sublumbar nodes. Extension from sublumbar nodes to the lumbar spinal cord can lead to **posterior paralysis**. Retrobulbar lymph node enlargement is another common finding. An **alimentary form** usually involves the wall of the abomasum and associated lymph nodes. Myocardial invasion, particularly of the right atrium, is common, and can lead to signs of heart failure. Bovine leukaemia virus can cause generalized lymphoma in sh eep and goats.

Ovine Leukaemia

Ovine leukaemia is caused by **ovine leukaemia virus**, which is related to bovine leukaemia virus. The virus has been recovered f rom sheep su ffering from lymphoma.

Porcine Leukaemia

Porcine leukaemia virus is **a C-type virus** associated with lymphoma in young pigs. Porcine lymphoma is usually multicentric with extensive replacement of lymph nodes, and invasion of the liver, spleen, and kidneys. Primary enteric lymphoma also occurs in pigs.

Diseases caused by Avian Type C Oncoviruses
Leukosis/Sarcoma Group of Diseases

The l eukosis/sarcoma g roup of d iseases o f the chicken comprises lymphoid, erythroid and myeloid l eukoses, a variety of o ther tumours, su ch as fibrosarcomas, h aemangiomas and nephroblastomas, and the bone d isorder, osteopetrosis (see **Table 6**). These conditions are caused by a group of related retroviruses, which are different from those which cause reticuloendotheliosis and lymphoproliferative disease of turkeys.

Table 6. Neoplasms caused by viruses of Leukosis/Sarcoma Group

Neoplasm	Synonyms
Leukoses	
Lymphoid leukosis	Big liver disease, lymphatic leukosis, visceral lymphoma, lymphocytoma, lymphomatosis, visceral lymphomatosis
Erythroblastosis	Leukaemia, erythroleukosis, erythroid leukosis, e rythromyelosis
Myeloblastosis	Leukaemic myeloid leukosis, myelomatosis, myeloid leukosis, myeloblastosis

| Myelocytomatosis | Myelocytoma, myelomatosis, aleukaemic myeloid leukosis |

Connective tissue tumours
- Fibroma and fibrosarcoma
- Myxoma and myxosarcoma
- Histiocytic sarcoma
- Chondroma
- Osteoma and osteogenic sarcoma

Epithelial tumours

| Nephroblastoma | Embryonal nephroma, renal adenocarcinoma, cystadenoma |
| Nephroma | Carcinoma of the kidney, papillary cystadenoma |

- Hepatocarcinoma
- Adenocarcinoma of the pancreas
- Thecoma (a tumour of the ovary)
- Granulosa cell carcinoma

| Seminoma | Adenocarcinoma of the testis |
| Sqamous-cell carcinoma | |

Endothelial tumours

| Haemangioma | Endothelioma, haemangioblastoma, haemangio-endothelioma |

- Angiosarcoma
- Endothelioma
- Mesothelioma

Related tumours

| Osteopetrosis | Marble bone, thick leg disease, sporadic diffuse osteoperiostitis |

- Meningioma
- Glioma

Of the diseases produced, only lymphoid leukosis is sufficiently prevalent to be of economic importance. The other conditions, with some exceptions, occur only sporadically (i.e., in isolated cases). **More recently, subclinical infection by avian leukosis virus, without the occurrence of neoplastic disease, has been found to depress egg production**.

Apart from their importance in causing poultry disease, the leukosis/sarcoma group of viruses **are of importance and interest in biomedicine**. Erythroid leukosis was the first leukaemic disease shown, by Ellermann and Bang in 1908, to be caused by a virus. An avian sarcoma was the first solid tumour shown by Rous in 1911 to be transmitted by a virus. Proof of the viral aetiology of lymphoid leukosis was provided by Burmester and his associates in 1947. **These diseases have become widely used as model systems for viral oncogenesis**.

Aetiology

The **avian leukosis/sarcoma viruses (ALSV)** are placed in **a subgroup of avian type "C" oncoviruses** of the Family **Retroviridae**. Retroviruses are approximately 100 nm in diameter and have a glycoprotein envelope that surrounds a capsid containing the viral RNA genome. As discussed earlier, within the virion of all retroviruses is present the enzyme "**reverse transcriptase**" (RNA-dependent DNA-polymerase). This enzyme catalyzes the transcription of an RNA molecule into DNA. That is, the reverse of what occurs in most biological systems. This phenomenon of **reverse transcription** is reflected in the family name Retroviridae. As mentioned, the retrovirus genome consists of two exactly similar strands of single-stranded, positive RNA.

The viral genome of **lymphoid leukosis virus (LLV)** is diploid and has three genetic regions in the sequence **5'- *gag-pol-env* 3'**, which encode the viral internal group-specific antigens, RNA-dependent DNA-polymerase (reverse transcriptase) and viral envelope glycoprotein, respectively. **This genetic make-up is associated with slow cell transformation and tumour development over several months**. Other avian oncoviruses cause **rapid neoplastic transformation** and tumour development within a few weeks. **These acutely transforming viruses possess additional genes**, called "***onc* genes**", responsible for oncogenic transformation. These genes originate by **transduction** (i.e., incorporation) **of normal cellular genes**. For example, Rous sarcoma virus has the genetic sequence **5'-*gag-pol-env-src*-3'**. The "*src*" **gene** has been derived originally from a cellular gene.

Virus Subgroups

ASLV are classified into six subgroups - A, B, C, D, E and J - on the basis of differences in their **viral envelope glycoprotein antigens.**

Endogenous and Exogenous Leukosis Viruses

In almost all chickens are present **leukosis viral genes**, which may be partially or completely expressed as infectious virus. These genes are carried as proviral DNA sequences integrated into somatic and germ-line cells. These are termed "**endogenous leukosis viruses**", and as they have viral envelope properties, they are placed in **subgroup E. Endogenous leukosis viruses have little or no oncogenicity for chickens. "Exogenous leukosis viruses",** which infect birds from outside, belong to subgroup **A, B, C, D, or J.**

Epidemiology

Exogenous ALSV are worldwide in distribution in commercial chickens. Subgroup A lymphoid leukosis virus is commonly found, whereas B subgroup of LLV is sometimes found. Subgroups C and D are very rare. **Endogenous subgroup** E viral loci are present in almost all chickens. **Subgroup J was**

reported in the U. K. in meat-type chickens and causes myeloid leukosis (myelocytomatosis). Most commercial chickens are exposed to and infected by the exogenous ALSV, and carry endogenous leukosis viruses, but only a few per cent develop LL or other tumours. Sometimes losses up to 30% can occur. Economic losses occur mainly from mortality from LL between 5-9 months of age in egg-laying and breeding stock. The other neoplastic diseases occur more sporadically. Subclinical infections by LLV have adverse effects on egg production, egg size, fertility, hatchability and growth rate.

Virus Replication

Discussion of viral replication is necessary to get a better grasp of the neoplastic transformation of the cell, described next. Penetration of the host cell by a retrovirus occurs through the receptors present on the cell membrane. Viral RNA is released in the cytoplasm, and under the influence of the **reverse transcriptase**, a strand of negative viral DNA is synthesized on the template of viral RNA. Reverse transcriptase then synthesizes a complementary strand of positive viral DNA. Both the strands get covalently linked to produce linear double-stranded viral DNA, referred to as a "**provirus**" or "**proviral DNA**". The linear viral DNA (proviral DNA) then migrates to the nucleus and becomes integrated into the host-cell DNA under the influence of the enzyme "**integrase**", present in the *pol* gene of the virus. The proviral genes (i.e., proviral DNA) are integrated in the same order as their RNA copies in the virion (i.e., *gag*, *pol*, and *env*) and are flanked on either side by exactly similar sequences of nucleotides termed "**long terminal repeats (LTRs)**" (**Fig. 3.**) (discussed next).

Formation of new virions is the result of transcription and translation of proviral DNA. After integration, the proviral DNA is transcribed by the cell's own machinery to form viral messenger RNA (mRNA) and genomic RNA. The genomic RNA is incorporated into new virions. The mRNAs are translated to produce the protein and enzyme products of the *gag*, *pol*, and *env* genes which form the "**virion**". These products localize at the plasma membrane of the cell and transform into spherical (rounded) virions.The envelope is acquired by budding through cell membranes.

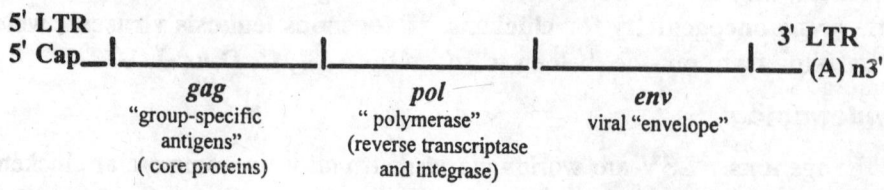

Fig. 3. Diagram showing the gene sequence of the proviral DNA of a standard replicatively competent retrovirus.

The figure shows genomic organization of a typical oncogenic retrovirus. Note that the three genes *gag*, *pol*, and *env* that make the virus are flanked by long terminal repeat (LTR) sequences of nucleotides on either sides. These contain elements that promote and enhance transcription of the viral genome.

As shown in Figure 3, the three genes that make the **proviral DNA** (*gag*, *pol*, and *env*) are required for viral multiplication. These are flanked on the 5' and 3' ends of the genome by sequences of nucleotides referred to as "**long terminal repeats**" or "**LTRs**". These LTRs contain exactly similar sequences, but the left 5' LTR enhances and promotes transcription of proviral DNA to viral RNA (i.e., acts as promoters), whereas the right 3' LTR specifies the site of polyadenylation of the mRNA transcript, which prevents it from being rapidly destroyed in the cytoplasm. The *gag* (core protein) transcript contains a **protease**, whereas the *gag-pol* **polyprotein** is eventually split and processed to form the **reverse transcriptase** and **integrase** required for integration of proviral DNA into host-cell DNA. These final events are mediated by virally encoded protease after the viruses have been assembled.

Neoplastic Transformation and Tumour Formation

As this topic is important and complicated, to get a better understanding, different mechanisms by which oncogenic retroviruses cause neoplastic transformation are discussed first, and then the transformation brought about by the avian leukosis viruses. The oncogenic retroviruses can be divided into two distinct types based on the rapidity with which they transform cells. These are: 1) **Rapidly or acutely transforming retroviruses**, and 2) **Slowly or slow transforming retroviruses**. These viruses represent the two different types of mechanisms. **Both the mechanisms are involved in tumour transformation by avian retroviruses.**

Rapidly or Acutely Transforming Viruses

These viruses produce tumours rapidly. They are responsible for naturally occurring tumours of animals. **Each virus in this group contains a viral oncogene (v-oncogene), which was acquired originally from a host-cell proto-oncogene** by recombinant events at some earlier time in evolution of the virus. There are about 30 known retrovirus oncogenes which have genetic similarity with avian and mammalian proto-oncogenes. All oncogene-containing retroviruses, **except that of Rous sarcoma (Fig. 4A) are "defective"** in replication. This is because they have acquired the oncogene at the expense of one of the three genes (*gag*, *pol*, *env*) essential for viral replication (**Fig. 4B**). **Therefore, these defective viruses require a helper virus to replicate.** The helper retrovirus, when it infects a cell containing a defective retroviral genome, provides the missing gene product needed for the defective oncogenic retrovirus to replicate. **Rous sarcoma virus is the only rapidly transforming retrovirus that is not defective. It contains all three genes** (*gag*, *pol*, *env*) **required for replication of the virus**, plus a viral oncogene known as *v-src* sarcoma (**Fig. 4A**).

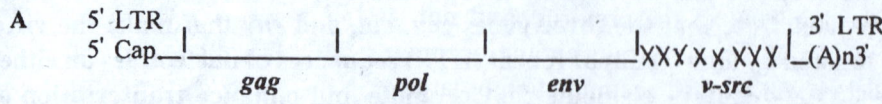

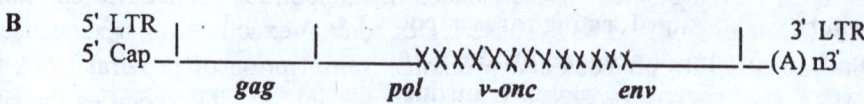

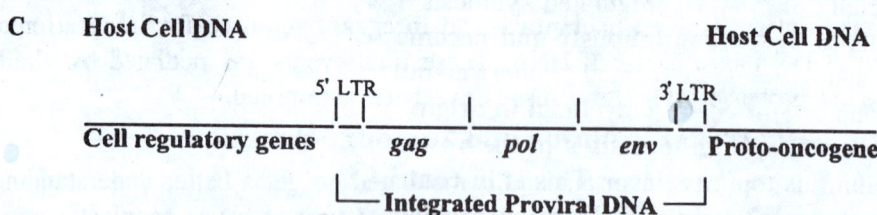

Fig. 4. Diagram s howing proviral g enome of r apidly transforming a nd slowly transforming retroviruses. **A.** Genomic organization of **Rous sarcoma virus**. This is t he only r eplicatively competent r apidly transforming retrovirus (i.e., non-defective). N ote that t he virus **has all the three genes** (*gag, pol, env*), but in addition it has acquired the **oncogene** *v -src*, derived from t he proto-oncogene *src*. **B** . Genomic organization of **a typical "defective" rapidly transforming retrovirus**. These viruses have a cquired a v-oncogene f rom proto-oncogene, but in doing so **they have lost a portion of** *pol* **and** *env* **genes** which are required for viral replication. **C.** The diagram shows **integration of t he proviral D NA of a slowly transforming retrovirus into the host cell DNA**. N ote that t he proviral D NA is i nserted at a site b etween a n ormal cell p roto-oncogene and its regulatory sequences. This results in the proto-oncogene coming under the control of the promoting and enhancing sequences of the 3'LTR of the virus. **This results in unregulated production of the proto-oncogene product and malignant transformation.**

The transforming capacity of the rapidly t ransforming retroviruses does not depend on the proviral DNA at a **specific site** within the host cell DNA, **as occurs in the case of slowly transforming retroviruses. In fact, every cell that is infected with a rapidly transforming virus becomes transformed.**

This is because transcription of the integrated proviral DNA is under the control of the left LTR of the provirus, **and not host regulatory genes**. As a result, transcription of the viral genome occurs **more or less continuously** in the infected cell with the accumulation of large quantities of viral oncogene product within the cell. For example, the *src* gene of Rous sarcoma virus encodes a transformation-specific phosphoprotein, **p60**, in the infected cell with protein kinase activity. Morphological change associated with high levels of p60 is believed to be responsible for the transformed state. The *v-onc* genes associated with other acute transforming viruses encode other transformation-associated proteins. In general, **oncogene products fall into four classes: growth factors, growth factor receptors, signal transducers, and DNA transcription factors.**

There are no negative feedback mechanisms that control v-oncogene expression, as they are in the case of proto-oncogene expression in unaffected cells. The unregulated synthesis of viral oncoprotein causes infected cells **to divide continuously and become immortalized**. Because many cells in a host are transformed soon after infection, the tumours caused by this group of viruses are **polyclonal in origin**. This means that the proviral DNA is integrated at **random sites** in the host-cell DNA in the population of cells making up the neoplasm. **This is in contrast to what is found in cells transformed by slowly transforming retroviruses.**

Slowly Transforming Retroviruses

These retroviruses **do not contain viral oncogene** (i.e., *v-onc* gene), and include **lymphoid leukosis** and many of the avian leukosis viruses, feline leukaemia viruses, and bovine leukaemia viruses. These viruses produce tumours after a **long latent period**. They have a full complement of *gag, pol*, and *env* genes, and are therefore capable of replicating on their own (Fig. 4C). These viruses cause neoplastic transformation by the phenomenon of **"insertional mutagenesis"** or **"downstream promotion of a proto-oncogene"**. For neoplastic transformation to occur, integration of the proviral DNA has to be immediately upstream of a normal cellular proto-oncogene. Integration at such a specific site is purely a chance event and therefore occurs in a small number of infected cells. **This accounts for the long latent period between infection and development of a neoplasm.**

Two events occur when a provirus DNA molecule integrates upstream from a cellular proto-oncogene. **Firstly**, the insertion (integration) of the provirus DNA immediately adjacent to a proto-oncogene **removes the proto-oncogene from control by its normal host cell regulatory genes. Secondly**, the promoting and enhancing sequences of the 3'LTR of the proviral DNA cause **continuous and unregulated expression of the neighbouring proto-oncogene**, leading to increased synthesis of gene product. **This results in uncontrolled proliferation and malignant transformation (Fig. 4C).**

Tumours caused by **slowly transforming retroviruses**, because they result **from the progeny of a single transformed cell, are monoclonic in origin**. This means that all cells making the neoplasm have the proviral DNA integrated **at exactly the same site** within the tumour-cell DNA.

To conclude, slowly transforming viruses transform cells indirectly by activation of a proto-oncogene. **Recent molecular studies** indicate that the avian leukosis virus (ALV) provirus becomes integrated within the host *c-myc* **proto-oncogene**, which is then expressed under the influence of the viral LTR promoter sequence. The increased expression of the *c-myc* gene by this 'promoter insertion' is believed to initiate the neoplastic transformation of the cell. However, multiple activation of other transforming **genes** such as *b-lym* and *c-bic* may be necessary for the full development of lymphoid leukosis.

Spread

Exogenous ALVs are transmitted in two ways: vertically from hen to progeny through the egg, and **horizontally** between birds by direct and indirect contact. Although usually only a small number of chicks are infected vertically, this route is important **because it maintains the infection from one generation to the next**. Majority of the chicks become infected by close contact with vertically infected chickens during rearing. The infection does not spread readily from infected birds to birds in indirect contact, i.e., in separate pens or cages. This is because of the relatively short life of the virus (a few hours) outside the bird.

Vertical infection occurs from hens which shed ALSV from the oviduct into the egg albumen, from where it passes into the chick embryo. **The virus is produced by albumen-secreting glands of the oviduct**, mainly in the ampulla and magnum of the oviduct. **Transovarian infection is not important.** Also, the embryos do not become infected from the male (cock). Congenitally infected chicks develop immunological tolerance to the virus and fail to develop virus neutralizing antibodies, **but are viraemic**. Hens of this class have a high levels of virus in the blood and tissues (highest in oviduct) and **an absence of antibodies (virus +ive, antibody -ive). Such hens shed the virus to most of their eggs and their embryos.**

Chicks infected horizontally develop a brief viraemia and then develop virus neutralizing antibodies **without viraemia (virus -ive, antibody +ive)**. Such birds are usually virus carriers and shedders. On the other hand, **vertically infected chicks that have high levels of virus in the blood and tissues and an absence of antibodies (virus +ive, antibody -ive) are several times more likely to develop lymphoid leukosis than are virus -ive and antibody +ive birds**. However, not all eggs that have ALV in the albumen give rise to infected embryos or chicks. Only about one-half to one-eighth of embryos are infected from eggs with virus in the albumen. This intermittent congenital transmission may be due to neutralization of virus by antibody in the yolk. The incidence of leukosis decreases if horizontal infection occurs after the first few weeks of life. Virus is present in the saliva, faeces and feather debris of infected birds, **but as its survival outside the body is short, ALSVs are not very contagious.**

Immunity

Virus-neutralizing antibodies from infected hens are passed through the yolk to chicks, and provide a passive immunity against contact infection which lasts for 3-4 weeks. Actively acquired humoral and cell-mediated immune responses following infection similarly help in reducing virus replication and neoplasia.

Genetic Resistance

Two types of genetic resistance to the ALSV group are recognized: 1. **Resistance to virus infection**, and 2. **Resistance to tumour development**. **Susceptibility genes** encode for the presence of **receptors** through which the virus gains access to the cell. **These receptors are either decreased in number, or are absent, in resistant cells.** Resistance to tumour development has been studied mainly with Rous sarcoma virus-induced sarcomas.

Signs

The **signs** in chickens affected with leukosis are **non-specific**. The bird may be anorectic, weak, and emaciated, diarrhoea may occur, and the wattles may be pale. In lymphoid leukosis, the enlarged liver and bursa may be palpable. Osteopetrosis is readily noticeable from thickening of the long bones.

Diagnosis

Diagnosis involves **pathological** and **virological examinations** to determine 1) the **type of neoplasm** responsible for mortality, and 2) which **viruses are present** in a flock. Because exogenous ALSV is almost ubiquitous (existing everywhere) in commercial flocks, its isolation does not prove that it caused the tumour. This would require transmission experiments in which the tumour is reproduced by the virus isolate.

Pathological Diagnosis

Identification of the neoplasm is made by **gross and histopathological examination**. Cytological examination of May-Grunwald-Giemsa stain impression smears of fresh tumour tissue is a useful aid to diagnosis. The set of tissues to be examined should include liver, spleen, bursa of Fabricius, thymus, bone marrow, gonads, sciatic, brachial and coeliac nerves, and any other tumour tissue. Differentiation of lymphoid leukosis from Marek's disease is important (see Marek's disease).

Virological Diagnosis

The presence of infection can be demonstrated easily by detecting **neutralizing antibodies in serum**. Viruses can be detected in and isolated from serum, plasma, tumor tissue, normal parenchymatous tissue (e.g., liver, vaginal and cloacal swabs, egg albumen and embryos). Because the viruses are thermolabile (destroyed by heat) at room temperature, samples should be collected from freshly killed birds, or from newly laid eggs, and stored and transported at -70° C.

The main techniques for ALSV detection are the ELISA test, non-producer (NP) cell activation tests, phenotypic mixing (PM) test, complement fixation avian leukosis virus (COFAL) test, resistance-inducing factor (RIF) test, and chick and chick embryo inoculation tests for ALSV.

Lymphoid Leukosis (LL)

Lymphoid leukosis is the commonest neoplasm caused by the ALSV. It is **characterized usually by enlargement of the liver by infiltrating lymphoblasts.** LL appears between the **14th and 30th week of age**. In field outbreaks, cases mostly occur after 14 weeks of age. However, **incidence is usually highest at about sexual maturity.** Spread has been discussed under general considerations of ALSV.

Pathogenesis

Three lines of evidence indicate that lymphoid leukosis is a malignancy of the bursa-dependent lymphoid system. 1) The first is that **removal of the bursa prevents LL.** The treatments which effectively destroy the bursa of Fabricius and thus prevent LL are: Surgical bursectomy, treatment of embryos or hatched chicks with androgens either by inoculation or in feed, chemical bursectomy with cyclophosphamide, and infection with infectious bursal disease virus (IBDV). **Thymectomy has no effect on the course of the disease.** 2) **Histopathological examination of the bursa** has provided the second line of evidence. Changes in the **bursal lymphoid follicles** can be observed as early as 2 weeks of age. Most tumour nodules originate from transformation of a limited number of cells, i.e., **they are clonal.** As transformed cells proliferate, affected follicles become engorged with **uniform blast-like cells.** Abnormal follicles expand and displace adjacent normal bursal follicles until a gross tumour of the bursa is visible. Necropsies performed on chickens dying with LL have revealed **macroscopic tumours of the bursa in almost every case.** 3) The third line of evidence has been provided by the **immunofluorescence studies.** Cells of LL tumours, transplantable tumours, and lymphoid cell lines cultured *in vitro* all have **B cell markers** (i.e., they are B-lymphoytes) and IgM on their surface.

Although target cells are transformed in the bursa of most birds, **only a** few birds develop LL. Thus, some early tumours must be regressing. Other tumours must be enlarging and their cells entering into the vascular system and producing metastatic foci in other visceral organs. **At about the time of sexual maturity (16-24 weeks of age), tumour involvement is so extensive that birds die.** Recent studies have revealed that though ALVs multiply in most tissues and organs, **the infection persists longer in bursal lymphocytes than in other tissues, and that cells of the bursa of Fabricius are the target cells that are neoplastically transformed.** Molecular biology studies indicate that a viral promoter gene activates a host *c-myc* gene in **B cells**, and this results in neoplastic transformation of B cells. The *c-myc* host gene also interferes with the normal intraclonal switch of B cell immunoglobulin production from IgM to IgG. **This is the reason why tumour cells have only IgM on their surface, and not IgG or IgA.** The *c-myc* host gene is present in all chickens.

Signs

External signs of disease are not specific. The comb may be pale, shrivelled, and cyanotic. Anorexia, emaciation, weakness and diarrhoea occur usually. The abdomen is often enlarged. Enlargement of liver, bursa of Fabricius and kidneys can often be detected on palpation. **The incubation period** from infection to the developed disease and death is **4 months or more.**

Gross Lesions

Grossly visible tumours almost always involve **liver, spleen,** and **bursa of Fabricius.** Size of tumours is highly variable as are number of organs affected. These include, in addition to liver and spleen, kidney, lung, gonad, heart, bone marrow, and mesentery. Tumours are soft, smooth, and glistening. A cut surface appears slightly greyish to creamy white, and rarely has areas of necrosis. Growth may be nodular, granular (miliary), or diffuse, or a combination of these forms. In the **nodular form,** lymphoid tumours (0.5 mm - 5 cm in diameter), usually spherical, may occur singly or in large numbers. The **granular or miliary form** consists of numerous small nodules (less than 2 mm in diameter) uniformly distributed throughout the parenchyma. In the **diffuse form,** the organ is uniformly enlarged, and usually very friable.

Microscopic Lesions

As tumour cells proliferate, they displace and compress cells of the organ rather than infiltrate between them. **Microscopically,** the lesions consist of diffuse areas or coalescing foci of extravascular lymphoid cells. The cytoplasm of most tumour cells contains a large amount of RNA, indicating that the cells are **immature and rapidly dividing. The main cell is a lymphoblast.** They have **B cell markers** and carry **surface IgM.**

Erythroblastosis (Erythroid Leukosis)

Erythroid leukosis is a rare and sporadic disease, affecting mainly **adult chickens**. There is always **anaemia**, which is associated with the **presence of a large number of immature red cells in the blood**. The disease originates in the bone marrow and a leukaemia is present from the outset. **It is a peculiarity of this disease that the malignant cells remain within the blood vessels throughout the course of the disease**. This leads to **erythrostasis** in sinusoids in organs such as the liver, spleen, and bone marrow, giving them a cherry-red colour which characterizes this condition at **postmortem**. The liver and spleen are moderately enlarged.

Myeloblastosis (Myeloid Leukosis)

Myeloblastosis involves an extravascular proliferation of cells of the granulocytic series. It is a sporadic disease mainly of **adult chicks**. It may occur as a myeloblastosis, originating in the bone marrow and involving **immature cells**. In diffuse myeloblastosis, the liver and spleen are diffusely and greatly enlarged. The liver usually has a granular appearance.

Myelocytomatosis

Myelocytomatosis, like myeloblastosis, also originates in the bone marrow, but in this condition the **cells affected are more mature**. The tumours of myelocytomatosis\are discrete (separate) and nodular, and have a yellowish-white colour. The tumours may occur in a wide range of organs, including the liver, spleen, and kidney; and they have a predilection for the visceral surface of flat bones such as ribs, skull, sternum and pelvis.

Other Tumours

Solid tumours which can be caused by ALSV include fibrosarcoma, chondroma, endothelioma, haemangioma, nephroblastoma, hepatocarcinoma and several others (see Table 6). They usually **occur sporadically** in young or older chickens and show features characteristic of their cellular origin.

Osteopetrosis

This is a bone disorder affecting mainly the **long bones**, particularly of the legs and wings. Excessive osteoblast proliferation and bone formation result in **gross thickening of the diaphyses of the long bones**. Occlusion of the marrow cavity may eventually give rise to **anaemia**.

Reticuloendotheliosis

Reticuloendotheliosis (RE) includes a group of pathological syndromes caused by **retroviruses** of the reticuloendotheliosis virus (REV) group. **The disease syndromes include: 1) acute reticulum cell neoplasia, 2) a runting disease syndrome, and 3) chronic neoplasia of lymphoid and other tissues**.

Natural i nfections by REVs o ccur i n chickens, t urkeys, d ucks, g eese, and Japanese quail. The REV group are **avian C-type oncoviruses** of the family **Retroviridae**, but are distinct from viruses of the leukosis/sarcoma group.

The virus i s **transmitted** by contact with i nfected chickens and t urkeys **(horizontal transmission)**. Virus is present in the faeces, and in body fluids of affected birds. Virus shedding occurs mainly during periods of active viraemia. **Vertical transmission** of REV has been reported in both chickens and turkeys, usually at very low rates. **There are no characteristic signs of the disease**. The l esions include: 1) **acute reticulum cell neoplasia** in newly hatched chickens causing high mortality. Affected birds have enlarged livers and spleen. 2) **chronic lymphoid neoplasia**. This is of **two types - lymphomas of large uniform lymphoreticular cells, and bursa-dependent B cell lymphomas. 3) a runting disease syndrome**. This syndrome includes **several non-neoplastic lesions**. REV infection can also cause **immunosuppression**. The presence of infection in a flock can be determined by examination of sera for antibodies, using the ELISA test, agar gel precipitin test, plaque reduction test, or fluorescent antibody test.

Lymphoproliferative Disease of Turkeys

Lymphoproliferative disease (LPD) of turkeys was first reported from UK in 1972. LPD is caused by **a type C retrovirus** of the Family **Retroviridae** which is distinct serologically and genetically from other avian retroviruses. The infection can **spread horizontally** between turkeys. **Vertical transmission has not been reported.**

The disease is seen mainly in growing turkeys, and sometimes in adults. Affected birds die suddenly. Up to 20% of the flock may be affected. Lesions comprise marked enlargement of the spleen, and moderate enlargement of the liver with miliary greyish-white foci. Miliary tumour infiltration may also occur in kidney, gonad, intestinal wall, pancreas, lungs, myocardium, and thymus. The tumour infiltration c onsists of p leomorphic cells, i ncluding lymphocytes, lymphoblasts, reticulum cells, and plasma cells. **Diagnosis** of LPD is based on gross and microscopic lesions in affected birds, and detection of LPD virus in tissues by immunofluorescence, or in plasma by an ELISA test.

Type B Oncoviruses

Mouse Mammary Tumour

It was observed that offspring of hybrid mice produced by pairs from two inbred strains had an increased incidence of certain mammary tumours, if their mothers were descendants of strains in which the incidence of tumours was high. In 1936, Bittner demonstrated that a factor in the milk of the mice from the affected strains was responsible f or the production of **mouse mammary tumours**. The mammary-tumour milk agent (**Bittner's factor**) is now known to be **type B oncovirus**. The virus, which is transmitted in milk, infects infant mice while nursing, whether or not the mother has mammary cancer. This is because infected m ice may be "**latently**" infected and e xcrete v irus i n t he absence of disease.

Not all mammary tumours in mice are related to this virus. There are several transplantable tumours in mice which are free of the milk agent. The murine (mouse) mammary tumour associated with the milk agent **is of much interest in experimental oncology**, as it provides a link in the chain of evidence towards the viral aetiology of neoplasia.

Type D Oncoviruses

Type D oncoviruses have been shown t o be of pathologic i mportance **only in sheep**, in which a type D virus is associated with **jaagsiekte**.

Jaagsiekte

Also known as "**ovine p ulmonary adenoma**", "**ovine pulmonary adenomatosis**", and "**pulmonary carcinoma of sheep**", jaagsiekte is **a neoplastic disease of older sheep**. The name "**jaagsiekte**" is derived from **Afrikaans** (a language developed from Dutch, spoken in South Africa) in which it means a "**driving sickness/disease**" (jaagt = drive; siekte = sickness). The disease was so named because the animal f irst manifests t he disease by dyspnoea (difficult breathing) after the stress of strenuous exertion, **such as a long drive**. Besides South Africa, the disease has been reported from many other countries of the world, **including India**. O ver the years, several different v iruses have b een suggested as the cause of jaagsiekte, but now **a type D oncovirus (a retrovirus)** has been implicated as the cause. However, the virus has not yet been cultured. **In India**, there are reports of the occurrence of jaagsiekte **in goats** at very low prevalence r ates.

Spread

The natural mode of transmission is by **droplet infection** from respiratory secretions, which are copious **in sheep** with clinical disease. When sheep are kept in close contact, the d isease gets transmitted by inhalation of infected droplets. Experimentally, j aagsiekte can be transmitted t o susceptible sh eep by intratracheal or intrapulmonary injection of affected lung tissue from sheep with the disease.

Pathogenesis

The virus replicates in the type II pneumocytes in the alveolus. **Type II pneumocytes and Clara cells in the terminal bronchioles are transformed, and their growth produces intra-alveolar and intra-bronchiolar polypoid ingrowths**. These cells are surfactant-producing secretory cells, and there is also c opious production o f fluid. T he excessive s urfactant-like protein p ro-duced (in the tumour), pro vides a stimulus for the accumulation of macrophages, seen in this disease. The **adenomatous ingrowths of alveolar epithelium** encroach gradually upon alveolar space so that **a noxic anoxia** occurs. The lesions produced by experimental inoculation are similar to those of the naturally occurring disease.

Signs

The incubation period in natural cases is 1-3 years. Clinical disease is rare in sheep younger than 2 years, and is most common at 3-4 years of age.The disease runs a progressive afebrile course of several months or longer. **Clinical signs are not noticeable until a significant proportion of the lung is affected by the tumour. Occasional coughing and some panting after exercise are the earliest signs,** but coughing is not a prominent sign in this disease. Emaciation, dyspnoea, lachrymation, and a **profuse watery discharge from the nose** follow. Jaagsiekte has a **prolonged clinical course,** and is **always fatal.** Death occurs within 6 weeks to 4 months after the onset of symptoms. Moist crackles (a series of sharp sounds) can be heard over the affected lung areas. Even they can be heard at a distance so that a group of affected animals are said to produce a sound like slowly boiling porridge. There is no rise of body temperature unless there is secondary infection. Pasteurellosis is a common complication and often the cause of death.

Lesions

The lesions consist of multiple foci of neoplastic alveolar type II cells in acinar and papillary patterns. The result is a pronounced thickening of the alveolar walls, and partial obliteration of the alveolar spaces by **small adenocarcinomas.** However, their malignancy is not clear. A certain number of mononuclear cells and lyphocytes fill the alveoli, and along with a few neutrophils, appear as an exudate in some of the bronchi. However, there is never any exudate similar to that seen in the acute exudative pneumonias. The peribronchiolar lymph nodules are hyperplastic and markedly enlarged. **Metastatic lesions** consisting of adenomatous foci in bronchial and mediastinal lymph nodes, similar to those seen in the lung, have been reported. A few reports have described extrathoracic metastases to sites such as muscle and kidney. **The proliferative nature of the pulmonary lesion together with metastases is strong evidence that jaagsiekte is neoplastic and malignant.**

Diagnosis

Both jaagsiekte and maedi/progressive pneumonia are chronic lung diseases with long incubation periods. Maedi/progressive pneumonia is not neoplastic and is characterized by interstitial pneumonia and marked lymphocytic nodular hyperplasia. Jaagsiekte has many points of similarity to Marsh's ovine progressive pneumonia, but one difference is the **large amount of catarrhal nasal discharge which is characteristic of this disease.** A diagnostic test in this disease is to hold the sheep up by the hind legs. In affected animals a quantity of watery mucus (up to about 200 ml) runs from the nostrils (**"wheelbarrow test"**).

Diseases caused by Lentiviruses

Lentiviruses have come from obscurity into the forefront with the discovery that the cause of acquired immunodeficiency syndrome (AIDS) of humans is a **lentivirus**, known as **"human immunodeficiency virus (HIV)"**. Lentiviruses affecting animals include the viruses of visna and maedi (which are very similar), caprine arthritis-encephalitis virus, feline immunodeficiency virus, bovine immunodeficiency virus, simian immunodeficiency virus, and equine infectious anaemia virus (see Table 5). Lentiviruses produce a chronic persistent infection with a long incubation period. In 1954, the term "**slow virus infections**" was introduced to describe chronicity of visna and maedi. The term is now used for other lentiviruses also, as well as some other chronic non-lentiviral diseases, such as scrapie. **Lentiviral infections persist even though they initiate humoral and cellular immune responses**. A number of hypotheses have been put forward to explain persistence, but the mechanism these viruses use to escape elimination is largely unclear. Lentiviruses share the characteristics with other retroviruses, **but differ antigenically. They do not require dividing cells for replication**, and transcription and translation occur from non-integrated viral DNA.

Pathologically, lentiviruses establish themselves in **macrophages and lymphocytes**, and **interfere with immune functions**. For this reason more recent isolates have been termed **immunodeficiency viruses**, following the nomenclature of human immunodeficiency virus. The **lesions** caused by different lentiviruses may vary, but most cause some combination of these: 1) lymphadenopathy with marked follicular hyperplasia. This may proceed to lymphoid depletion, 2) lymphocytic infiltration, 3) interstitial pneumonia, 4) encephalomyelitis, or 5) arthritis. In severely immunodeficient animals, **opportunistic infections** may develop (especially true for HIV), and may dominate the pathological findings and be the immediate cause of clinical signs, or death.

Visna-Maedi

In 1935, a chronic viral encephalomyelitis of sheep was reported from Iceland. It was named "**visna**". "**Visna**" is an Icelandic word and means **shrinkage** or **wasting**. The name was used to indicate one clinical feature of the disease (**wasting**) in the paralyzed sheep. Then, in 1939, a chronic, progressive pneumonia was recognized, again in Iceland, and was named "**maedi**". "**Maedi**" is also an Icelandic word and means dyspnoea. **It is now believed that visna and maedi are caused by the same virus**. The same or similar virus appears to cause the **Marsh's progressive pneumonia** described first in Montana, USA, in 1923. **The virus of visna/maedi is closely related to the** lentivirus of goats which causes caprine arthritis-encephalitis. The synonyms for visna-maedi are "ovine progressive pneumonia", "lymphoid interstitial pneumonia", and "chronic viral encephalomyelitis of sheep". Visna-maedi are different clinical manifestations of the same viral infection. The 'visna syndrome' is a slow, progressive demyelination, whereas the 'maedi syndrome' is a slowly progressive interstitial pneumonia. A mixed syndrome has recently been observed. All syndromes invariably terminate fatally. In India, maedi of sheep has been reported from different parts of the country.

Spread

Infection is mainly spread by the respiratory route. Mononuclear cells in the colostrum and milk of infected ewes are infected with virus. These cells may pass through the intestinal wall to infect the lamb.

Pathogenesis

Replication of the virus occurs mainly in the macrophages. This leads to cell-associated viraemia, and dissemination of the virus to the brain and other organs. Pulmonary secretions and milk containing infected macrophages are the main source of virus for natural transmission. Diseases such as jaagsiekte (pulmonary adenomatosis), which increase the number of macrophages in lung secretions, facilitate spread of visna-maedi virus.

Visna-maedi virus avoids destruction by antibodies through antigenic variation. In visna-maedi infections, neutralizing antibodies are produced very slowly. As a result, these antibodies are inefficient in selecting antigenically different viruses and therefore they are unable to reduce the viral burden in infected sheep. These antibodies have a very low affinity for their epitopes and take at least 20 minutes to bind to the virus and 30 minutes to neutralize it. In contrast, it takes only 2 minutes for this virus to infect a cell. Thus, the virus can spread between cells very much faster than it can be neutralized.

Signs

Due to the long interval between infection and development of clinical disease (i.e., incubation period), which is usually 2-3 years but may be as long as 8 years, these disorders are seen only in adult sheep. Goats are susceptible, but usually they suffer from their own lentiviral infection, caprine arthritis-encephalitis. The clinical signs develop insidiously (gradually without being noticed) and progress slowly. The initial signs are listlessness (having no energy) and loss of body condition which progress to emaciation. Signs of respiratory involvement are not noticeable in the early stages. Dyspnoea develops later. There is no evidence of excess fluid in the lungs. There may be coughing and some nasal discharge. Clinical disease lasts for 3-10 months and the disease is always fatal. In some sheep, clinical respiratory disease is minimal and the major manifestation is wasting, and the thin ewe syndrome.

The involvement and induration (hardening) of the **mammary glands** are also insidious in onset, and ewes are usually in their third or later lactation by the time the disease is fully manifest. **In advanced cases the udder is enlarged and very firm.**

Lesions of Visna

Originally, when discovered, the virus appeared to affect either the central nervous system, or the lungs. **It is now clear that both systems may be affected in the same animal.** The lesions in the **central nervous system** consist of zones of **demyelination** with destruction of paraventricular white matter in the cerebellum and cerebrum. Similar lesions occur in the spinal cord. The demyelinated zones are surrounded by gliosis and lymphocytic infiltration. The meninges of both brain and spinal cord are usually infiltrated by lymphocytes and other mononuclear cells. The lesions in the CNS result in greatly increased numbers of cells in the spinal fluid (**pleocytosis**). This is of help in differentiating the clinical disease from scrapie, which does not result in pleocytosis.

Lesions of Maedi/Progressive Pneumonia

The **gross lesions** of the **pulmonary form** of this disease (maedi) are **quite characteristic. The lungs do not collapse fully when the thorax is opened.** They have a dense, rubbery consistency, but are not consolidated. All lobes have a uniform greyish colour, and are of uniform consistency. This is in marked contrast to the differences between normal and consolidated areas in the usual type of acute pneumonia. The lungs are distended, appear large, **and weigh 2-5 times as much as normal adult sheep lungs (normally 300-500 g).** The cut surface is dry and exudate cannot be squeezed.

The **microscopic lesions** show that the loss of elasticity and compressibility and the greyish colour **are caused by a great increase in the thickness of the alveolar walls. The thickening may be so great that the alveolar spaces are obliterated.** The thickening is caused by proliferation and infiltration of reticulo-endothelial or mesenchymal cells that invade the septa everywhere. The cells vary from large round mononuclear forms, some of which appear to be macrophages, to short fibroblastic cells. Hyperaemia of the inter-alveolar capillaries occurs in early stages. Lymph nodules occur along the course of the bronchi and bronchioles. A few large mononuclear cells contain one or more peculiar cytoplasmic inclusions, 1-3 mm in diameter, which take a bluish-grey colour with Giemsa's stain. **These are probably specific for the disease.** There is generalized follicular hyperplasia in **lymph nodes** and spleen, and lymphoid infiltrations are found in almost any organ. The polyarthritis is characterized by villous hyperplasia of the synovial membrane and an extensive lymphocytic and plasma cell infiltration.

Diagnosis

There are several chronic pneumonias which need to be differentiated from maedi, including jaagsiekte, in which the microscopic picture is quite different. Also, profuse nasal discharge and the flow of fluid with the wheelbarrow test in jaagsiekte are the common signs, and there is a shorter course.

Caprine Arthritis-Encephalitis

In 1974, **a new disease of goats** was described in the United States, which is now known as "**caprine arthritis-encephalitis (CAE)**", and recognized as **one of the most important diseases of goats**. It is caused by a **lentivirus related to the visna/maedi virus**, which is distributed worldwide with prevalence rates of up to 80% in some herds. However, the number of infected animals with clinical disease is usually 25%, or less. **Sheep can be infected with the virus**. The disease is characterized by **arthritis in adult goats** and **encephalomyelitis in young goats. The disease has been reported from India.**

Spread

The main route of infection is through colostrum or milk. More than 75% of kids born to infected dams may acquire infection through the colostrum and milk. The virus can be isolated both from the cells in the milk, and from cell-free milk from infected dams. The disease can be transmitted by contact both during and after the perinatal period. **The mechanism of transmission is not known.**

Pathogenesis

Animals infected at birth remain persistently infected for life, although only some develop clinical disease. **The virus infects cells of the monocyte-macrophage type**. Shedding of the virus occurs as infected monocytes mature to macrophages. Disease is the result of inflammation resulting from the reaction of the host immune system to expressed virus. **The lesions are lymphoproliferative in nature.**

The virus of CAE tries to avoid the immune system of the host through antigenic variation. As a result, although infected animals mount an immune response to CAE virus, the antibodies formed are unable to neutralize the virus. Goats with CAE make large amounts of antienvelope antibodies, but they develop insignificant levels of neutralizing antibodies. This is because goats fail to recognize and respond to the virus-neutralizing epitopes **due to antigenic variation of the virus.**

Signs

The **encephalitic form** of the disease is usually seen **in young goats** 1-4 months of age. This is in contrast to most lentiviral infections. Affected kids have difficulty in abducting (taking away) the hind limbs and become ataxic (i.e. unable to coordinate the muscular movements). An ascending paralysis progresses to total posterior paralysis, and ultimately tetraparesis (paralysis of all four limbs). There may be torticollis (twisted neck), and the head is held upward, or at another angle. There is only mild fever, but interstitial pneumonia can occur and be noticeable clinically.

The **arthritic form** is seen **in adult goats**. It is usually a chronic, slowly progressive disorder, developing over months. All joints are affected, but swelling of the carpal (**big knee**), hock, and stifle joints is most noticeable.

Lesions

Central nervous system lesions are confined to the white matter, and are characterized by disseminated perivascular accumulations of mononuclear cells and demyelination. The mononuclear cuffs are composed of lymphocytes, macrophages, and large reticulum cells. The **articular lesions** are characterized by a villous proliferative synovitis with extensive lymphocytic infiltration. Similar lesions are present in tendon sheaths and bursae. In the lung, there is an interstitial pneumonia with pronounced lymphoid hyperplasia.

Diagnosis

Diagnosis is based on clinical signs, lesions and serology. An agar gel immunodiffusion test (AGID) is widely used for detection of infection. Other serological tests include ELISA and dot ELISA. Identification of CAE is usually provided by isolation of the virus into tissue culture.

Feline Immunodeficiency Virus Infection

Feline immunodeficiency virus (FIV) is a **lentivirus**. It was first isolated in 1987 from domestic cats (in the United States) having an immunodeficiency syndrome. The virus has since been identified in cats throughout the world. FIV bears many similarities to HIV. **It is tropic for T lymphocytes, macrophages and astrocytes.**

Spread

The virus is shed mainly in the saliva, and it is transmitted primarily through bites. Accordingly, the highest incidence is in the free-roaming (wild and pet) male and aged cats (i.e., in cats living outdoors). Very often FIV-infected cats are also infected with feline leukaemia virus (FeLV). However, **cats are more adapted to FIV than are human to HIV**, and that **FIV is less immunosuppressive than HIV.**

Signs

Following infection, there is a low-grade fever, generalized lymphadenopathy, and sometimes, diarrhoea. This is mostly seen **in young cats**, and usually persists for 2-4 weeks, although lymphadenopathy may persist for several months. This is followed by clinically normal interval of 1-2 years during which there is depression of the CD4+ to CD8+ T cell ratio. Afterwards, infected cats may develop recurrent fever, lymphadenopathy, anaemia, diarrhoea, and weight loss. **Chronic secondary infections**, especially gingivitis, dermatitis and upper respiratory disease, and **opportunistic infections** may occur at the final stages of disease. Opportunistic infections include toxoplasmosis, calicivirus infection, feline herpesvirus infection, candidiasis, cryptococcosis, haemobartonellosis, mycobacteriosis, and others. Several neurological abnormalities, including dementia, twitching, tremors and convulsions, may also occur.

Lesions

Lesions basically reflect those of opportunistic infections. Encephalitis, characterized by perivascular mononuclear infiltrations and glial nodules, is most likely a primary FIV lesion, comparable to the encephalitis seen in AIDS. Care must be taken to rule out toxoplasmosis, or other agents that can lead to encephalitis. **Microscopically**, the lymphadenopathy is characterized by early follicular hyperplasia which may later progress to marked lymphoid depletion.

Cats remain infected for life. The presence of serum antibodies is directly correlated with the ability to isolate virus from blood cells and saliva.

Bovine Immunodeficiency Virus Infection

Bovine immunodeficiency virus (BIV), a lentivirus, is one of the three bovine retroviruses. The others are **bovine leukaemia virus** (a type C oncornavirus), and **bovine spumavirus** (a foamy virus). **BIV was the first of the bovine retroviruses to be isolated**. This happened in the course of the search for the cause of bovine leukaemia in the 1960s. Since BIV did not prove to be the cause of bovine leukaemia, the virus remained unstudied until the recognition of HIV as the cause of AIDS in humans. BIV was the third of the lentiviruses to be discovered, preceded by equine infectious anaemia virus and the ovine lentivirus of visna-maedi and ovine progressive pneumonia.

The original BIV isolate was recovered from a Holstein **cow** in Louisiana, USA, which had lymphocytosis and a gradually weakening condition. Since then, several additional isolates have been obtained. Studies have revealed that the infection is life-long and associated with lymphocytosis or lymphopaenia, generalized lymphadenopathy, and multiple **grossly visible** subcutaneous nodules of lymphocytes. Lymphocytic cuffing in the brain and lymphocytic meningitis also occur along with neuronal degeneration and lymphocytic infiltration of the neuropil (complex network of processes of neurons and neuroglial cells).

Clinical findings include lethargy, mastitis, pododermatitis (dermatitis of foot), pneumonia, mycotic abomasitis, and abscessation and lymphosarcoma. Persistent infection with BIV predisposes to the effects of bovine leukaemia virus. Some infected cattle can be detected by serological tests for viral antibodies. Virus isolation from blood appears to be the most accurate way to detect infected animals.

Equine Infectious Anaemia

Also known as "swamp fever", equine infectious anaemia (EIA) is **an important viral disease of horses, mules and asses (donkeys).** It is caused by **a lentivirus,** and has a worldwide distribution. **The virus shares serological reactivity with the human AIDS lentivirus (HIV).** EIA was first recognized in France in 1943. It is not only a serious economic problem, but also a useful model for the study of mechanism involved in the persistence of virus in the host, and its pathogenic effects. Once the virus enters into a susceptible animal, it can be demonstrated in the blood **as long as the animal lives. Despite the immune response, the virus persists like other lentiviral infections.** The disease was first **recorded in India in 1987** in an equine stud at Bangalore. Serosurveillance of EIA carried out in recent years by the National Research Centre of Equines, Hisar, Haryana, found a number of horses positive in different states of India, particularly in Haryana and Maharashtra.

EIA infection may be almost **subclinical,** or it may be **acute** with febrile manifestations, **and a rapidly fatal outcome.** But infected horses have lived up to 18 years with few signs. However, at any time, minute amounts of their blood injected into normal horses induces acute infectious anaemia. Horses which appear recovered from the acute disease may suddenly show severe symptoms, and die after exposure to some harmful influence, such as hard work. It appears that host and parasite, under some conditions, maintain a delicate balance.

Spread

The virus is transmitted mechanically by the bite of mosquito (Culex sp.) or biting fly (***Stomoxys calcitrans,* Tabanus** sp.) It can even be transmitted iatrogenically (i.e., by a clinician) by the transfer of a minute amount of blood from an infected horse to a normal horse by the use of **unsterilized hypodermic needles,** tattoo needles, curry combs, or items of equipment, such as harness, bit, or saddle. **The disease is not spread by ordinary contact.**

Pathogenesis

The virus localizes in many organs, especially spleen, liver, kidney and lymph nodes. It can be detected there in greatest quantity when a severe clinical attack is present. It disappears from tissues in periods between attacks. Although there is persistent viraemia, probably throughout the horse's life, the level is low except during periods of clinical activity, so that it is at these times that the animal is most infective. **Pathogenesis** of EIA involves primary entry and infection of macrophages; destruction of macrophages and release of virus; production of antibodies to antigenic components; formation of antigen-antibody complexes, which induce fever, glomerulitis, and complement depletion; specific complexes cause haemolysis or phagocytosis by activating the reticulo-endothelial system; pathological processes subside, as virus-neutralizing antibodies prevent viral multiplication in macrophages; and the horses become permanently asymptomatic. The animal can be said to have achieved an appropriate level of immune response sufficient to protect it against antigenic epitopes which are common to all EIA virus strains. **Life-long viral persistence is due to a virus-induced defect of the macrophages.**

The EIA virus tries to avoid host's immune system by undergoing rapid antigenic variation. The EIA virus, like other lentiviruses, undergoes random mutation at a high rate, **and new antigenically different variants are produced.** Their survival depends on the presence of neutralizing antibodies in the horse's serum. As variant strains of the virus are produced, the infected horse makes neutralizing antibodies to that variant. As a result, that period of viraemia ends. However, variants of the EIA virus appear rapidly and randomly. **The appearance of a new non-neutralizable variant leads to clinical relapse.**

The **anaemia** which appears intermittently **is caused mainly by destruction of red blood cells by means of an immunologically mediated mechanism.** Erythrocytes of infected horses are coated with **antiviral antibodies** and **complement 3.** This binding to the cell surface results in increased osmotic fragility (i.e., easily damaged), shortened half-life, and **erythrophagocytosis.** Plasma haemoglobin level increases and serum haptoglobin level decreases. Haptoglobin is a glycoprotein synthesized in the liver. It binds free haemoglobin released from intravascular haemolysis. The **haemoglobin-haptoglobin complex** is rapidly removed from the circulation by the Kupffer cells. These findings suggest **haemolysis as a key factor in genesis of the anaemia.** Another less important factor is depression of the bone marrow during acute episodes.

Renal glomeruli are affected in horses with active disease. The glomeruli have thickened basement membranes and mesangium cells are increased in number, and neutrophils are present. Immunoglobulin G (IgG) and complement 3 (C3) can be demonstrated in the mesangium and on basement membranes. It appears that this **glomerulitis is the result of deposition of virus-antibody complexes** which have been demonstrated in the peripheral circulation. Immunological factors may also be involved in the production of lesions in other organs, such as the liver.

Signs

The **clinical disease** is usually divided into **three types: acute, subacute, and chronic.** However, usually cases fall into two or more of these groups, and may even pass through all the three. **Acute cases** are characterized by rapid onset of high fever (up to 108 ° F) after an incubation period of 1-3 weeks. The fever is accompanied by extreme weakness, excessive thirst, anorexia, depression, oedema of the lower abdomen, and sublingual (beneath the tongue) or nasal haemorrhages. **Death may occur within a month. If the animal survives, disease takes up the subacute or chronic form.** Anaemia is not a prominent feature at the onset, but there is a gradual reduction in circulating red blood cells. **The normal count of 8 million/mm3 drops to about 4 million/ mm3 in most cases.**

In the **subacute form,** the disease is manifested by relapsing (recurring) fever and recurrence of other symptoms at regular intervals. Other symptoms are similar to those of the acute type, but less severe. The attacks may increase in severity, with gradual weight loss, debility, oedema of dependent parts, and unsteady gait. Death may occur during any of these recurrent attacks. Pallor (paleness) of mucous membranes indicates the loss of circulating erythrocytes, **which may fall as low as 1.5 million/mm3. The sedimentation rate is greatly increased.**

The **chronic form** may develop after the animal has passed through an acute infection. It may even occur in the absence of an obvious attack. Some animals appear to be in good health except for mild fever at intervals. Others remain thin despite a good diet, and sometimes show oedema under the thorax and abdomen. The red cell count is usually 2-3 million/mm3 below normal.

Lesions

The nature of the lesions depends to a large extent on the clinical type of disease and the duration of illness. In other words, an animal which dies during an attack, after several aggravations characteristic of the chronic disease, shows different changes than one that dies after a single acute attack. **Therefore, the lesions are described in relation to the clinical type of the disease.**

Acute Disease

Jaundice, oedema and haemorrhages are the main gross findings at necropsy. Oedema is most prominent in the ventral wall of the abdomen, at the base of the heart, and perirenal fat. The haemorrhages are petechial, or less often ecchymotic, and are found in the oedematous areas, or in the pleura and peritoneum. The **heart** is enlarged; the myocardium is pale and flabby. Haemorrhages and oedema occur in the epicardium and pericardium. Pericardial sac may contain excessive amounts of clear or sanguineous fluid. **Microscopically,** oedema and haemorrhages are found. The **liver** may be grossly enlarged, red to dark brown, and may show haemorrhages. **The spleen is nearly twice normal size.** The capsule is tense and may show petechiae. The cut surface is dark red and somewhat granular. Haemorrhagic infarcts may be present. **Microscopically,** the red pulp is increased in volume which results from infiltration of the cords of Bilroth with mononuclear cells. These cells are believed to arise in the reticulo-endothelium and to be **immature lymphoid cells.**

The **lymph nodes** may be enlarged, and their changes are similar to those of the spleen. The **bone marrow** is strikingly red as the normal fatty marrow is replaced by areas of active haematopoietic marrow. The **kidneys** are usually oedematous. There is intense infiltration of immature lymphoid cells into the interstitial stroma of both cortex and medulla. Immunoglobulins and complement have been demonstrated with immunofluorescent techniques. All organs and tissues of the body may show evidence of the reticulo-endothelial hyperplasia described in spleen, lymph nodes, liver and kidney, **but these changes are not constant.**

Subacute Disease

Oedema and haemorrhages may occur, but they are less prominent than anaemia. **Microscopically**, in the myocardium, some muscle bundles show hyaline degeneration and leukocytic (mainly lymphocytic) infiltration. The **liver** is enlarged, dark brown, and firm. On the cut surface, the lobular markings are more marked than the normal organ. **Microscopically**, the central veins are congested, and sinusoids dilated and filled with lymphocytes, plasma cells, macrophages containing haemosiderin, and reticulo-endothelial cells. The reticulo-endothelial cells often form small nodules within the sinusoids. Affected livers show haemosiderosis. The **spleen** is enlarged. The trabeculae are widely separated, as are the splenic corpuscles, which are enlarged and **clearly visible in some gross specimens. Microscopically**, reticulo-endothelial hyperplasia in the cords of Bilroth, similar to that observed in the acute form, is the cause of its gross appearance. In **lymph nodes**, replacement of normal structures by reticulo-endothelial and lymphoid cells is more pronounced. The centres of **long bones** contain large areas of red, and sometimes haemorrhagic-appearing marrow. In **kidneys**, lymphoid cells are present in smaller numbers.

Chronic Disease

Hypertrophy of the **spleen** and **bone marrow** may be the only pathological change present. Changes in the spleen and lymph nodes are similar to those described for the subacute disease. The **bone marrow** in long bones, even in aged horses, is markedly red rather than fatty. This hyperplasia of the haematopoietic marrow is more noticeable in the gross specimens than in microscopic sections. **Microscopically**, myeloid and erythroid elements are in about normal proportion, indicating that haematopoiesis is not depressed but rather stimulated, as a result of destruction of erythrocytes.

Haematological Changes

The anaemia is normocytic and normochromic. The anaemia occurs from a combination of haemolysis, erythrophagocytosis, and a decreased production of erythrocytes. Thrombocytopaenia is a usual finding. Serum levels of immunoglobulin are usually increased in the acute stages, and the Coombs' test results are positive.

Diagnosis

A presumptive diagnosis can be made during the acute disease from the clinical signs and also from the characteristic gross and microscopic lesions at necropsy. Confirmatory diagnosis, however, depends on specific identification of the virus, either in the affected animal, or after isolation in horse leukocyte culture. **An agar-gel immunodiffusion (AGID) test, developed by Coggins in 1972 in USA, is particularly useful in detecting humoral antibodies in the serum of infected horses.** A precipitin line develops in the presence of humoral antibodies to tissue culture-derived antigen. The presence of these antibodies is consistently associated with virus. **Therefore, the test (Coggins' test) is a useful method to detect the virus.** Fluorescein-labelled immunoglobulins are useful to demonstrate viral antigens in infected tissues.

Spumaviruses

Spumaviruses, or foamy viruses, are retroviruses. They are found in a number of mammals, including cats, cattle, primates, and humans. **The infection persists for the lifetime of infected hosts,** and the viruses are shed orally. The incidence of infection is high, but **infection is asymptomatic. To date, no specific disease has been associated with the foamy viruses.**

Caliciviridae

Viruses of this family were once included in **Picornaviridae.** Now they are classified as a separate group. **Caliciviruses** are slightly larger than picornaviruses, and virion has 32 **cup-shaped** surface depressions. This gives rise to their name (G. calyx, calix, calici = cup). There are **only two important viruses in this group**: the virus of vesicular exanthema of pigs, and the calicivirus of cats.

Diseases caused by Caliciviruses

Vesicular Exanthema of Swine

Vesicular exanthema is **an acute, febrile, infectious disease of pigs** caused by a calicivirus. It is characterized by fever and vesicle formation, and is indistinguishable clinically from foot-and-mouth disease in pigs, vesicular stomatitis, and swine vesicular disease. The disease was first reported in 1935 from California, USA. Except for isolated outbreaks in Hawaii and Iceland, **the disease has remained confined to the United States.**

Spread

The virus appears to be **transmitted by feeding uncooked garbage to pigs.** It was found that in California, the sea lion virus in the aborted sea lion foetuses appeared to be identical to the calicivirus of vesicular exanthema. **It is thought that sea lion carcasses fed to pigs caused the initial porcine infection**, and that the disease was spread widely by uncooked pork scraps (leftover small pieces) taken from railway dining cars and fed to other pigs. **Thus, raw garbage containing infected pork scraps is the most common medium of spread from farm to farm**. The sources of infection are infected live pigs and infected pork. On infected premises, the disease spreads by direct contact.

Pathogenesis

There is a viraemia lasting for 72-84 hours. The virus then localizes in the buccal mucosa and skin above the hooves.

Signs

There is an initial high fever (106°-107° F) followed by the development of vesicles in the mouth, on the snout, on teats and udder, and on the coronary skin, the sole, the heel bulbs and between the claws, and accompanied by complete anorexia. **Vesicles are full of clear fluid**. The vesicles rupture easily leaving raw, eroded areas. Rupture usually occurs about 24-48 hours after they appear, and is accompanied by a rapid fall of temperature. Secondary crops of vesicles often follow. The affected feet are very sensitive and there is severe lameness. Healing of the oral vesicles occurs rapidly. Recovery in uncomplicated cases is usually complete in 1-2 weeks. Actually, **vesicular exanthema runs a mild, rapid course of about 10 days, and is almost never fatal**.

Lesions

A sudden rise in temperature to as high as 107° F, is accompanied by the appearance of **small vesicles filled with clear fluid**. The vesicles appear in the epithelium of the snout, nose, lips, gums, tongue, and between digits, around the coronary band, on the ball of the foot, or even in the dew-claws. Vesicles may develop on the udder and teats of nursing sows. Vesicles sometimes coalesce. **Rupture of all vesicles occurs after a few days, and is followed by healing**. After 7-10 days, only slightly scarred areas are left. Ulceration and secondary bacterial infections of lesions on the feet may make animals lame for some time. The cutaneous lesions are indistinguishable from the intraepithelial lesions of foot-and-mouth disease, but systemic lesions are not seen in vesicular exanthema.

Diagnosis

Diagnosis of vesicular exanthema depends on complement-fixation test, animal inoculation, or virus isolation and identification. These are necessary to distinguish it from foot-and-mouth disease, vesicular stomatitis, or swine vesicular disease.

Feline Calicivirus Disease

Feline calicivirus causes **an acute respiratory disease** characterized by fever (often biphasic), depression, anorexia, dyspnoea or polypnoea (very rapid breathing, panting), pulmonary rales; and **vesicles** resulting in ulcers of the nostrils, tongue or hard palate. Sneezing may occur, but nasal or conjunctival discharge is not an important feature.

Lesions

Important lesions include vesicles of the nostrils, tongue, oral mucosa, or hard palate. These vesicles are followed by further necrosis of cells in the epithelium, leaving sharply demarcated ulcers that heal slowly. Viral antigen can be demonstrated in cells at the margin of these ulcers by immunofluorescence technique.

In the **lung**, the virus has a **tropism for alveolar type I epithelial cells**, which become necrotic and initiate a pulmonary inflammatory response. This is followed by adenomatous proliferation of type II alveolar lining cells, with eventual shedding of these cells into the alveoli. These changes result in sharply demarcated, irregularly outlined **gross lesions** in the lungs. The lesions are solid dark purple, often located near the periphery of the lung. **Ultrastructurally**, virions are seen in relation to smooth endoplasmic reticulum, often in vesicles.

Viral invasion of enterocytes of the small intestine also occurs and causes **enteritis**. **Arthritis** has also been attributed to feline calicivirus.

Diagnosis

Diagnosis is made by isolation or immunological means. The disease should be differentiated from feline viral rhinotracheitis, which is usually more severe and in which typical herpesvirus intranuclear inclusion bodies occur. The oral ulcers in calicivirus infections are much smaller than those seen in feline viral rhinotracheitis.

Picornaviridae

The Family Picornaviridae includes a large number of viruses (Table 7). The family is **so named because the viruses are small in size and contain RNA** (L. pico = small; rna = ribonucleic acid).

Table 7. Diseases caused by viruses of Picornaviridae family

Enterovirus
Porcine encephalomyelitis
Swine vesicular disease
Avian encephalomyelitis
Avian nephritis
Duck hepatitis
Turkey viral hepatitis

Cardiovirus
Viral encephalomyocarditis of pigs

Rhinovirus
Human rhinovirus infection
Bovine rhinovirus infection
Equine rhinovirus infection

Aphthovirus
Foot-and-mouth Disease
(Aphthous fever)

The viruses of this family are serologically different, but similar in their morphology and physical and chemical properties. They are responsible for a wide range of illnesses in humans and animals. Viruses of this family have an icosahedral (i.e., having 20 faces) capsid 25-30 nm in diameter, and are **non-enveloped**. The viral nucleic acid consists of a single linear molecule of **positive-sense single-stranded RNA**.

The Family Picornaviridae has four genera which contain animal pathogens. These are **enterovirus, cardiovirus, rhinovirus,** and **aphthovirus.** The only physical difference between these genera is about their pH stability. **Enteroviruses** in the beginning infect the oropharynx. But because of their stability at a low pH, they pass through the stomach to the intestines, where replication occurs, probably in lymphocytes. Subsequent viraemia allows dissemination to other target organs, such as the central nervous system. Members of the genus **rhinovirus** are susceptible to low pH, and include pathogens for humans, cattle, and horses. They are highly specific. These viruses replicate in the upper respiratory tract, which is their primary and definitive (final) site of localization. The genus **aphthovirus** contains the virus of only foot-and-mouth disease (7 serotypes and 53 subtypes). These viruses are inactivated at a pH of less than 7. Primary replication occurs in the pharynx after inhalation of aerosols (suspended viral particles in the air), or ingestion of contaminated materials. This is followed by viraemia and spread of virus to other organs and tissues. Encephalo-myocarditis virus is the only member of the **cardiovirus** genus. The final site of localization of this virus (definitive tropism) is either the central nervous system, or the myocardium.

Diseases caused by Enteroviruses

Porcine Encephalomyelitis

Several enteroviruses have been recovered from **pigs**. One of these, termed **porcine enterovirus** 1, causes encephalomyelitis. **Porcine encephalomyelitis** is also known by several other names. The first of these was **"Teschen disease"**, so named after the province of Czechoslovakia in which the first outbreak was identified. Other names include **poliomyelitis suum, Talfan disease**, and **benign enzootic paresis. The disease is similar to poliomyelitis of humans** in that the virus can be isolated from the alimentary tract, and the ventral columns of grey matter in the spinal cord are consistently affected. However, in the porcine disease, the lesions in the cerebral cortex and cerebellum are much more extensive and randomly located than in poliomyelitis.

Pathogenesis

Infection occurs by **ingestion,** or even by the **respiratory route.** The virus multiplies mainly in the intestinal tract, but also in the respiratory tract, and may invade to produce viraemia. Invasion of the central nervous system may follow depending upon the virulence of the strains and the age of the pig at the time of infection.

Signs

Following an incubation period of 10-20 days, the onset is usually accompanied by fever (104°-105° F), anorexia, lassitude (fatigue, lethargy), depression, and sometimes slight incoordination, particularly of the hind limbs. Recovery may occur, or these symptoms may be followed by irritability, stiffness of the extremities, and in severe cases by tremors, violent convulsions, prostration (lying down), and coma. A sudden drop in temperature followed by paralysis and death within 3-4 days after onset is the usual course. Some animals may even die within 24 hours.

Lesions

There are **no specific gross lesions. Microscopic lesions are limited to the central nervous system.** The virus attacks neurons of **brain and spinal cord.** The changes produced are linked to the destruction of these cells. The lesions have a specific distribution. **The spinal cord is constantly affected,** the changes being limited to the ventral columns of the grey matter. The Purkinje, molecular and granular layers of the **cerebellum** are also involved, in order of decreasing severity. The leptomeninges over the cerebellum are heavily infiltrated with lymphocytes. The thalamus also suffers considerable damage. Lesions of decreasing intensity occur in the basal nuclei, the base of the brain, olfactory bulbs, hippocampal gyrus, and the pons and medulla.

In affected sites, **multipolar nerve cells undergo degeneration of varying degrees, including necrosis.** This is accompanied by neuronophagia, inflammatory or glial nodules, occasional haemorrhage, and diffuse infiltration of leukocytes, mainly lymphocytes. Accumulations of lymphocytes in the perivascular (Robin-Virchow) spaces are often seen. They are usually close to lesions in the grey matter, and may extend into the white matter. **Otherwise, the white matter is not involved. Ultrastructurally** (i.e., electronmicroscopically), there is extensive vesiculation (dilation) of neuronal (of neuron's) endoplasmic reticulum cisternae (spaces).

Diagnosis

The demonstration of typical microscopic lesions in the brain and spinal cord is sufficient for presumptive diagnosis. The definitive diagnosis requires that the virus be isolated and identified, or that specific antibodies be demonstrated in increased quantities in the serum of recovered pigs.

Swine Vesicular Disease

This is **a new disease of pigs** that is spreading rapidly throughout the world. **The disease is of considerable importance as it is clinically indistinguishable from foot-and-mouth disease.** The disease was first recognized in 1966, in Italy, as a febrile illness accompanied by vesicle formation on the mouth, snout, and feet. Lameness and ulcerations followed the early vesiculation (vesicle formation). All these features were indistinguishable from the signs of foot-and-mouth disease. The disease is caused by **a specific enterovirus.** This makes it possible to differentiate this infection from vesicular exanthema (**calicivirus**), foot-and-mouth disease (**aphthovirus**), or vesicular stomatitis (**vesiculovirus**).

Spread

Infection generally occurs **through minor abrasions on the feet**, but may occur through other routes. The virus is excreted in oral and nasal secretions and in faeces. The vesicular fluid and shed vesicular epithelium are potent sources of infection. **Transmission occurs by direct contact** or contact with infected food, or water, or infected faeces, and the disease spreads rapidly between pigs within the same group. Air-borne transmission of the virus is not a feature, and the spread between groups of pigs is less rapid than that which occurs with foot-and-mouth disease.

Pathogenesis

There is variation in the susceptibility of different sites of the body to invasion by the virus. In natural outbreaks initial infection occurs mostly through damaged skin. Once infection is established in a pig, virus excretion is so massive as to result in infection of others through the tonsil of gastrointestinal tract, as well as through skin abrasions. Infection is followed by **viraemia**, and the virus has a special affinity for epithelium of the coronary band, tongue, lip and snout, and for myocardium. Lesions in the brain are seen microscopically, but nervous signs are not a common clinical finding.

Signs

The incubation period varies from 2-14 days. A transient fever (104°-105° F), lameness, arching of the back and other signs of foot discomfort are seen, **but are less severe than with foot-and-mouth disease**. Characteristic vesicles occur usually **on the coronary band of the claws, especially at the heel**. In severely affected pigs, the lesions encircle the coronary band, and the horn may be shed as in foot-and-mouth disease. Lesions also occur on the tongue, lips and snout, and the skin of the legs and belly. The course of the disease is generally 2-3 weeks. **Mortality is very uncommon**.

Lesions

Changes in the stratified epithelium are most evident in the skin of the coronary band of the hoof. Coagulative necrosis in the Malpighian layer results in vesiculation and sloughing. This is followed by regenerative pseudo-epitheliomatous hyperplasia. Similar lesions develop on the snout, lips and tongue.

Zoonotic Importance

The swine vesicular disease virus resembles closely coxsackie virus B, a common pathogen to humans. **The swine virus is suspected of infecting laboratory workers**, who have been in contact with it. Coxsackie virus B has been associated with aseptic meningitis, encephalitis, myositis, orchitis, myocarditis, diarrhoea, respiratory disease, and vesicular and papular rash in humans.

Diagnosis

The occurrence of vesicles differentiates this disease from other non-vesicular diseases of pigs. Foot rot in pigs is associated with lesions on the sole and horn of the claw, rather than the epithelial areas of the coronary band. The differentiation of swine vesicular disease from other vesicular diseases depends on various laboratory tests (ELISA and others) and virus identification.

Avian Encephalomyelitis (Epidemic Tremor)

Avian encephalomyelitis (AE) is an infectious viral disease of young chickens, turkeys, pheasants, and quail. It is characterized by ataxia and rapid tremors, especially of the head and neck. Because of this it was often called "**epidemic tremor**". AE occurs worldwide. The diameter of the virus ranges from 20-30 nm. It is a **single-stranded RNA (ssRNA) virus**. All strains appear to be antigenically uniform, but there are variations in neurotropism and virulence. Field strains are mainly **enterotropic**, whereas egg-adapted strains are mainly **neurotropic**.

The **immune status** of the affected bird appears to be the main factor influencing the outcome of infection. Antibodies are transferred to progeny from the dam through the egg, and can be demonstrated in egg yolk. **Maternal antibodies** can protect young birds against systemic infection. It becomes increasingly difficult to produce disease in chicks as they become older. **This is due to increasing immuno-competence with age, and the development of a protective humoral response**.

Spread

Under natural conditions, AE is basically an enteric infection. **Ingestion is the usual route of entry.** Exposure through the respiratory tract may be unimportant, except through the coincident exposure of the alimentary tract. Virus is shed in the faeces for a period of several days, and because it is **quite resistant to environmental conditions**, it remains infectious for long periods of time. It appears that some birds are **enteric carriers** and excrete virus in their droppings. Infected litter is a source of the virus which is easily **transmitted horizontally** by fomites and mechanical carriers. **Vertical transmission is a very important means of virus dissemination.** Transmission of the virus occurs through the egg, from infected to susceptible stock. Egg transmission occurs during the period from the infection of susceptible laying hens to the development of immunity, a period of 3-4 weeks.

Pathogenesis

There are significant differences between egg-adapted and field strains of the virus in the pathogenesis of the disease. In young chicks exposed orally to **field strains**, primary infection of the alimentary tract, especially duodenum, is rapidly followed by a viraemia, and subsequent infection of the pancreas and other visceral organs (liver, heart, kidney, spleen) and skeletal muscle, and finally the central nervous system. Viral antigen is abundant in the CNS, where Purkinje cells and the molecular layer of the cerebellum are favoured sites of virus replication. Persistence of the viral infection is common in the CNS, alimentary tract, and pancreas. CNS and the pancreas are the only sites uniformly infected by egg-adapted strains.

Age at exposure is especially important in the pathogenesis. Birds infected at 1 day of age generally die, whereas those infected at 8 days develop paresis (partial paralysis), but usually recover. Infection at 28 days causes no clinical signs. Bursectomy (surgical removal of bursa of Fabricius), but not thymectomy (surgical removal of thymus) abolished (ended) the age resistance. **This indicated that humoral immunity was the basis of age resistance.** It is found that young age (thus immunological incompetence) correlates with prolonged viraemia, persistence of virus in the brain, and development of clinical disease. **The immune response of an immunologically competent bird stops the spread of infection before it reaches the CNS.**

Signs

AE usually makes its appearance when chicks are 1-2 week of age. Affected chicks first show a slightly dull expression of the eyes. This is followed by a progressive ataxia from incoordination of the muscles, which may be detected readily by exercising the chicks. As the ataxia becomes more pronounced, chicks show an inclination to sit on their hocks. Finally, they come to rest, or fall on their sides. **Fine tremors of the head and neck may**

become noticeable. Their frequency and intensity may vary. Ataxia usually progresses until the chick is incapable of moving about, and this stage is followed by inanition (loss of vitality from lack of food and water), prostration (lying down), and finally death. Some chicks may survive and grow to maturity. Survivors may later develop blindness from an opacity giving a bluish discoloration to the lens.

As mentioned under pathogenesis, there is a marked age resistance to clinical signs in birds exposed after they are 2-3 weeks of age. Mature birds may experience a temporary drop in egg production, but do not develop neurological signs.

Lesions

The only **gross lesions** in chicks are whitish areas in the muscles of ventriculus, which are due to masses of infiltrating lymphocytes. In adult birds, no changes have been described except the lens opacities.

Microscopically, the **main changes are in the CNS, and some viscera**. The peripheral nervous system is not involved. In the CNS, the lesions are those of a disseminated, non-purulent **encephalomyelitis**, and a **ganglionitis** (inflammation of a ganglion) of the dorsal root ganglia. The most common finding is a striking perivascular infiltration in all portions of the brain and spinal cord, except cerebellum. Infiltrating small lymphocytes pile up several layers to form a conspicuous cuff. Microgliosis occurs as diffuse and nodular aggregates. The glial lesion is seen chiefly in the cerebellar molecular layer. In the midbrain, **two nuclei - nucleus rotundus** and **nucleus ovoidalis - are always affected** with a loose microgliosis which is considered pathognomonic. Another lesion of **pathognomonic** importance is central chromatolysis (axonal reaction) of the neurons in the nuclei of the brain stem, particularly those of the medulla oblongata. The dying neuron is surrounded by satellite oligodendroglia. Later, microglia phagocytize the remains. The central chromatolysis is never seen without an accompanying cellular reaction.

Visceral lesions appear to be hyperplasia of the lymphocytic aggregates. In the **proventriculus**, there are normally only a few small lymphocytes in the muscular wall. In AE, these become dense lymphocytic foci (aggregates). **This lesion is pathognomonic**. Similar lesions occur in the ventriculus muscle, but unfortunately they also occur in Marek's disease. In the **pancreas**, circumscribed lymphocytic follicles are normal, but in AE the number increases several times. In the **myocardium**, particularly in the atrium, there are aggregates of lymphocytes. These are considered to be the result of AE.

The recovered birds develop circulating antibodies capable of neutralizing the virus. **Humoral, and not cellular, immunity is important in restricting infection.**

Diagnosis

The **clinical signs, absence of gross lesions**, and **microscopic findings** in the brain, spinal cord and visceral organs, together with the absence of other virus infections and nutritional deficiencies affecting the nervous system, are used for routine presumptive diagnosis. A definitive diagnosis requires demonstration of the virus by isolation and identification, or by other means. Examination o f s mears f rom t he b rain, or cryostat sections s tained b y direct immunofluorescence may also be used to demonstrate virus; positive results are confirmatory. A number of serological tests are available for determining the presence of infection. These include virus n eutralization (VN) test, an indirect immunofluorescence test, and an ELISA test. Because of the specificity and sensitivity, rapidity of performance and usefulness in large-scale screening, **the ELISA₁ has replaced other tests for antibody assessment**, including the assessment of efficiency of vaccination.

In **differential diagnosis**, A E should n ot be c onfused w ith o ther a vian diseases manifesting s imilar clinical signs. These i nclude Ranikhet disease, nutritional encephalomalacia, a nd Marek's disease. Certain l esions are s pecific to AE; central chromatolysis as opposed to peripheral chromatolysis of Ranikhet disease, gliosis in the nucleus rotundus and nucleus ovoidalis which is not observed in Ranikhet disease, lymphocytic foci in the muscular wall of the proventriculus, and circumscribed lymphocytic follicles in the p ancreas. Ranikhet disease rarely c auses an interstitial pancreatitis. Encephalomalacia usually appears 2-3 weeks later than AE. **Microscopically**, i t causes se vere degenerative lesions in no way similar to AE. Marek's disease, which occurs still later, presents no difficulty. The p eripheral nerve involvement and lymphocytosis of the visceral organs are two criteria not seen in AE.

Avian Nephritis

Avian nephritis, caused b y an e nterovirus, is **a n acute, highly contagious, typically subclinical disease of young chickens that produces lesions in the kidneys.** The v irus, called " **avian nephritis virus (ANV)**", was first described in Ja pan in 1 979. **It is a single-stranded RNA (ss RNA) virus**: morphology b eing 30 nm small round particles. ANV is d istinct from avian encephalomyelitis virus and duck hepatitis viruses.

Spread

ANV is distributed worldwide in the domestic fowl. Transmission readily occurs by direct or indirect contact. The most common method is probably through **ingestion** of f aecally contaminated m aterial. Egg t ransmission (vertical transmission) has been suggested on the basis of field observations.

Pathogenesis

Only young chickens are known to develop clinical disease and distinct kidney lesions when exposed to ANV. Following infection, the virus is first detected in faeces within 2 days, with maximum virus shedding at 4-5 days. The virus is widely distributed, with maximum titres in the kidney and jejunum and lower titres in the bursa of Fabricius, spleen, and liver. The virus is consistently isolated from kidney, jejunum, and rectum, but not from brain and trachea.

Signs

The clinical sign in 1-day-old chicks is only transient diarrhoea, but not all chicks show the signs. Weight gain is depressed. In the broiler chickens, symptoms vary from none (subclinical) to outbreaks of the so-called "**runting syndrome**" and "**baby chick nephropathy**".

Lesions

Gross lesions in dead chicks are mild to severe discoloration and swelling in the kidneys, and **visceral urate deposits**. Chalk-like urate crystals are seen on the surface of the peritoneum and liver. The heart is white due to heavy urate deposits on the epicardium. **Microscopically**, the primary changes consist of necrosis and degeneration of epithelial cells of the proximal convoluted tubules with infiltration of granulocytes. The degenerating epithelial cells show **acidophilic granules of various sizes in the cytoplasm**. Also, there is interstitial lymphocytic infiltration and moderate fibrosis. In the later stages, lymphoid follicles develop. Virus particles and viral antigens can be demonstrated in the degenerating epithelium by electron microscopy, and also by immunofluorescence.

Diagnosis

Antibodies against the virus can be detected by indirect immunofluorescence, serum neutralization tests, and ELISA. Of these serum neutralization is the most sensitive, but is costly and laborious. For isolation and identification of the virus, samples of faeces and/or kidney should be inoculated into cultures of chick kidney cells, or into chick embryos.

In **differential diagnosis**, certain nephrotoxic strains of infectious bronchitis virus cause interstitial nephritis. It is difficult to separate the two conditions on the basis of the microscopic lesions. However, with infectious bronchitis there are some changes in the trachea, and infections in kidneys are usually preceded by respiratory signs.

Duck Hepatitis

Duck hepatitis (DH) is **a highly fatal, rapidly spreading viral infection of young ducklings** characterized primarily by **hepatitis**. It can be caused by any of three different viruses, namely, duck hepatitis virus (DHV) types 1, 2, and 3. **They are serologically distinct**. DHV type 1 is 20-40 nm in size, **contains RNA**, and has been classified as an **enterovirus**.

Spread

The natural infection has been reported only in ducks. The virus remains viable for many weeks in faeces. It is therefore thought that infection occurs following the **ingestion** by susceptible ducklings of virus-carrying particles from the environment. Spread between places is by means of contaminated equipment, vehicles, and personnel. Egg transmission is not thought to occur. Within a flock the disease spreads rapidly to all susceptible ducklings.

Pathogenesis

In natural outbreaks, DH type 1 occurs **only in young ducklings**. Adults apparently do not become ill and continue in full production. **Chickens and turkeys are resistant**. Ducklings after oral exposure, have mottled livers, and enlarged gallbladders and spleens. Duck hepatitis virus type 1 can be isolated from livers up to 17 days.

Signs

Signs are peracute, and death usually follows within an hour of their onset. Affected birds are often in good condition, but start to fall behind the main flock. Soon they fall over on their sides and, after a short struggle with paddling movements of the legs, the birds die. The head is usually stretched upwards and backwards (**opisthotonus**). Morbidity is 100% and mortality rate may be over 90% of the flock. However, in the endemic situation a 5-10% loss is more common. The highest losses occur in duckling below 7 days of age.

Lesions

The **main lesions** are in the **liver**, which is enlarged and has a number of petechial and ecchymotic **haemorrhages**. In addition, fatty kidneys described as "**duck fatty kidney syndrome**", may be caused by duck hepatitis virus. **Microscopically**, primary changes in the acute disease consist of necrosis of hepatic cells. Survivors with more chronic lesions show widespread bile duct hyperplasia. **Inclusion bodies are not found**.

Diagnosis

The sudden onset of a disease causing high mortality in young ducklings, the opisthotonus of the dead bird, and the characteristic liver haemorrhages, are sufficient to justify the diagnosis of duck virus hepatitis. Laboratory diagnosis is based on virus isolation and identification. Rapid diagnosis using the direct FA technique can be made on the livers of affected duckling.

Turkey Viral Hepatitis

Turkey viral hepatitis (TVH) is **a highly contagious usually subclinical**

disease of turkeys, characterized by multifocal hepatic necrosis, with or without pancreatic necrosis. Outbreaks are usually seen in turkeys under six weeks of age. **Transmission** of infection occurs by both direct and indirect contact. **Faeces** from infected turkeys is believed to be the main source of virus transmission. **Vertical transmission probably occurs**.

The disease is usually diagnosed only at postmortem examination, when lesions are seen in the liver and sometimes the pancreas. **Liver lesions** are macroscopic pale foci 1-2 mm in diameter, occurring on the surface and in the parenchyma. Foci represent focal necrosis of hepatocytes and infiltration with mononuclear cells. The liver is usually enlarged. Electron microscopic examination of degenerating hepatocytes has revealed the presence of intracytoplasmic aggregates of **enterovirus-like viruses**.

Turkey viral hepatitis is often subclinical, but disease, may be precipitated by stress. Depression, anorexia and increased mortality are the **main signs**. Morbidity can be very high but mortality is usually low. Infection of laying turkeys may impair reproductive performance, but deaths are not seen in birds over 6 weeks of age.

Diagnosis

Presence of lesions in both liver and pancreas is highly suggestive of turkey viral hepatitis. Liver is the best tissue for viral isolation.

Disease caused by Cardiovirus

Viral Encephalomyocarditis of Pigs

Pigs from 3-16 weeks are affected with **myocarditis** and **encephalitis**. The virus produces a fatal myocarditis and the disease may occur as outbreaks with high rates of morbidity and mortality. It is now known that the virus may also cause reproductive failure in gilts and sows characterized by stillbirths and mummified foetuses. The cause is a **cardiovirus** which is primarily a pathogen of **rodents** (chiefly wild rats), in which the infection is inapparent. But the virus has the ability to produce the disease in domestic animals and **man**. Infected rodents excrete the virus for a long period, **and the disease in pigs is probably due to the close association of these two species**.

The virus is now considered **a major cause of reproductive failure in swine herds**. The clinical course is short. **Signs** include inappetence (lack of desire for food), depression, trembling, incoordination, and dyspnoea. Usually the pigs are found dead. Death appears to result from **cardiac failure**, and clinical signs from encephalitis are rare. The reproductive form of the disease is characterized clinically by inappetence, fever, abortion, and stillbirth. **The principal lesion is interstitial myocarditis**. The heart is usually dilated, and there is some slightly blood-tinged pericardial effusion. Sometimes, bilateral hydrothorax and pulmonary oedema are observed. **Micro-scopically**, there is necrosis of myocardial fibres and intense infiltration with polymorphonuclear and mononuclear cells.

Encephalomyelitis virus infection must be differentiated from **gut oedema** and **mulberry heart disease** in growing pigs, and the peracute bacterial septicaemias in suckling pigs. The myocardial lesion in suckling pigs has similarities to that produced by foot-and-mouth disease in this age group.

Diseases caused by Rhinoviruses

Rhinoviruses cause the common cold in humans. More than 100 different rhinoviruses have been identified from humans. However, **very few have been recognized as causes of disease in domestic animals**. The human isolates do not infect domestic animals. Distinct rhinoviruses that cause mild respiratory disease in horses and cattle have been identified. The infection is of little importance. However, it can predispose the infected animal to other respiratory pathogens. **The equine rhinovirus is reported to infect humans**.

Diseases caused by Aphthovirus

Foot-and-Mouth Disease (Aphthous Fever)

Foot-and-mouth disease (FMD) is **an extremely contagious, acute viral disease of all cloven-footed animals**, characterized by fever and vesicular eruption in the mouth and on the feet and teats. **It is rarely fatal except in very young animals**. However, because of the speed with which it spreads, the trade sanctions imposed on countries in which it occurs, and the loss in production by affected animals, FMD is one of the world's most important animal diseases. **The disease has a special place in the history of virology, for it was the first animal virus to be recognized**. It was also with FMD virus that different serotypes between strains of an animal virus were first recognized.

Cause

The disease is caused by an **aphthovirus**, which is a **non-enveloped, single-stranded RNA (ssRNA) virus**, between 22-30 nm in diameter, with strong epitheliotropic features. The disease occurs in cloven-hoofed animals, the most important being **cattle, sheep, goats**, and **pigs**. It may also affect ruminants such as deer and antelope, and under some conditions, ruminants act as reservoirs for the infection. **In wildlife**, FMD has been reported in camel, wild buffalo, bison, waterbuck, wild boar, elephant, yak, llama and giraffe. The virus occurs in **seven principal antigenic types**. These are designated in the international nomenclature as O, A, C, SAT 1, SAT 2, SAT 3, and **Asia 1** ('O' from the department of Oise; 'A' from Allemagne, 'C' from a revised classification where Ó and A were termed A and B; and **SAT 1, SAT 2** and **SAT 3** from South African Territories). Although the symptoms and lesions produced by each virus type are basically similar, **infection with one virus does not immunize against the others**.

Only four types, namely, O, A, C, and Asia 1 are prevalent in India. In cattle, type O is the predominant type, followed by **Asia 1**. Severe outbreaks of the disease **in goats and sheep** are also caused mainly by serotype O and Asia 1. However, type A and C have been reported to be associated with the disease. **FMD, in adult goats is very mild**, but it may cause **severe mortality in young kids because of tigroid heart necrosis**. In recent years **numerous subtypes** have been identified, which are also antigenically distinct.

Spread

An important feature of the disease is the **extreme infectiousness of the virus**, and the ease with which it is carried, not only by infected animals and their products, **but also mechanically by humans and animals**. The virus may be transported on the shoes or clothing of humans, in or on the bodies of migratory birds or animals, and in such products as raw hides, milk, bedding, and forage (i.e., fodder). Recovered cattle can carry the virus for periods of **up to 2 years**, and recovered sheep may carry it for up to **6 months**. The virus apparently does not persist in recovered pigs. **Infection is spread mainly by the air-borne route.**

Pathogenesis

After entry, the primary viral replication occurs in the pharynx or respiratory tract. Once infection gains access into the bloodstream (**viraemia**), the virus is widely disseminated throughout the body, probably in mononuclear cells, and produces lesions, chiefly in epithelial tissues. Gross lesions develop only in areas subjected to mechanical trauma, or unusual physiological conditions, such as the epithelium of the mouth and feet, and to a lesser extent, the teats. **In young animals**, the virus usually causes **necrotizing myocarditis**. This lesion may be seen also in adults infected with some strains of the virus, **particularly type O**.

Signs

In typical field cases **in cattle**, the onset begins by a **sudden fall in milk yield** and a **high fever** (104° - 106° F), accompanied by severe dejection and anorexia, followed by the appearance of an acute painful stomatitis. **The signs are directly related to the lesions**. Those in the oral mucosa produce excess salivation and make eating painful. This causes the infected animal to refuse food and water. The saliva hangs in long, ropy strings. Smacking (opening and closing) of the lips and tongue is characteristic. **Vesicles and bullae** (1-2 cm in diameter) appear on the **buccal mucosa**, and on the **dental pad** and the **tongue**. These rupture within 24 hours, **leaving a raw painful surface**. Along with the oral lesions, **vesicles** appear on the **feet**, particularly in the **clefts** and **on the coronet**. Rupture of the vesicles causes acute discomfort and produces

lameness. The animal is often recumbent, with a marked, painful swelling of the coronet. **Secondary bacterial infection** may interfere with healing. **Vesicles** may occur on the teats, the vulva, and the conjunctiva. When the teats orifice is involved, severe mastitis often follows. Abortion and subsequent infertility are common sequels. Very rapid loss of condition and fall in milk yield occur during the acute period.

Young calves and **lambs** are **more susceptible than adults**, and during an outbreak heavy mortality may occur in them as a result of **severe myocardial damage**, even when typical vesicular lesions are absent in the mouth and feet. A sequel to FMD in cattle, due probably from endocrine damage, is a chronic syndrome of dyspnoea, anaemia, overgrowth of hair, and lack of heat tolerance described as '**panting**'. **Diabetes mellitus** has also been observed as a sequel in cattle. Occasional cases show localization of virus in the alimentary tract with dysentery or diarrhoea, indicating the presence of **enteritis**. Ascending posterior paralysis may also occur.

Lesions

In cattle, the distribution of vesicular lesions is characteristic. The oral mucosa over the lips, dorsum of the tongue, and palate is mostly severely involved. Lesions occur in the skin near the coronary band adjacent to the inter-digital space. They are also common in lightly haired areas, such as the vulva, teats, and udder. The conjunctiva may be affected, as also the part of the forestomach that is lined by squamous epithelium (rumen, reticulum, and omasum). Small epidermal vesicles may also occur in grossly normal skin of the brisket, abdomen, hock, and perineum. Mucosa of the abomasum and small intestine may show punctate haemorrhages, or diffuse oedema. The mucosa of the large intestine may be hyperaemic and blue-red.

The specific lesions in their **early stages are microscopic**, and are limited to the epithelium at the site of predilection. The lesion begins as a localized "**balloon degeneration**" of cells in the middle of the stratum spinosum of the epithelium. The inter-cellular prickles are lost, and the epithelial cells become round and detached from one another. Their cytoplasm takes an intensely eosinophilic stain, and their nuclei are pyknotic. Oedematous fluid containing bits of fibrin accumulates between the cells and separates them. Neutrophils infiltrate the epithelium at this stage. Liquefactive necrosis and accumulation of serum and leukocytes produce **vesicles**. The vesicles are roofed over by the compressed stratum corneum, lucidum, and granulosum, and extend down to the basal layer, which usually remains in place over the heavily congested dermis. These **small vesicles (aphthae)** coalesce to form **large vesicles (bullae)**, which cause large areas of epithelium to be easily shed or rubbed off. Loss of epithelium is most common on the dorsal surface of the anterior two-thirds of the bovine tongue, which is separated by a transverse notch from a dorsal eminence occupying the posterior third of the tongue. The entire epithelium over the anterior area may be lost, leaving a raw, red surface that oozes blood. **The pain from this denuded area explains the severe anorexia.** Apart from the virus, the vesicles contain necrotic epithelial cells, leukocytes, occasional erythrocytes, and, in the late stages, bacteria.

Lesions in the myocardium are most common in the fatal disease in very young calves or lambs, but also occur in pigs and young goats. The lesions observed in the wall and septum of the **left ventricle,** and seldom in the atria, appear as small, greyish foci of irregular size, which give the myocardium a somewhat **striped appearance** - so-called **"tiger heart". Microscopically,** hyaline degeneration and necrosis of muscle fibres are accompanied by an intense lymphocytic, occasionally neutrophilic, infiltration. In the **skeletal muscles,** lesions similar to those in the myocardium may be observed. Sharply defined areas of necrosis are seen grossly as grey foci of various sizes, and microscopically, as necrosis of muscle bundles associated with intense leukocytic infiltration.

Zoonotic Importance

Natural infection may occur in humans. However, in humans, the disease is usually mild and limited to acute fever associated with the appearance of vesicles on the hands, feet, and oral mucosa.

Diagnosis

In differential diagnosis of FMD, it is necessary to consider all other so-called **"vesicular diseases",** such as vesicular exanthema, swine vesicular disease, and vesicular stomatitis. These cannot be differentiated with absolute certainty by their symptoms and lesions. It is necessary, therefore, to isolate and identify the virus, or to demonstrate complement-fixing or virus-neutralizing antibodies in recovered animals. The agar gel diffusion reaction is also useful in detecting antigenic relationships. Immunofluorescent methods are used to detect viral antigen in cells. **Under Indian conditions,** FMD has to be differentiated from rinderpest, bluetongue, and peste-des-petits-ruminants (PPR). The laboratory diagnosis is based on virus isolation and identification by micro-complement-fixation test (micro-CFT), virus-neutralization test (VNT), and sandwich ELISA. In recent years, subtype analysis by Mab (monoclonal antibody) profiling and molecular studies, including the genetic mapping of this virus, have been carried out. **DNA probes** and the **polymerase chain reaction (PCR)** are newer methods that are now being applied to virus in tissues.

Diseases caused by Double-Stranded RNA (dsRNA) Families

Birnaviridae

The Family **Birnaviridae** has only one genus "**Birnavirus**". Viruses of this family have genomes consisting of two (L. birna = two) segments of double-stranded RNA (dsRNA), hence the name birnaviruses. It is a non-enveloped virus. The family has **only one important disease, infectious bursal disease (Gumboro disease).**

Birnavirus

Infectious Bursal Disease (Gumboro Disease)

Also known as "infectious bursitis", infectious bursal disease (IBD) is **an acute, highly contagious infection of young chickens,** caused by a **birnavirus.** It is an important viral disease of poultry throughout the world. **The disease is also widely prevalent in India, and every year takes a heavy toll of chicken lives.** In the beginning the name "**Gumboro disease**" was given to this condition, because it was first recognized in the Gumboro district of Delaware, a state of USA. **Lymphoid cells, especially B cells, are the primary target cell.** The lymphoid tissue of the bursa is most severely affected. The disease is of great economic importance for two reasons: 1) Due to the **heavy mortality in chickens 3 weeks of age, and older**, and 2) Due to a severe prolonged **immunosuppression** of chickens infected **at an early age.** Immunosuppression can lead to vaccination failures, *Escherichia coli* infections, gangrenous dermatitis, inclusion body hepatitis-anaemia syndrome.

In 1962, IBD was described as a specific new disease by Cosgrove in USA, and was referred to as "**avian nephrosis**" because of the extreme kidney damage found in birds that succumbed to infection. In 1970, Hitchner proposed the term "**infectious bursal disease**" on the basis of specific pathognomonic lesions of the bursa. In 1972, Allan and his associates reported that IBD virus (IBDV) infections at an early age were **immunosuppressive.**

Aetiology

The viruses can be divided into **two main serotypes (serotype 1 and 2)** by virus-neutralization (VN) tests and electrophoresis of viral RNA and proteins. But they are not distinguishable by fluorescent antibody tests, or enzyme-linked immunosorbent assay (ELISA). Infections with **serotype 1 IBDV** are worldwide in distribution. Within the serotype 1 group, antigenic variants exist. There is also a **considerable variation in virulence, from apathogenic strains to highly virulent strains,** which cause up to 50% mortality. These viruses, in contrast to serotype 2 viruses, have a tropism for B lymphocytes of the bursa and cause depletion of this organ. **Serotype 2 IBDV infections are** also widespread a nd occur in chickens, t urkeys, and d ucks. **However, no serotype 2 isolates have been demonstrated to be either pathogenic or immunosuppressive. Both serotype 1 and 2 viruses infect turkeys and ducks but cause no disease in these species.**

Spread

IBD is highly contagious. The affected birds excrete the virus in faeces **for 10-14 days.** The virus is very stable, and remains highly infectious in the poultry environment **for many months** (up to 122 days). **Water, feed, and droppings in the infected pens remain infectious even after 52 days.** The **hardy nature of this virus** is responsible for its persistent survival in poultry houses, even w hen t horough cleaning a nd disinfection procedures a re followed. **Resistance of the virus to heat and disinfectants** accounts for its survival in the environment between outbreaks. **Mechanical vectors** such as wild birds, humans, and vermin (insects) are likely to play a part in the spread of the virus. Meal worms and litter mites have been shown to be infective for up to 8 weeks. **There is no evidence that the virus is transmitted through the egg, or that a carrier state exists in recovered birds.**

Young chicks with maternally derived antibody (MDA) are immune to infection while their antibody levels are high. However, they become susceptible when antibody titres drop. **Some of the more recent high virulent strains appear capable of breaking through MDA at an early age.** Some breeds, such as L eghorns, a re m ore s usceptible to d isease t han others a nd have the highest mortality rates. **Older birds,** when the bursa has i nvoluted (regressed, reduced i n size) a ppear **more resistant** to i nfection and d o n ot develop clinical d isease.

Pathogenesis

The most common route of infection is oral, but **conjuctival** and **respiratory routes** may also be important. Four to five hours after oral infection, virus can be detected in **macrophages** and **lymphoid cells** in the caeca, duodenum, jejunum, a nd Kupffer c ells of t he liver. T he virus f irst reaches t he liver. It then enters t he bloodstream, where it is distributed to other t issues including the bursa. That is, **bursa is infected through the bloodstream,** and a **viraemia** occurs when the virus infects other organs including the spleen, the Harderian gland, and the thymus. **The bursal infection is followed by a second massive viraemia.** Viral antigen c an be found in the bursa u p to 9 days post-infection. The virus affects lymphoid tissue, causing **destruction of lymphoid cells within the bursa of Fabricius, spleen, and caecal tonsils. B lymphocytes and their precursors are the main target cells,** although virus may be f ound in m acrophages. T l ymphocytes are r elatively unaffected. I n some b irds the kidneys may a ppear swollen a nd may c ontain urate d eposits and cell d ebris. This i s probably t he result o f blockage o f the u reters by a severely swollen bursa. The cause of muscle haemorrhage is unknown. Recently it has been suggested that haemorrhages may be because **IBD virus interferes with the normal blood clotting mechanism.**Bursal depletion from virulent virus infection in early life can result in impaired immune responses. **The consequences of immunosuppression are lowered resistance to disease and suboptimal (inadequate) responses to vaccines given during this time**.

The period of greatest susceptibility is between 3 and 6 weeks of age. Susceptible chickens **younger than 3 weeks** do not exhibit signs, but have **subclinical infections** which are economically important due to severe immunosuppression of the chicken. The reason for the **age susceptibility** has been the subject of research regarding the pathogenesis of IBDV infections. 3-day-old chicks treated with cyclophosphamide (**chemical bursectomy**) are refractory (resistant) to disease when challenged at 4 weeks of age. Similar results are obtained with birds **surgically bursectomized** at 4 weeks of age. When they were challenged immediately, there was no clinical disease, **whereas 100% of control non-bursectomized chickens died**. Bursectomized chickens challenged with virulent virus produced 1000 times less virus than control birds and very mild necrosis of lymphatic tissues.

Several studies conducted on the pathogenesis of IBDV infections have revealed that haemorrhagic lesions result from the **formation of immune complexes**. Microscopic lesions in the bursa resemble an **Arthus reaction**, characterized by necrosis, haemorrhage, and large numbers of polymorphonuclear leukocytes. This reaction (**type III hypersensitivity**) is a localized immunological injury caused by **antigen-antibody-complement complexes** which induce chemotactic factors. The chemotactic factors, in turn, cause haemorrhage and leukocyte infiltration. It was found that both 2-week and 8-week old chicks produced high levels of antibody following infection, **but 2-week-old chicks did not develop the Arthus-type lesions**. 2-week-old chickens had very little complement compared with 8-week-old chickens. It is believed that the reason 2-week-old chickens did not develop Arthus-type lesions **was a lack of sufficient complement**.

Increased clotting times in affected chickens have led to the suggestion that such **coagulopathies** (disorders of coagulation) may contribute to the haemorrhagic lesions observed with this disease. It was found that 17-day-old chickens did not show clotting defects, but at 42 days had markedly increased clotting times, became clinically ill and several died. The key to pathogenesis of IBD in birds of different ages may lie with the factors involved in the clotting of blood and/or an immunological injury. The pathogenesis is certainly not straightforward and simple.

Signs

The severity of clinical signs depends upon age, breed, and maternally derived antibody (MDA) level of the chick, as well as the virulence of the virus.

The **acute form** is **seen in chicks between 3-6 weeks of age** after an incubation period of 2-3 days. Signs include depression, white watery diarrhoea, soiled vents, anorexia, ruffled feathers, reluctance to move, closed eyes, and death. Morbidity ranges from 10%-100% and mortality 0%-20%, sometimes reaching 50%. **Strains of very virulent IBDV (VVIBDV) cause 90%-100% mortality.** The **milder form** of disease may result in little or no signs except suboptimal growth, and sometimes an increase in other diseases and reduced response to vaccines.

The **course of the disease** in the individual chick is short, leading to death or recovery. However, in a flock where protective MDA levels vary it is prolonged, with chicks succumbing when their antibody levels drop. **On the flock basis mortality reaches a peak 3-5 days after infection.**

Lesions

Gross Lesions

The carcasses are dehydrated. There are **haemorrhages in the thigh and pectoral muscles**, and sometimes on the mucosa of the proventriculus. **Haemorrhages of leg muscles are typical of IBD.** There is increased mucus in the intestine. The **bursa** is first **enlarged, inflamed, oedematous** and **cream coloured**. After about 3-8 days, it **atrophies. Haemorrhages** may be seen on the internal and serosal surfaces, and **a caseous core** is formed within the lumen from sloughed epithelial tissue. The **liver** may be swollen and show **peripheral infarcts**. In some cases **splenomegaly** occurs. The **swelling and white appearance of the kidneys**, and **dilatation of the tubules with urates** and cell debris are seen in some outbreaks, but do not appear to be a consistent finding.

Microscopic Lesions

Microscopic changes occur mainly in the lymphoid structures, i.e., bursa, spleen, thymus, Harderian gland, and caecal tonsil. Changes in the **bursa** comprise the initial inflammatory response with hyperaemia, oedema, and infiltration of heterophils, **accompanied by B lymphoid cell necrosis.** There is hyperplasia of reticulo-endothelial cells and inter-follicular tissue. With the decline in the acute inflammatory response, the cortico-medullary epithelium proliferates and cystic cavities develop in the medullary areas of the follicles. In the **spleen** there is some necrosis of lymphoid cells. The **thymus** and **caecal tonsils** show some cellular reaction in the lymphoid tissues in the early stages, but the damage is less extensive. There may be plasma cell depletion in the Harderian gland. Microscopic lesions of the **kidney** are non-specific. The **liver** may show slight perivascular infiltration of monocytes.

Diagnosis

The history, clinical signs and gross lesions are adequate for the diagnosis of **acute disease**. In the case of **subclinical IBD**, differential diagnosis may be necessary and this should include coccidiosis, Ranikhet disease, haemorrhagic syndrome of muscles and other haemorrhages, avitaminosis A, fatty liver and kidney syndrome, water deprivation with swollen kidneys, and excess renal urates.

Diagnosis can be confirmed by using macerated bursa as antigen in a gel diffusion test, or in an ELISA test, against a known positive antiserum; by microscopic examination of tissues for typical lesions, or the presence of antigen following immunoperoxidase staining. The detection of antigen by immunofluorescence in frozen bursal sections, or smears, may also be used.

Virus isolation is rarely used for diagnosis, as it is time consuming. Bursa is the most commonly used tissue for isolation and identification of the causative agent. Most strains can be grown on the chorio-allantoic membrane of 10-11 day-old embryonated eggs. Some strains grow in chick embryo fibroblast, vero cells, or certain lymphoblastoid cell cultures. Antibodies which can be detected by neutralization, ELISA, or precipitation tests develop following infection. These can be used for diagnosis where MDA has declined below detectable levels.

Nucleic acid probes, and **antigen-capture ELISA using monoclonal antibodies** to detect IBD virus directly in tissues, are useful for rapid diagnosis of field viruses. However, **polyclonal antibodies were found more sensitive than monoclonal antibodies**, and embryo inoculation was more sensitive than antigen-capture ELISA. The **polymerase chain reaction (PCR)** is also useful for detection of the virus. Reverse transcription with PCR followed by restriction endonuclease analysis is used.

Reoviridae

The Family **Reoviridae** contains **six genera, three of which infect animals**: 1) **orthoreovirus (reovirus)**, 2) **orbivirus**, and 3) **rotavirus**. The original isolates were called "reovirus", an acronym for "*respiratory enteric orphan virus*", because they were not associated with any disease. (An **acronym** is a word formed from the **first letters** of a group of words). In fact, most reoviruses of the genus orthoreovirus are non-pathogenic. **The most important pathogens are in the orbivirus genus**, which includes **bluetongue virus** and **African horse sickness virus**. The rotaviruses cause enteritis in many different species. **All reoviruses** are **non-enveloped** icosahedral (having 20 faces) of 60-80 nm in size, which contain segmented **double-stranded RNA (ds RNA)**.

Diseases caused by Orthoreoviruses (Reoviruses)

Generally the term "reovirus" is used for members of this group, **most of which are non-pathogenic**. There are three serotypes (1, 2, and 3). The reoviruses have been used extensively to study viral replication, viral genetics, and viral pathogenesis. Otherwise, the viruses as a group remain relatively unimportant as natural pathogens. Reoviruses have been associated with gastrointestinal and respiratory disease in **cats** (type 3), **dogs** (types 1 and 2), and **horses** (type 3).

Avian Reoviruses

Reoviruses have been associated **in the chicken** with **ulcerative enteritis, acute and chronic respiratory disease, pericarditis and hydropericardium, anaemia, inclusion body hepatitis, and death**. Reoviruses have also been associated with **tenosynovitis** (inflammation of a tendon sheath), or **viral arthritis**. This produces **lameness** and the birds are reluctant to move.

Orbiviruses

The genus **"orbivirus"** (L. orbi=ring, a small circle) contains viruses which multiply in arthropods (insects) as well as in vertebrates. Thus, these are **arboviruses** (arbo = arthropod-borne), but this is no longer used in classification of viruses. **Bluetongue virus is the type species**. This virus has **double-stranded RNA (dsRNA)**. The virion is **non-enveloped** and contains a virus-specific transcriptase. **The virions are assembled in the cytoplasm of host cells.**

Bluetongue of Sheep

Also known as **"catarrhal fever of sheep"** and **"soremuzzle"**, bluetongue (BT) is a viral disease of **sheep**, and occasionally **cattle** and **goats**, transmitted by insect vectors. The disease is characterized by catarrhal stomatitis, rhinitis, enteritis, and lameness. **Bluetongue virus is an arthropod-borne orbivirus in the Family Reoviridae.**

The disease was first recognized in South Africa in 1902. It is now reported to occur worldwide in tropical, subtropical and temperate climates. **Bluetongue is endemic in India.** In the recent past incidence of bluetongue in **sheep, cattle** and **buffaloes** has increased manifold in our country. In a recently carried out survey by the National Dairy Development Board, Anand, Gujarat, a large number of animals were found to be positive for bluetongue antibodies. **The rate of positivity in buffaloes was higher than in cattle,** and the incidence was higher in males than in females. There are **24 different serotypes of bluetongue virus (BTV)**, which are only variably cross-protective. **BT is most severe in sheep.** The severity of the disease depends on the strain of virus and breed of sheep. Most domestic species are highly susceptible. Cattle, goats, and deer are also susceptible to infection. **In cattle, the infection is usually not much noticeable.** It may resemble a mild version of the disease in sheep. Cattle may carry the virus for long periods of time, with the development of sporadic viraemia adequate for insect transmission. **The virus has also been recovered from bovine semen.**

Spread

Bluetongue is transmitted by biting insects of the genus **Culicoides**. Other vectors may transmit the disease mechanically, but are unlikely to be of major significance. Infection has been transmitted by insemination from an infected bull, **since the virus is present in the semen**.

Pathogenesis

Following infection, viral replication is believed to initially occur in haematopoietic cells. This results in **viraemia** and subsequent replication in endothelial cells throughout the body. **Endothelial cell damage is responsible for the widespread gross and microscopic lesions.** Endothelial cells become swollen and later become necrotic, causing oedema, haemorrhage, thrombosis, and infarction.

Signs

High fever (105° F) is the first sign, with associated reddening of the nasal and oral mucosa and excessive salivation. A watery discharge from the nostrils later becomes mucous, and may dry to form crusts. **Oedematous swellings** appear in the lips, tongue, ears, face, and inter-mandibular space. **Oedema and cyanosis of the tongue (bluish) are so striking that they have given the disease its name.** However, they are not always present. **Petechiae** soon appear on the oral and nasal mucosa, where the epithelium becomes thickened and is shed, leaving excoriations (abrasions) and bleeding points. As the fever subsides, flushing (redness) of the skin and feet appears, and the coronets become warm and tender. This results in stiffness and **lameness**.

The disease may terminate in severe emaciation, prostration (lying down), and muscular weakness (sometimes with torticollis, i.e., twisted neck drawing the head to one side), which may last 3 weeks or more. **This is followed by pulmonary oedema and death from pneumonia.** The morbidity rate in mild outbreaks is usually about 50%, and the mortality rate is about 7%. **In severe outbreaks, however, losses from death may reach 50%.** Sheep of all ages are susceptible, but adults seem to be affected more often than lambs.

Lesions

As indicated, the **lesions of bluetongue originate from replication of the virus in endothelial cells,** and are characterized by oedema, hyperaemia, haemorrhage, and infarction. There is extensive oedema of the subcutis around the head and neck. Changes around the mouth, which characterize the clinical disease, consist of hyperaemia, oedema, cyanosis, and multiple haemorrhages, especially on the muzzle, tongue, and cheeks, with erosion and even ulceration of the epithelium. The dental pad, hard palate, gums, oesophagus, reticulum and rumen may have similar lesions.

Microscopic examination o f the skin near t he hoof reveals, intense hyperaemia of the corium, mostly concentrated at the tips of the dermal papillae, and associated with oedema and infiltration with neutrophils. The musculature (muscles) usually contains foci of gross haemorrhage, which are associated with microscopic evidence of necrotic changes in muscle bundles. Haemorrhage and necrosis also occur in the myocardium, particularly in the papillary muscles of the left ventricle.

Bluetongue virus infection during pregnancy may result in foetal infection, which causes severe cerebral abnormalities in both **sheep** and **cattle**. The nature and severity of the disease depend on the **stage of pregnancy**. In ewes exposed at 40-60 d ays of pregnancy and cattle of 60-120 days, a severe necrotizing encephalopathy occurs, which at birth is seen as **hydranencephaly (hydrocephalus)**. Later in pregnancy, focal necrotizing lesions develop, which are seen as **porencephaly** (cavities in brain) **at birth**. Lamb foetuses exposed after 100 days of gestation develop a focal encephalitis with glial nodules. A necrosis of the retina also develops, which causes lambs or calves to be born with **retinal dysplasia** in addition to the cerebral abnormalities.

Diagnosis

The clinical diagnosis can be made from the symptoms and gross lesions, but b luetongue must b e d ifferentiated f rom photosensitization, c ontagious ecthyma, foot-and-mouth disease, *Oestrus ovis* infestation, ulcerative dermatitis, and sheep-pox. In **cattle**, t he disease must be d ifferentiated from f oot-and-mouth disease, rinderpest, vesicular stomatitis, infectious rhinotracheitis, mycotic stomatitis, and the bovine-virus d iarrhoea disease complex.

Isolation and identification of the virus (from blood or spleen) are necessary to confirm diagnosis. D iagnostic techniques b ased o n serology i nclude agar-gel immunodiffusion (AGID) test, complement fixation test (CFT), and ELISA. Serotyping is carried by plaque inhibition or polyacrylamide gel electrophoresis (PAGE). Fluorescent antibody technique (FAT) has been found useful for the d etection o f group s pecific antigen. N ewer d iagnostic tests, including those using Mab (monoclonal antibody) in competitive ELISA (C-ELISA), h ave been employed. **PCR (polymerase chain reaction)** b ased techniques may h ave important p ractical application. H owever, these t echniques are yet to be made available for routine use.

African Horse Sickness

African horse sickness is **a highly fatal, infectious disease of horses, mules, and donkeys,** caused by an **orbivirus**. Even goats and dogs may be infected. The disease was originally present in South Africa, but in recent years, it has crossed the boundaries of other countries. This disease is at present not prevalent in India, **but in 1960 India had experienced the worst outbreak of Afri-**

can horse sickness. The disease had inflicated heavy mortality reaching up to 90%. It is therefore vital that we remain on our guard. The outbreak was first recorded in Rajasthan, and had then spread to Maharasthtra, Madhya Pradesh, Punjab, Bihar, Orissa and Andhra Pradesh. **Since 1963 no case has been reported from the country.**

Several different serotypes of the virus have been identified, which are not completely cross-protective. Native horses are the most susceptible, and morbidity and mortality are very high. The disease in mules is somewhat less severe than in horses, but more severe than in donkeys. A variety of laboratory animals may be infected.

Spread

The disease is spread by biting insects, mainly by several species of **Culicoides. The virus is present in all body fluids and tissues of affected animals from the onset of fever until recovery**. The disease is spread by the passive transfer of very small quantities of blood by biting insects. Spread does not occur between animals in direct contact unless the necessary insect vectors are present. The **mosquitoes Anopheles, Culex** and **Aedes** sp. have been shown to be **true biological carriers**.

Pathogenesis

African horse sickness is a disease of vascular endothelium, with various serotypes affecting endothelium in different organs. This results in **a variety of "forms" of the disease**. The **pulmonary form** is caused by damage to vascular endothelium in the lungs, and the development of pulmonary oedema. The development of various forms of the disease depends on the envelope chemistry of the individual strain of the virus. The chemistry dictates the tissue to which the serotype will be directed. The virus is present in the blood from the first day of clinical illness, and persists for about 30 days and up to 90 days. It can be recovered from blood by intracerebral inoculation into infant mice.

Signs

Clinically, the disease may occur in one of the **four forms** : 1) **acute pulmonary form**, 2) **subacute cardiac form**, 3) **a mild form**, known as **horse sickness fever**, and 4) **a mixed form**. An intermittent fever of 105°-106° F is characteristic of all forms.

Acute pulmonary form is the **most common**. It is characterized by an incubation period of 3-5 days, sudden onset of fever (105°-107°F), and severe dyspnoea caused by pulmonary oedema, often with frothy exudate in the nostrils. Sweating and coughing may occur, and **death** usually results **within a few hours** of onset of the pulmonary oedema. This form has been described in dogs as well. In the **subacute cardiac form** the incubation period and course are usually longer than in the pulmonary form. It is characterized by the occurrence of oedema of the head, neck, lips, eyelids, cheek, and tongue. The most characteristic is the oedematous bulging of the supraorbital fossa. Petechiae may appear on the ventral aspect of the tongue. Abdominal pain and paralysis of the oesophagus may occur. Death is usually caused by cardiac failure and hypoxia. The **mixed form** is a combination of pulmonary and cardiac lesions found at necropsy. This form is not common in field outbreaks. The **mild form**, also known as "**horse sickness fever**", is the least serious. It is usually seen in partially immune animals, particularly donkeys. Clinical signs include mild fever, anorexia, dyspnoea, and an accelerated heart rate. Rapid recovery follows.

Lesions

Lesions at necropsy can usually be correlated with the clinical form of the disease. The most prominent changes are seen in the respiratory system. Hydrothorax usually accompanies severe oedema, which involves the subpleural and interlobular stroma, and fills alveoli in many lobules. Frothy fluid usually fills the bronchi, trachea, and rest of the upper respiratory tract. **Microscopically**, fibrin, leukocytes and proteinaceous material are present in the oedematous tissues. The **cardiac lesions** are also significant. Hydropericardium is usually present, along with petechiae and inflammatory oedema in the epicardium. **Microscopically**, foci of myocardial necrosis are seen. Spleen and lymph nodes usually show depletion of lymphocytes, and reticulo-endothelial and plasma cells are usually increased in number. However, the spleen is usually not enlarged. Some lymph nodes may be grossly haemorrhagic. In the gastrointestinal tract, oedema around the pharynx may account for the paralysis of the oesophagus. Haemorrhage is common in the gastric mucosa. The liver is usually only congested. Haemorrhage and oedema may occur in the kidneys, particularly in the peripelvic fat.

Diagnosis

A presumptive diagnosis can be made from the clinical features and necropsy findings, **but should be confirmed by recovery and identification of the virus**. A number of serological tests are available. These include agar gel immunodiffusion (AGID), indirect fluorescent antibody (IFA), complement fixation (CF), virus neutralization (VN), and ELISA tests. All the tests have their own strengths and weaknesses. However, all are effective. For accurate identification of the virus strain, the serogroup-specific, enzyme-linked immunosorbent ELISA test is mostly used, and is specific and sensitive.

The disease must be differentiated from equine viral arteritis, because both diseases are characterized by oedema and haemorrhage in the subcutis, heart, and lungs. The specific lesions in the musculature of arterioles in equine viral arteritis are helpful in the differential diagnosis, but isolation and identification of the virus should also be carried out.

Diseases caused by Rotaviruses

Members of the genus "rotavirus" are important causes of **diarrhoea in young animals and children** throughout the world. The virions have a characteristic appearance. The sharply defined outer capsid resembles a **wheel** (L. rota = wheel). They are icosahedral, and about 70 nm in diameter. Most rotaviruses share common inner capsid antigens (**Group A rotavirus**). However, recently, isolates which are serologically distinct have been obtained. These are known as "**para-rotaviruses**" or "**novel rotaviruses**" (**Group B rotavirus**). Rotavirus diarrhoea or enteritis occurs in infant children, calves, lambs, pigs, dogs, foals, mice and other animals. **Rotaviruses are not highly species specific**. The pathogenesis and lesions are similar in each species. **In India**, rotavirus has been found to be associated with **diarrhoea in foals.**

Neonatal Calf Diarrhoea (Scours)

This serious disease of **calves** appears during the **first 2 weeks of life**. It affects most of the animals in the herd, and causes death of up to half of infected animals. The **principal sign** is the appearance of **yellowish, watery faeces**, which soon leads to severe dehydration. This syndrome has been known for many years, but was usually attributed to enteric bacteria, such as *Escherichia coli*. Although multiple factors may be involved, which are not clearly understood, it is clear that **rotaviruses are the essential aetiological factor**. In India, rotavirus is one of the major pathogens responsible for **high morbidity and mortality in neonatal calves.**

Spread

A large number of viral particles are shed in the **faeces**, which is the main source for dissemination of the disease, either through direct contact, or by contamination of water supplies and by airborne spread. The virions are highly resistant to drying, high temperatures, and other environmental conditions, and can remain infectious for months.

Pathogenesis and Lesions

After ingestion, the low pH-stable rotaviruses infect epithelial cells of the **small intestine**, producing lesions first in the anterior portion of the intestine which later progress distally. **Only differentiated columnar epithelial cells lining the apical halves of villi are susceptible.** That is, only mature enterocytes toward villous tip are preferentially affected. Entry and replication does not occur in immature or proliferating cells in the crypts (**Fig. 5A**). **These cells lack receptors for the virus.** Lesions and signs follow an extremely short incubation period, and develop within hours. **The first changes are visible under the electron microscope**. Epithelial cells develop cisternae (wide spaces) in the endoplasmic reticulum and swollen mitochondria. **Viral particles** appear in the distended cisternae and lysosomes. There is loss of microvilli. **Microscopically**, epithelial cells become vacuolated and shed prematurely. Villi thus become atrophic and shortened. **With para-rotaviruses an additional lesion is the formation of multinucleated cells or syncytia**. These cells are formed by fusion of enterocytes on the surface of villi (**Fig. 5B**).

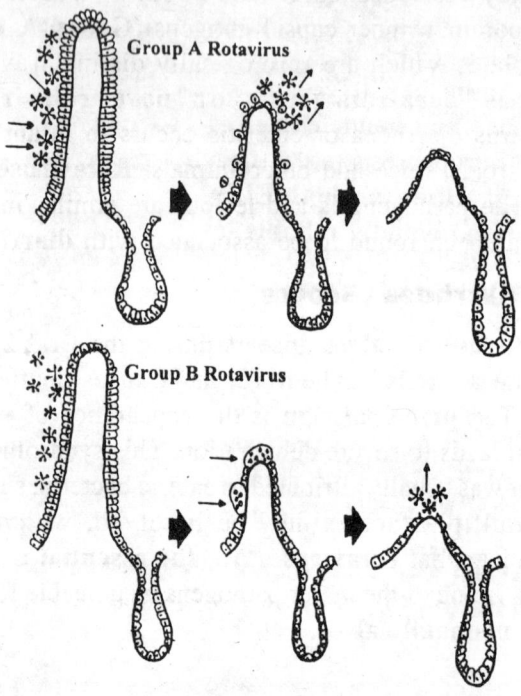

Group A Rotavirus

Group B Rotavirus

Fig. 5 **A. (Group A rotaviruses)** Mature enterocytes toward villous tip are preferentially affected leading to necrosis, sloughing, stunted villi, and hypertrophy of enterocytes in crypts.

B. (Group B rotaviruses) Para-rotaviruses are more often associated with multinucleated cells, or syncytia on surface of villi (arrows in middle diagram).

In surviving animals, villi return to normal in 3-4 weeks. **In all species,** rotaviral enteritis is much more severe when complicated by simultaneous infection with enterotoxigenic *Escherichia coli*. Reduced levels of disaccharides have been demonstrated. These cause reduction in lactose digestion and promotion of bacterial growth. This results in an osmotic effect which further contributes to **diarrhoea**.

Diagnosis

Several laboratory tests are available for detection of rotaviruses in the faeces and intestinal contents and tissues. The most common is the use of **immunofluorescent staining** of desquamated epithelial cells in the faecal specimens to demonstrate the presence of virus. However, this is now getting replaced by the **electron microscopic examination of faecal material**. This is because the fluorescent antibody technique (FAT) will detect the virus within epithelial cells in the faeces only 4-6 hours after the onset of diarrhoea. **With electron microscopy**, the virus can be detected for up to 6-10 days after the onset of diarrhoea. However, the enzyme-linked immunosorbent assay (**ELISA**) has been found more sensitive and simple than complement fixation, immunofluorescence on inoculated cell cultures, or electron microscopy. A counter-immunoelectrophoresis test is also available, and compares favourably with the ELISA test. **However, both ELISA test and electron microscopy of faeces are considered equally reliable in detecting the rotavirus.**

Porcine Rotaviral Enteritis

A syndrome of enteric disease is recognized clinically in **piglets 1-4 weeks of age**. The **principal signs** are diarrhoea, anorexia, depression, and sometimes vomiting, with a mortality rate between 7-20%. The syndrome is often referred to as **"milk scours"**, **"white scours"**, or **"three-week scours"**. One of the causative agents is a **porcine rotavirus**. This virus should be differentiated from the virus of transmissible gastroenteritis, porcine enterovirus, and enteropathogenic *Escherichia coli* (colibacillosis).

Lesions

The lesions are those of typical rotaviral enteritis described above. In pigs affected with para-rotaviruses, syncytial cells may be seen.

Diagnosis

The diagnosis can be done by isolation and identification of the virus in tissue cultures or by direct demonstration of viral antigen in intestinal epithelial cells, using immunofluorescent methods. The differentiation from the virus of transmissible gastroenteritis (a coronavirus) is important.

Diseases caused by Avian Rotaviruses

Rotaviruses are also now known to infect a number of avian species, including chickens, turkeys, ducks, and pigeons. Rotavirus infection occurs worldwide in domestic poultry. The infection has been associated with **outbreaks of enteric disease**. Rotaviruses possess a **double-stranded RNA (dsRNA) genome**.

Spread

Rotaviruses are stable viruses which are **excreted in large numbers in the**

faeces. This leads to heavy and persistent environmental contamination. Horizontal transmission occurs readily between birds in direct and indirect contact. Egg transmission of rotaviruses has not been demonstrated.

Pathogenesis and Lesions

Rotavirus infection is confined to the intestinal tract. The virus grows mainly in the mature villous epithelial cells of the small intestine. Some isolates may also replicate to a lesser extent in the large intestine. Infected epithelial cells are **destroyed**, resulting in **villous atrophy**. Compensatory crypt hypertrophy occurs, resulting in **decreased villous:crypt length ratios**. Pathogenesis of rotavirus infection in avian species is similar to that in mammalian species, that is, replacement of mature epithelial cells by immature cells deficient in digestive enzymes and in their ability to transport water and electrolytes leading to a malabsorption-type diarrhoea.

Signs

Watery droppings, lasting 2-5 days, are observed, and may be accompanied by litter eating, vent pecking, abnormal thirst, and stunting growth. There may be lesions on the breast (**breast burns**), legs, (**hock burns**), and plantar surfaces of the feet. However, in chickens and turkeys, rotavirus infections are **usually subclinical**. Most infections occur in young birds in the first 5 weeks of age. However, there is no age resistance to infection, and rotavirus-associated diarrhoea has been recorded in 92-week-old birds.

Diagnosis

The clinical signs of rotavirus infection are not pathognomonic. Direct electron microscopic, or immunoelectron microscopic examination, is used extensively to detect **rotaviruses in avian faeces**. However, this is time-consuming and expensive. Recognition of rotavirus RNA in faecal extracts subjected to polyacrylamide gel electrophoresis (PAGE) is almost as sensitive as electron microscopy. Attempts to isolate rotaviruses in chick embryo liver and cell cultures are usually unreliable, and are selective for group A rotaviruses. Most group A rotaviruses are non-cytopathic and are detected by immunofluorescence. **In general, ELISAs meant for detection of group A mammalian rotaviruses are not efficient in detecting group A avian rotaviruses**, and also fail to detect the more numerous rotaviruses belonging to the other groups. Antibodies to rotavirus are widespread in the domestic avian species. In view of this, **serology is not used routinely for diagnostic purposes**.

Rotaviruses are usually not the only entero-pathogens detected in the faeces of chickens and turkeys **with diarrhoea**. Enterovirus-like viruses, reoviruses, adenoviruses, astroviruses, and potentially entero-pathogenic bacteria may also be present. **It may therefore be difficult to decide which agent is primarily responsible for the disease.**

Diseases caused by Single-Stranded DNA (ss DNA) Families

Circoviridae

Circoviridae is a new virus family. It has **only one genus "Circovirus"**, which **contains three viruses**: 1) **chicken infectious anaemia virus** (chicken anaemia virus), 2) **porcine circovirus**, and 3) **psittacine beak and feather disease virus**. Circoviruses are characterized by having **circular single-stranded DNA (ssDNA)**. It is because of this characteristic circular DNA that the family is called **Circoviridae** (L. circo = circular). All circoviruses are **non-enveloped**. **Only chicken infectious anaemia virus is important.**

Diseases caused by Circovirus

Chicken Infectious Anaemia (Chicken Anaemia Virus)

Chicken infectious anaemia (CIA) is **a disease of young chickens** caused by a unique small (25 nm) virus. The disease is characterized by **a plastic anaemia** and **generalized lymphoid atrophy**, with an accompanying **immunosuppression**. As a result, CIA is usually complicated by secondary viral, bacterial, or fungal infections.

The agent was first reported from Japan in 1979 and was called **"chicken anaemia agent (CAA)"**. Following its characterization as a non-enveloped virus containing a single-stranded circular DNA, it was renamed as **"chicken anaemia virus (CAV)"** and classified under **Circoviridae** along with the two other small viruses (mentioned above), which had similar structure. Because the disease caused by it is commonly called chicken infectious anaemia, the virus is **now called "chicken infectious anaemia virus (CIAV)"**. **CIAV is a remarkably resistant virus**, its infectivity resists heating at 80° C for 15 min, and exposure to pH 3. **Serological surveys indicate that CIAV infection is common in chickens throughout the world**. It is not known if avian species other than domestic fowl are infected. All isolates of CIAV isolated to date belong to a **single serotype**.

Spread

The virus spreads both horizontally and vertically. Vertical transmission through the hatching egg is considered to be most important means of dissemination. Embryo infection can also be caused by **semen of infected cocks**. The virus is present in high concentrations in the **faeces** of chickens 5-7 weeks after infection. **Horizontal infection** by direct or indirect contact usually occurs through the **oral route** by ingesting infected material, but infection through the respiratory route may also be possible.

Pathogenesis

Anaemia and other pathological changes associated with CIAV occur in neonatal, fully susceptible (i.e., having no maternal antibody) chicks. Chicks infected by contact shed virus. **Maternal antibody is protective. Chicks with maternal antibody usually show no disease or anaemia, but may shed the virus.**

Dual (double) infection of CIAV and immunosuppressive viruses such as virulent Marek's disease virus, infectious bursal disease virus, and reticuloendotheliosis virus enhances the pathogenicity of CIAV. This results in greater mortality and more persistent anaemia and microscopic lesions. **In such dual infections, the protective effect of maternal antibody may be overcome**. In chicks dually infected with CIAV and IBD virus, the age resistance is overcome and contact-infected chicks also develop anaemia. **CIAV** has recently been shown to be **immunosuppressive**. Functional changes were detected in splenic lymphocytes and splenic and bone marrow macrophages, from both clinically affected and subclinically infected chicks. **The main sites of CIAV replication are precursor T cells in the thymic cortex and in haemocytoblasts in the bone marrow.** However, the virus also replicates in all lymphoid aggregates throughout the body. **Destruction of these cells accounts for the immunosuppression and anaemia.**

Signs

Disease occurs in the progeny of breeder flocks which are infected for the first time with the virus after they come into lay. **CIAV is vertically transmitted to the progeny.** No clinical signs are seen in the parents. However, **around 2 weeks of age**, the young chicks show variable mortality. The mortality may go even up to 60%, but usually averages around 10%. The **most characteristic changes** are anaemia, aplasia of the bone marrow, and atrophy of the thymus, spleen, and bursa of Fabricius. **Anaemia** is characterized by haematocrit values ranging from 6-27%. Affected birds are depressed and more or less pale. **Haemorrhages** may occur under the skin and throughout the skeletal muscles. Enlarged livers and gangrenous dermatitis may also be present. Other names (synonyms) for this condition are **anaemia dermatitis syndrome, infectious anaemia syndrome, haemorrhagic syndrome**, and **blue-wing disease.**

Surviving chicks completely recover from anaemia by 20-28 days after infection. However, retarded recovery and increased mortality may be associated with **secondary bacterial and viral infections**. Secondary infections cause more severe clinical signs. **Subclinical infection** of the progeny of **immune breeder flocks** is common. This occurs soon after maternally acquired antibodies have disappeared at about 3 weeks of age.

Gross Lesions

Thymic atrophy is the m ost consistent l esion. However, **bone marrow atrophy is the most characteristic lesion**. Femoral bone marrow is fatty, and yellowish or pink. Thymic atrophy may result in a complete regression of the organ. As infected chicks develop a ge resistance, t hymic atrophy is a much more consistent lesion than grossly visible bone marrow lesions. Bursal atrophy is less noticeable. **Haemorrhages in t he p roventricular mucosa**, and subcutaneous a nd m uscular haemorrhages are sometimes associated with severe a naemia.

Microscopic Lesions

In t he anaemic chicks, microscopic c hanges have b een characterized as **panmyelophthisis** (wasting away o f the bone marrow), a nd **generalized lymphoid atrophy**. In the bone marrow, atrophy and aplasia involve all compartments a nd all h aematopoietic cells. **H aematopoietic cells are replaced by adipose tissue or proliferating stroma cells. Severe lymphoid depletion** is seen in the thymus, bursa of Fabricius, spleen and caecal tonsils, as well as in a wide range of o ther tissues. T he thymus c ortex and m edulla b ecome equally atrophic. Lesions in the bursa o f Fabricius consist of atrophy of t he lymphoid follicles. **In the spleen also**, there is atrophy of lymphoid tissue. In the liver, kidneys, lungs, proventriculus, duodenum, and caecal tonsils, **lymphoid foci are depleted of cells.**

Haematology

Blood of severely affected chicks is more or less **watery, the clotting time is increased**, a nd the blood p lasma is paler t han normal. **Low haematocrit values** (may even d rop to 6% in moribund, i.e., dying b irds) are d ue to **pancytopaenia**, with markedly decreased numbers of erythrocytes, white blood cells, and t hrombocytes.

Haemorrhagic-Aplastic Anaemia Syndrome

Outbreaks of infectious anaemia in f ield flocks are mostly associated with so-called "**haemorrhagic syndrome**", with or without **gangrenous dermatitis.**

Diagnosis

Presumptive diagnosis is based on the characteristic signs and pathology. Laboratory diagnosis is based on immunofluorescent or immuno-cytochemical detection of CIAV antigens in thymus or bone marrow. Viral DNA can also be detected in thymus or bone marrow by *in situ* hybridization, dot blot hybridization, or **polymerase chain reaction (PCR)**.

Virus isolation is not recommended because it is slow and expensive. Serum antibody t o CIAV c an be d etected by a variety o f serological t ests.

These are serum neutralization (SN), indirect immunofluorescence and ELISA.

Diseases caused by Parvoviruses

Parvoviridae

The Family **Parvoviridae** (L. parvo = small) is made up of unique DNA viruses which have a genome consisting of **single-stranded DNA (ss DNA)**. **Three genera make up this family: 1) Parvovirus, 2) Dependovirus,** and 3) **Densovirus**. Of these only genus **Parvovirus** contains viruses which cause disease in animals (**Table 8**). **Parvoviruses are the smallest viruses of vertebrates**, measuring about 18-26 nm in diameter. They are of icosahedral symmetry and are **non-enveloped. A unique feature of parvoviruses is that they depend on cell proliferation for viral DNA synthesis to occur. This restricts lesions to those tissues in which cells are undergoing mitosis,** and explains the difference in **cell tropism** seen in foetal, neonatal, and adult animals. The clinical signs of most parvovirus infections of animals are due to their replication in the gastrointestinal tract, bone marrow, or foetus.

Parvoviruses are highly stable, resistant to chemical and physical reagents, and are not affected seriously by heat at 60° C for an hour. **Thus, the environment may remain contaminated long after diseased animals have been removed.**

Table 8. Diseases caused by Parvoviridae

Virus	Disease	Species
Feline panleukopaenia	Feline panleukopaenia Cerebellar hypoplasia	Cats
Canine parvovirus 2	Enteritis, myocarditis	Dogs
Bovine parvovirus	Diarrhoea	Cattle
Porcine parvovirus	Infertility, foetal death and maceration	Pigs

Feline Panleukopaenia

Also known as "**feline distemper**", "**feline enteritis**", and "**agranulocytosis**", feline panleukopaenia is **a highly contagious and usually fatal febrile disease of cats** (and **other felidae,** such as wild cat, **cheetah, leopard** and **tiger**), caused by a **parvovirus.** Feline panleukopaenia virus is closely related antigenically to canine parvovirus type 2.

Spread

The virus is present in all secretions and excretions of affected animals.

Virus may be shed in the urine and faeces up to 6 weeks after recovery. The virus may survive for years. **Infection spreads by direct contact or through fomites.** M ost free-roaming c ats are e xposed to t he virus d uring their f irst year.

Signs

The d isease is characterized by s evere **panleukopaenia** (abnormal d ecrease in all types of leukocytes), **fever**, and **enteritis**, which result in extreme dehydration. The disease runs a rapid course. Its onset is marked by lassitude (tiredness, lack of energy), and sudden rise of temperature to between 104° - 105° F. **The fever is diphasic (biphasic).** It falls after about 24 hours and rises about 48 hours later. **Severe leukopaenia**, involving all the granulocytic series (agranulocytosis) a nd all o ther leukocytes, i s a **constant feature**. Vomiting and intractable (uncontrollable) diarrhoea may also be observed. **Death** usually occurs soon after the second peak of temperature.

Lesions

The **gross lesions** consist o f extreme dehydration a nd emaciation, w ith mucopurulent exudate on the nasal and lachrymal mucosa. The mucosa of the ileum is c overed w ith haemorrhagic exudate. Mesenteric l ymph n odes a re oedematous and enlarged. The bone marrow in the long bones is often yellowish or white, and semi-fluid. **There is lack of haematopoietic marrow.**

The main microscopic lesions are found in the gastrointestinal tract. Here, the virus replicates in the diving cells in the crypts. (The virus requires actively diving cells for replication. Tissues undergoing the most rapid mitotic a ctivity a re damaged most severely). The superficial l ayers o f t he mucosa in the **small intestine** are eroded, and the remaining epithelium undergoes proliferation. The crypts are dilated with mucus, and lined with i rregular, hyperplastic e pithelial c ells. I n some cases granular, e osinophilic **intranuclear inclusion bodies** are seen in the lining epithelium remaining at the sites of erosion. **These inclusions, when present, are helpful in diagnosis.**

Lesions always occur in lymphoid organs, which are the site of initial viral replication before dissemination to gastrointestinal e pithelium, or other tissues. In the beginning, **lymph nodes** are oedematous and hyperaemic, and histiocytes proliferate. This is followed by **necrosis of lymphocytes** in follicular and paracortical r egions in lymph nodes, t he Malpighian c orpuscles of t he spleen, the cortex of the thymus, and Peyer's patches. **Intranuclear inclusion bodies are sometimes present in the histiocytes.** In animals surviving infection, marked regenerative hyperplasia of lymphocytes occurs. The bone marrow is markedly h ypocellular (i.e., h aving reduced number of c ells). This r esults from necrosis of all stem-cell populations. This, too, is followed by hyperplasia in surviving animals. **Inclusion body myocarditis,** as seen in canine parvovirus infection, is not a usual feature of feline panleukopaenia.

Diagnosis

A presumptive diagnosis can usually be made from symptoms and agranulocytosis. Demonstration of **intranuclear inclusion bodies** in the epithelial cells of the small intestine is helpful in postmortem diagnosis, but unfortunately inclusions are not always present. **The inclusion bodies are best demonstrated in tissues fixed in acidic fixatives, such as Zenker's or Bouin's fluids.** Confirmatory diagnosis requires use of serum neutralization, haemagglutination-inhibition, or ELISA, and even these are not always reliable.

Panleukopaenia and Cerebellar Hypoplasia

The virus of feline panleukopaenia can produce cerebellar hypoplasia in **kittens.** The virus invades cells of the external germinal layer of the foetal cerebellum, produces **intranuclear inclusion bodies** and necrosis, and causes gross or microscopic **"hypoplasia" of the cerebellum in the newborn kitten.**

Canine Parvovirus Infection

Canine parvovirus was first recognized in 1978, when it was found associated with a disease of dogs. **The virus is more than 98% identical in DNA sequence to the virus of feline panleukopaenia.** In contrast to the feline panleukopaenia virus, **canine parvovirus causes disease only in dogs.** It does not replicate in cats. Since its recognition in 1978, the canine parvovirus has undergone two evolutionary changes. The virus present worldwide today is different from the original virus.

The infection produces **two different clinico-pathological forms of the disease.** 1) an **intestinal form,** which is the main form, and 2) a **cardiac form.**

Intestinal Form

This form **occurs in dogs of all ages,** but is most severe in **dogs older than 6 weeks.** It is characterized by vomiting, diarrhoea, and dehydration. There may be fever and leukopaenia. **Microscopically,** there is a necrotizing enteritis of the small intestine like that of feline panleukopaenia, with dilated crypts and regeneration of epithelium. **Intranuclear inclusion bodies** are found in **intestinal epithelial cells** as often as they are in cats with panleukopaenia. Lesions in lymphoid organs resemble those seen in feline panleukopaenia. There is lymphopaenia and neutropaenia resulting from necrosis of precursor cells. These signs and lesions may occur together with the cardiac form.

Cardiac Form

The cardiac form is confined to puppies of **2-8 weeks of age, i.e., in younger dogs.** This form may exist with, or without, signs or lesions in the small intestine. **Clinically, death may be sudden**, or follow a brief period of dyspnoea and sometimes signs of enteritis. **Microscopically**, there are multiple foci of myocardial necrosis associated with a mononuclear cellular infiltration. **Intranuclear inclusion bodies are present in muscle fibres**. At times, canine parvovirus in neonates may cause generalized infection with necrotizing lesions and inclusion bodies in tissues other than the gastrointestinal tract and heart, such as brain, liver, lungs, kidneys and adrenal cortex. Vascular endothelium is severely affected, causing the lesions to be haemorrhagic.

Diagnosis

This depends on the lesions and isolation of virus. The myocardial form is typical, but the intestinal form can be confused with other causes of enteritis, such as coronavirus infection. The latter is usually not milder clinically, and is not associated with leukopaenia, or significant necrosis of intestinal epithelium.

Bovine Parvovirus Infection

Bovine parvovirus has been isolated from the **intestinal tract of young calves** suffering from a severe but brief **diarrhoea**. Each of several isolates is closely related and is believed to be the same agent, which is immunologically different from parvovirus of any other species.

Although the virus is widely distributed and infection is common, **bovine parvovirus rarely causes serious disease**. Oral infection of **newborn calves** results in mucoid to watery diarrhoea in 24-48 hours. Intestinal cells of all levels become infected, but those of the **small intestine** are most clearly involved. **Viraemia** lasts for 4-6 days, but virus may be isolated from faeces for up to 11 days. The illness is usually transitory (brief), but could be severe if complicated by other viral or bacterial infections. **Lesions** are similar to those seen in feline panleukopaenia, but less severe. The **diagnosis** depends on isolation and identification of the virus in cultures of bovine cells, or on demonstration of specific immunofluorescence, or ultrastructurally typical virions in affected cells.

Porcine Parvovirus Infection

Parvovirus is widespread in pigs, as judged by the demonstration of antibodies and recovery of strains of agent. **The main effects of the virus are on reproduction**. It causes **intrauterine death of foetuses**. Rarely **abortion** occurs. Infected pig foetuses undergo maceration (softening into fluid, liquefaction) or mummification (drying and shrivelling), but are not usually expelled prematurely. The only noticeable sign of infection may be **infertility**. The macerated or mummified foetuses contain the virus. The virus is easily demonstrated with fluorescent antibody staining technique. **Porcine parvovirus is not known to cause disease in non-pregnant adult pigs**.

Diseases caused by Double-Stranded DNA (ds DNA) Families

Herpesviridae

The Family **Herpesviridae** is divided into **three subfamilies**: 1) **Alphaherpesvirinae** (Genus: **Alpha-herpesvirus**), 2) **Betaherpesvirinae** (Genus: **Beta-herpesvirus**), and 3) **Gammaherpesvirinae** (Genus: **Gamma-herpesvirus**). The word "**herpes**" is of Greek origin and means **to creep** (G. herpes = to creep). The family was so named presumably because these viruses enter or advance gradually (**creep in**) so as to be almost **unnoticed**.

Alpha-herpesviruses are citocidal viruses (i.e., cause cell death), their main pathological effect being **necrosis**. They have a broad host range, and wide cell tropism. Disease may be localized and transient (brief), or generalized and fatal. The outcome depends on the species affected, and the age and immune status of the host. **Recovery is followed by lifelong latent infection**, usually in the nerve ganglia. Recurrence of active disease is common.

The **beta-herpesvirus group** consists of "**cytomegaloviruses**". These viruses have a very restricted host range. The infected cells become very large, and show intranuclear and sometimes cytoplasmic inclusion bodies ("**cytomegalic inclusion body disease**"). The cells ultimately undergo lysis from the effects of viral replication, or host immune response. **Recovery is followed by persistent or latent infection in a variety of tissues**. These include secretory glands (especially salivary glands), kidneys, and lymph nodes. As with alpha-herpesviruses, recurrent infection is common.

Gamma-herpesviruses are lymphotropic herpesviruses, tropic for either B or T lymphocytes. Their host range is narrow, and **infection is followed by lifelong latency in lymphocytes**. Pathological effects may vary from no visible disease to **lymphoma**.

The nucleic acid of herpesviruses is **double-stranded DNA (ds DNA)**, and the capsid is icosahedral in shape, about 100-200 nm in diameter. **The virions are surrounded by an envelope**, acquired by budding through the inner lamella of the nuclear membrane.

Most of the herpesviruses have been given species names, on the basis of their host. **Table 9** presents a list of the more important herpesviruses, their hosts, species names and the diseases they cause.

Table 9. Diseases caused by Herpesviruses

Virus	Host(s)	Disease
Alpha-herpesviruses		
Herpesvirus simplex, type1	Humans, apes, monkeys	Herpes simplex, usually oral; generalized in monkeys
H. simplex, type 2	Humans, apes, monkeys	Genital herpes
H. varicella-zoster	Humans	Varicella (chicken pox), and zoster (shingles)
H. simiae, "B-virus"	Monkeys, humans	Herpesvirus B
H. canis	Dogs	Canine herpes
H. suis	Pigs, cattle	Pseudorabies (Aujeszky's disease)
Bovine herpesvirus, type1	Cattle	Infectious bovine rhinotracheitis, infectious pustular vulvovaginitis, infectious balanoposthitis, viral abortion
Bovine herpesvirus, type 2	Cattle	Herpesvirus mammillitis
Equine herpesvirus, type 1 (EHV-1, subtype 1)	Horses	Viral abortion, rhinopneumonitis, neonatal death, neurological disease, enterocolitis
Equine herpesvirus, type 4 (EHV-1, subtype 2)	Horses	Rhinopneumonitis, viral abortion
Equine herpesvirus, type 3	Horses	Coital exanthema
H. felis	Cats	Infectious rhinotracheitis
Avian herpesvirus, type 1	Birds	Infectious laryngotracheitis
Duck herpesvirus (probably alpha ?)	Ducks	Duck virus enteritis
Pigeon herpesvirus (most probably alpha ?)	Pigeons	Pigeon herpesvirus infection
Beta-herpesviruses		
Porcine cytomegaloviruses (CMVs)	Pigs	Inclusion-body rhinitis, generalized CMV infection

Cytomegaloviruses (CMVs) of bovines, equines, apes, monkeys, guinea-pigs, rats and others	Host-specific	No visible disease
Gamma-herpesviruses Epstein-Barr virus	Humans	Infectious mononucleosis, Burkitt's lymphoma and nasopharyngeal carcinoma
Malignant catarrhal fever virus	Cattle	Malignant catarrhal fever
Marek's disease virus	Chickens	Marek's disease, avian lymphomatosis

Diseases caused by Alpha-herpesviruses

Most **alpha-herpesviruses** produce **localized cytolytic lesions** on mucosal surfaces of the mouth, respiratory or genital tract, skin, or eye. Primary infection often goes **unnoticed**, but may be characterized by **vesicles, pustules, and ulcers**. During this phase, **progeny virus enters naked nerve endings in the epidermis**, and travels centripetally (towards centre) to sensory neurons in respective ganglia. (A ganglion is a mass of mainly nerve cell bodies, lying outside the brain or spinal cord). By multiplying in ganglia, virions travel centrifugally (away from the centre) down axons, and protected from humoral antibodies, enter epithelial cells at sites served by the ganglion. This extends the duration and extent of the acute primary infection. Following healing of the primary lesion by action of humoral and cellular immune mechanisms, **viral DNA remains latent in neurons for life**. Lesions may recur in response to a variety of stimuli. **Latent virus then becomes active**, spreads down axons (still protected from antibodies), to re-enter epithelial cells and repeat the lytic cycle.

In young animals, particularly neonates (newborns), primary infection may become widespread, and necrotizing lesions may appear in many organs and tissues. Systemic spread is also seen in immuno-compromised (immunologically damaged) individuals. Virus may also be transported by way of mononuclear cells to the placenta, leading to abortion or neonatal infection.

Spread of alpha-herpesviruses is by contact and droplets.

Herpesvirus Simplex Infection in Monkeys and Humans

Herpesvirus simplex infection **is one of the oldest viral diseases known to humans**. Herpesvirus simplex is also an important spontaneous disease of **monkeys, gibbons** (a small ape, i.e., monkey, with long arms), and chimpanzee (a type of small African ape).

Disease in Humans

Humans are the natural host and reservoir for herpesvirus simplex. Humans play a role similar to that of the rhesus monkey with herpesvirus B, and p igs with h erpesvirus suis. T wo antigenically d ifferent herpes s implex viruses infect humans. **Type 1 usually affects the lips and oral mucosa, whereas type 2 causes lesions on the genital mucosa of both sexes, and is transmitted by coitus.** Infection with type 1 v irus occurs m ainly in young children, taking the form of an acute gingivo-stomatitis, which heals with no serious side e ffects. By e arly adulthood, 9 0-95% of a ll individuals b ecome infected, as evidenced by the presence of serum-neutralizing antibodies. Many people, despite the presence of antibodies, suffer from periodic recurrence of secondary herpes simplex infection for much of their lives, often with several episodes occurring each year. **Recurrent lesions are due to activation of a latent infection which persists in all infected individuals for life.**

Recurrent **lesions** are c haracterized by s mall c lusters of v esicles which rupture, leaving **erosions** or **ulcers** that heal in 5-10 days. The mucocutaneous junction of the lip is the most common site. **Microscopic features** are ballooning degeneration, necrosis, intracellular oedema, multinucleated giant cells, and **intranuclear inclusion bodies.** There is a strong association between **type 2 genital infection and carcinoma of the cervix in women**, but a causative role has not been proved.

Disease in Monkeys

In monkeys, chimpanzee, gibbon, and probably other apes, herpes simplex **infection** is similar to that in humans, **usually remaining localized and resolving**. Recurrence of both oral and genital lesions has been described in chimpanzees. **In monkeys**, following an incubation period of about 7 days, a short clinical course occurs, characterized by oral and labial ulceration, ulcerative dermatitis, conjuctivitis, anorexia, weakness, and incoordination. Death is the usual outcome in 2-3 days. A **presumptive diagnosis** of herpes simplex infection in monkeys can be made on the basis of history and pathological changes. **Definitive diagnosis**, however, requires viral isolation and identification.

Herpesvirus Varicella Zoster

These two seemingly completely different disorders of humans are **both caused by the varicella-zoster virus (VZV), and are therefore closely related.**

Varicella (Chickenpox)

Chickenpox, also known as **"varicella" is one of the most common childhood infections**. It i s characterized by a **papulo-vesicular rash** (eruption), beginning on t he trunk a nd spreading t o head a nd limbs. T he virus e ~~~~ **through the respiratory mucosa**, and after viraemia, localizes and rep' in reticulo-endothelial tissues. After a second phase of viraemia, virus localizes in dermal capillary endothelial cells, and then spreads to the epidermis. **Microscopically**, the epidermal lesions are similar to those of the herpes simplex infection.

Zoster (Shingles)

Zoster, also known as 'shingles', **represents activation of latent varicella infection**, and is characterized by **vesicular dermatitis along** the distribution of **peripheral or cranial nerves**. Although associated with **severe pain** and hyperaesthesia (increased sensitivity to sensory stimuli, such as pain), it usually resolves. Lesions in the skin resemble varicella.

Herpesvirus B Infection of Monkeys
(Herpes-B, Herpesvirus simiae, B-virus)

In 1934, a virus was isolated from the brain of a human patient who died after being bitten by an apparently normal rhesus monkey. Further investigations revealed that most species of macaques (Old World monkeys), especially rhesus monkeys, were found to be the natural reservoir hosts for the virus. The virus was named "**herpesvirus B**".

Disease in Monkeys

Most of the knowledge on herpesvirus B comes from studies on rhesus monkeys, in which the infection is very similar to herpes simplex infection in humans. **Clinically**, the disease is characterized by **vesicles** and **ulcers**, particularly on the dorsal surface of the tongue and on the mucocutaneous junction of the lip. These lesions heal in 7-14 days. The disease is rarely fatal. **Microscopically**, the lesions are characterized by ballooning degeneration and necrosis of epithelial cells and the presence of **intranuclear inclusion bodies**. Once a monkey is infected with herpesvirus B, the animal probably **remains infected for life** with persistent infection in ganglia. However, recurrent lesions are not common.

Disease in Humans

The importance of herpesvirus B is not because of its danger to the reservoir host monkey, **but due to the fatal disease the virus produces in humans**. Although the rate of morbidity is low, **most cases have proved fatal**. Infections usually follow a **monkey bite**. The disease is characterized clinically and pathologically by encephalomyelitis. Focal necrosis may occur in the liver, spleen, lymph nodes, and adrenal glands. **Intranuclear inclusion bodies** may be found in any affected tissue, but have not been demonstrated in all cases. A **presumptive diagnosis** can be made from the characteristic lesions. However, definitive diagnosis requires isolation and identification of the virus.

Herpesvirus Canis Infection of Dogs

Herpesvirus canis was first isolated and characterized in 1965. It was identified as the cause of a fatal systemic infection of **neonatal (newly born) puppies**. It is now known that **dogs are the natural and reservoir hosts** for this herpesvirus, just as humans are for herpesvirus simplex, monkeys for herpesvirus B, and pigs for herpesvirus suis. Although adult dogs carry the virus as a latent infection, it has been shown to cause a mild tracheo-bronchitis. The occurrence of fatal infections in neonatal puppies appears similar to the parallel condition of fatal herpesvirus simplex in infants, or fatal herpesvirus suis in piglets. Each is an example of fatal disease in the host which usually carries the virus as a latent infection.

Puppies are infected *in utero*, **or during birth**, by exposure to the virus in the vagina. The infection results in either stillbirth, or an acute fatal disease in the first 3 weeks of life. The most striking **gross lesion** is haemorrhage, especially in the renal cortex and lungs, but the stomach, intestine, and adrenals may also have haemorrhages. Sero-sanguineous fluid is usually present in the thoracic and abdominal cavities. Splenomegaly and enlargement of lymph nodes are noticeable. **Microscopically**, the lesions in all tissues are characterized by focal necrosis, and the presence of **intranuclear inclusion bodies**. Inclusion bodies may be difficult to demonstrate, unless an acid fixative such as Zenker's fluid is used. The characteristic necrotizing lesions and intranuclear inclusion bodies help in making a **presumptive diagnosis**. **Definitive diagnosis** requires virus isolation and characterization. Dogs are natural hosts for this virus and subject to latent infection. Therefore, virus isolation in the absence of characteristic histopathological lesions must be interpreted with caution.

Pseudorabies

Also known as "infectious bulbar paralysis", "Aujeszky's disease", and "mad itch", pseudorabies is a disease to which many species are susceptible. It is caused by a virus of herpes group called **herpesvirus suis**. The disease was first described in 1902 by Aujeszky in Hungary, but is now known to occur in many parts of the world, **including India**. Natural infection occurs in pigs, cattle, dogs, cats, sheep, and rats, **but it is of greatest importance in cattle, in which the disease is almost always fatal. In wildlife**, pseudorabies has been reported in deer and fox. The infection is similar concerning its epizootiology, clinical signs, and pathological changes to certain other herpesvirus infections, such as herpesvirus B and herpesvirus simplex.

Spread

Pigs and probably **rats** serve **as the natural and reservoir hosts for herpesvirus suis**. The virus is present in the nasal discharge and in the mouth of affected pigs on the first day of illness, and for up to 17 days after infection.

Transmission is primarily **by direct contact** but can also occur through contaminated drinking water and feed. Spread of the virus within and between farms can occur mechanically. **Virus is also excreted in the milk of infected sows**, and *in utero* infection occurs. Young and adult pigs may excrete the virus in the absence of clinical disease, a situation similar to herpesvirus simplex in humans. This may represent **activation of a latent infection maintained in ganglia. Pigs serve as the source of infection for cattle and sheep**, usually when housed together, but transmission can take place even if the animals are separated by fencing.

Pathogenesis

The route of entry is through the damaged skin, or through the intact nasal mucosa. The virus is **pantropic**, and affects tissues derived from all embryonic layers. **In the pig**, there is a short period of **viraemia** with localization of the virus in many organs. However, **multiplication occurs mainly in the respiratory tract**. Spread to the brain occurs by way of the olfactory, glosso-pharyngeal, or trigeminal nerves. When the virus enters through a skin abrasion, it quickly invades the local peripheral nerves, passes along them centripetally (i.e., towards centre), and causes damage to nerve cells. It is this form of progression which causes local **pruritus** (intense itching) in the early stages of the disease, and **encephalomyelitis** at a later stage when the virus has invaded the central nervous system. **In cattle**, pruritus of the head and neck is usually associated with respiratory tract infection, and perianal pruritus is usually due to vaginal infection. **The virus can invade the uterus** and infect pre-implanted embryos, which can lead to degeneration of the embryo and **reproductive failure**.

Signs

Pigs are susceptible to infection, but adult animals rarely exhibit symptoms, or die from the disease. **In adult pigs**, a mild, febrile, non-fatal disease may occur, **but recovery is the rule. In piglets, the infection is more severe**. It occurs as an acute illness, which may lead to death in 24-48 hours without specific clinical signs. Piglets more than 4 weeks of age may show signs of involvement of the central nervous system, usually as incoordination of the hind quarters, tremors, convulsions, and paralysis. Although it is uncommon, older pigs may develop encephalitis and die of the infection. Intrauterine infection can occur, resulting in abortion and stillbirth.

Intense itching develops in the skin of the cattle at the point of contact after about 50 hours. Severe scratching of this area by the animal causes ulceration of the skin, and secondary infection results. Paralysis may develop, and cattle may die rather suddenly with indication of bulbar involvement (i.e., of medulla oblongata), hence the name **"bulbar paralysis"**. The disease affects **cattle** of all ages, **and is almost always fatal**. The course in affected **dogs and cats** is similar, and also rapidly fatal.

Lesions

After infection, herpesvirus suis reaches central nervous system by travelling up nerve fibres. Lesions occur in the nerve fibres, ganglia, and central nervous system in all species. Their extent and distribution depend on the duration of the illness and species of the animal. In general, lesions are most extensive in the spinal ganglia, temporal cerebral cortex, and basal ganglia of the brain. **In cattle and sheep**, there is intense inflammation of para-vertebral ganglia. Lesions in the brain vary. Moderate perivascular cuffing of lymphocytes and some foci of microglial proliferation are seen, but most neurons are normal, or exhibit only mild chromatolysis. **Intranuclear inclusion bodies are present in neurons and glial cells.**

In pigs, the lesions in the CNS may be **very mild**. There are vascular, perivascular and interstitial lesions with slight nerve cell degeneration. **Inclusion bodies** are present, but may be few in number. Besides nervous system, lesions are also present in other organs and tissues. Focal necrosis of pharyngeal mucosa, tonsils, lymph nodes, lungs, liver, and adrenal cortex, associated with intranuclear inclusion bodies, is usually seen in young piglets. Necrotizing placentitis with intranuclear inclusion bodies in trophoblast and mesenchymal cells precedes abortion in pigs.

Zoonotic Significance

Care should be taken during postmortem examination, as infection of humans may occur **through skin wounds.**

Diagnosis

Pseudorabies may be suspected in outbreaks in which animals die soon after showing severe pruritus limited to a specific area of the skin. Cattle or sheep with the disease have always been closely associated with pigs. The microscopic lesions in the skin and spinal ganglia may be of some help in presumptive diagnosis, but the final diagnosis depends on reproduction of the disease in experimental animals. This is done by the subcutaneous injection of rabbits with suspension of nervous tissue from diseased animals. Rabbits show intense itching, with characteristic local inflammation of the skin. Death is caused by respiratory failure, and the main lesions are necrotic changes in ganglion cells.

The main serological tests for detection of specific antibodies are the serum neutralization test and the enzyme-linked immunosorbent assay (ELISA). The serum neutralization test has been widely used because of its sensitivity and specificity. However, an indirect ELISA has been found to be a more rapid and convenient procedure, offering many advantages over the serum neutralization test for routine sero-diagnostic work. Commercial ELISA kits are available. In infected pigs, the virus is usually present in nasal secretions for up to 10 days. A common method for the diagnosis of pseudorabies in sows is to take swabs from the nasal mucosa and vagina. The virus can be demonstrated in nasal cells by immunofluorescence and immunoperoxidase techniques.

Infectious Bovine Rhinotracheitis

Infectious bovine rhinotracheitis (IBR) is **a highly infectious viral disease of cattle**. IBR is also known by a variety of other names: **infectious pustular vulvovaginitis, coital exanthema, vesicular venereal disease, vesicular vaginitis, coital vesicular vaginitis, coital vesicular exanthema**, and **red nose**. First isolated in Colorado, USA, virus of IBR is now recognized as **a herpesvirus of cattle of worldwide distribution. IBR has been reported in India**. The virus is termed '**bovine herpesvirus type 1 (BHV-1)**". After recovery of the animal from disease, **the virus remains latent in sciatic and trigeminal ganglia**, and sheds periodically in a manner similar to that seen with herpesvirus of humans (herpesvirus simplex), monkeys (herpesvirus B), and dogs (herpesvirus canis). The virus is responsible for a variety of clinico-pathological manifestations, **in addition to upper respiratory disease**. These include conjunctivitis, encephalitis, mastitis, infectious pustular vulvo-vaginitis and balanoposthitis (inflammation of the glans penis and prepuce), abortion, and systemic infection in calves. It appears that different viral strains are responsible for the various clinico-pathological manifestations. **Infectious bovine rhinotracheitis and infectious pustular vulvovaginitis are the most common manifestations.**

Spread

The main sources of infection are the nasal exudate and coughed-up droplets, genital secretions, semen and foetal fluids and tissues. **Aerosol (droplet) infection** is considered to be the method of spread of the respiratory disease. **Venereal transmission** is the method of spread of the genital diseases. **The IBR virus may survive for up to 1 year in frozen semen.**

Pathogenesis

In the respiratory disease the virus multiplies in the nasal cavities and upper respiratory tract, resulting in rhinitis, laryngitis and tracheitis. There is extensive loss of cilia in the trachea. This leaves the tracheal epithelium covered with microvilli. **This has an adverse effect on the defence mechanisms of the respiratory tract**. Spread from the nasal cavities to the ocular tissues occurs through lachrymal ducts, and causes conjuctivitis. Spread from the nasal mucosa through the trigeminal peripheral nerve to the trigeminal ganglion may occur, resulting in a non-suppurative encephalitis. Systemic invasion by the virus is followed by localization of the virus in several different tissues. The virus may be transported by peripheral leukocytes to the placenta, and transferred to the foetus to cause abortion. **The foetus is highly**

susceptible to the IBR virus.

Signs

These are described under various clinical forms.

Respiratory Form

Young cattle are most susceptible. The disease is highly infectious, with morbidity approaching 100% and mortality up to 10% of infected animals. The symptoms begin with fever, anorexia, and a mucous nasal discharge, which later becomes mucopurulent. Respiratory distress is noticeable by dilated nostrils, mouth breathing, dyspnoea, and coughing. Conjunctivitis often accompanies the respiratory form. The course is usually about 10 days.

The gross lesions are limited to the nasal passages, paranasal sinuses, trachea, and bronchi. Nasal and turbinate mucosae are congested and oedematous and contain thick mucopurulent exudate. Lining of all paranasal sinuses is congested, has excess mucus, and sometimes shows petechiae. The tracheal mucosa is similarly congested, oedematous, and covered with mucopurulent exudate. Severe oedema in the wall of the trachea may cause the wall to become as much as 2 cm thick, thereby decreasing the diameter of the lumen. Stenosis (narrowing) of the trachea contributes to the respiratory distress, and may result in **death from asphyxia, or bronchopneumonia. Microscopically,** there is necrosis of the respiratory tract mucosa with intense neutrophilic and mononuclear infiltration of the submucosa. The mucosa becomes ulcerated and has fibrin and necrotic debris. **Intranuclear inclusion bodies are present in epithelial cells.**

Neonatal Form

During an outbreak of IBR, the infection in **very young calves** may become generalized. The condition is acute and usually fatal, with no signs of respiratory system involvement. Lesions consist of widespread focal necrosis in the respiratory epithelium, liver, kidney, spleen, lymph nodes, oesophagus, and forestomachs. **Intranuclear inclusion bodies** have been described in each of these tissues.

Genital Form

In 1957, it was discovered that IBR virus also causes another bovine disease with very different manifestations. This disease, "**infectious pustular vulvovaginitis**", has been known for many years under such names as **coital exanthema, vesicular venereal disease, vesicular vaginitis, coital vesicular vaginitis,** or **coital vesicular exanthema.** This **infection involves mainly the female genital tract,** but lesions may occur on male genitalia as well. **Clinical signs** in the cow appear within 24-72 hours after coitus with an infected bull. The mucosa of the vulva becomes reddened with dark red punctate (pinpoint) foci, which quickly form **vesicles** and **pustules** (0.1-5.0 mm in diameter). The pustules soon form a membrane by fusion. The membrane soon gets detached and presents an underlying zone of ulceration. Vulva may be swollen. Affected bulls may have similar lesions on the penis and prepuce. Healing of all these lesions is complete in about 2 weeks. However, recurrent attacks may occur due to the recurrence of latent infection, as seen in herpes simplex type 2 infections in humans. **Cows and bulls can carry the virus in the absence of visible lesions. Microscopically**, the lesions consist of foci of necrosis of the mucosal epithelium with an associated inflammatory reaction. **Intranuclear inclusion bodies** develop within epithelial cells.

Abortion

The IBR virus is also an important cause of abortion in cattle. The abortion usually occurs after the rhinotracheitis form of the disease, and **up to 60% of pregnant cows in a herd may abort.** Although abortion may occur at any stage of pregnancy, it is most common in the third trimester (i.e., last three months). At the time of abortion, there is no visible clinical disease in the dam. Advanced postmortem autolysis is the most striking gross finding in the foetus, which is expelled 24-36 hours after intrauterine death. **Microscopically**, characteristic lesions in the foetus consist of focal necrosis in the liver, lymph nodes, spleen and kidney. **Intranuclear inclusion bodies** are found in these tissues. However, they may be difficult to demonstrate due to the extensive autolysis.

The pattern of IBR abortion and the foetal lesions are remarkably similar to equine rhinopneumonitis abortion in mares. Both diseases are caused by herpesviruses.

Diagnosis

A presumptive diagnosis of any form may be made on the basis of characteristic clinical signs, and demonstration of necrotizing lesions containing **intranuclear inclusion bodies**. The diagnosis may be confirmed by isolation and characterization of the virus. The virus can be detected in nasal swabs by the use of an enzyme-linked immunosorbent assay (ELISA) test, direct and indirect immunofluorescence techniques, immunoperoxidase, and by electron microscopic examination which may reveal herpes-like viral particles. Several serological tests are available for the detection of antibody, which include the ELISA test, the indirect or passive haemagglutination test, and the virus neutralization test.

Bovine Ulcerative Mammillitis

Also known as '**bovine herpesvirus mammillitis**' (**mammillitis** is inflammation of teats), bovine ulcerative mammillitis is a viral disease of cattle characterized by **severe ulceration of the skin of the teats and udder**. This specific ulcerative disease of the bovine teat was first reported in 1964, and is caused by **bovine herpesvirus 2 (BHV-2).**

Lesions

The lesions are mostly confined to the teats, although they may spread to the skin of the udder and perineum, and to the face and oral cavity of nursing calves. **Lesions** begin as local areas of erythema and oedema, and progress to **vesicles**, which rupture, leaving ulcers. Healing usually occurs in 10-18 days. **Microscopically,** the changes resemble other localized herpesvirus-induced lesions, i.e., lesions of herpesvirus simplex B. In the epidermis, ballooning degeneration, intercellular oedema, and necrosis lead to vesicle formation. Multinucleated giant cells form within the epidermis. **Intranuclear inclusion bodies** are numerous in epithelial cells and giant cells. A cellular inflammatory response develops in the dermis.

Diagnosis

The disease must be differentiated from cowpox, pseudo-cowpox, and lumpy skin disease. Microscopically, the presence of giant cells and **intranuclear inclusion bodies** differentiate the herpes infections from poxvirus infections, **which are characterized by cytoplasmic inclusions**. Viral isolation and identification confirm the diagnosis.

Equine Alpha-Herpesvirus Infections

Horses are subject to three alpha-herpesviruses: 1) **equine herpesvirus type 1** (equine herpesvirus-1, subtype 1). This is an important cause of abortion, neonatal (newborn) death, respiratory disease, and neurological disease. 2) **equine herpesvirus type 4** (equine herpesvirus-1, subtype 2). This mainly causes acute respiratory disease in young horses (**equine viral rhinopneumonitis**), but may also cause abortion. 3) **equine herpesvirus type 3**. This causes **equine coital exanthema. Equine herpesvirus type 2 is a beta-herpesvirus (cytomegalovirus).**

Virtually nothing is known about the latency, or recurrence of the equine herpesviruses. Infection with the viruses EHV-1 and EHV-4 is universally common in horses, **including India.**

Spread

The disease is highly infectious, and **spread occurs by the inhalation of infected droplets**, or by the **ingestion** of material contaminated by nasal discharges, or aborted foetuses.

Equine Herpesvirus Abortion

This disease is caused by herpesvirus equi type 1, and is characterized by intra-uterine death of near-term equine foetuses. It is a particular hazard in horse breeding establishments. **In India,** EHV-1 causing **abortion in mares** was recorded in 1975.

Signs

Infection of the foetus has some characteristic features, by which a presumptive diagnosis can often be made. The disease affects the foetus during the 8th to 11th months of pregnancy. **The majority of abortions occur in the 9th and 10th month.** The foetus is expelled from the uterus immediately after death. Complications such as retained placenta, delayed involution, and post-parturient (after parturition) metritis are rare. The mare usually recovers promptly. A storm of abortions may occur. As many as 90% of the pregnant mares in a band (group) may be affected. Neonatal infection may lead to fatal generalized disease.

Lesions

Lesions in the **aborted foetus** are typically found in the lungs, liver, and lymph nodes. Changes in the **liver** are seen grossly as tiny grey subcapsular foci. **Microscopically**, these foci consist of aggregations of necrotic liver cells. Liver cells surrounding the foci of necrosis often contain small **eosinophilic intranuclear inclusion bodies.** In the **lung,** interlobular oedema and excessive pleural fluid are constant gross lesions. The microscopic lesions consist of cellular debris in the lumen of the bronchi and bronchioles, and erosion of adjacent epithelium. In epithelial cells near the eroded areas, the nuclei contain eosinophilic inclusion bodies similar to those in liver cells. Similar intranuclear inclusions and foci of necrosis are found in the **spleen** and **lymph nodes** in many cases.

Equine Viral Rhinopneumonitis

The causative agent of rhinopneumonitis of horses is **"herpesvirus equi type 4"**, a virus closely related to the herpesvirus of **"equine herpesvirus abortion"**. In India, equine rhinopneumonitis caused by EHV-1 was recorded in 1975.

Signs

In young horses of 1-4 years, fever develops with a sudden onset. Slight congestion of nasal and conjunctival mucosa occurs, and a dry hacking cough may develop. The fever usually subsides in 2-4 days, and the animal recovers soon. In complicated cases, severe respiratory symptoms may appear, particularly when beta-haemolytic streptococci are also involved. **Death may result from pneumonia**, or in a few cases from streptococcal septicaemia. One late complication (sequel) is damage to the left recurrent laryngeal nerve, which produces paralysis of the vocal cords, causing characteristic sounds with each inspiration (**"roaring"**). Rarely, the virus may also cause late abortion.

Lesions

Most horses recover. In those which succumb lesions are often complicated by haemolytic streptococci and other bacteria. In fatal cases lesions are haemorrhagic or purulent bronchopneumonia or even disseminated abscesses. The virus attacks the respiratory epithelium, resulting in lysis and **intranuclear inclusion bodies**, which are usually only a few at this stage of the disease. The main lesions are purulent rhinitis, tracheitis, and pneumonia.

Equine Coital Exanthema

This disease more or less resembles infectious pustular vulvo-vaginitis. It is caused by **herpesvirus equi type 3**, which is different from other equine herpesviruses. The disease is characterized by vesicles, pustules, erosions, and ulcers of the vagina, vulva, perineum, penis and prepuce, and less often on the teats and lips. The lesions heal without complication. The virus does not cause abortion. **In India**, equine coital exanthema was reported for the first time from Karnataka in 1987 and then from Haryana and Punjab in the same year.

Equine Herpesvirus Associated Meningo-encephalomyelitis

A syndrome of ataxia (muscular incoordination) and paralysis has been reported in horses following epizootics (outbreaks) of herpesvirus abortion or respiratory disease (probably caused by equine herpesvirus 1). **Clinically,** there is sudden onset of foreleg and/or hindleg lameness, causing ataxia. This may rapidly progress to paralysis of legs and even to complete quadriplegia (paralysis affecting all four legs) and recumbency (state of lying down) often causing death. The nature of the meningo-encephalomyelitis is not similar to that caused by other alpha-herpesviruses. **Inclusion bodies are absent,** and it is difficult to recover virus. **Microscopically,** lesions in the brain, spinal cord, and meninges consist of arteriolitis (inflammation of arterioles) characterized by mononuclear cuffing and infiltration, medial necrosis, endothelial hyperplasia, and necrosis and thrombosis. The pathogenesis of the vasculitis is not understood, but an immune complex-mediated disease has been suggested.

Diagnosis of Alpha-Herpesvirus Infections

The clinical picture of a mild upper respiratory infection in horses, with a high incidence of abortions in mares, and characteristic lesions in the aborted foetuses, are virtually diagnostic of equine viral rhinopneumonitis. As an upper respiratory tract infection it must be differentiated from strangles, with its catarrhal rhinitis and lymph node abscessation; from the more severe equine viral arteritis in which there are no lesions in aborted foetuses, and from equine influenza. Until proved to be otherwise, all abortions in mares should be considered as being caused by equine herpesvirus 1.

Of the serological tests available, the immunofluorescent test is most sensitive. An ELISA test has been established, and a **polymerase chain reaction (PCR)** is a sensitive technique for the detection of equine herpesviruses in such specimens as naso-pharyngeal swabs. The virus can be isolated in tissue culture, chick-embryos and hamsters, from either nasal washings, or aborted foetuses.

Feline Viral Rhinotracheitis

This disease is caused by a herpesvirus called **"feline herpesvirus 1"**. The disease is manifested by sudden onset of sneezing, and copious discharge of a mucous nasal exudate. This exudate may be seen sticking to the nostrils. Ulcerative glossitis often occurs. A transient fever occurs in the early stages. Young recently weaned kittens are particularly susceptible, but the disease may affect cats of all ages.

Lesions

Lesions are confined to the nasal cavity, tongue, pharynx, larynx, and trachea, only rarely involving the lungs. The virus attacks the respiratory and oral epithelium, resulting in necrosis of cells, and in the early stages presence of **intranuclear inclusion bodies**. Necrosis in the epithelium is followed by ulceration and leukocytic infiltration.

The virus may also cause abortion, and systemic disease of the neonate (newborn) in a manner similar to other herpesvirus infections such as herpesvirus simplex, herpesvirus canis, and infectious bovine rhinotracheitis.

Infectious Laryngotracheitis

Also known simply as "**laryngotracheitis (LT)**", infectious laryngotracheitis (ILT) is **a viral respiratory tract infection of chickens which may result in severe production losses due to mortality and/or decreased egg production**. The disease is caused by an **alpha-herpesvirus**, and was first reported from the USA in 1925. ILT occurs worldwide, **including India. The virus appears to infect naturally only the fowl**, and sometimes the pheasant. **The virus affects only the respiratory tract and conjunctiva**, and strains vary in virulence. **Fowls of all ages are susceptible.** Although greatest susceptibility occurs in the **very young chicks (and broilers)**, the disease is mostly seen in the field in birds from 3-9 months old. In endemic areas, older birds are usually immune. In general, males are more susceptible than females, and the heavier breeds more susceptible than light. The disease is aggravated by concurrent infection with a variety of other pathogens, such as the viruses of Ranikhet disease, infectious bronchitis and fowlpox, and also *Haemophilus paragallinarum* and *Mycoplasma gallisepticum*. Deficiency of vitamin A and excess ammonia in the atmosphere may also predispose to a more severe disease.

Aetiology

ILT virus is an **enveloped, double-stranded DNA (dsDNA) virus**. The complete virus particle has a diameter of 195-250 nm. The **envelope** contains fine projections representing **viral glycoprotein spikes** on its surface. Replication of ILT virus is similar to that of other alpha-herpesviruses, such as pseudorabies virus and herpes simplex virus. **ILT virus strains vary in virulence from highly virulent strains** which produce high morbidity and mortality **to strains of low virulence** which produce mild-to-inapparent infection. **Antigenically the virus strains appear to be homogeneous** based on virus neutralization, immunofluorescence tests, cross-protection studies, and ELISA. The virus can survive away from the host for **several weeks** under farm conditions, and longer when the environment is very cold.

Spread

Transmission through the egg is not known to occur. The virus is present mainly in the exudate from the nares, oropharynx, trachea, and the conjunctiva. Infection is spread in **aerosol (droplets)** form from infected birds, i.e., **through the upper respiratory and ocular routes**. It enters the body through the upper respiratory tract and conjunctiva. **Ingestion** can also be a mode of infection. However, exposure of nasal epithelium following ingestion is required with this route. Among recovered birds, the virus can become latent and the birds carriers. Thus, birds which appear healthy may excrete the virus for long periods, **perhaps for several years**. However, spread occurs more readily from acutely infected birds than through contact with clinically recovered carrier birds. Because of the survival of the virus outside the body of the host, **fomites**, such as infected crates, receptacles, equipment and buildings, and **mechanical carriers**, such as people, wild birds, vermin (insects), and cats and dogs can be transmitters of the virus.

Pathogenesis

The virus initiates infection by **attachment to cell receptors**. This is followed by fusion of the envelope with the host cell plasma membrane. The nucleocapsid is released into the cytoplasm and transported to the nuclear membrane. Viral DNA is released from the nucleocapsid, and migrates into the nucleus through nuclear pores. **Transcription and replication of viral DNA occur within the nucleus**. Infection of the upper respiratory tract is followed by **intense viral replication**. Infectious virus is usually present in tracheal tissues and secretions for 6-8 days, and at very low levels up to 10 days. **Virus multiplication is limited to respiratory tissues, with no evidence of viraemia**. From trachea the virus spreads to trigeminal ganglia 4-7 days after tracheal exposure. Reactivation of latent virus from the trigeminal ganglia after long periods has been recorded. More recently, with the use of polymerase chain reaction (PCR) technology, **it has been confirmed that the** trigeminal ganglion is the main site of virus latency.

Clinically inapparent infection of the respiratory tract is a major feature of virus persistence. Studies have revealed a "field" carrier rate of about 2% for periods up to 16 months after a disease outbreak. Other studies have revealed latent tracheal infections for similar periods in 50% or more of infected chickens.

Signs

The period of incubation is about 6-12 days. Infection may result in **peracute, acute, mild, or asymptomatic disease**. In the **peracute form**, the bird may be found dead without prodromal (warning) signs; or show sudden acute dyspnoea with severe coughing and expectoration of mucus, and blood-stained exudate and blood clots, followed by death in 1-3 days. In the **acute form** dyspnoea is a feature, but it is not as sudden in onset, or as severe as in the peracute form. **Obstruction of the trachea with exudate causes the bird to breathe with long drawn-out gasps, with a wide open beak**. In some birds, there may be nasal discharge and conjunctivitis with frothy exudate at the canthus of the eye. In birds which are severely dyspnoeic, there is cyanosis of the face and wattles, and death usually occurs in 3-4 days. In other birds, dyspnoea increases and then subsides, and recovery occurs in 2-3 weeks. In the **mild form**, the signs include moist rales, slight coughing and head shaking, nasal exudate and conjunctivitis. **Egg production is affected and may stop completely for a time,** but in those birds which recover, egg production returns to normal. The **asymptomatic form** occurs without clinical signs. Its presence in a small flock may be undetected.

Gross Lesions

The **gross lesions vary with the severity of the disease**. In most cases they are restricted to the upper respiratory tract. In the **peracute form**, there is **haemorrhagic tracheitis**. The trachea contains blood casts, or is filled with blood-stained mucus. There is respiratory obstruction. In the **acute form** caseous, diphtheritic exudate, mucus and some haemorrhage occur in the trachea, and usually cause obstructive plugs in the laryngeal and syrinx regions. The trachea is often very congested and cyanotic. In the **mild form**, there may be excess mucus with or without diphtheritic exudate in the trachea. Conjunctivitis is the most common ocular lesion. The lungs and airsacs are rarely affected, but there may be congestion of the lungs, and some thickening of the airsac walls and caseous exudate in the lumen.

Microscopic Lesions

Early microscopic changes in tracheal mucosa include loss of goblet cells and infiltration with inflammatory cells. As the infection progresses, **cells enlarge, lose cilia, and become oedematous. Multinucleated cells (syncytia)** are formed, and lymphocytes, histiocytes and plasma cells migrate into the mucosa and submucosa after 2-3 days. Later, cell destruction and desquamation result in a mucosal surface lacking any epithelial covering. Haemorrhage may occur in cases of severe epithelial destruction and desquamation with exposure and rupture of blood capillaries. **Intranuclear inclusion bodies** are found in the epithelial cells by 3 days. They are generally present in the early stages of infection (1-5 day). They disappear as infection progresses due to the necrosis and desquamation of epithelial cells.

Diagnosis

Usually diagnosis of ILT requires laboratory help, as other respiratory pathogens can cause similar clinical signs and lesions. Only in cases of severe acute disease with high mortality and expectoration of blood can ILT be diagnosed reliably on the basis of clinical signs. Laboratory diagnosis is based on **demonstration of intranuclear inclusion bodies**, virus isolation, detection of ILT virus antigens in tracheal tissues or respiratory mucus, detection of ILT virus DNA, or serology.

ILT is characterized by the development of **pathognomonic intranuclear inclusion bodies** in respiratory and conjunctival epithelial cells. A variety of different procedures have been described for rapid diagnosis of ILT, including fluorescent antibody (FA) procedures, an immunoperoxidase (IP) procedure, enzyme-linked immunosorbent assays (ELISA), electron microscopy, DNA hybridization techniques, and PCR techniques. Techniques for demonstration of ILT virus antibodies in serum include agar-gel immunodiffusion (AGID), virus neutralization (VN), indirect fluorescent antibody (IFA) test, and ELISA.

Duck Virus Enteritis

Also known as "**duck plague**", duck virus enteritis (DVE) is **an acute contagious disease of ducks, geese, and swans** caused by **a herpesvirus**, probably alpha type. The disease was first reported from The Netherlands in 1949. The disease at times has resulted in heavy losses in ducks and geese.

Spread between birds is rapid, transmission being direct from bird to bird, or indirect from the contaminated environment. Vertical transmission through the egg has been shown experimentally.

Signs

The incubation period following exposure is 3-7 days. In adults, a serious drop in egg production may occur. Ataxia is common. Birds use their wings to aid walking or swimming. Photophobia, pasted eyelids, nasal discharge, inappetence, thirst, soiled vents, and diarrhoea are usually seen.

Lesions

Multiple tissue haemorrhages are seen as well as free **blood in body cavities and lumen of the gut**. Petechial and larger haemorrhages may be seen on the heart, liver, pancreas, intestines, lungs, and kidneys. In the adult female the ovarian follicles may be deformed and discoloured. **Microscopically**, the disease in its early stages is one of vascular damage, and later, areas of necrosis are seen. Intranuclear inclusion bodies can be seen.

Mortality following the clinical signs is usually rapid (1-5 days) and may exceed 90%, particularly in adult birds.

Diagnosis

A presumptive diagnosis can be made on the basis of gross and histopathological lesions. Isolation and identification of virus confirms the diagnosis even in the absence of typical lesions. Serological procedures for detecting antibodies include a reverse passive haemagglutination test and enzyme-linked immunosorbent assay (ELISA).

Pigeon Herpesvirus Infection

This infection is caused by **pigeon herpesvirus 1** (most probably alpha), which is antigenically different from duck virus enteritis agent.

Spread

Susceptible pigeons can be infected **through direct contact** with infected birds. Egg transmission of the virus seems unlikely. Mature pigeons in infected flocks are asymptomatic carriers of the virus, and some of them may shed virus from time to time.

Signs

Clinical disease is observed mainly in young pigeons not protected by maternal antibodies. In the **acute form**, pigeons sneeze frequently and show conjunctivitis, and nostrils become obstructed with mucus and moisture. In the **chronic form**, sinusitis and intense dyspnoea may be observed.

Lesions

Grossly, mucous membranes of the mouth, pharynx and larynx are congested and covered with foci of necrosis and small ulcers. The mucous membrane of the pharynx may be coated with diphtheritic membranes. In generalized infection (**viraemia**), foci of necrosis can be observed in the liver. **Microscopically**, foci of necrosis are observed in the lining epithelium of pharynx, larynx, and trachea. In generalized infections, pigeons show hepatitis. **Intranuclear inclusion bodies are found in many hepatic cells widely throughout the organ.**

Diagnosis

Diagnosis is based on isolation and identification of the causative agent, and demonstration of sp ecific antibodies by serological tests, which include virus neutralization test, indirect immunofluorescence, and counter-immunoelectrophoresis.

Diseases caused by Beta-Herpesviruses

Cytomegalic Inclusion Diseases

"Cytomegalic inclusion diseases" affect a variety of animal species, including h umans. These are caused by **host-specific viruses called "cytomegaloviruses", which are classified within the beta-herpesvirus group**. The characteristic feature of these viruses is that thay induce the **formation of extremely large cells (megalocytes)** of up to 40 μm in diameter, which carry **large intranuclear inclusion bodies.**

In contrast to alpha-herpesviruses, cytoplasmic inclusion bodies are also often present. These represent accumulations of mature virions in cyto-plasmic vesicles. Most of the cytomegaloviruses have a peculiar affinity for the salivary glands. The infection is usually latent or su bclinical, but under proper c ircumstances, generalized a nd often f atal infection m ay develop. Specific cytomegaloviruses have been isolated from humans, pigs (**inclusion body rhinitis**), cattle (**bovine herpesvirus 3**), horses (**equine herpesvirus 2**), cats, guinea-pigs, mice, rats, monkeys, and ground squirrels. **In most species, the infection is of little importance.** As with most herpesviruses, incidence of infection is very high, and remains latent for life with periodic shedding, usually in the urine. O nly cytomegalic inclusion disease of pigs will be considered, since in other species no visible disease occurs in response to localized or generalized i nfection.

Inclusion Body Rhinitis of Swine

Also known as "**porcine h erpesvirus 2 infection**" and "**generalized cytomegalic inclusion body disease of swine**", inclusion body rhinitis of pigs is a cytomegalovirus disease first described in Great Britain in 1955. The disease mainly occurs in **piglets** of 2-3 weeks, and produces a mild catarrhal to purulent rhinitis. Morbidity is high, but mortality is low, unless complicated by more serious secondary p athogens. **As in humans,** the porcine virus can cross the placenta and cause foetal death, or generalized disease in neonates (newborns).

Microscopically, the picture is dominated by **intranuclear inclusion body containing megalocytes** in the glandular epithelium of the nasal cavity. Recovery is uneventful. Inclusion-bearing megalocytes have also been described in the kidney and salivary gland. The **diagnosis** is usually made from demonstration of **typical intranuclear inclusion bodies** in tissue sections. Inclusion bodies can also be demonstrated in exfoliated cells obtained from nasal swabs of live pigs. Antibody to infection can be detected by indirect immunofluorescent techniques and ELISA test.

Diseases caused by Gamma-Herpesviruses

These herpesviruses are **lymphotropic. Only two gamma-herpesviruses are important in veterinary medicine:** 1. The virus of **malignant catarrhal fever,** and 2. The virus of **Marek's disease.** Marek's disease virus appears to be gamma-herpesvirus on the basis of its lymphotropism, but its genome more closely resembles an alpha-herpesvirus.

Malignant Catarrhal Fever

Also known as **"bovine malignant catarrh (BMC)", "malignant head catarrh"** and **"snotsiekte",** malignant catarrhal fever (MCF) is **an acute, highly fatal, infectious disease of cattle caused by a gamma-herpesvirus.** BMC is also an important disease of deer and wild ruminants. The disease is characterized by catarrhal and mucopurulent inflammation of the eyes and nostrils, erosions of the nasal mucosa, rapid emaciation, enlargement of lymph nodes, corneal opacity, and nervous symptoms. The disease has a worldwide distribution. Its existence has been reported **in India.**

Spread

In Africa, the virus is carried by **wildebeest** (a wild animal, gnu) which serves as the source of infection for **cattle** (the "**wildebeest-associated**" **virus**). In the United States, sheep carry ("**sheep-associated virus**), and are the source of this infectious agent. The disease is not transmissible between infected cattle.

Signs

Infection is followed by high fever (106^0-107^0 F) and catarrhal conjunctivitis and rhinitis, which are accompanied by mucopurulent discharge from the eyes and nose. This exudate characteristically flows from the eyes and nostrils, but soon dries and sticks. The eyes are sensitive to strong light. The cornea becomes opaque in the final stages. Emaciation develops rapidly. The skin of the muzzle is eroded, and the nasal passages are obstructed by mucopurulent exudate. In some cases, erosions develop inside the cheeks and on the roof of the mouth. **These are grossly indistinguishable from the erosive oral lesions of rinderpest.** Diarrhoea is common, and nervous manifestations are seen in the final stages. In mild forms of the disease, skin lesions may be observed. These consist of thickening and peeling, particularly of the skin of the neck, axillae, and perineum. The **lymph nodes** are swollen, which is an almost constant sign. Those lymph nodes which appear as small subcutaneous nodules form a chain along the jugular groove of the neck.This can be observed clinically. **The disease is almost always fatal.**

Lesions

The most constant lesion is a marked **perivascular and intramural infiltration of mononuclear cells, mainly monocytes.** Arteries and arterioles in almost all organs are affected, and often there is medial necrosis and endothelial swelling. This change may be responsible for the inflammatory and necrotizing lesions seen grossly and m icroscopically.

Lymph nodes are always swollen, and the cut surface appears granular. The **main microscopic changes** are d ilation of lymphatic channels, and severe oedema and proliferation of reticulo-endothelial cells and lymphocytes. Changes in t he heart and skeletal m uscles are p erivascular infiltrations b y lymphoid cells. In the **nostrils**, irregularly-shaped erosions of the mucosa are covered with a mucopurulent exudate. **Microscopically**, these lesions are the result of necrosis of the epithelium and intense lymphocytic infiltration of the underlying stroma. S imilar lesions m ay develop i n the o ral and p haryngeal mucosa. Congestion, oedema, a nd erosions occur in the oesophagus, rumen, reticulum, and omasum. Erosions and ulcers may be present in the abomasum. The small and large intestines show hyperaemia and oedema.

In the **eye**, congestion and oedema are severe. The **liver** and **kidneys** are often g rossly enlarged a nd mottled. G rossly, t he renal c ortex m ay c ontain grey to w hite foci w hich resemble i nfarcts. **Microscopically**, t hese lesions consist of collections of mononuclear cells. Similar infiltrates are found in the periportal areas of the liver. In the **brain**, a "**cooked**" **gross appearance** and an odour resembling that of broth have been described. **Microscopic lesions** include oedema and lymphocytic infiltration in the meninges, and perivascular oedema and accumulation o f lymphocytes in t he m edulla, pons, olfactory bulb, a nd hippocampus, a s well a s in t he cerebrum, c erebellum, and s pinal grey matter.

Although the disease is caused by a herpesvirus, behaviour of the virus is unlike cytocidal herpesviruses, such as those of bovine viral rhinotracheitis, feline viral rhinotracheitis, or equine abortion. The behaviour of the virus does, however, resemble lymphotropic herpesvirus, such as the Epstein-Barr virus of humans. **No free virus is present in tissues of affected cattle and virions cannot be recovered; the virus is associated with lymphocytes**; in affected c attle t here are **n o inclusion bodies or syncytial giant cell formation**; the disease is not contagious among cattle; t he incubation p eriod is variable; and t he main p athological features a re lymphocytic p roliferation and i nfiltration and v asculitis. **The pathogenesis of the disease remains to be worked out**. It may be lymphoproliferative disease like that caused by Epstein-Barr virus of humans, or a n immune-mediated l ymphoproliferation and v asculitis directed a gainst viral antigens in infected cells.

Diagnosis

The diagnosis of the disease is often difficult. It should be differentiated from rinderpest by the greater infectivity and shorter course of rinderpest and its more prominent gross intestinal lesions. The microscopic changes in the mucosa and lymph nodes are also helpful in differentiating these two diseases. Until recently the virus neutralization test was the only serological test available for the presumptive diagnosis. Tests for the detection of immunofluorescent antibodies and complement-fixing antibodies have now been developed, and an ELISA test is now available for the wildebeest-associated virus. The sheep-associated virus is undetectable serologically.

Marek's Disease

Marek's disease (MD) is **a lymphoproliferative disease of chickens caused by a herpesvirus**. It is characterized by a mononuclear infiltration of the peripheral nervous system, and to a lesser degree, other tissues and visceral organs. Marek's disease virus (MDV) is **a cell-associated herpesvirus** with lymphotropic properties similar to those of **gamma-herpesviruses**. However, its molecular structure and genomic organization are similar to those of **alpha-herpesviruses**. Marek's disease exists in poultry-producing countries throughout the world, **including India**.

The disease was first described by the Hungarian veterinarian Jozsef Marek in 1907, after whom it is named "**Marek's disease**". Neural involvement, leading to paralysis, was the most visible symptom, and the names of **polyneuritis, fowl paralysis, range paralysis**, and **neurolymphomatosis** were commonly applied.

Aetiology

Marek's disease virus (MDV) is **an enveloped DNA virus**. The DNA of MDV is **a linear, double-stranded molecule (ds DNA)**. The MDV and related herpesviruses have been **classified into three serotypes**. Type-specific monoclonal antibodies are used to determine virus serotypes. **Serotype 1** comprises oncogenic strains of MDV. **Serotype 2** is a group of naturally apathogenic (non-pathogenic) strains of MDV. **Serotype 3** is the apathogenic and antigenically related herpesvirus of turkeys (HTV). Thus, it can be seen that **virulence or oncogenicity is associated only with serotype 1 viruses. Serotype 2 and 3 are non-pathogenic**. However, within serotype 1, a wide variation in pathogenic potential is recognized. **Serotype 1 strains have been subdivided into three pathotypes: 1. Mildly virulent (mMDV), 2. Virulent (vMDV), and 3. Very virulent (vvMDV). Virus infectivity *in vivo* and *in vitro* is strictly cell-associated except in the feather follicle epithelium, where cell-free virus is produced.**

Spread

The virus spreads rapidly from infected to uninfected birds. The virus is present in desquamated feather follicle epithelial cells, and in oral, nasal, and tracheal secretions. **The feather follicle cells are the most important source of infection**, and are responsible for the infectivity of dander (minute scales from feathers or skin), poultry house dust, and litter. **Infectivity in these materials can last for at least one year at room temperature**. Direct or indirect contact between birds spreads the virus. **Airborne spread of virus and infection through the respiratory tract is considered to be the most important route**. Beetles can carry the virus, but insects are not considered to be an important means of spread of infection. **The virus is not transmitted through the egg, and thus chicks are hatched free of infection.**

Once contracted, the infection persists throughout the life of the chicken, and infected birds continue to contaminate the environment by shedding the virus.

Epidemiology (Factors Influencing the Disease)

There are a number of factors which influence the clinical picture and severity of Marek's disease in an individual chicken, and the severity of an outbreak in a flock. The **genetic constitution** of the chicken greatly influences the incidence and pathology of the disease. The genetic resistance is not resistance to infection, but resistance to the development of disease after infection. **Genetic resistance is of two types**: 1. One is associated with a **major histocompatibility complex allele (B21)**. It is thought to be the result of a **superior immune response**. 2. The second type is independent of the histocompatibility locus. It is determined by **susceptibility of T cells to transformation**.

The **sex of the chicken** also influences the incidence of the disease. **Females are more susceptible than males**. The **age at infection** and **immune status of the chicken** are also important. Resistance to the development of disease increases with the age. Chickens with passive or active immunity are more resistant.

The **strain of virus** is also important. The more pathogenic strains have a greater chance of producing the disease. Also important is that infection with a non-pathogenic or mild strain may occur first. This would result in the development of immunity against the effects of later infection with a pathogenic strain. Apart from this, **stress** is the main environmental factor associated with increased incidence of the disease. Movement, vaccination against other diseases, handling, beak trimming, and changes of food are stresses which are of potential importance.

MD Virus-Cell Interactions

For a better understanding of the **pathogenesis**, it would be helpful if we discuss first **virus-cell interactions.**These **are of three types**: 1. **Productive**, 2. **Latent**, and 3. **Transforming**.

In the **productive infection**, replication of the viral DNA occurs and virus particles are produced. The number of genome copies (i.e., virus particles) per cell can e xceed 1200. T here are t wo **types of productive infection**: 1 **Fully productive infection** with virus in the feather follicle epithelium (FFE) results in the development of a large number of **enveloped, fully infectious virions**. 2. **In productive-restrictive infection** also virions are produced, but most of the virions are **non-enveloped**, and therefore **non-infectious**. In all types of cells, **productive infection is lytic** and leads to intranuclear inclusion body formation, cell destruction, and formation of frank necrotic lesion. Because of this, **productive infection** has been termed **cytolytic**, and the terms are used synonymously.

Latent infections are **non-productive**, i.e., no virus particles are produced. Latent infection can be detected only by hybridization with DNA probes. At least two cytokines help in maintaining latency. One of this has been identified and is **interferon**. Interferon suppresses production of viral particles in latently infected l ymphocytes.

Transforming infection occurs in cells transformed by serotype 1 Marek's disease virus. Unlike latent infection, in which the viral genome (virus) is present but is expressed only to a very limited degree, the t ransforming infection is characterized by more extensive expression of the viral genome, sometimes resulting in viral particle production. Transformed cells contain about 5-15 copies of viral genome (viral particles). A **Marek's disease tumour-associated surface antigen (MATSA)** develops on cells of MD lymphomas and lymphoblastoid cell lines derived from lymphomas. This antigen is not present on the surface of productively infected cells. However, MATSA was also detected on lymphocytes from c hickens vaccinated w ith herpesvirus o f turkeys (HVT), and non-oncogenic strains of MDV. Subsequent studies with monoclonal antibodies revealed MATSA to be present on activated T cells from uninfected chickens. Thus, **MATSA is now considered to be a host antigen and is not tumour-specific. It is simply a marker for activated T cells.**

Pathogenesis

Pathogenesis of Marek's disease can be described in **four phases of infection**: 1. **Early productive-restrictive virus infection**, causing mainly degenerative (cytolytic) changes, 2. **Latent infection**, 3. **A second-phase of cytolytic, productive-restrictive infection** coinciding with permanent immunosuppression, and 4. **A proliferative phase involving non-productively infected** lymphoid cells which may or may not progress to lymphoma formation.

The virus enters through the respiratory tract, where it is picked up by the phagocytic cells. **An acute phase of the disease follows** within 3-4 days, characterized by **cytolytic infection** of the lymphoid system, most marked in the bursa of Fabricius, thymus, and also spleen. **The primary target cells in all these organs are B cells,** although some activated T cells become infected and undergo degeneration as well. Resting T cells are resistant to infection. The necrotizing effects of this early infection provoke an acute inflammatory reaction with infiltration of macrophages, granulocytes, and lymphocytes. Infected birds normally recover from the acute phase of the disease and after 6-7 days the infection becomes latent.

At about 6-7 days, the infection switches to latency. This coincides with the development of **immune responses.** Cell-mediated immunity (CMI) has been shown to be important. **Most latently infected cells are T cells, although B cells can also be involved.** The virus is spread throughout the body by infected lymphocytes, and a persistent, cell-associated viraemia is present. A secondary cytolytic infection occurs in the FFE two weeks after primary infection and infectious cell-free virus is produced and shed into the environment in feather debris and dander. **The latent infection is persistent, and can last for the life of the bird.**

Infection in genetically resistant birds does not progress beyond the second phase (latency). Susceptible birds, on the other hand, develop **a second wave of cytolytic infections** after the second or third week coinciding with **permanent immunosuppression.** The lymphoid organs are again involved, and foci of infection occur in tissues of epithelial origin in various organs (e.g., kidney, pancreas, adrenal gland, proventriculus etc.), and especially in the **skin,** where a prominent infection of the feather follicle epithelium (FFE) occurs. **Infection of FFE is unique in that it is the only known site of complete virus replication.** There is focal necrosis, and inflammatory reactions develop around affected areas.

Lymphoproliferative changes constitute the final response and may progress to tumour development. Transformed T cells proliferate in peripheral nerves and other tissues and organs, leading to type A nerve infiltrations and lymphoma formation. Transformed T cells contain viral genome, but the synthesis of viral particles is severely restricted. Death from lymphomas may occur at any time from about 3 weeks onward.

Lymphomas

The composition of lymphomas is complex. They consist of a mixture of neoplastic, inflammatory, and immunologically active cells. **Both T and B cells are present, but the former predominate.** The usual target cells for transformation are CD4+ activated T cells, probably **T- helper cells**. As mentioned, a normal antigen (**MATSA**) found on some populations of non-infected, activated T cells may be marker since it is present on tumour cells, **but is not tumour-specific**. More recenly it has been proposed that MD tumours are of **clonal origin**.

Vaccination alters the pathogenesis of infection by severely reducing or eliminating the early cytolytic phase. Also, the level of latent infection is markedly reduced. Moreover, neither late cytolytic infection nor immunosuppression occurs. Vaccinal immunity and embryonal bursectomy both suppress the active viral infection, thereby prevent an inflammatory reaction, and both reduce the incidence of tumours.

Clinical Signs

Marek's disease affects chickens from about 6 weeks of age. It occurs usually between 12 and 24 weeks of age, but older chickens may also be affected. The incubation period may be as short as 3-4 weeks in some, and several months in others. **Clinical disease occurs in several forms**.

Classical Marek's Disease

Mortality is variable, but rarely exceeds 10-15%. In some outbreaks, mortality is confined to a few weeks, while in others a low incidence continues over many months. **The signs depend on the peripheral nerves affected**. Involvement of **brachial and sciatic nerves** is common, and leads to progressive **spastic paralysis** (i.e., paralysis accompanied by muscular rigidity) **of the wings and legs**. Sometimes, when the **cervical nerves** are involved, there may be **torticollis** (twisting of the neck); and if the **vagus** and **intercostal nerves** are affected, **respiratory signs** may develop. The interval between onset of signs and death varies from a few days to several weeks. **Rarely birds may recover**.

Acute Marek's Disease

Mortality in this form is usually much higher than in the classical form. Mortality of 10-30% of the flock is common, and outbreaks involving up to 80% of the flock are recorded. Many birds die suddenly without preceding symptoms. Others appear depressed before death, and some show paralytic signs similar to those seen in the classical form.

Transient Paralysis

This is an **uncommon** encephalitic manifestation of Marek's disease in birds between 5 and 18 weeks of age. Birds suddenly develop varying degrees of paresis (partial paralysis) or paralysis of the legs, wings and neck. Mortality is low. The disease is characterized by recovery, and signs usually disappear within 24-48 hours.

Gross Lesions

In classical Marek's disease, the characteristic lesion is enlargement of one or more peripheral nerves. Affected nerves are up to 2-3 times the normal thickness. The normal striated and white glistening appearance is lost, and the nerve may appear greyish and sometimes oedematous. Nerves commonly affected are the brachial and sciatic plexi (singular, plexus = a network of nerves), coeliac plexus, abdominal vagus, and intercostal nerves. Some paralysed birds show no visible nerve enlargement at necropsy, but characteristic nerve lesions are found microscopically. Sometimes, lymphomas are present in addition to nerve lesions. These tumours occur usually in the ovary, and are mostly small, soft, and grey in appearance, or rarely large, yellowish, and lobulated. Lungs, kidney, heart, and liver are sometimes affected by lymphomas.

Acute Marek's disease is characterized by diffuse lymphomatous involvement, and enlargement of the liver, gonads, spleen, kidneys, lungs, proventriculus and heart. Sometimes, lymphomas also arise in the skin in association with feather follicles (known as "skin leukosis" in the USA), and in the muscles. In younger birds liver enlargement is moderate, but in adult birds the liver is greatly enlarged, which is similar to that in lymphoid leukosis. Most birds have some degree of lymphoid infiltration of the nerves, while some adults do not.

Microscopic Lesions

The basic pathological process is the same in classical and acute Marek's disease. The disease begins as a proliferation of lymphoid cells. Proliferation is progressive in some cases, and undergoes regressive changes in others. In the classical form regressive changes are more common than in the acute form, in which the lymphoid proliferation leads to widespread tumour formation.

In the nervous system, peripheral nerves are affected by proliferative, inflammatory or chronic but minor lesions, termed type A, B, and C, respectively. Type A lesion consists of proliferating lymphoid cells, lymphoblasts, and small, medium and large lymphocytes. Type B lesion is characterized by inter-neuritic oedema, Schwann cell proliferation, and light to moderate infiltration of mainly small lymphocytes and plasma cells. A primary cell mediated demyelination occurs in the type A and B nerves, causing paralysis. Type C lesion consists of lightly scattered lymphocytes and plasma cells.

Type A lesion is the primary reaction and is seen most commonly in chickens dying early in the disease. It is usually associated with lymphoid tumours than the type B lesion. Type B lesion follows type A, and is usually seen in chickens with disease of longer standing. Type C lesion is seen in infected birds which show no clinical signs. Lesions of the CNS include proliferative lymphoid lesions of the type A, but inflammatory lesions characteristic of a viral encephalomyelitis are more common. **The most prominent change is perivascular cuffing**, but microgliosis and endotheliosis may also occur.

The most common lesions in visceral organs are lymphoid tumours. These are made up of cells similar to the type A lesion of peripheral nerves. **The malignantly transformed cell is a thymus-dependent lymphocyte (T cell), and the lymphoma** consists of a mixture of malignant T cells and reactive, bursa-dependent lymphocytes (B cells), T cells, and macrophages. Although proliferative lesions are seen in the bursa of Fabricius, degenerative changes are also seen in this organ as well as in the thymus. In both these organs, there may be hypoplasia. In the bursa of Fabricius cysts are also seen.

Immunity

Importance of the immune response in Marek's disease is **due to four reasons**: 1. MD can be immunosuppressive, 2. Immunological response is the basis of resistance to MD, 3. Vaccinal immunity is the most important means of control, and 4. Immunological response contributes to the cellular mass of the lymphoma (see pathogenesis).

Immunosuppression

Impairment of the immune response can result directly **from lytic infection of lymphocytes,** or indirectly from activity of **suppressor cell populations.** Probably both are important. Permanent immunosuppression correlates with eventual tumour development. **Both humoral immunity and cell-mediated immunity are depressed.** Thus, MD virus infection can increase susceptibility of birds to infection with coccidia. It is emphasized that while there is depression, there is not a total loss of function.

Immune Responses

Both humoral and cell-mediated immunity develop in competent birds after infection with MD virus. Humoral immunity is due to the development of precipitating and virus-neutralizing (VN) antibodies. Since antibodies are not required in immune resistance of MD, it is believed that cell-mediated immunity (CMI) is important. **Thus, functional T cells are required for resistance, as well as vaccinal immunity.**

Vaccinal Immunity

This is immunological in nature. Regarding the **other resistance mechanisms, mac** ophages may be involved in resistance by restricting virus replication directly, or in association with antibody. Immune B cells and macrophages can interact to inactivate cell-free virus. **Various cytokines may** be important in MD, particularly **interferon.** Interferon has been shown to be important in the development and maintenance of latency. Innate (inherent) resistance in the form of **natural killer (NK) cells** could also be important.

Diagnosis

Diagnosis is made on clinical signs, and gross and microscopic lesions. Infection not accompanied by the clinical disease, is detected by viral isolation, or by demonstration of viral antigen in feather tips by agar-gel precipitation tests, or antigen in serum. The most commonly used method for isolation of MD virus is inoculation. of susceptible tissue cultures with blood lymphocytes. **However, it is emphasized that diagnosis of clinical disease cannot be made by virological and serological tests alone.**

By using **viral markers in tissues**, presence of viral infection in chicken can be detected without isolating the virus in culture. Viral antigens can be detected in feather tips and feather follicle epithelium, infected lymphoid tissues, or infected cell cultures with appropriate antibodies (monoclonal) by fluorescent antibody (FA) tests, immunoperoxidase tests, agar-gel precipitation (AGP) tests, and enzyme-linked immunosorbent assays **(ELISA)**. **Polymerase chain reaction (PCR) assays** have the potential to detect viral DNA in lymphomas. Methods utilizing **DNA probes** for the detection of MD virus DNA in feather tip extracts have been described. Also, herpesvirus particles can be detected in the FFE and other tissues by **electron microscopy**. Tests for identifying the presence of specific antibodies in the serum are useful, and include AGP, FA, ELISA, and virus neutralization. Finally, **tumour-associated markers** have been found useful. Even though **MATSA** is considered as a host antigen associated with activated T cells, this and other host cell markers have diagnostic value.

Differentiation of Marek's disease from lymphoid leukosis is important. **The main differentiating features are presented in Table 10.**

Table 10. Features useful in differentiating Marek's Disease from Lymphoid Leukosis

Feature	Marek's disease	Lymphoid leukosis
Susceptible age	6 weeks or older	Not less than 16 weeks
Symptoms	Usually paralysis	Non-specific
Incidence	Usually above 5% in unvaccinated flocks	Rarely above 5%
Gross lesions		
Neural enlargement	Frequent	Absent
Bursa of Fabricius	Diffuse enlargement or atrophy	Nodular tumours

Tumours in skin, muscle, and proventriculus	May be present	Usually absent
Microscopic lesions		
Neural involvement	Yes	No
Liver tumours	Usually perivascular	Focal or diffuse
Splenic changes	Diffuse	Often focal
Bursa of Fabricius	Interfollicular tumour and/or atrophy of follicles	Intrafollicular tumour
Central nervous system	Yes	No
Lymphoid proliferation in skin and feather follicles	Yes	No
Cytology of tumours	Pleomorphic lymphoid cells, including lymphoblasts, small, medium, and large lymphocytes and reticulum cells. Rarely can be only lymphoblasts	Lymphoblasts
Category of neoplastic lymphoid cell	T cell	B cell

Diseases caused by Poxviridae

Poxviridae

Viruses of the Family Poxviridae cause infections in humans, animals, and birds. These viruses produce generalized disease with **pustular** (Anglo-Saxon word pock = pustule) **lesions**, or **benign tumours of the skin. The pox viruses are the largest animal viruses.** They have complex, brick-shaped virions measuring up to 450 nm by 260 nm. Virions contain single, linear molecules of **double-stranded DNA (ds DNA)**, and **multiply and mature in the cytoplasm of host cells.** Sites of multiplication are visible by light microscopy as **inclusion bodies.** The virions contain several enzymes, including a DNA-dependent transcriptase. Mature virions may be released by budding in which case they are **enveloped**, or after cell lysis, in which case they **lack an envelope. Five genera contain pathogens for animals**, but several viruses have not been classified (**Table 11**).

Table 11. Diseases caused by Poxviridae

Genus	Disease
Ortho-poxvirus	Smallpox (variola)
	Vaccinia
	Cowpox
	Buffalopox
	Camelpox
	Monkeypox
	Rabbitpox
	Mousepox (ectromelia)
Capri-poxvirus	Sheep-pox
	Goatpox
	Lumpy skin disease
Sui-poxvirus	Swinepox
Avi-poxvirus	Fowl pox
	Pigeon pox
	Turkey pox
	Canary pox
Lepori-poxvirus	Myxomatosis of rabbits
	Shope fibroma of rabbits
	Hare fibroma
Para-poxvirus	Contagious pustular dermatitis
	Bovine papular stomatitis
	Pseudo-cowpox (Milker's nodules)
Unclassified	Molluscum contagiosum of human
	Ulcerative dermatosis
	Yaba poxvirus
	Horsepox

Diseases caused by Ortho-Poxviruses
Smallpox (Variola)

This **human disease, no longer in existence**, was a highly infectious viral infection with a febrile onset followed in a few days by characteristic cutaneous eruptions. Beginning as **macules** (discoloured spots), these lesions soon become **papules**, then **vesicles**, and finally, within about 10 days, **pustules**, which undergo typical umbilication (having a depression or pit like an umbilicus). **Microscopically**, epidermal cells swell, are separated by fluid, and eventually become necrotic. Before necrosis occurs, the epithelial cells contain basophilic or eosinophilic **cytoplasmic inclusion bodies**, known as **"Guarnieri bodies"**, composed of innumerable minute spherical granules, and **"Borrel"** or **"Paschen bodies"**, believed to be the elementary visible form of the virus. As necrosis progresses in the epithelium, a clear **vesicle** forms and soon gets filled with neutrophils (i.e., becomes a **pustule**). This pustular lesion, 2-4 mm in diameter appears grossly elevated above the skin surface. The contents of the pustule become desiccated, producing an umbilicated lesion. Healing follows, and a deep pitted (having a pit, depression) **scar** is left.

Vaccinia

Vaccinia is the virus used for immunization of humans against small-pox. The origin of the virus is not well understood. It is considered to have been derived from cowpox, but continuous passage over many years through humans, laboratory animals, and tissue culture, has resulted in the **"creation"** of a laboratory virus, which, although infectious to a wide range of animals, **does not exist as a natural disease**. There are two major types of vaccinia (virus), a **dermatotropic strain** and a **neurotropic strain**. These are the properties developed on the basis of propagating the virus in rabbits. The vaccinia virus, or closely related viruses, have been isolated from natural diseases in several animal species. Some of the pox viruses discussed may not be distinct entities, but rather vaccinia infections. Vaccinia is known to be infectious for rabbits, mice, cattle, sheep, pigs, monkeys, and humans. The lesions produced in each of these species are similar to those described for smallpox.

Cowpox

Cowpox is caused by a virus with an unusually wide host range. It is **closely related to, but different from, variola and vaccinia viruses. The disease, which is not common, is mild and self-limiting**. Its lesions are found only on the **teats and udder. Microscopically**, the lesions resemble smallpox, with vesicle formation and cytoplasmic inclusions. The disease is spread by milking. **Human infection may occur, with lesions usually limited to the hands.**

Cowpox, or a very similar virus, causes in **cats**, in certain European countries, lesions in the mouth, conjunctivitis, and sometimes, pneumonia. **The disease is transmissible from infected cats to humans**. Cowpox virus can infect large cats (e.g., lions, cheetahs) and elephants, where the virus often causes severe and fatal pneumonia. The reservoir of cowpox virus is believed to be wild rodents, which serve as the source of infection for other species. The disease in cows must be differentiated from **pseudo-cowpox**, and **bovine herpesvirus 2** (bovine mammillitis). Cattle are also susceptible to vaccinia. Infection usually occurs from exposure to a person recently vaccinated.

Buffalopox

This contagious disease of buffaloes, which has been reported from **India**, Indonesia, Pakistan, Egypt, Italy, and Russia, is caused by a virus similar to vaccinia virus. **Lesions occur mainly on the teats and udders of milking buffaloes.**

Camelpox

Camelpox is a debilitating, often fatal poxvirus infection of camels. It occurs in Africa and south-western Asia, including **India**. Mortality may be high, and the lesions are generalized in **young camels**. A milder, localized form of the disease develops in **older camels**. Humans are not susceptible.

Monkeypox

Monkeypox was first identified in a colony of monkeys in Denmark, in 1958. Since then it has been reported from many countries of the world. The disease has also been recognized as **a rare zoonosis, occurring sporadically in humans in Africa**. Monkeypox is characterized by a generalized cutaneous rash and pocks. These eruptions are most common on the hands, feet, legs, and buttocks. Generalized fatal infection can occur, particularly in infant monkeys, with necrotizing lesions in many visceral organs. **Microscopically,** the lesions resemble those described for smallpox. The presence of cytoplasmic inclusion bodies helps in the diagnosis.

Rabbitpox

Rabbitpox virus is indistinguishable from vaccinia. The disease may become generalized, with necrotizing lesions in visceral organs, in addition to cutaneous pocks. **The skin lesions lack the vesicular character.** Inclusion bodies have not been reported.

Mousepox (Infectious Ectromelia)

Mousepox occurs in Europe, and has caused serious outbreaks in laboratories in the United States. The **clinical disease** occurs in **two forms**: 1. A **rapidly fatal form**, with a few or no cutaneous lesions, 2. A **chronic form**, characterized by ulceration of the skin, particularly the feet, tail and snout. In the fatal form, mortality ranges from 50-100%, and varies with the strain of mouse. If death does not occur, during the stage of virus multiplication in the spleen and liver, **recovery usually follows**.

Diseases caused by Capri-Poxviruses

Three diseases which occur from infection by the viruses **of this genus** (Capri-poxviruses) are: **sheep-pox, goatpox, and lumpy skin disease. Whether they represent three different, but immunologically related viruses, is uncertain**. They may be variants of a single virus with varying degrees of species pathogenicity.

Sheep-Pox

Sheep-pox is a serious disease with cutaneous lesions appearing particularly in areas devoid of wool, such as the cheeks, lips, nostrils, and under the tail. Sheep-pox is prevalent in Asia, and Southern Europe. **It is endemic in**

India, and inflicts serious economic losses. The disease has a tendency to become generalized. **Mortality may reach 50% in adults and approach 100% in lambs.** There is variation in breed susceptibility. Merino sheep are highly susceptible, whereas Algerian sheep are comparatively resistant.

Sheep-pox is highly contagious, and in most cases **spread** appears to occur by **contact** with infected animals and contaminated articles. However, spread by **inhalation** also occurs. During an initial viraemia, the virus is deposited in most tissues, including the skin. There is an incubation period of 2-14 days. **Clinically,** in lambs the malignant form is more **common.** There is marked depression and prostration, a high fever, and discharges from the eyes and nose. Affected lambs may die during this stage before **typical pox lesions** develop. They **commence as papules, then become nodular, vesicular, pustular, and finally scabs.** Some of them progress from nodules to tumour-like masses. Skin lesions appear on unwoolled skin, and on the buccal, respiratory, digestive, and urogenital tract mucosa. In the mouth, ulcerative lesions on the tongue, gums, and cheeks are common. **The mortality rate in this form of the disease may reach 100%. In the benign form,** common in adults, only skin lesions occur, particularly under the tail, and **there is no systemic reaction.**

The **lesions in the epidermis** are similar to those of other poxviruses. Localized acanthosis (thickened epidermis) and hyperplasia are followed by **vesiculation (vesicle formation),** beginning in the middle layers of epithelium. The underlying oedematous dermis and subcutis contain many distinctive cells called **"cellules claveleuses"** of Borrel, or **"sheep-pox cells".** These cells are concentrated mainly around vessels and between collagen bundles. They contain nuclei with marginated chromatin, nucleoli, and large vacuole in the centre of the nucleus. The cytoplasm of these cells varies in shape, and may resemble that of monocytes or macrophages. Some cells are fusiform (tapering at both ends, spindle-shaped), and resemble fibroblasts. Most of the cells contain **cytoplasmic eosinophilic inclusion bodies. These bodies,** as seen under the electron microscope, **are sites of viral replication.** Similar inclusions are seen in infected keratinocytes.

Severe necrotizing vasculitis involves dermal and subcutaneous blood vessels. This results in ischaemic necrosis, and intense infiltration by neutrophils in and around the affected blood vessels. **Pneumonia,** with "sheep-pox cells" **and inclusion bodies** in alveolar septal cells, is the most important visceral lesion. Foci of necrosis and "sheep-pox cells" may also develop in the heart, liver, kidneys, adrenals, pancreas, and elsewhere.

Diagnosis

The lesions are characteristic of the disease. Confusion with contagious pustular dermatitis and bluetongue can occur, but differentiation on the basis of clinical signs and lesions is usually not difficult. Direct fluorescent antibody test is used to detect the presence of virus in the oedema fluid. Serological tests, such as indirect fluorescent antibody (FAT) test and an immunodiffusion technique are also used. A large number of characteristic "**sheep-pox cells**" containing inclusion bodies can be demonstrated in the skin.

Goatpox

The disease exists in **India**, North Africa, the Middle East, and parts of Europe. **Goatpox has been reported from most of the Indian states.** It is usually benign compared to sheep-pox. **The virus is immunologically related to and possibly the same as that of sheep-pox.** Rarely, the goatpox virus has been **reported to infect men** who are in close contact with goats. The disease has a somewhat longer incubation period, and is less severe than sheep-pox. Goatpox is very similar clinically to sheep-pox. **Young kids** suffer a systemic disease with lesions generally spread over the skin, and on the respiratory and alimentary mucosa. The skin lesions are smaller in goatpox, and are rarely haemorrhagic. In adults, the disease is mild and lesions are occasional only.

Lumpy Skin Disease

Lumpy skin disease (LSD) is a highly infectious disease of cattle and buffaloes caused by a capri-poxvirus (Neethling virus). It is characterized by the appearance of **nodules on all parts of the skin**. The disease was first seen in Zambia (formerly Northen Rhodesia) in 1929, and is restricted to Africa. **The virus of LDS is related to the viruses of sheep-pox and goatpox.** It is **spread by insect vectors,** mainly **flies. Clinically,** the disease is characterized by a generalized cutaneous eruption of **round, firm nodules,** varying from 0.5 cm to 5.0 cm in diameter. Nodules may also appear on oral, nasal, and genital mucous membranes, and there is enlargement of the superficial lymph nodes. The mortality rate is usually low, but may approach 10%.

Microscopically, the nodule is characterized by the inflammatory reaction in the dermis. The nodule is oedematous, and is composed of perivascular collections of lymphocytes, macrophages, plasma cells, and neutrophils; and proliferating fibroblasts. There is **acanthosis** (thickened epidermis), **parakeratosis** (thickened stratum corneum containing pyknotic nuclei), and **hyperkeratosis** (thickened stratum corneum) of the epidermis followed by necrosis and **vesicle formation. Eosinophilic cytoplasmic inclusion bodies** form in keratinocytes, fibroblasts, and macrophages. Necrosis of the entire nodule is followed by healing, which usually occurs within 3-5 weeks, but some nodules may persist for months.

The rapid spread of the disease and the sudden appearance of **lumps in the skin** after an initial fever make this disease very different from any other affliction of cattle. **Diagnosis** depends on finding of **eosinophilic cytoplasmic**

inclusion bodies in sections of skin lesions, and in tissue cultures of the virus. Electron microscopy is used in demonstrating the characteristic pox virions in the lesions. Virus can be cultured from lesions. Fluorescent antibody and serum neutralization tests are used extensively.

Diseases caused by Sui-Poxvirus

Swinepox virus is the only member of this genus.

Swinepox

Swinepox is usually a benign disease characterized by the appearance of typical pox lesions on the **ventral abdomen**. The virus of swinepox (**sui-poxvirus**) is not related to vaccinia, although pigs are also susceptible to vaccinia virus. The disease occurs in most countries where pigs are raised, **including India**. In some outbreaks the **mortality in young suckling pigs may be heavy, but older animals suffer little ill-effect**. The virus of swinepox may be transmitted by the swine louse, *Haematopinus suis*. However, a vector is not necessary for transmission. Solid immunity occurs after infection with the virus.

The incubation period is 5-7 days, after which erythematous areas, and then papules 4-5 mm in diameter, may appear. **Papules** pass through the vesicular stage very quickly with the formation of red-brown, round **scabs**. Scabs drop off and healing occurs. These **lesions** usually are limited to the underside of the body (belly) and inside the upper limbs, but may involve the back and sides, and sometimes spread to the face. A slight febrile reaction may occur in the early stages in young animals, and in suckling pigs some deaths are observed. **Eosinophilic cytoplasmic inclusion bodies** develop in epithelial cells. Distribution of the pox-like lesions, and the association of the disease with louse infestations, suggest the **diagnosis**.

Diseases caused by Avi-Poxviruses

Diseases caused by avi-poxviruses are fowl pox (avian pox, contagious epithelioma), pigeon pox, turkey pox, and canary pox. It was with the agent of fowl pox that in 1930 Woodruff and Goodpasture demonstrated that a single elementary body (**Borrel body**), i.e., virus particle, separated from the inclusion body (**Bollinger body**) was capable of causing typical infection. **Only fowl pox is described**.

Fowl Pox

Fowl pox is a disease characterized by cutaneous lesions. It is a slow-spreading disease accompanied by the development of discrete (separate), **nodular, proliferative skin lesions** on the non-feathered parts of the body (**cutaneous form**), or fibrino-necrotic and proliferative lesion in the mucous membrane of the upper respiratory tract, mouth, and oesophagus (**diphtheritic form**). **Fowl pox virus infects birds of both sexes, and of all ages and breeds**. The disease is prevalent in most poultry-producing countries. **In India the disease is endemic, and of considerable economic importance**. Research using fowl pox virus has contributed much to the field of virology. **It was the first virus to be grown on the chorio-allantoic membrane (CAM) of the embryonated chicken egg**. The presence of virus was easily determined by growths, or "**pocks**" on the membrane. The viral particles in these lesions were so large that they could be stained and seen under the light microscope. These particles were called "**Borrel bodies**", after the name of their discoverer. They are mainly present in a structure in the cytoplasm of the infected cell called a "**Bollinger body**", later called 'inclusion body'. These inclusion bodies are eosinophilic and can be identified microscopically. The virion (virus particle) has since been shown to be **the largest known, and contains the most DNA of any virus**. More recently, **fowlpox virus is being used as a vector for producing new types of vaccine**. The theory is that protective immunity to a pathogen can be produced during the replicative cycle of a vector which contains the relevant immunogen gene(s) from this pathogen.

Aetiology

Fowl pox is the largest virus known in birds. The mature virus (elementary body) is brick-shaped, with dimensions of 300 x 250 x 100 nm. Tubular structures are wound round the surface which give the virus its characteristic appearance. The viral genome is a single linear, **double-stranded DNA (ds DNA)** molecule. The virus enters the cell by a process of **endocytosis**. Once inside the host, cellular enzymes degrade the structural proteins. This frees the viral DNA and viral enzymes. The viral enzymes use the DNA as a template to initiate the cycle of replication, which produces all the necessary viral proteins, enzymes and DNA for new infectious virions. **Fowlpox virus is unusual, because it is a DNA virus which is capable of replication in the cell cytoplasm. Complete virions accumulate within the inclusion body,** which is composed of a morphous (shapeless) material, surrounded by an outer membrane. Some virus leaves the cell by budding, in which case it acquires an outer membrane. **However, most of the virus remains in the inclusion body**. When the infected cells die and are sloughed off into the environment in the scab, the virus remains in the inclusion and is resistant to desiccation (drying).

Spread

Fowl pox virus does not penetrate intact skin. Some break in the skin is required for the virus to enter the epithelial cells, replicate, and cause disease. Spread of the virus from one bird to another by direct contact is a major factor in the spread of disease. **Individuals handling birds at the time of vaccination may carry the virus on their hands and clothing, and may un-**

knowingly deposit the virus in the eyes of susceptible birds. The virus may reach the laryngeal region through the lachrymal duct to c ause infection of the upper respiratory tract. In a contaminated environment, the aerosol (droplets) generated by feathers and dried scabs containing poxvirus particles provides suitable conditions for both cutaneous and respiratory infection. **Cells of the mucosa of the upper respiratory tract and mouth appear to be highly susceptible** to the virus. This is because infection may occur in the absence of apparent trauma or injury. However, it has now been shown that certain biting insects, such as **mosquitoes**, transmit the disease. In warm climates this can result in a rapid spread of disease. It is possible that fowl pox could also be transmitted by the respiratory route, such as in smallpox and mousepox.

Pathogenesis

Virus enters an epithelial cell, and then spreads from cell to cell. This is helped by the production of **epidermal growth factor**, which causes proliferation of cells. Some virus enters the blood to cause **viraemia**. Although the virus s preads to i nternal organs, no gross p athological changes are seen. However, it is likely that there is some viral multiplication in certain organs, such as the liver and spleen, and a secondary viraemia occurs. Virus can again localize in the epithelium, and a generalized disease can be produced. However, this is rare.

Signs

The disease may occur in one of the two forms: cutaneous or diphtheritic, or both. The **cutaneous form** is usually the most noticeable in disease o utbreaks. Cutaneous lesions appear on the unfeathered skin of the head, neck, legs, and feet. Its onset in the flock is often gradual, and it may not be noted until the lesions are seen. The disease usually spreads slowly through the flock. In some cases this may last several weeks. Sometimes the disease may show a mild reduction in the rate of weight gain, or a lack of vigour in the flock. **Fowl pox can cause a drop in egg production in laying birds**. The c uatneous **lesions** can **vary in appearance**. First, there is a **papule**, which rapidly progresses through t he **vesicle to pustule**, a nd finally to the c rust or scab stage. I n most o utbreaks, the t erminal scab stage is present on some of the birds presented for diagnosis. After about 2 weeks, the scab drops off, and a healed lesion is left, which may or may not leave a scar. **In the cutaneous form, mortality is usually low**. However, it can be high when the disease is complicated by other infections.

In the **diphtheritic form ("wet pox")** small white **nodules** are observed in **the upper respiratory and digestive tracts**. These nodules coalesce (fuse) to form raised yellow plaques on the mucous membranes. Most lesions are found in the mouth, but o thers are present in the larynx, trachea, and oesophagus. These lesions c an give r ise to i nappetence (lack o f desire f or food) a nd/or difficulty in breathing (dyspnoea). Lesions in nares can give rise to nasal discharge. Those on the conjunctiva give rise to ocular discharge, and in rare cases, result in blindness. **Mortality as high as 50% has been reported with the diphtheritic form,** but it is usually low.

Gross Lesions

The characteristic lesion of the **cutaneous form is a local epithelial hyperplasia** involving epidermis and underlying feather follicles, with formation of **nodules**. Other features of the cutaneous lesions have been described under 'Signs'. In the **diphtheritic form**, slightly elevated, white opaque **nodules** develop **on the mucous membranes**. Nodules rapidly increase in size, and often coalesce to become a yellow, cheesy, necrotic pseudo-diphtheritic or diphtheritic membrane. If the membranes are removed, they leave bleeding erosions.

Microscopic Lesions

The most important lesion, regardless of the form, is **hyperplasia of the epithelium** and enlargement of the cells, with associated inflammatory changes. **Characteristic eosinophilic cytoplasmic inclusion bodies (Bollinger bodies)** are seen by light microscopy. Microscopic changes in tracheal mucosa include initial hypertrophy and hyperplasia, with subsequent enlargement of epithelial cells which contain eosinophilic cytoplasmic inclusion bodies. **The inclusion body may occupy almost the entire cytoplasm, with resulting cell necrosis.**

Immunity

Actively acquired immunity against fowl pox occurs after recovery from naturally occurring infection, or vaccination. **Cell-mediated and humoral immunity provide protection.** Cell-mediated immunity develops earlier than the humoral antibody response.

Diagnosis

Diagnosis can be made on the basis of the **clinical signs.** The presence of **cutaneous lesions** is suggestive of fowl pox. Even in the diphtheritic form, there are some chickens with cutaneous lesions. Microscopic examination of lesions will reveal **intracytoplasmic eosinophilic inclusion bodies.** Material can be scraped from the lesions, and smears made on glass slides. Using the appropriate stain, the virions (**Borrel bodies**) can be seen under the light microscope. **The diphtheritic form is more difficult to diagnose on clinical signs alone.** The lesions are adherent, **and if removed leave ulcers.** This fact helps in differentiating it from infectious laryngotracheitis and avitaminosis A. However, in both forms, confirmation can be made by detection of the virus from the lesion. Ground-up scabs inoculated onto the chorio-allantoic membrane of 9-12 day-old embryonated eggs produce characteristic pock lesions. Microscopically, inclusion bodies can be identified in pock lesions. Material can also be inoculated into susceptible chickens. The routes of inoculation can be the wing web, scarification of the comb, or into feather follicles. Characteristic lesions develop 5-7 days after inoculation.

Infection can also be determined by serological means. Various tests have been used to detect fowl pox specific antibodies. These include the agar gel precipitation test (AGPT), passive haemagglutination, serum neutralization (SN), indirect fluorescent antibody, immunoperoxidase, and ELISA. The antibodies detected by the AGPT are transitory (of short duration). SN bodies are usually low in titre. **The most sensitive test is the ELISA.**

Diseases Caused by Lepori-Poxviruses

Infectious Myxomatosis of Rabbits

Infectious myxomatosis of **rabbits** is characterized by the appearance of **firm, raised nodules in the skin**, particularly in the vicinity of the eyes, mouth, nose, ears and genitalia. **The disease runs a rapid, highly fatal course**, with death occurring a week or two after onset of symptoms. The causative agent is a **lepori-poxvirus**, which can be readily transmitted to susceptible rabbits. Its relationship with the Shope fibroma virus is indicated by the immunity of rabbits against myxomatosis after infection with the fibroma virus. Most of the nodules are firm and solid, but those near the genitalia may be oedematous. **Vesicle formation** (vesiculation) soon occurs, and vesicles are replaced by crusts. **Diagnosis** is made on the basis of clinical features, and the gross and microscopic lesions, which are characteristic of the disease.

Shope Fibroma of Rabbits

Fibromas in the skin of rabbits were described by Shope in 1932, as being caused by a filterable virus. The virus is now classified as a **lepori-poxvirus**, and is related to that of infectious myxomatosis. The fibroma virus produces an effective immunity to subsequent infection by myxomatosis, otherwise there is no similarity between the two diseases. The **lesions** are often multiple, and occur as elevations of the skin by a fibrous mass. The overlying epidermis is thickened and sends proliferating epithelium deep into the tumour. The tumours are benign proliferations of fibroblasts which eventually regress. **Large eosinophilic cytoplasmic inclusion bodies** occur in the affected keratinocytes.

Diseases caused by Para-Poxviruses

Contagious Pustular Dermatitis

Also known as "**contagious ovine ecthyma**", "**infectious labial dermatitis**", "**scabby mouth**", "**sore mouth**", and "**orf**", contagious pustular dermatitis is **a highly infectious viral disease of sheep and goats** characterized by the development of pustular and scabby lesions on the muzzle, lips, oral mucous membranes, udder, and rarely feet. **The disease is widely prevalent in India.**

Several outbreaks occur throughout the year, but are more common in spring and summer. The disease affects equally both young and adult animals, and is **more common in goats**. The virus is immunologically related to the viruses of bovine papular st omatitis and pseudo-cowpox. The virus also a ppears to be related to the virus of ulcerative dermatosis of sheep.

Spread

Spread in a flock is very rapid, and occurs by **contact** with other affected animals, or inanimate objects, such as ear-tagging pliers and castrators. The scabs remain highly infective for long periods. The virus withstands drying and is capable of surviving at room temperature for **at least 15 years**.

Pathogenesis

Damage to the skin is essential for the establishment of infection and development of lesions. Following infection, the virus replicates in the cells of a replacement epidermal layer, which lies under epidermis and is derived from the walls of the wool follicles. Virus can first be detected in the centre of the newly differentiated epidermis. The infection then spreads laterally from the new epidermis, and afterwards throughtout the entire depth of the epidermis. The skin reaction consists of a cellular response with **necrosis and sloughing of the affected epidermis. Immunity is solid**, but lasts for only about 8 months. The immune response is mainly humoral, but recovery appears to be the result of cell-mediated immune m echanisms.

Signs

Lesions develop as **papules** and then become **pustules**. After this the stages are not usually observed. F inally lesions become as thick, tenacious s cabs covering a raised a rea of u lceration, granulation, and inflammation. Lesions first develop at the **oral muco-cutaneous j unction**, usually at the **oral commissures**. From here, they spread on to the muzzle and nostrils, the surrounding haired skin, and to a lesser extent, on the **buccal mucosa**. They may appear as d iscrete (separate), thick scabs 0 .5 cm in diameter, or are packed together as a continuous plaque. **Fissuring occurs and the scabs are painful to the touch**. A ffected lambs su ffer a se tback because of restricted sucking and g razing. Rarely s ystemic invasion o ccurs, and l esions appear o n the coronets and ears, around the anus and vulva or prepuce, and on the nasal or buccal mucosa. There is a severe systemic reaction, and extension down the alimentary tract may lead to a severe gastroenteritis, and extension down the trachea may be followed by bronchopneumonia. M ortality is low unless complicated b y screw-worm larvae, or b acterial infection (*Fusobacterium necrophorum*). The **disease is most severe in lambs and kids**. Usually t he lesions resolve in 2-4 weeks, but can persist for several months.

Lesions

The gross lesions appear as **raised papules, vesicles, and then pustules,** with necrosis and eventual sloughing of the affected areas. **Microscopically,** the lesions are sharply defined. The affected epidermis overlies a densely cellular dermis, richly vascular, oedematous, and infiltrated with leukocytes. The epidermis proliferates, and becomes several times its normal thickness with long extensions into the dermis. Although **hyperplasia** of the epidermis is seen in most poxvirus infections, it **is particularly striking in ecthyma.** The epidermis undergoes degenerative changes consisting of vacuolation, ballooning degeneration, vesicle and pustule formation. **Eosinophilic cytoplasmic inclusion bodies** are present in keratinocytes, but they are of short duration.

Zoonotic Importance

The disease is also transmissible to humans. Mild transitory (of short duration) **pustular lesions,** particularly on the forearm, characterize the human disease. The disease usually occurs after contact with **infected sheep.** Infection has been reproduced in sheep with material taken from such human lesions. In slaughterhouse workers it is commonest in those handling wool and skins. In man typical lesions occur at the site of infection, usually an abrasion infected while handling diseased sheep, or by accidental means when vaccinating. **The lesions are very itchy and respond poorly to local treatment.**

Diagnosis

Diagnosis is based on the **characteristic lesions,** and **isolation and identification of the virus.** The disease must be differentiated from sheep-pox and ulcerative dermatosis. The virus is immunologically different from sheep-pox virus. And, although related, it is separable from the virus of ulcerative dermatosis. The downgrowth of the basal layer of epidermis into the dermis does not occur in sheep-pox or ulcerative dermatosis. This is a differentiating feature. The widespread cutaneous distribution of the lesions of sheep-pox, and the preputial lesions of ulcerative dermatosis, also help in differential diagnosis. Recovered animals have a high level of neutralizing antibodies in their serum, and this is detectable by agar-gel diffusion test (AGPT). Techniques for complement fixation test and tissue culture on lamb testicular tissue are also available. Electron microscopic identification of the virus is the quickest and most reliable method of diagnosis.

Bovine Papular Stomatitis

Also known as "**infectious ulcerative stomatitis and oesophagitis**", bovine papular stomatitis is **a mild viral disease of young cattle characterized by papules** on the **muzzle, inside the nostrils,** and in the **oral cavity.** The disease does not cause serious illness, but is important because of the confusion it creates, such as foot-and-mouth disease, vesicular stomatitis, mucosal disease, and viral diarrhoea. The virus (a **para-poxvirus**) is closely related to, and may be the same as, pseudo-cowpox virus (discussed next). The disease mostly affects **young calves**. **The clinical signs are mild**. Fever is usually not seen, although viraemia occurs.

Lesions

Usually lesions are found on the lips, muzzle, nostrils, gingivae, tongue, and oral mucosa. Lesions also occur in the oesophagus, rumen, reticulum and omasum. **Grossly**, the earliest lesions are small foci of hyperaemia on the lower margin of nostrils, on the palate, or inner surface of the lips. In about a day, these foci form a whitish papule. **Microscopically**, the epidermis is focally hyperplastic, and contains focal areas of hydropic degeneration. Nuclei are pyknotic and may undergo karyorrhexis. As the disease progresses, the hydropic lesions move toward the surface. The affected keratinocytes often contain spherical **eosinophilic cytoplasmic inclusion bodies** which are 10 μm or more in diameter. The lesions may become infiltrated with neutrophils and finally progress to erosions or ulcers. Healing is usually uneventful.

Zoonotic Significance

The virus also infects humans. It produces mild erythematous papules on the hands and arms, similar to "**milker's nodules**", which are associated with pseudo-cowpox virus.

Pseudo-Cowpox

The virus of pseudo-cowpox is called **paravaccinia**, but is **not related to vaccinia or cowpox**. It is **closely related to contagious pustular dermatitis virus and bovine pustular stomatitis virus**. The lesions are limited to the **teats** and udders of milking cows, and appear as **red papules** and **vesicles**. **Microscopically**, there is hyperplasia of squamous epithelium, proliferation of the sub-epithelial capillary network, vesicular degeneration of the epithelium, and **eosinophilic cytoplasmic inclusion bodies**. Infection does not confer immunity.

Zoonotic Significance

The disease is transmissible to humans. The infection usually results in the development of "**milker's nodules**" on the **hand**. Milkers' nodules are clinically indistinguishable from human lesions caused by contagious pustular dermatitis virus. The lesions vary from multiple vesicles to a single, indurated nodule.

Diseases caused by Unclassified Poxviruses

Molluscum Contagiosum

This is a disease of humans caused by a different poxvirus. The lesions

are characterized by epithelial hyperplasia, and **extremely large** (up to 35 μm) **eosinophilic cytoplasmic inclusion bodies ("molluscum bodies")**, which enlarge and eventually occupy the whole cell. A disease microscopically similar to molluscum contagiosum has been described in **horses**, and chimpanzees. In **horses**, the lesions are microscopically similar to those seen in humans and are usually localized in the muzzle, penis, and prepuce.

Ulcerative Dermatosis

Also known as **"lip and leg ulcerations"**, **"ulcerative vulvitis"**, and **"infectious balanoposthitis"** (inflammation of the glans penis and prepuce), ulcerative dermatosis is a disease of **sheep** and **goats** characterized by an **ulcerative dermatitis of the lips, legs, feet, prepuce, and vulva.** The virus is a member of the poxvirus group, and is immunologically related to the virus of contagious pustular dermatitis. **Microscopically**, the lesions lack the hyperplasia of epidermis seen in contagious pustular dermatitis.

Yaba Poxvirus

Yaba poxvirus affects many species of Asian and African **monkeys**, as well as **humans**. The **lesions are tumour-like masses** in the subcutis. This disease resembles lumpy skin disease of cattle. The lesions are not true tumours, and eventually regress.

Horsepox

Horsepox is a benign disease characterized by the development of typical **pox lesions** either **on the limbs**; or on the **lips, nose, oral mucosa,** and **genitalia**. It is believed to be caused by an immunologically different virus. However, the relationship of the horsepox virus to other poxviruses is not known.

Adenoviridae

Many adenoviruses (G. adeno = gland), differentiated from one another by immunological methods, have been isolated from mammals. However, **except canine hepatitis, most are not serious causes of disease** unless animals are immuno-compromised (i.e., immunologically damaged). The Family **Adenoviridae** contains **two genera: 1. Mast-adenovirus** (G. masto = mammal), and 2. A **vi-adenovirus** or a **vian adenovirus** (L. avi = bird). All are **unenveloped** (non-enveloped) icosahedral viruses, 70-90 nm in diameter, with 252 capsomeres. Of these 240 are hexons (hexamers; G. hexa = six) and 12 are pentons (pentamers; G. penta = five). **The pentons have been shown to be toxic to cells, and may represent a "viral toxin".** The **nucleic acid** consists of a single linear molecule of **double-stranded DNA (ds DNA), which is replicated in the nucleus, where a characteristic inclusion body is produced**. Although suspected, a causal relationship of these viruses to spontaneous neoplasms has not been established. **Adenoviruses are highly species specific.**

Adenoviruses of several serotypes have been recovered from many species, which include cattle, sheep, pigs, horses, dogs, and rats. These viruses are currently identified by the species of origin and a number (e.g., bovine adenovirus type 3). **Diseases caused by Adenoviridae are listed in Table 12.**

Table 12. Diseases caused by Adenoviridae

Virus	Disease	Species
Genus: Mast-adenovirus		
Canine adenovirus-1	Infectious canine hepatitis	Dogs
Canine adenovirus-2	Upper respiratory disease	Dogs
Bovine adenoviruses types 3 and 5	Bovine adenoviral infections	Young calves
Ovine adenoviruses several different serotypes	Ovine adenoviral infections	Sheep
Equine adenovirus	Equine adenoviral infection	Horses
Porcine adenovirus	Porcine adenoviral infection	Pigs
Simian adenoviruses	Simian adenoviral infections	Monkeys
Murine adenovirus	Murine adenoviral infections	Mice
Genus: Avi-adenovirus (Avian adenovirus)		
Group I (Conventional avian adenoviruses)	Inclusion-body hepatitis Respiratory disease Falls in egg production Viral arthritis/tenosynovitis	Chickens
Group II (comprises type II avian adenoviruses)	Turkey haemorrhagic enteritis Marble spleen disease Avian adenosplenomegaly	Turkeys Pheasants Chickens
Group III (includes haemagglutinating adenoviruses)	Egg drop syndrome 1976	Chickens, ducks, geese

Diseases caused by Mast-Adenoviruses

Infectious Canine Hepatitis

Also known as "**hepatitis contagiosa canis**", "**Rubarth disease**", and "**canine adenovirus infection**", infectious canine hepatitis (ICH) is a contagious disease of dogs caused by **canine adenovirus-1**, which is antigenically related only to canine adenovirus-2. Although ICH was recognized for many years, it was not established as a separate disease until the classical report of

Rubarth in 1947, from Sweden. Rubarth pointed out that fox encephalitis virus, infective for dogs, was the same as the virus of canine hepatitis. **This has since been confirmed**. The disease occurs worldwide, **including India**, with signs that vary. **In wildlife**, the disease has been reported in **foxes**.

Spread

The disease is spread mainly by **excretion of virus in the urine**, and is **acquired as a naso-oral infection**, after causing pharyngitis and tonsillitis as initial signs. Ingestion of urine, faeces, or saliva from infected animals is another route of infection. Virus may be excreted in the urine for as long as 30 days.

Pathogenesis

Initial infection occurs in the tonsillar crypts and Peyer's patches, followed by **viraemia** and infection of endothelial cells in many tissues. This initiates infection of visceral organs. Liver, kidneys, spleen, and lungs are the main target organs. Chronic kidney lesions and corneal clouding ("**blue eye**") result from immune-complex reactions following recovery from acute disease.

Signs

The disease affects mainly **young dogs**. The infection is common, but usually goes unnoticed, or is not manifested. When clinical disease occurs, its course is rather variable. However, it is **often peracute**, with the first signs seen only a few hours before death. Usually, however, the illness is manifested for several days before death, or recovery occurs. The disease begins with apathy (lack of interest, listlessness), followed by anorexia (loss of appetite), and intense thirst. Severe subcutaneous oedema of head, neck, and ventral aspects of the trunk is prominent, but is a rare manifestation. **Other signs** include vomiting, diarrhoea with haemorrhage, abdominal pain expressed by moaning sounds, and fever (104° F) at onset, but may fall suddenly to subnormal levels as death approaches.

Central nervous system signs are uncommon. When seen they comprise clonic spasms of the extremities and neck, paralysis of the hindquarters and extreme agitation. The mucous membranes appear anaemic, even slighly icteric, but rarely deeply jaundiced. Tonsils are reddened and swollen, and tonsillitis is often the initial diagnosis. Copious lachrymation with hyperaemic conjunctiva is common. Sometimes, diffuse, opaque cloudiness of the cornea ("**blue eye**") develops 1-3 weeks after initial signs. **In the urine, albumin may be present in significant amounts**. Other clinico-pathological findings include neutropaenia and lymphopaenia during the course, with lymphocytosis during recovery; prolonged bleeding and coagulation times; and elevation of SGOT and SGPT.

Lesions

The virus has an affinity for parenchymal and Kupffer cells of the liver, and endothelial cells generally. A ffected cells develop sp ecific **basophilic intranuclear inclusion bodies**, and become necrotic. Reticulo-endothelial cells and sometimes other cells, such as renal tubular epithelium, may be affected. **Gross lesions** are dominated by h aemorrhage, m ainly of the stomach and serosal su rfaces, resulting f rom endothelial damage and l oss of c oagulation factors o f hepatic origin. The **spleen** and **lymph nodes** are oedematous and congested; **liver** congested and enlarged; and the **gallbladder** wall oedematous and thickened.

The most characteristic microscopic lesion is **focal hepatic necrosis, particularly in the periportal region.** Hepatocytes become **acidophilic**, lose their outline, a nd u ltimately disppear, to b e r eplaced by dilated sinusoids. **Intranuclear inclusion bodies are prominent,** u sually in cells adjacent t o areas of n ecrosis. The inclusion body, w hich almost f ills the n ucleus, has a rather indistinct outline, and takes basophilic colour in sections with H & E. Similar i nclusions may be found i n the e ndothelial cells a nd Kupffer cells. Recovery is followed by c omplete regeneration of the liver. Intranuclear inclusion bodies also occur in the reticulo-endothelial cells and endothelial cells of the spleen. In the kidney, intranuclear inclusions may be found in endothelial cells of the glomerular tufts.

The lesions in the **brain** are directly related to the changes in the capillary endothelium. The endothelial cells may contain intranuclear inclusions. Many of the capillaries are surrounded by a small collar of haemorrhage.

Diagnosis

Diagnosis in the living animal is difficult because of the non-specific nature of the symptoms. Microscopic demonstration of intranuclear inclusion bodies in surgically r emoved tonsils, o r liver b iopsy specimens, c onfirms the presumptive clinical diagnosis. P ostmortem diagnosis i s not a problem. It is established b y the **d emonstration o f typical lesions and characteristic intranuclear inclusion bodies.** The diagnosis can also be confirmed by virus isolation and immunofluorescence. This disease can occur in association with canine distemper, or leptospirosis, and has to be differentiated.

Canine Adenovirus-2

First isolated in 1962 in Canada from **dogs with laryngotracheitis**, this virus is different from the virus of infectious canine hepatitis. The virus is now recognized as a cause of conjunctivitis, upper respiratory disease, and sometimes, pneumonia. It has also been a ssociated with enteritis. However, mild infections a re more c ommon. The i nfection also o ccurs along w ith a m ore serious disease like canine distemper. It is considered to be one of the causes of kennel cough. **Clinical signs** include fever, nasal discharge, coughing, and dyspnoea. Mortality is very low. The mucosae of the larynx, pharynx, trachea, and bronchi are hyperaemic, and sometimes ulcerated and covered with a purulent or fibrinous exudate. The principal microscopic lesions are necrosis of respiratory epithelium, and the presence of **intranuclear inclusion bodies**.

Bovine Adenoviral Infections

Bovine adenoviruses are of several serotypes. Some of them (**types 3 and 5**) are more pathogenic than others to **young calves**, producing disease of the respiratory and gastrointestinal tracts. Serological surveys of cattle indicate that infection is widespread, but rarely leads to clinical disease.

Signs

Clinical signs include fever, kerato-conjunctivitis, gastrointestinal tract involvement with tympany, colic, and diarrhoea. In calves, systemic infection with oedema and haemorrhage around joints, has been described as "**weak calf syndrome**". Morbidity and mortality are low.

Lesions

The lesions may be **generalized, or limited to the respiratory or gastrointestinal tracts**. The characteristic gross lesion in the respiratory tract is the presence of mucinous or mucopurulent exudate in the nasal passages. Other lesions include diffuse congestion, haemorrhage and areas of consolidation in lungs; haemorrhage and oedema in the lymph nodes related to the respiratory tract; petechiae and oedema in the kidneys, adrenal cortex, myocardium, and wall of the intestine. Petechiae and oedema are especially prominent around major joints in outbreaks in which lameness is a common sign.

Microscopically, respiratory tract lesions are characterized by necrosis of respiratory epithelium with the presence of **characteristic intranuclear inclusion bodies** in epithelial and endothelial cells. Interstitial pneumonia may occur. In the gastrointestinal form, the virus invades enterocytes of villous epithelium leading to necrosis and blunting of villi. Inclusion bodies occur within affected enterocytes. In the systemic disease, necrosis, oedema, and haemorrhage are accompanied by intranuclear inclusion bodies, especially in the intestine, kidneys, and joints.

Ovine Adenoviral Infections

Several different serotypes of ovine adenoviruses have been identified. **Even bovine adenoviruses have been recovered from sheep with respiratory tract disease**. As in cattle, ovine adenoviruses are associated with conjunctivitis, respiratory tract disease, and enteritis. Respiratory lesions comprise epithelial necrosis and **typical intranuclear inclusion bodies**, followed by epithelial hyperplasia. Ovine adenovirus type 6 causes marked cytomegaly (enlargement of cell) of respiratory epithelial cells. Type 6 also causes focal hepatic n ecrosis with i ntranuclear inclusion b odies in h epatocytes. T ype 5 causes nephritis with intranuclear inclusion bodies in endothelial cells. Morbidity and mortality in ovine adenoviral infections are usually low.

Equine Adenoviral Infection

Adenoviral infection is associated with respiratory d isease in **foals**. B ut like other species the infection is usually not manifested clinically. The **clinical signs** include sudden onset of fever with m ucopurulent nasal d ischarge, cough, dyspnoea, i ncreased respiratory r ate, and sometimes, death. **L esions** are usually confined to the respiratory tract, and include mucopurulent rhinitis, tracheitis, a nd consolidation o f dependent portions of the lungs. **B asophilic intranuclear inclusion bodies** occur in e pithelial cells along the entire respiratory tract. These inclusions may also be found in association with focal necrosis in epithelial cells lining the renal pelvis, ureter, urinary bladder, and urethra. Sometimes focal lesions are found in the gastrointestinal tract, particularly the small intestine.

Porcine Adenovirus

Porcine adenovirus infection is widespread, and virus can be isolated from faeces. Clinical and pathological changes are uncommon. But there are reports of spontaneous pneumonia, enteritis, and encephalitis. Epithelial necrosis and **intranuclear inclusion bodies** in the respiratory tract and small intestine are the most common findings.

Diseases caused by Avi-Adenoviruses (Avian Adenoviruses)

Avian adenoviruses are **divided into three groups**: 1. **Group I** contains the c onventional group I adenoviruses (**Table 12**). T hese avian a denovirus group I i solates from b irds share a common group antigen. 2. **Group II** comprises the so-called type II avian adenoviruses and includes turkey haemorrhagic enteritis (THE) virus and marble spleen disease (MSD) virus of pheasants, and a vian adenovirus g roup II splenomegaly v irus of c hickens. **These viruses share a common group antigen which is different from the group I viruses. 3. Group III** are the haemagglutinating viruses a ssociated with egg d rop syndrome 1 976 (EDS 7 6) (**Table 12**). T hese viruses **only partially share the group I common antigen.**

Group I Adenovirus Infections

In marked contrast t o the c lear association o f group I I and g roup III adenoviruses with disease, **the role of group I adenoviruses as pathogens is not well understood**. The majority of them have a limited role as pathogens. Some, however, appear to be primary pathogens. But they do play a role as secondary pathogens i n **chicken infectious anaemia (CIA)** and i nfectious **bursal disease (IBD).** Group I adenoviruses are further classified into **serotypes** using the neutralization test. Currently **at least 12 serotypes of fowl adenoviruses** are recognized. Group I adenoviruses are widely distributed throughout the world.

Spread

Vertical transmission through the embryonated egg is very important. This is the main method of spread from one generation to the next. Afterwards, **horizontal spread** by contact with infected faeces occurs. Virus is present in faeces, tracheal and nasal mucosa. Therefore virus could be spread in all excretions, but highest levels are found in the faeces. Horizontal spread appears to be mainly by direct faecal contact. Aerial spread between farms does not appear to be important, but spread by fomites, personnel, and transport can be very important.

Disease

As mentioned, **the role of group I adenoviruses as primary pathogens is not clearly established.** Furthermore, adenoviruses are widely distributed **in healthy birds**, and are even commonly isolated from them under all systems of management. This does not mean they do not cause disease, but it does mean that isolation of adenoviruses from diseased birds forms no basis to believe that they are the cause of the disease.

Adenoviruses have been isolated from virtually every clinical condition. However, they are most commonly associated with **inclusion body hepatitis, falls in egg production, respiratory disease, diarrhoea, poor growth and reduced feed conversion, and tenosynovitis** (inflammation of a tendon sheath). It has been reported that adenovirus infection **causes a 10% fall in egg production, or affects eggshell quality.** Also, there are reports of adenovirus infection resulting in decreased food consumption and **growth retardation.** More recently, it has been found that group I adenoviruses are associated with a **"hydropericardium syndrome"** of chickens reported from Pakistan in 1987; and more commonly known as **"Angara disease".** However, there is evidence that another agent may also be involved. There are similarities between the signs and pathology of this syndrome and inclusion body hepatitis, but it is not clear if they are different.

Inclusion Body Hepatitis

This disease is **usually seen in meat-producing chickens 3-7 weeks of age,** but has been reported in birds as young as 7 days old, and as old as 20 weeks. **The disease is characterized by a sudden onset of mortality.**

Aetiology

The aetiology of this disease has not been properly established. There is **no separate inclusion body hepatitis (IBH) virus.** Virtually every serotype **of adenovirus group I** has been isolated from the naturally occurring disease.

Furthermore, all the known adenovirus serotypes produce hepatitis when very young chicks are inoculated parenterally. **Most experimental infections produce basophilic intranuclear inclusion bodies in the hepatocytes, whereas most natural cases produce eosinophilic intranuclear inclusion bodies**. If adenoviruses are involved in producing IBH, they appear to act with some other factor. It has been suggested that **immunosuppression** produced **by infectious bursal disease (IBD)** helps adenoviruses in producing IBH. However, many flocks undergoing combined infections with these viruses remain healthy. Moreover, both Northern Ireland and **New Zealand outbreaks** of IBH occurred in chickens before IBD was present in the country. Some outbreaks described as IBH closely resemble haemorrhagic syndrome/infectious anaemia caused by chicken anaemia virus.

Outbreaks of IBH which occurred in **Australia** during the last decade, differ significantly from the above. They have occurred in much younger chicks (i.e., under 3 weeks of age), have caused higher mortality, and mainly **basophilic inclusion bodies** are present in hepatocytes. Adenoviruses have been isolated from field cases and the disease reproduced experimentally in chickens. **In India**, the disease has appeared as seasonal, especially after monsoon, in the cold season. The **mycotoxin stress** seems to be another predisposing factor besides IBD.

Signs

The disease is characterized by sudden onset of mortality, reaching highest after 3-4 days, and dropping on the 5th day, but sometimes continuing for 2-3 weeks. Morbidity is low. Sick birds adopt a crouching position with ruffled feathers, and die within 48 hours, or recover. **Mortality may reach 10%, and sometimes as high as 30%.** Overall feed conversion and weight gain are usually decreased. Anaemia, jaundice of the skin and subcutaneous fat, haemorrhages in various organs, especially the muscles, and bone marrow degeneration are usually present, but vary in severity. In some outbreaks the bone marrow lesions are most prominent, and it has been suggested that the disease should be called "**hepato-myeloporetic disease**".

Lesions

The main lesions are **pale, friable, swollen livers. Petechial or ecchymotic haemorrhages** may be present in the **liver** and **skeletal muscles. Microscopically**, there is a diffuse and generalized hepatitis, with **intranuclear inclusion bodies in the hepatocytes**, which are often **eosinophilic**, or **sometimes basophilic**. In the **Australian outbreaks**, basophilic inclusions predominated. **Virus particles were detected only in cells with basophilic inclusions. Eosinophilic inclusions were composed of fibrillar granular material.** In the New Zealand outbreaks, inclusions were eosinophilic.

Respiratory Disease

Adenoviruses a re frequently i solated from airsacs, lungs a nd trachea of birds with respiratory disease. It is unlikely that they are primary pathogens. However, they do appear **important as secondary pathogens.**

Falls in Egg Production

It is likely that exposure of laying fowls to an adenovirus may result in a fall in egg production. However, falls in egg production due to conventional (Group I) adenovirus infection appears to be unimportant.

Viral Arthritis/Tenosynovitis

Adenoviruses have been usually isolated from joints or tendons of birds having arthritis or tenosynovitis. However, poor success has been achieved in experimental reproduction o f this disease using adenoviruses.

Diagnosis

This depends on **isolation and identification o f the virus, a nd on serological tests.** Specimens of choice are faeces, pharynx, kidney, and a f-fected organs, e.g., livers. **Isolation** is done on either chick embryo liver cells, or chick kidney cells. **Antibody** to the conventional adenovirus group antigen can be d etected using t he double immunodiffusion (DID) t est. The i ndirect immunofluorescent test is much more sensitive and rapid, and is inexpensive. ELISA h as been u sed to d etect group a ntibodies, and i t is e xpensive and sensitive. The main problem with any serological test is in the. interpretation of r esults. Antibodies a re common i n both h ealthy and diseased birds, a nd birds are frequently infected with a number of serotypes. On the other hand, demonstration of **eosinophilic intranuclear inclusion body** in H and E staining in the hepatocytes of chickens in naturally occurring inclusion body hepatitis, is **diagnositc.**

Group II Adenovirus Infections

There are **three diseases** caused by the group II adenoviruses (**Table 12**). These are: 1. **Turkey haemorrhagic enteritis (THE)**, 2. **Marble spleen disease (MSD) of pheasants**, and 3. **Avian adenovirus group II splenomegaly (AAS)**, also known as avian adenosplenomegaly o f chickens. **Haemorrhagic enteritis (HE)** is an acute viral disease of **turkeys 4** weeks of age, and older. It i s characterized by depression, b loody droppings, a nd death. **Microscopically**, nuclei of infected cells in the spleen contain characteristic **intranuclear inclusion bodies.**

Marble spleen disease is a condition affecting **pheasants 3-8 months of age.** The c ausative virus i s serologically i ndistinguishable from t hat of H E virus. The clinical disease, however, is mainly respiratory in nature, with death occurring as a result of asphyxia. MSD virus also produces **intranuclear inclusions** and splenic lesions similar to those of HEV.

Avian adenosplenomegaly is observed as **splenomegaly in young or mar-ket-age broilers,** or **as splenomegaly** with pulmonary congestion and oedema **in mature birds**. Death of chickens i n peracute or acute c ases results f rom asphyxia. Therefore, s igns may c onsist of depression, weakness, d yspnoea, and finally a sphyxia. The v irus also p roduces **intranuclear inclusions** and splenic lesions similar to those of HEV.

Group III Adenovirus Infection
Egg Drop Syndrome

Since its initial description in 1976 by Dutch workers, egg drop syndrome 1976 (EDS 76) has become **a major cause of loss of egg production throughout the world**. It is caused by **an adenovirus belonging to group III**. EDS 1976 is characterized by **otherwise healthy birds** producing **thin-shelled,** or **shell-less eggs**.

Cause

The **EDS adenovirus differs from conventional (group I) serotype 1 adenoviruses**. Although EDS virus shares the conventional avian adenovirus group I antigen, this can be detected only by indirect means. **In fact, EDS virus is a naturally occurring adenovirus of ducks and geese which has infected fowl**. It grows best in duck and geese cell cultures, but also well in chick embryo liver and chick kidney cells. **All EDS virus isolates belong to one serotype.**

Spread

EDS outbreaks are divided into **three types**: 1. In the **classical form,** primary breeders are infected and the main method of **spread is vertical through the embryonated egg**. Although the number of infected embryos is low, **spread is very efficient**. 2. The second pattern is the **endemic form**. Probably originating from the classical form, virus has become established in some areas in commercial egg-laying flocks. **In India, 32.6% of poultry flocks were found to be infected**. This endemic form results from **lateral spread between flocks**. This form is often associated with a common egg-packing station. Both normal and abnormal-shelled eggs, laid during the period of **virus growth in the pouch shell gland of the oviduct**, contain virus both on the exterior and interior. This l eads to c ontamination of e gg trays. D roppings also contain virus, b ut this is d ue t o c ontamination of f aeces b y o viduct exudate. L ateral spread between f locks through c ontaminated personnel o r fomites, o ther than e gg trays, can occur, but d oes not a ppear to be a major risk. Other methods o f spread could b e c ontaminated needles, a nd perhaps, biting i nsects. 3 . T he third type is the **sporadic form**. This form results from introduction of infec-tion from ducks, geese, or any infected bird, either through direct contact, or indirectly through d rinking water contaminated with droppings.

Pathogenesis

Following infection of laying hens, the virus grows to a limited extent in the nasal mucosa. This is followed by **a viraemia** with **virus replication in lymphoid tissue throughout the body,** e specially **spleen** and **t hymus**. The infundibulum of the oviduct is consistently affected. At 8 days after infection, there is massive v iral replication in the **pouch shell glands** and, to a m uch lesser extent, in other parts of the oviduct. This coincides with the production of eggshell changes. Both normal and affected eggs contain virus, both externally and internally, for the next two weeks. Chicks hatched from these infected eggs usually do not develop antibody, and may be latently infected.

Signs

The first signs are loss of shell strength and pigmentation. This is followed by **thin-shelled, soft-shelled, and shell-less eggs.** Eggshells may show mineral deposits. However, ridging and mis-shapen eggs are not a feature. **There is a drop in egg production.** The birds are normally healthy, but sometimes they appear slightly depressed. Diarrhoea may be due to an excess of oviduct se-cretion in d roppings. Classical E DS is manifested by **a sudden fall in egg production around peak production,** or b y a f ailure to achieve o r hold expected p roduction.

Gross Lesions

Inactive ovaries and atrophied oviducts are o ften the only recognized lesions, and these are not consistently present.

Microscopic Lesions

The main pathological changes occur in the **pouch shell gland of oviduct.** Virus replicates in epithelial cell nuclei, and produces **intranuclear inclusion bodies.** Many affected cells are sloughed into the lumen. There is a severe in-flammatory response involving macrophages, plasma cells, and lymphocytes, together with variable numbers of heterophils in the lamina propria and epithelium.

Diagnosis

The combination of a **sudden fall in egg production,** associated with thin-shelled a nd shell-less e ggs in a flock of apparently healthy birds, **is almost diagnostic.** Virus isolation can be difficult because it is difficult to identify the correct bird to sample. The easiest method is to feed affected eggs to susceptible hens. Once they produce abnormal eggs, the pouch shell gland is harvested, and samples i noculated into either duck k idney, or f ibroblast cell c ultures, or embryonated eggs. Virus growth is d etected by t esting for haemagglutinins. Detection of a ntibodies to E DS virus by the **h aemagglutination inhibition (HI) test** using fowl erythrocytes i s sensitive and easy. **ELISA** is now a lso used.

Iridoviridae

African swine fever virus is the only member of this family which affects mammals. Iridovirus virions replicate in the cytoplasm of infected cells, although the nucleus is required for replication. **Poxviridae** are the only other DNA viriuses which assemble in the cytoplasm. Virions are released either by budding, in which case they obtain an envelope, or through lysis. The latter particles a re u nenveloped, b ut i nfectious. T he genome i s made o f a s ingle linear molecule of **double-stranded DNA (ds DNA).**

African Swine Fever

Also k nown as "**warthog disease**", a nd " **African pig disease**", African swine fever is **a highly contagious disease of domestic pigs** caused by an **iridivirus**.

Spread

Ticks are the biological vectors, and serve as the primary means of maintaining the i nfection, and s preading it t o domestic p igs. T ransmission also follows **ingestion** of uncooked infected pork products. Once introduced into pigs by ticks, or infected meat, t he virus s preads readily **b y contact. C urrently, the disease appears to be confined to Africa**. Multiple strains of virus of varying virulence now exist. Wild warthogs (African wild pigs) and bush pigs act as asymptomatic carriers.

Pathogenesis

The virus invades through the tonsils and respiratory tract, and replicates in the draining lymph nodes prior to the occurrence of generalized **viraemia** which can occur within 48-72 hours of infection.

Signs

The disease occurs in **two forms: acute** and **chronic**. In the **acute form** disease begins with a high fever (105^0 F). However, during this febrile period, the a ffected pigs m ay appear w ell and have a g ood appetite. T hen, in their final 48 h ours, they b ecome depressed, w eak, cyanotic; d evelop cough and dyspnoea; and then die. Vomiting and diarrhoea may be observed, and there may be haemorrhage from the nose a nd anus. P regnant sows m ay abort. In the **chronic form**, the course of the disease is prolonged. **Some pigs recover and act as carriers of the virus.**

Lesions

Gross changes are similar in many respects to those of swine fever, **but are more severe**. Lymph nodes a re d iffusely haemorrhagic. O ther l esions include pulmonary oedema; petechiae and ecchymoses in the pleura, pericardium, and peritoneum; oedema and congestion in gallbladder; haemorrhages in the renal cortex; and catarrhal enteritis. The spleen is engorged and swollen. Pathogenesis of the haemorrhage is not understood. **African swine fever virus does not affect endothelial cells as does the virus of swine fever.** The **microscopic vascular lesions** are similar to those of swine fever, but result in more severe circulatory disturbances, e.g., oedema, haemorrhage, infarction.

Diagnosis

The lesions are helpful in acute cases. The prolonged cases and latent infections require **isolation and identification of the virus** in appropriate tissue cultures. Immuno-histochemical techniques have been used to identify viral antigens in tissues of affected pigs.

Papovaviridae

The Family **Papovaviridae** was created by the **grouping of three different viruses** leading to the **acronym** (a word formed from the first letters of a group of words) **"papova"** from **papilloma virus**, **polyoma virus**, and vacuolating agent. Papovaviruses are small (45-55 nm in diameter), **non-enveloped**, icosahedral virions. The genome consists of one molecule of **double-stranded DNA (ds DNA).** The family contains **two genera: papillomavirus** and **polyomavirus**, which are immunologically distinct. **Only papillomaviruses are of veterinary importance.**

The **genus Papillomavirus** contains viruses responsible for **benign papillomatosis** (e.g., **warts**, verrucae vulgaris) **in humans and other animals.** The viruses are **highly species-specific**, with the exception of bovine papillomaviruses. As with oncogenic DNA viruses, viral replication does not occur in the transformed, rapidly dividing cells. Therefore, viral particles and viral antigens are not demonstrable in cells of the germinal layer. However, the cells of the upper layers, i.e., the epidermis, are permissive for viral replication, and viral particles can be localized here. **Basophilic intranuclear inclusion bodies** may, sometimes, also be seen in these cells. Only human and bovine papillomaviruses have been characterized in any detail. The genus **Polyomavirus** (G. poly = many; G. oma = tumour) is made up of several **viruses of scientific interest**, because of their oncogenic and transforming effects on mammalian cell systems. **Their pathogenicity in nature is negligible.** The viruses of this genus include SE polyoma virus of mice, K virus of rats, simian virus 40 (SV 40), and rabbit vacuolating virus.

Diseases caused by papillomaviruses are presented in **Table 13**.

Table 13. Diseases caused by Papillomaviruses

Virus	Host(s)	Disease
Bovine type 1	Cattle	Cutaneous fibropapilloma
	Horses	Equine sarcoid
Bovine type 2	Cattle	Cutaneous fibropapilloma
	Horses	Equine sarcoid
Bovine type 3	Cattle	Cutaneous papilloma
Bovine type 4	Cattle	Alimentary tract papilloma
Bovine type 5	Cattle	Teat fibropapilloma
Bovine type 6	Cattle	Teat papilloma
Equine papillomavirus	Horses	Cutaneous papilloma
Canine oral papillomavirus	Dogs	Oral papilloma
Ovine papillomavirus	Sheep	Cutaneous papilloma
Caprine papillomavirus	Goats	Cutaneous papilloma
Porcine papillomavirus	Pigs	Genital papilloma
Monkey papillomavirus	Monkeys	Cutaneous papilloma
Rabbit papillomavirus	Wild rabbits, domestic rabbits, hares	Cutaneous papilloma (may progress to squamous-cell carcinoma)
Rabbit oral papillomavirus	Domestic rabbits	Oral papilloma

Bovine Cutaneous Papillomatosis

In cattle, cutaneous papillomatosis is more common than in any other domestic animal. The disease affects young animals more often and more severely, but may affect cattle of all ages. At least **six distinct (separate) bovine papillomaviruses** have been recognized (**Table 13**). The most common form is caused by types 1 and 2. It differs from papillomas of other species in that there is a **marked proliferation of connective tissue,** the lesion being known as "**fibropapilloma**". These are mostly found around the head and neck, but may also occur on the udder and external genitalia. The disease is usually self-limiting and recovery may occur without treatment. However, when lesions are on the genitalia, they interfere with reproduction.

Grossly, **fibropapilloma is a rough, cauliflower-like mass.** It is of varying size, irregular in shape, elevated, and attached by either a narrow stalk, or a broad base. The lesions are numerous, closely spaced, round and smooth, but soon become rough and horny. **Microscopically,** the lesions are made up of greatly thickened epidermis, which is both acanthotic and hyperkeratotic, supported by a core of hyperplastic dermis. Sometimes, overgrowth of the connective tissue of the dermis is a dominant lesion. Epithelial cells of the stratum spinosum may contain **intranuclear eosinophilic** homogeneous structures, which are **viral inclusion bodies.**

More **classical papillomas** with only a moderate amount of connective tissue support are caused by **bovine papillomaviruses type 3** (skin) and **type 5** (teat). These are smaller and less pedunculated. **Type 4 virus** causes papillomas of the oesophagus, forestomach, and urinary bladder. With the consumption of bracken fern, these papillomas may progress to squamous-cell carcinoma. It has been experimentally demonstrated that the bovine papilloma virus can produce fibromas and polyps of the bovine urinary bladder similar to the naturally occurring tumours associated with chronic enzootic haematuria.

Equine Sarcoid

Bovine papillomaviruses 1 and 2 cause equine sarcoid (Table 13). This cutaneous growth peculiar to equines is called "**sarcoid**" because **microscopically it resembles a sarcoma** of moderate malignancy. The lesion is often multiple and usually occurs on the lower legs, head, and prepuce. It is **more common in mules and donkeys than in the horse. Microscopically**, the growth is made up mainly of interlacing bundles of **spindle-shaped cells**, which may form whorls and bundles suggestive of a neurofibrosarcoma. The real **difficulty is in distinguishing the sarcoid from a sarcoma.** Usually there is less anaplasia of nuclei and fewer mitoses than in a sarcoma, but in borderline cases differentiation may not be possible on histological grounds alone. Metastasis, however, does not occur.

Equine Cutaneous Papillomatosis

Common warts are usually found on the **nose, muzzle, and lips** of horses during their first and second years of life. The papillomas are usually small, discrete and attached by a narrow stalk. Sometimes, they are very numerous and may be confluent. **Small papillomas** appear as raised nodules with a smooth surface. The **larger papillomas**, however, have the rough surface characteristic of warts in other species. **Microscopically**, hyperplastic, folded layers of squamous epithelium are supported by a thin core of connective tissue which is continuous with the dermis. **Acanthosis** and **hyperkeratosis** are prominent features in the affected epidermis.

Canine Oral Papillomatosis

Infectious papillomas occur in the oral cavity of young dogs. These lesions are transmissible by contact, **but will grow only on the oral mucosa.** Skin and other epithelial surfaces are resistant to infection. The duration of oral papillomas is usually from 3-5 months. The **lesions** may be single, but are usually mutiple. Sometimes, they are so numerous as to interfere with mastication and deglutination. They occur anywhere on the oral mucosa, such as cheeks, tongue, palate, or pharynx, but do not extend below the epiglottis, or into the oesophagus. Papillomas are sharply defined, single or confluent, cauliflower-shaped masses with a roughened surface, raised from the oral mucosa. **Microscopically**, the earliest lesion is a hyperplastic epithelium in which mitotic figures are common. The prickle-cell layer then becomes gradually thicker. Other lesions include hyperkeratosis, and enlargement of the squamous cells, their cytoplasm being filled with albuminous material. In older lesions, a few **cytoplasmic inclusions** may be seen just under the keratin layer. These are keratohyaline masses. In some cases, **basophilic inclusions** fill nuclei of epithelial cells. Viral particles have been demonstrated in epithelial nuclei. The underlying dermis is relatively unchanged.

Ovine and Caprine Papillomatosis

Papillomas in sheep and goats are rare. In sheep, they occur as fibropapillomas, or squamous papillomas, on face, ears or limbs. Malignant transformation has been described. **In goats**, two forms have been described, one limited to the teats and udder, and a cutaneous form found around the head, face, shoulder, and neck. **Malignant transformation to squamous-cell carcinoma may occur**.

Porcine Genital Papilloma

A transmissible papilloma of the genital tract of **pigs** has been described. However, it is an uncommon disease.

Papillomatosis of Monkeys

Papillomas are rare in monkeys. Regression of the lesion occurs, and there is no evidence of malignancy.

Cutaneous Papillomatosis of Rabbits (Shope Fibroma)

An infectious papillomatosis of wild cottontail rabbits was originally described by Shope in 1933. Hence it is often referred to as **"Shope fibroma"**, or **"Shope papilloma"**. The **warts** are usually found on the inner surface of the thighs, abdomen, or neck and shoulders. The lesions are black or grey, and covered with a thin layer of keratin. They may become malignant. **Domestic rabbits are rarely affected naturally**, but can be experimentally infected, in which case the papillomas may progress to squamous-cell carcinoma and metastasize.

Oral Papillomatosis of Rabbits

In 1943, Parson and Kidd described spontaneous papillomatosis of the oral cavity in domestic rabbits, and demonstrated it to be caused by a virus. The viral agent is different from the Shope fibroma (papilloma) virus, which affects the epithelium of the skin, but not the mouth. The papillomas are small, discrete, greyish-white nodules, either sessile or pedunculated. Usually multiple and sometimes numerous, they always occur on the undersurface of the tongue, sometimes on the gums, and rarely on the floor of the mouth. **Microscopically,** the lesions comprise thickened, folded, hyperplastic epithelium, supported by stroma which may form delicate papillae.

Diseases caused by Unclassified Viruses

In Domestic Animals

Borna Disease

Borna disease is **an infectious, progressive immune-mediated polio-encephalomyelitis** (inflammation of the grey matter of the brain and spinal cord) of **horses and sheep** in Europe. It is caused by **a single-stranded, negative-sense RNA (ss RNA) virus**, which has not yet been visualized, and therefore **remains unclassified**. The disease derives its name from **Borna in Saxony, Germany**, where a severe attack was described in 1885. An insect vector is not needed for spread. **Spread** is through saliva and nasal secretions; possibly through colostrum and milk from infected horses with clinical disease; or through individuals with a persistent infection, who serve as carriers of the virus.

Clinically, affected horses develop a slight fever, followed by lethargy (a lazy state), ataxia (muscular incoordination), circling, paralysis, and death in most animals. The virus replicates in neurons, astrocytes, and oligodendrocytes, and has a predilection for grey matter of the cerebrum and brain stem. The cerebellum is spared. **Microscopically**, the encephalitis is characterized by marked cuffing with lymphocytes, along with some macrophages and plasma cells, and gliosis. **Acidophilic intranuclear inclusion bodies** are present within neurons, particularly of the hippocampus. These are termed as **"Joest bodies"** or **"Joest-Degen bodies"**, after the names of their discoverers. **They are specific for Borna disease**. The pathogenesis of the encephalitis is believed to be mainly immune-mediated. **Diagnosis** is made microscopically by the demonstration of Joest bodies. Specific diagnosis can be made with such techniques as *in situ* hybridization and polymerase chain reaction (PCR) viral amplification. Using these techniques, viral RNA can be demonstrated in neurons, astrocytes, and Schwann cells.

In Poultry

Hydropericardium-Hepatitis Syndrome (Angara Disease)

Hydropericardium-hepatitis syndrome (HHS) is **an acute, infectious disease of chickens** characterized by high morbidity, excessive pericardial fluid, and multifocal hepatic necrosis. Although the specific aetiology of HHS has yet to be defined, it appears that the condition is caused by **a pathogenic group I adenovirus, a non-enveloped double-stranded DNA (ds DNA) virus**. Other agents may act as potentiators and increase the severity of the disease. Role of intercurrent immunosuppressive diseases, such as infectious bursal disease, Marek's disease, and chicken infectious anaemia may be significant.

HHS syndrome was first recognized in flocks in Angara Goth near Karachi, Pakistan, in late 1987. Hence the name **"Angara Disease"**. **In India**, outbreaks have occurred in the northern states of Jammu and Kashmir, Punjab, and Delhi. **The disease in India has been called as "Leechi Disease"**, because the heart looks like a leechi fruit. Although 3-5 week-old broilers are usually affected, the condition has been recorded in young broiler breeds, and also in commercial layers.

Spread

Since group I adenoviruses appear to be involved in the aetiology, it is presumed that the disease can be **spread both vertically and horizontally**. Adenoviruses may remain latent in breeding stock until onset of maturity, and then be shed following immunosuppression, or stress. After 3 weeks of age, progeny of infected parent stock may excrete virus for up to 14 weeks. **Viral replication in the intestinal tract** suggests that faecal contamination of clothing, footwear, and equipment, including transport crates and vehicles, may spread infection under commercial conditions.

Signs

Non-vaccinated broilers and young breeder flocks can have mortality up to 80% if they are also exposed to velogenic Ranikhet disease, highly pathogenic infectious bursal disease, and erosive infections such as mycoplasmosis. The disease usually lasts 9-14 days with morbidity of 10-30%, and daily mortality of 3-5%. Flocks show **no specific signs**. However, the disease is characterized by sudden onset of mortality, lethargy, huddling with ruffled feathers, and yellow, mucoid droppings. Affected birds have decreased haemoglobin, packed cell volume, erythrocytes, and total leukocytes. **Decreased albumin production** because of liver damage is considered to be responsible for the **hypoproteinaemia** in affected birds, which probably contributes to development of hydropericardium.

Lesions

The most striking gross lesion is the presence of up to 10 ml of clear transudate in the pericardial sac. Generalized congestion and pulmonary oedema are evident and the liver and kidneys are usually enlarged, pale, and friable. **Microscopic lesions** consist of myocardial oedema, degeneration, and necrosis with mild, mononuclear cell infiltration and extravasation of erythrocytes. Liver shows multifocal coagulative necrosis with mononuclear cell infiltration, and **basophilic intranuclear inclusion bodies in hepatocytes**. There may also be extensive areas of necrosis in renal epithelium.

Diagnosis

Hydropericardium together with microscopic demonstration of **basophilic intranuclear inclusions in hepatocytes** is highly suggestive of Angara disease. To confirm the diagnosis, a denovirus can be isolated by infecting embryonic chick liver cells. The presence of adenovirus in tissue culture is indicated by characteristic cytopathology. Adenoviruses can be demonstrated by negative-stain electron microscopy, and identified by a serum neutralization test.

Infectious Stunting Syndrome

In 1976, a new disease was recognized in broiler chickens in the USA and Europe. It was characterized by birds becoming severely stunted and growing poorly. However, the birds were not ill. They were active with great appetites. Despite this the financial losses were considerable due to excess culling rates, poor feed conversion, reduced weight for age, and greater than expected variations in weight at slaughter. The disease has now been reported from most broiler-growing countries of the world, **including India**.

"**Infectious stunting syndrome (ISS)**" is also known by several other names. These are: "**runting and stunting syndrome**", "**malabsorption syndrome**", "**broiler runting syndrome**", "**pale bird syndrome**", "**infectious runting**", and "**helicopter disease**" or as "**helicopter feathering**". There is also a stunting disease in turkeys, known as "**turkey stunting syndrome**". It is characterized by enteritis and diarrhoea.

Cause

Infectious stunting syndrome is probably **caused by a number of viruses**, which include **calicivirus, enterovirus, parvovirus, coronavirus, FEW virus, reovirus, or togavirus**. Recent studies have revealed **picornavirus-like particles** in the cytoplasm of degenerate enterocytes and associated macrophages in acute intestinal lesions. All breeds and strains of chickens are susceptible, **but suppression of growth is most noticeable in broilers because of their rapid growth rates**.

Pathogenesis

Following infection, the lesions are most pronounced in the mid-jejunum. **Picornavirus-like particles are detected in the cytoplasm of enterocytes on the villi**. These viruses are associated with necrosis of enterocytes, and there is marked infiltration of macrophages and lymphocytes into the villus. The viruses are then spread through macrophages to the lamina propria surrounding the crypts, and multiplication of the virus in crypt enterocytes leads to **necrosis and loss of crypts**. At this stage there is significant villus atrophy. By 2 weeks, the lost enterocytes are replaced through crypt cell proliferation, but the villi are populated by biochemically immature enterocytes. This results in impaired digestive capability, and **leads to poor growth, the characteristic feature of the disease**. Retarded feathering is probably the result of reduced digestion and absorption of sulphur-containing amino acids.

Signs

The prevalence of stunted (small) birds in an affected flock ranges from 1-75%. At 4-8 days, the stunted chickens are characterized by the **retarded feathering on their heads and necks**, and **pendulous abdomens**. At this stage, they eat well and are very active. At about 2 weeks, affected chickens are often called as "**yellow heads**" because of the prominence of the retained down feathers on the head and neck. Broken and displaced primary wing feathers have given the disease names like "**helicopter feathering**" or "**helicopter disease**". At 2-4 weeks clinical signs include lameness due to secondary osteodystrophy, poor weight gain, opisthotonus (stretching of the head upwards and backwards), and **pale shanks**. Pale shanks are an important feature in some strains given high carotenoid diets. **Feed conversion rates are poor**. One of the important features of the disease is the presence of **severely stunted (runted) chickens, which remain small despite their huge appetites**. However, their incidence is low, usually 1-5%. If allowed to live to 6 weeks, they weigh only 100-200 g. These small chickens become more noticeable after 2 weeks when the unaffected chickens grow rapidly.

Gross Lesions

The subcutaneous fat is pale compared to normal, hence the name "**pale bird syndrome**". They are not anaemic. Intestines are distended and pale with poorly digested contents. This phenomenon has been referred to as "**malabsorption syndrome**". The intestines may contain clear watery fluid, described as "**mucoid**" or "**catarrhal enteritis**". The thymus is reduced to a chain of small dark lobes, and the bursa of Fabricius is usually swollen. The pancreas may be hard and white. During a normal postmortem, the hips are disarticulated, but in infectious stunting syndrome, this usually results in the **separation of the head of the femur** from the underlying growth plate (physis). This occurs in chickens with osteodystrophy **because the physis is weaker than the ligaments**. This lesion is a traumatic separation of the femoral head, and should not be described as "**femoral head necrosis**". The parathyroids are more prominent than normal.

Microscopic Lesions

Intestinal lesions include villus atrophy, and necrosis and degeneration of enterocytes on the sides of villi and crypts, associated with significant infiltration of lymphocytes and macrophages into the villus and lamina propria. Lesions are most pronounced in the mid-jejunum. Enterocytes and degenerate macrophages reveal **small cytoplasmic inclusions**.

Diagnosis

The aetiological agent has not been characterized, and serological tests are not available. Therefore, diagnosis depends upon characteristic features of the disease, namely, severely stunted (runted) but active chickens with retained down feathers on the head and neck at 2-3 weeks of age; and poor growth in a variable percentage of the remaining flock at 2-4 weeks.

Big Liver and Spleen Disease

Big liver and spleen disease (BLS) is **an infectious, transmissible disease, probably of viral aetiology**. It is characterized by decreased egg production, increased mortality, and enlargement of the liver and spleen of mature chickens. **The disease occurs mainly in broiler breeders**, and less commonly, egg layers. The condition was first recognized in Australia in 1980. The cause of BLS is considered to be **a virus**. However, so far it has not been possible to isolate or identify the agent. **Spread** occurs by horizontal transmission among flocks, and faecal-oral route has been suspected. The possibility of vertical transmission during clinical infection of the hens, has been suggested.

Morbidity and mortality are low. Affected flocks usually appear normal. **Clinical signs** vary considerably from inapparent infection, general poor performance, delayed maturity, and failure to attain peak production to definite egg drops. Small eggs with thin, poorly pigmented shells are produced. At necropsy, **the most common gross lesion is an enlarged spleen, 2-3 times that of normal**. Multiple pale foci on splenic capsular and cut surfaces may be present. Usually, the liver is also enlarged and may have a large number of small subcapsular haemorrhages. Other lesions are variable. **Microscopically**, there is proliferation of lymphoid tissue in spleen and liver initially. **In liver**, lymphoid follicles and perivascular lymphoid tissue are increased. When signs develop, there is widespread necrosis of lymphoid tissue **in the spleen**, and in tissues where lymphoid hyperplasia had occurred earlier.

Diagnosis

Presumptive diagnosis is based on typical clinical signs in mature chickens, with **enlarged livers and spleens (spleen:bodyweight ratios greater than 0.001)**. Detection of antigen and/or antibody will confirm the diagnosis. Agar-gel immunodiffusion tests have been used to detect antigen and antibody. However, they are less sensitive than ELISA tests. Currently, ELISA tests are used for detection of antibodies and antigen, using purified antigen extracted from spleen and liver of affected birds, or monoclonal/polyclonal antibodies, respectively. Immunofluorescence can be used for identifying antigen in frozen tissue sections.

2

Prion Diseases

"**Prions**" are the most recent addition to the class of **pathogens** causing diseases in domestic animals and humans. "**Prion**" is a proteinaceous infective particle. Recent work has revealed that prion is a heavily glycosylated specific protein (a polypeptide) of 30 kilodaltons (30-kD), called "**prion protein (PrP)**". Since it is a proteinaceous particle closely associated with infectivity, the term "**proin**" was coined from "**pro**teinaceous **in**fective particle". The word "**proin**" thus formed from "**pro**" and "**in**" was changed to "**prion**" to sound rhythmic.

Although both "**prions**" and "**viruses**" replicate, their properties, structure, and modes of replication are fundamentally different. **Prions lack nucleic acid (RNA or DNA),** and also do not produce any inflammatory or immune reaction in the host. **Thus, prions are the most unconventional agents**. Because they lack nucleic acids, prions are remarkably resistant to many agents that normally inactivate viruses, such as ultraviolet light and standard disinfectants. In fact, they can be classified as an entirely separate category. **For his discovery of "prions", Stanley Prusiner,** Professor of Biochemistry at the University of California, San Francisco, USA, **won the 1997 Nobel Prize** in Physiology and Medicine. The diseases caused by prions are called "**prion diseases**". B oth, in domestic animals and humans, prions cause a group of diseases known as "**transmissible spongiform encephalopathies (TSEs)**". These will now be discussed.

Transmissible Spongiform Encephalopathies (TSEs)

These diseases are so named because they all are characterized microscopically by a spongiform change in the grey matter of brain (**encephalopathy**), and are caused by **transmissible agents**. A lso, they all share an aetiological basis that distinguishes them from other neurodegenerative and infectious diseases. They are all associated with abnormal forms of a specific protein termed "**prion protein (PrP)**". The **spongiform change,** also known as "**spongiosis**" or "**status spongiosus**", is characterized by the development of vacuoles or empty spaces (**vacuolation**) both in the neurons and the neuropil (i.e., complex tissue network of the cytoplasmic processes of neurons and neuroglia in the grey matter). Thus, TSEs are "**prion diseases,**" that constitute a distinct group of neurodegenerative disorders. They are all characterized by classical pattern of neurohistology (**spongiosis**) restricted to the central nervous system, an unusually long incubation period (**months to years or decades**), and a variable course associated with typical clinical signs.

Spongiform encephalopathies, **in animals**, comprise **scrapie** of sheep and goats, **transmissible mink encephalopathy (TME), transmissible feline encephalopathy (TFE), chronic wasting disease of mule deer and elk**, and the recently identified "**bovine spongiform encephalopathy (BSE)**". **In humans**, they include **Creutzfeldt-Jakob disease (CJD), kuru** (associated with cannibalism), **Gerstmann-Straussler-Scheinker syndrome (GSS)**, and **fatal familial insomnia**. Since they are all caused by the same class of pathogen - "**a prion protein (PrP)**", they are more accurately called as "**prion diseases**". All types of human and animal spongiform encephalopathy, including kuru, scrapie, and bovine spongiform encephalopathy, are experimentally transmissible in animals. With the arrival of BSE and its zoonotic potential, importance of TSEs has increased manifold. Therefore, scrapie and bovine spongiform encephalopathy are discussed at some length. Since scrapie is a prototype of TSEs (i.e., an original model), it is discussed first.

Scrapie of Sheep (Ovine Spongiform Encephalopathy)

Scrapie is the oldest of prion diseases, the earliest record of its occurrence in Britain being in 1732. Between 1878 and 1900, at least 17 countries reported the disease. Australia, which had recognized it earlier became free later on. On the other hand, Japan which was free for several decades, was invaded in 1990. **Scrapie is the most intensively studied prion disease**, and several aspects of scrapie research have shed considerable light on multiple parameters, such as the characteristics of the causative agent, concepts of infectivity and pathogenesis, histopathological hallmarks, transmissibility, and characterization of the so-called "**scrapie-associated fibrils**".

Scrapie is best known as a disease of **sheep**, but it also occurs in **goats**. The name is derived from almost continuous **scraping** (rubbing) of the skin against any stationary object because of the intense pruritus (severe itching) the animal suffers, which often results in loss of wool in sheep.

Aetiology

The precise nature of the transmissible agent in TSEs remains elusive. Like a virus it is filterable, but lacks many of the features of ordinary viruses. Unlike conventional viruses, the agent is unusually resistant to many chemical agents, including formalin, chloroform and ether; also to heat, ultraviolet and ionizing radiation, ultrasonication, proteases and nucleases. Also, no structures resembling virions can be detected ultrastructurally (i.e., by an electron microscope).

The current belief is that the agent is a proteinaceous infective (prion). Much recent work has focussed on a heavily protein (a poplypeptide) of 30 kilodaltons called **"prion protein (PrP)." Prions contain no nucleic acid (RNA or DNA), and also do not produce any inflammatory or immune reaction in the host**. Immune B c ell a nd T cell functions are intact.

Transmission

The principal means of transmission is from infected ewes to their lambs early in life. The placenta is infectious. Thus, prenatal transmission may also be important. Owing to the resistance of prions to physical and chemical agents, environmental contamination probably persists for long periods. The incubation period is long (from 2-5 years), **restricting the clinical disease to adult sheep**.

Pathogenesis

Pathogenesis of TSEs involves complex molecular mechanisms, and is still not fully understood. Most of the information is derived from work on natural scrapie, and experiments in mice. The results of a genetic linkage, and open reading frame sequencing studies in humans and mice, suggest that amino acid substitution in PrP may modulate the development of prion diseases.

It is n ow known that prion p totein (PrP) o ccurs normally in the central nervous system of all domestic animals and also humans, **bound to the surface of neurons**. A nimals susceptible t o prion d isease(s) bear a gene (PrP gene). This gene encodes for normal " **prion protein (PrP)**", also known a s **"cellular prion protein (PrPc)."** P rP is attached t o the o uter l eaflet of the plasma membrane lipid bilayer of the neurons. Although its normal function is n ot known, in a **modified form**, i t is associated with the pathogenesis o f TSEs. In other words, in all TSEs, a normal non-infectious PrP of the host is slowly and progressively converted to an abnormal form of PrP **(PrPsc)**. That is, **in spongiform encephalopathies, an abnormal isoform (similar type) of PrP, termed "scrapie PrP" or "PrPsc" or "scrapie-associated fibril protein (SAF)" is generated, which accumulates in and around neurons as large aggregates of polymerized macromolecular fibrils similar to amyloid protein**. The fibrils are resistant to proteases, whereas normal PrP is not. It is these fibrils of prion protein which make u p the **"amyloid plaques"** seen in spongiform e ncephalopathies. In o ther words, **the abnormal form (PrPsc) has a high beta-pleated sheet conformation (structure) characteristic of amyloid protein**, and spontaneously forms neurotoxic amyloid fibrils, which accumulate i n the b rain. The a bnormal form o f PrP is also e ncoded by the same gene which encodes for normal prion protein PrP.

To put it more simply, **PrP is a normal cellular protein present in neurons**. Disease o ccurs when t he prion p rotein undergoes a conformational change (i.e., change i n shape o r form) f rom its n ormal alpha-helix i soform **(PrPc)** to an abnormal beta-pleated sheet isoform, known as either **PrPsc (for scrapie)** or **PrPres (for protease resistant)**. **With the conformational change,** the prion protein becomes resistant to digestion with proteases. Accumulation of PrPsc (PrPres) in neural tissue appears to be the cause of the pathology in prion diseases, but how this material causes the development of cytoplasmic vacuoles and eventual death of the neurons, is still unknown.

It is believed that following oral infection at an early age, there is a long eclipse phase of about one year, before the infective agent (prion protein) can be detected in the animal. At this time the infective agent is present in low concentrations in the tonsils, supra-pharyngeal lymph node, and lymphoid tissue of the intestine. Infective agent then spreads to other lymph nodes and spleen. The infective agent continues to replicate in the extra-intestinal and intestinal lymphoid tissues for even a year or more before it reaches the CNS, which is the target organ. The CNS in sheep is infected probably by haematogenous spread, although axonal spread may also occur. Infective agent first appears in the CNS in the medulla oblongata and diencephalon, when infected sheep are clinically normal. It then spreads to other parts of the CNS and replicates. Clinical disease usually occurs when sheep are 3-4 years of age, when high concentrations of the infective agent are present in the CNS. The pathogenesis of the disease in goats appears similar to that in the sheep.

However, it is still not clear by which mechanism the "infective prion agents" alter the normal PrP. Since both PrP and PrPsc are transcribed from the same gene, the disease-linked modification of the protein is considered to be a post-transcriptional event. That is, it occurs after the genetic information encoded in the DNA is transferred to messenger RNA. It is believed that this post-transcriptional modification occurs following infection (by the infective form), and may take a very long period. This may perhaps account for the unusually long incubation period of TSEs. The conversion of the normal PrP to abnormal form (PrPsc) is associated with the acquirement of infectivity. That is, normal PrP is not infective or pathogenic, whereas the abnormal form becomes infective or pathogenic, and produces characteristic neuropathology of the disease. The mechanism by which the abnormal form develops is still not fully understood. Recent studies suggest that it develops because of the substitution of one amino acid in the normal prion protein for another, at a given position in the nucleotide sequence. This involves substitution of histidine in place of tyrosine at position 155, and serine in the place of aspartic acid at position 143.

Clinical Signs

The signs, which appear in adult sheep, are characterized at the outset by restlessness and a startled look. The eyes have a wild and fixed expression. The pupils are dilated. The sheep may hold its head down and move it rapidly from side to side or up and down. Its movements are aimless, and stiffness of forelegs results in a trotting gait, The animal usually grinds its teeth. The voice may be altered. The skin irritation begins in the lumbar region, then may involve the rest of the body. **The intense pruritus causes the sheep to rub against objects continuously until the wool coat is almost completely lost.** Incoordination may be followed by paralysis and inability to stand, and finally the animal dies.

Lesions

No characteristic gross lesions are found in this disease. Microscopic lesions in sheep and goats are limited to the CNS. They usually occur in diencephalon, brain stem, and cerebellum, with variable lesions in the spinal cord. The cerebral cortex basically remains unaffected. The characteristic lesions include neuronal degeneration, astrocytosis, and **variable spongiosus (spongiosis) characterized by prominent neuronal and neuropil vacuolation, generally affecting the grey matter. Pronounced hypertrophy and hyperplasia of astrocytes are characteristic of scrapie.** Neuronal degeneration is characterized by shrinkage of neurons with increased basophilia and cytoplasmic vacuolation. Other changes, such as central chromatolysis and ischaemic cell damage, also variably occur. It was not known until recently whether the **pronounced astrocytosis** is a primary, or a secondary response. Recent studies have helped clarify this problem. **An abnormal protein (prion amyloid protein) first accumulates in astrocytes** in the brain during scrapie infection, which means that this cell is the primary site of replication. The **spongiform change** affects the grey matter, and results from dilatation of neuronal processes. Other causes, including vacuolation of neuronal and astroglial perikarya (cytoplasm around nucleus), swelling of astrocytic processes, and splitting of myelin sheaths, have also been reported. **Cerebrovascular amyloidosis** has also been detected in sheep.

Diagnosis

Diagnosis is made on the basis of the clinical signs, and is confirmed by microscopic examination of the brain and spinal cord. Specific diagnosis is now possible with antisera against purified prion protein, or scrapie-associated fibril protein, either on extracts of brain or on reaction with tissue.

Recently, **an eyelid test** has been developed in the United States to detect scrapie in the living animals suspected of the disease. It was discovered that, besides brain, PrP also accumulates in lymphatic tissue of the inner eyelid of sheep during incubation period of the disease. The lymphatic structure is present in sheep and cows, but not humans. A skin sample is taken from a sheep's eyelid and tested for PrP using a monoclonal antibody that binds tightly to the protein. The eyelid test has yielded encouraging results, and may make it possible to destroy scrapie-infected sheep before they have a chance to spread infection. The test could thus prove to be an important tool in the eradication of scrapie. **Work is now under way to find out whether the eyelid test also works in cows to detect BSE before they show symptoms.**

Another related test to detect scrapie in living animals is also under development. The test, from a Dutch team, involves extracting sheep's tonsils.

Bovine Spongiform Encephalopathy (BSE, Mad Cow Disease)

Bovine spongiform encephalopathy, commonly known as "**mad cow disease**", **is a more recent addition** to the group of transmissible spongiform encephalopathies. **It is a non-inflammatory, degenerative disease of CNS in cattle, which is invariably fatal**. BSE was first clinically suspected in April 1985 in British dairy herd. It was then identified and confirmed as a prion disease in November 1986. The disease was subsequently confirmed to exist in cattle in the Republic of Ireland. It was also identified in cattle **exported** from England to Oman, Italy, Denmark, Germany, Canada, and Falkland Islands. In France, Switzerland, and Portugal a limited number of cases have occurred in **native cattle**.

In Britain, BSE has emerged as a major agricultural and economic problem, and also as a potential hazard to public health. Restriction on the import of British beef by the European countries, coupled with a demand of slaughter of all affected cattle, present an alarming problem to British agriculture.

It is most unlikely that BSE or BSE-derived new variant CJD are prevalent in our country since no sheep meat meal and bone meal (scrapie infected) have been fed to cattle in India as a cheaper source of protein, as was done in Britain. **All the same, this anthropogenic (man-made) disease of Britain does have a message for us - to remain very vigilant and proceed with utmost caution, and also to refrain from any unnatural practices**.

Aetiology

BSE is caused by a prion protein (PrP). For details on the causative agent, refer to aetiology discussed under scrapie.

The incubation period is unusually long of about 4-5 years. All cases in British cattle (mainly Friesian/Holstein cows) have occurred in **adult animals**, with a peak incidence in those **between 3-5 years of age**. By April 1995, BSE had been confirmed in 53% British dairy herds, 15% of beef herds and 34% of all herds with adult breeding cattle. Since 1986 more than 1,70,000 cases of BSE have been confirmed in British cattle, and the animals slaughtered.

Transmission

In the early 1980s, in Britain, there was an increase in the use of protein derived from ruminants, as a cheaper source of protein for cattle feed. This was done following an increase in the world prices of protein supplements, such as fish meal and soyabeans. The epidemiological evidence strongly indicates that the disease was caused initially, during the early 1980s, by the feeding o f rations c ontaining meat a nd bone m eal supplements to cattle, **contaminated with the scrapie agent**. It appears that this happened because of a change from **high temperature** batch rendering (treatment) of sheep carcass material to **low temperature** continuous rendering. This changed process, introduced in the 1980s, **appears to have been less efficient in inactivating the scrapie agent**. When meat meal and bone meal processed in this manner were fed to cattle as part of their concentrate ration, **the agent got introduced into cattle**. The e pidemic then became amplified b y the s ubsequent recycling, through meat meal and bone meal, of infected cattle material within the cattle p opulation.

Pathogenesis

Pathogenesis of the disease involves conversion of **normal prion protein (PrP)** in the CNS, slowly and progressively, to an **abnormal form (PrPsc)** and this causes development of the disease. For details, refer to pathogenesis discussed under scrapie.

Symptoms

As already s tated, **BSE has a very long incubation period** (about 4 -5 years), and has an insidious onset. That is, it develops so gradually as to be well established before becoming apparent. The disease advances mercilessly, and there i s **an inevitable progression to death within weeks or months (usually six months)**. **Clinical signs include** behavioural, gait, and p ostural abnormalities which usually begin with apprehension, anxiety, and fear. That is, the affected cattle show a variety of nervous signs, mainly changes in behaviour, abnormalities i n posture a nd gait, and extreme sensitivity to so und and t ouch (hyperaesthesia). Following the onset of c linical signs, affected cattle lose weight until they die, or require euthanasia (painless killing). **This period ranges from 2 weeks to 6 months**. Slaughter of the affected animals becomes necessary because of their unmanageable behaviour, traumatic damage as a result of repeated falling, and prolonged recumbency. It is because of t his p eculiar a nd uncontrollable behaviour o f t he affected cow t hat t he disease has been termed **"mad cow disease"**. **Almost all cases have occurred in adult females, and not in adult males**. It has been suggested that this may be because only a small proportion of bulls are kept for breeding to reach the susceptible age (3-5 years) when the disease is manifested.

Histopathological Findings

BSE was initially diagnosed in 1986 by histological examination of sections of brain. (The changes described here should be read in context with the microscopic lesions described under scrapie). The characteristic changes comprise discrete (separate) ovoid and spherical vacuoles, or microcavities, in the neuropil (**Fig. 6**). This **spongiosis** (i.e., neuropil vacuolation) is a predominant form of vacuolar change observed, **and is a feature of TSEs**. Subsequently it was e stablished t hat the p athognomonic v acuolar changes are c onsistently present in the brain stem facilitating routine diagnosis of the disease. Neuronal perikarya and neurites (axons) of certain brain stem nuclei contain large well-defined intracytoplasmic vacuoles. These are single or multiple, and sometimes distend the soma (body) to produce **ballooned neurons** with a narrow rim of cytoplasm (**Fig. 6**). The contents of vacuoles, both in the neuropil and in neurons remain unstained and clear, after histological staining for glycogen in paraffin and for lipids in fixed cryostat sections. A mild gliosis sometimes accompanies the degenerative changes. The changes described in the brains of cattle affected with BSE are clearly pathological, and distinguishable from single large intracytoplasmic vacuoles recognized in healthy cattle. Also, now established as an additional diagnostic criterion for the spongiform encephalopathies is the detection by electron microscopy in extracts of affected brain of abnormal fibrils which have been called "**scrapie-associated fibrils**" (**Fig. 7**).

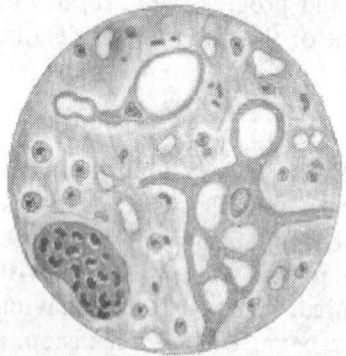

Fig. 6. Diagrammatic vacuolation in the grey matter of a BSE affected cow. Note vacuoles in the neuropil, multiple vacuoles in the cytoplasm and processes of the right neuron, ballooning of the upper neuron, and neuronophagia of the left necrotic neuron.

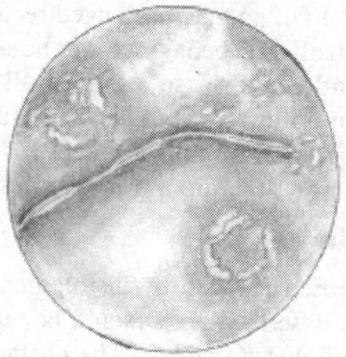

Fig. 7. Diagrammatic electron micrograph of negatively-stained "**scrapie-associated fibril**" from the brain of a BSE affected cow.

Diagnosis

There are at present no tests available for diagnosis of BSE before the death of the animal. Diagnosis is based on clinical signs, and **confirmed by characteristic pathological changes found in the brain of affected animals**. More specifically, it can be made through the use of antibodies to prion protein, or scrapie-associated fibrils.

More recently, in the United States and Germany, a test has been developed for diagnosing **"mad cow disease"** and its **human equivalent CJD in living subjects**. This raises hopes of an end to the slaughter of uninfected cattle. At present, the only way to confirm a case of BSE or CJD is at postmortem examination. The test relates to the proteins found in the cerebrospinal fluid of animals with spongiform encephalopathies and patients with CJD. The test has been developed to detect the characteristic proteins, designated as 130 and 131. **In humans**, the test has a sensitivity of more than 98% and a specificity of more than 99%. **Use of the test in cattle is still far away and requires much more work**.

Control

There is at present no specific evidence to suggest that BSE is transmitted by contact between cattle, or from mother to offspring. Artificial insemination and embryo transfer do not seem to transmit the BSE agent. Since there is no treatment, control measures should include immediate destruction of affected animals and ban on the feeding of ruminant tissues to livestock. Carcasses and all parts from affected cattle must be destroyed.

Zoonotic potential

BSE has now posed itself as a potential hazard to public health in Great Britain. There is a real fear in the mind of people that BSE may be transmissible to man.

The evidence that the agent causing BSE in cattle may cause neurological disease in beef eaters is now gaining momentum. It is likely that the prion protein responsible for BSE might **'jump species'**, and infect humans. Microbes are capable of rapid genetic adaptation. Prions may do likewise. Ever since humans made intimate contact with other animal species - by encroaching on their natural environment, eating them, or domesticating them - mutant strains of zoonotic agents have opportunistically become infectious agents in humans. Thus, we have acquired smallpox from cattle, measles from ungulates (i.e., hoofed animals, such as pigs, horses, ruminants) or dogs, influenza from pigs, and acquired immunodeficiency syndrome (AIDS) from monkeys. **As such it is likely that transmission may be happening with BSE and its human equivalent Creutzfeldt-Jacob disease (CJD).**

Recent sequencing of the prion protein in vertebrates indicates **an evolu-**

tionary connection between BSE and CJD in cattle and in humans. In other words, the nucleotide sequence of genes of naturally occurring prion proteins in a variety of animals has revealed **a unique genetic modification shared only by cattle and humans.** Although the prion protein in cattle closely resembled that in sheep, the cattle and human prions were found to be uniquely similar at two points in their genetic sequence. This genetic modification, found in cattle and human's prion sequence, occurs in a region known to be involved in the process of acquiring infectivity; and takes the form of a substitution of one a mino a cid in t he n ormal prion f or a nother at a given position in t he sequence, as discussed under pathogenesis of scrapie. **As the substitution is unique to cattle and humans, this finding could explain why humans may become infected with BSE, yet remain unaffected with scrapie.** Scrapie in sheep has been endemic in Britain for more than 200 years, yet not a single case of scrapie derived CJD has ever been reported in man.

Another event that has occurred is that **several British farmers have recently died from CJD** - an occupational association that is unlikely to have arisen by chance. Moreover, **these farmers had BSE infected cows in their herd.** All these findings have added new dimension to the fear that the agent responsible f or variant C JD could be transmitted t o humans from cattle i n-fected with BSE

Creutzfeldt-Jacob Disease (CJD)

CJD is the most important spongiform encephalopathy of human, and also the best characterized. It is now feared that people may contract this disease from eating beef. CJD has been in existence much before BSE was discovered. Typically, the **classical (sporadic, idiopathic) cases of CJD** begin in the sixth or seventh decade of life with amnesia (loss of memory), or less commonly, with behavioural changes, or higher cortical function disturbances such as dysphasia (impairment of speech), or dyslexia (difficulty in reading). With time, patients develop rapidly progressive dementia (mental deterioration) and myoclonus (i.e., twitching or clonic spasm of a muscle or group of muscles. A clonic spasm is characterized by muscular rigidity and then relaxation.) associated with various neurological signs. In about 10% of cases the initial clinical symptom is a behavioural disturbance or personality change often resulting in psychiatric problems. **Other signs include** abnormalities of vision or coordination, rigidity and involuntary movements. **Death occurs usually within six months,** and at autopsy, the brain shows **pathognomonic spongiosis** with neuronal loss and gliosis in the cortex, deep nuclei, and cerebellum. Amyloid plaques are found in only about 5% of cases.

Following the arrival of BSE, the above typical pattern of CJD has changed, and the disease has now started appearing in **two variant or atypical forms:** (1) CJD has now been reported in the **younger age group,** which never has been the case before. So much so that recently **even teenagers** have suffered from the disease and died. That is, the variant form of the disease affects teenagers and young adults. Moreover, the distribution of lesions differs from that of classical CJD. (2) **Clinically**, in marked contrast to classical CJD, **cases of new variant CJD (nvCJD) are characterized by psychiatric symptoms.** Since 1990, there has been a significant increase in the incidence of CJD in Britain in people under the age of 40.

New Variant or Atypical CJD (Will-Ironside Syndrome)

Usually, **patients of new variant CJD (nvCJD)** present severe depression or other psychiatric disorders, or sensory disturbances, such as disaesthesia (loss of sensation) or paraesthesia (abnormal sensation, such as numbness, prickling, and tingling), or both. However, recent studies of psychiatric symptoms in patients with the new variant disease indicate that there is no specific psychiatric picture **and that differentiation from common psychiatric conditions, such as depression may be impossible.** After a few months, the psychiatric symptoms are replaced by progressive and severe neurological dysfunction - including ataxia, cognitive impairment (i.e., damage to the mental processes of knowing, thinking or acquiring knowledge), and involuntary movements - **terminating in death**. The ill-defined early emotional and behavioural symptoms of the new variant CJD would mean examination of thousands of suspected cases of CJD over the next few years, and it will be a matter of great practical importance to screen them from imaginary cases. At present clinical diagnosis of the new variant CJD could be made during the psychiatric phase of the illness. Identification of these cases depends on the development of neurological signs, and in particular, on neuropathological examination, such as by brain biopsy. However, brain biopsy is difficult as a routine diagnostic tool in view of the risk of complications . There is therefore an urgent need for an early non-surgical diagnostic test.

Recently a new test for CJD, based on immunoassay of 14-3-3 protein in the cerebrospinal fluid, with high sensitivity and specificity, has been reported. Although this test has provided promising results, it is equally positive in both variant and the classical disease. At present definite diagnosis of both forms of CJD is possible only by neuropathological lesions, or PrP glycotyping on Western blot. More recently, single photon emission computed tomography, a neuroimaging technique that uses intravenously administered radioactive ligands to map different aspects of brain function, has been reported to be promising.

Because the new variant disease occurs in **younger patients, including teenagers**, it is essential to monitor the paediatric population. Moreover, **surveillance of classical CJD in elderly people suggests that the new disease needs to be monitored in this age group also.**

BSE and CJD

Clear evidence now exists that the variant form of CJD is caused by the same strain of agent which causes BSE, and that this strain differs from other strains isolated from cases of classical CJD. At present definite diagnosis of either form of the disease (new variant and classical CJD) **is possible only after death**. But the clinicians want the two forms to be differentiated **in the living subjects**, as early as possible.

Exposure of t he h uman p opulation i n Britain c ausing variant CJD occurred in the 1980s through beef products affected by BSE. Although so far there have been only about 30 cases of variant CJD, **it is impossible to predict how many people are now incubating the new variant form of the disease.** Cows infected with B SE entered the human food chain before the introduction o f control m easures in 1988. It i s estimated t hat about 1.8 million (18 lakhs) cows incubating BSE may have entered the human food chain between 1983 and 1999. The number of people w ho would have eaten this beef, and thus h ave had a theoretical e xposure to i nfection, may b e extremely l arge. **This could result in a possible "epidemic" of CJD.** There is also the possibility that the level of infectivity outside the nervous system may be higher in variant CJD than i n the c lassical disease. T his may i ncrease the r isk of a ccidental transmission by medical procedures. Preliminary data have shown that postmortem samples of **tonsils** from patients with variant CJD are loaded with the infective f orm of the PrP p rotein, while t hose of p atients with c lassical disease are not.

To conclude, it is now believed that human infection can occur from the ingestion of affected beef, o r even, t hough more u nlikely, from m ilk. However, **a great deal of work remains to be done in order to establish the final link between BSE and CJD.**

3

Bacterial Diseases

General Considerations

In contrast to viruses, **most bacteria are extracellular pathogens**, or facultative intracellular pathogens. That is, they are intracellular only under certain conditions, e.g., **Mycobacterium** and **Brucella** species. **All bacteria contain both DNA and RNA**, lack a nucleus, have few cytoplasmic organelles, and usually reproduce by **binary fission**. **They are classified on the basis of a large number of morphological, cultural, biochemical, antigenic, and nucleic acid parameters**. In **morphology**, they may be round (**micrococci**) (G. coccus = berry-shaped, i.e., spherical); in chains of cocci (**streptococci**); rod-shaped (**bacilli**) (L. bacillus = small rod, i.e., rod-shaped), or filamentous often with **branching** (G. actin = filament + G. myces = fungus, i.e., filamentous and branching like a fungus) (**actinomyces**). Some bacteria have cilia or flagella; others produce spores. On the basis of Gram's staining they can be divided into two groups: **Gram-positive** and **Gram-negative**. Other staining techniques can further distinguish certain groups, such as acid-fast staining of mycobacteria.

The virulence or pathogenicity of various bacteria and the mechanisms by which they cause disease are of different kinds. Some organisms, such as certain types of staphylococci and streptococci live in the nasopharynx and skin of normal animals, and produce disease only if introduced through a wound, or in immunosuppressed animals. Other strains of streptococci are not normal inhabitants, and if animals are exposed to them, they usually cause disease. These are always pathogenic. Certain bacteria are highly invasive. They multiply and spread rapidly throughout the body, producing **bacteraemia** or **septicaemia**. *Bacillus anthracis*, the cause of **anthrax**, is an example. Others tend to be **localized**, either at the point of entry, or at another site after systemic spread through bacteraemia. *Clostridium tetani*, the cause of tetanus, is an example of an organism which is not very invasive and remains at the site of entry; whereas **mycobacteria** may spread throughout the body and then get settled in localized lesions. Still other bacteria produce disease without invading the host at any time. **Botulism** and **staphylococcal food poisoning** are examples of bacterial diseases which result from the ingestion of toxins formed outside the body.

   The mechanisms whereby bacteria cause specific diseases are not always clear. Several different ways are, however, recognized. Many bacteria produce **toxins**. These can be divided into **exotoxins, endotoxins,** and **other bacterial products. E**xotoxins are harmful substances. They are often **enzymes** produced by bacteria, which interfere with host metabolism. **Exotoxins** are produced within bacterial cytoplasm. Some are secreted through the cell wall and are called "**extracellular toxins**", whereas others are released only on lysis of bacteria and are therefore called "**protoplasmic toxins or prototoxins**". Those that attack cells are called "**cytotoxins**", "**leukotoxins**" attack white cells, "**neurotoxins**" attack nerve cells, and so on. Some are highly specific, such as **tetanospasmin** (a prototoxin) produced by *Clostridium tetani.* It is a potent neurotoxin which blocks inhibitory transmitter substance. Likewise, the toxin of *Clostridium botulinum* is highly specific. It blocks cholinergic neuro-transmitters and causes paralysis. The dose of **botulinum toxin** needed to block nervous activity is extremely small. Only about eight molecules are required to block transmission by a neuron. **Alpha toxin of *Clostridium perfringens*** is an extracellular phospholipase (a lecithinase). It causes haemolysis and tissue destruction by disrupting the plasma membranes, and thus facilitates bacterial growth and spread. **Anthrax lethal toxin** works in yet a third way. It stimulates macrophages to produce oxidizing radicals and cytokines, such as interleukin-1-beta and tumour necrosis factor-alpha, which induce systemic shock and death. Thus, the diseases caused by these organisms **are entirely due to their lethal exotoxins.** The same is true for diphtheria *(Corynebacterium diphtheriae)* and cholera *(Vibrio cholerae)* in humans. Both diphtheria and cholera toxins cause ribosomal dysfunction; the former reduces the assembly of polypeptides on ribosomes, and the latter causes generation of excessive cyclic adenosine monophosphate (cAMP), which causes intestinal epithelial cells to secrete isosmotic fluid, resulting in voluminous diarrhoea and loss of water and electrolytes. One of the exotoxins of *Bacillus anthracis,* and the exotoxin of *Escherichia coli* also lead to ribosomal dysfunction, **resulting in an increase in cAMP.**

Endotoxins are complex lipopolysaccharides (LPS) which are components of the cell wall of Gram-negative bacteria, and are released on their disintegration. Lipopolysaccharide is composed of a long-chain toxic fatty acid (lipid A) connected to a core sugar chain. Both of these are the same in all Gram-negative bacteria. Attached to the core sugar is a carbohydrate chain (O antigen), which is used to serotype and differentiate various bacteria. Lipopolysaccharides have severe systemic effects which include fever, hypotension, haemorrhage, intravascular coagulation, and destruction of neutrophils with release of enzymes. Most of the biological activities of lipopolysaccharide, including the production of fever, macrophage activation, and B cell mitogenicity, come from lipid A and the core sugars, and are mediated by production of host cytokines, including interleukin-1 (IL-1) and tumour necrosis factor (TNF). LPS, in association with a circulating blood protein, binds as a complex to CD14 molecules on leukocytes (especially monocytes and macrophages), endothelial cells, and other cell types. (CD14 is a protein molecule found on monocytes and macrophages and acts as a ligand for LPS-binding protein complex). LPS-binding protein complex can then directly activate leukocytes and endothelial cells, or produce a series of cytokine mediators, which cause the pathological state (Fig. 8).

At low doses, LPS activates monocytes and macrophages, which are then able to eliminate invading bacteria. LPS can also directly activate complement, which contributes to bacterial removal. The mononuclear phagocytes, on activation by LPS, produce tumour necrosis factor (TNF), which, in turn, causes interleukin-1 (IL-1) synthesis (Fig. 8). TNF and IL-1 both act on endothelial cells to produce further cytokines (e.g., IL-6 and IL-8). Thus, the initial release of LPS results in a cytokine cascade intended to enhance the local acute inflammatory response and improve clearance of the infection. At higher levels of LPS (i.e., in moderately severe infections), cytokine-induced secondary effects (e.g., nitric oxide and platelet-activating factor) become important. (Nitric oxide, a free radical, is a soluble gas, and is produced by endothelial cells and macrophages. It is a powerful vasodilator). In addition, systemic effects of TNF and IL-1 begin to appear. These include fever, and increased synthesis of acute phase reactants. At still higher levels, LPS produces a syndrome of septic (endotoxic) shock. The same cytokine and secondary mediators now at high levels produce systemic vasodilation (hypotension), low cardiac output, and activation of the coagulation system, resulting in disseminated intravascular coagulation (DIC) (see Fig. 8).

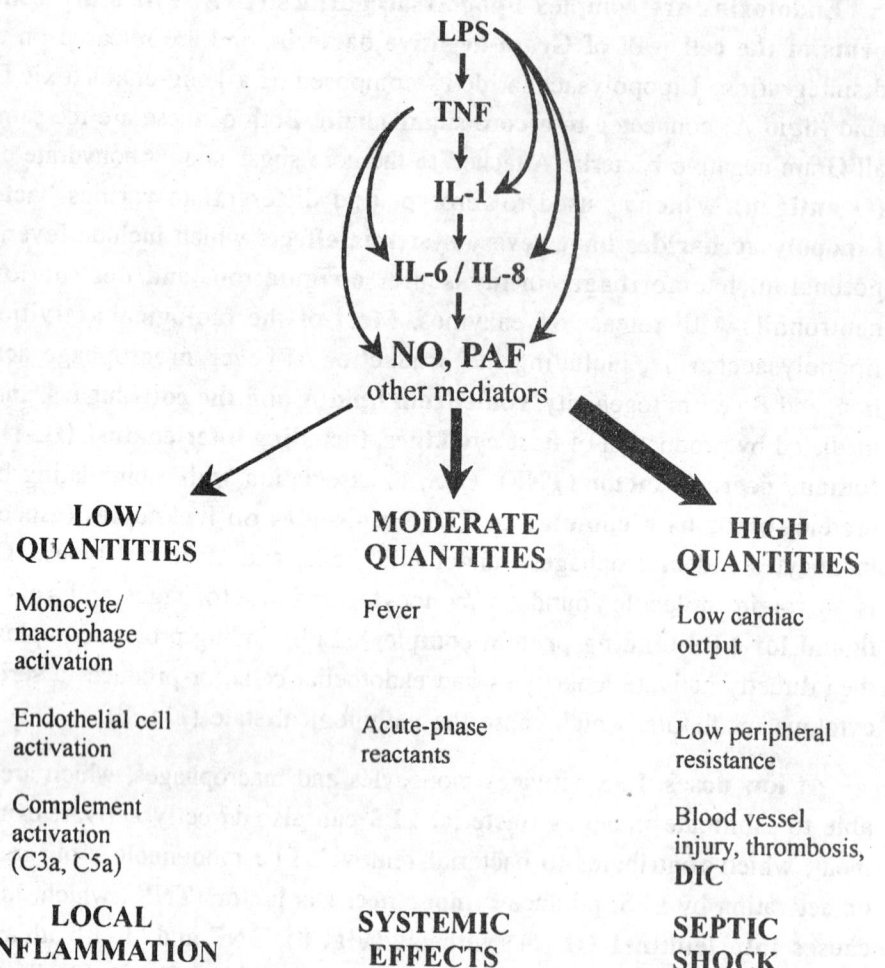

Fig. 8. Effects of lipopolysaccharide (LPS) and secondarily-induced effector molecules.

LPS = lipopolysaccharide   TNF = tumour necrosis factor

IL-1 = interleukin-1   IL-6 = interleukin-6

IL-8 = interleukin-8   NO = nitric oxide

PAF = platelet-   DIC = disseminated intravascular coagulation
activating factor

There are also various other products of bacteria. They include **haemolysins, fibrinolysins, coagulases, hyaluronidases,** and **other enzymes,** which are harmful to the host. In cases of severe septicaemia, bacterial products and waste products interfere with host metabolism, often fatally. Host responses also contribute to the mechanisms by which bacteria cause disease. **Pyogenic bacteria** cause the release of many chemical mediators responsible for fever and accompanying inflammation. **Cellular immune mechanisms (hypersensitivity)** contribute to the development of tuberculosis. Immune complex glomerulonephritis and immune-mediated arthritis may also be precipitated by bacterial infections.

Elements in the Production of a Bacterial Disease

Transmission (spread) of a bacterial disease occurs by **ingestion; inhalation; or mucosal, cutaneous, or wound contamination. Airborne infection** takes place largely through droplet nuclei (aerosol) which are **0.1 - 5 μm** in diameter. These are dried residue of droplets, **10-100 μm** in size, that originate from the respiratory tract. Particles of this size (**0.1 - 5 μm**) remain suspended in air and can be inhaled. Larger particles settle out but can be resuspended in the dust, which may also harbour infectious agents from non-respiratory sources (skin squames, faeces, saliva). **Arthropods** usually serve as mechanical carriers of pathogens.

Damage to host tissues depends on bacteria's ability to adhere to host cells, invade cells and tissues, and deliver toxic substances. Attachment and entry into the epithelial cell require interaction between the bacteria's **adhesins**, which are usually proteins, and the **epithelial cell receptors**, which are usually carbohydrate residues. Examples of bacterial adhesins are **fimbrial proteins** (*Escherichia coli*, Salmonella sp.) and lipoteichoic acids (some streptococci). **Fibrillae** covering the surface of **Gram-positive cocci**, such as **Streptococcus**, are composed of **M protein** and **lipoteichoic acids**. Lipoteichoic acids bind to the surface of all cells, although they have a higher affinity for particular receptors on blood cells and oral epithelial cells. **Fimbriae** or **pili** on the surface of **Gram-negative rods** and **cocci** are non-flagellar filamentous structures (**Fig. 9**). At the tips of the pili are minor protein components that determine to which host cells the bacteria will attach ("**bacterial tropism**"). In *Escherichia coli*, these minor proteins are antigenically different and associated with particular infections. For example, **type I proteins** bind mannose (host receptor) and cause urinary infections; **type P proteins** bind galactose and cause pyelonephritis; and **type S proteins** bind sialic acid and cause meningitis. A single bacterium can express more than one type of pili as well as non-pilar adhesins. Host receptor substances include **fibronectin** for some streptococci and staphylococci, and **mannose** for many *E. coli* strains. Adhesins often form fibrils (**fimbriae, pili**) on the bacterial surface (**Fig 9**). Attachment is inhibited by normal commensal flora which occupy or block available receptor sites, and prevent colonization by excreting toxic metabolites and bacteriocins. This **colonization resistance** is an important defence mechanism, and may be helped by mucosal antibody and other antibacterial substances (**lysozyme, lactoferrin, organic acids**).

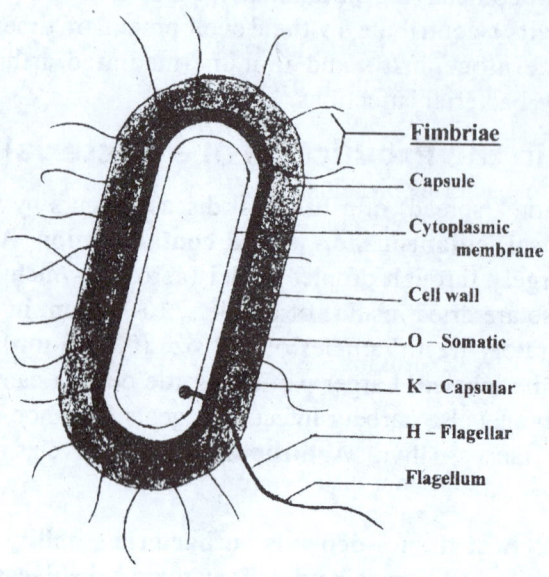

Fig. 9. *Escherichia coli* showing fimbriae.

Penetration of host surfaces is a requirement which varies among pathogens. Some bacteria, having reached the primary target cell population, do not penetrate further (enterotoxic *E. coli*, *Vibrio cholerae*), others cross surface membranes after endocytosis by epithelial cells, or go between these cells (**Salmonella, Brucella**). Inhaled facultative intracellular bacteria, like *Mycobacterium tuberculosis*, are taken up by pulmonary macrophages. They may multiply in macrophages and travel through lymphatics to lymph nodes and other tissues. Percutaneous penetration occurs through injuries, including insect bites. **Dissemination** occurs by extension, helped by bacterial enzymes, such as **collagenase, hyaluronidase**, and **others**. These are produced by many pathogens. **Growth** in host tissue is a prerequisite of pathogenesis for all pathogenic bacteria, except those which produce toxins in food stuffs prior to ingestion.

With **host defences neutralized, bacterial growth can proceed** if nutritional supplies are adequate, and the pH, temperature, and oxidation reduction potential (i.e., Eh) are appropriate. **Iron** is usually a limiting (restrictive) nutrient. Bacteria's ability to take away iron from iron-binding host proteins (**lactoferrin**) is a factor in virulence. **Gastric acidity** accounts for the resistance of the stomach to most pathogenic bacteria. The high body temperature of birds may explain their resistance to some infections (anthrax, histoplasmosis). Low Eh requirements account for the restriction of **anaerobic growth** in devitalized (i.e., non-oxygenated) tissues in which simultaneous aerobic growth has lowered Eh.

Pathogenic Action

Bacterial disease results from either direct damage to host by **exotoxins**, or damage to host reactions caused by **endotoxin or immune responses**.

Direct Damage

Exotoxins are bacterial proteins, which are freely excreted into the environment. **The differences between exotoxins and endotoxins are presented in Table 14.**

Table 14. Comparison of Exotoxins and Endotoxins

	Exotoxins	Endotoxins
Source	Secreted by living, usually **Gram-positive bacteria**, or from their cytoplasm on autolysis	Autolytic products from the cell walls of **Gram-negative bacteria**
Chemical composition	Protein	Lipopolysaccharide. Lipid A is the toxic component
Structure	Each is different according to its bacterial species	All are similar in structure and effect, regardless of the bacterial species
Effect	Produce a single specific effect	Produce a range of effects, mostly through host-derived mediators
Lethality	Potent toxins. Lethal in minute amounts	Lethal in large amounts. Stimulate interleukin-1 and tumour necrosis factor release
Stability	Heat labile	Heat stable
Antigenicity	Protein antigens (the toxic molecule is antigenic), neutralized by antibody	Poor antigens, poorly neutralized
Denaturation by formalin	Forms toxoid	No effect

Exotoxins are of two types. One acts **extracellularly, or on cell membranes**, attacking inter-cellular substances or cell surfaces by enzymatic mechanisms. It includes **bacterial haemolysins, leukocidins, collagenases, and hyaluronidases**. These play a supporting role in infections. **The other** type consists of proteins or polypeptides **which enter cells**, and enzymatically disrupt cellular processes. These exotoxins consist of an **A fragment**, which has enzymatic activity, and a **B fragment**, which is responsible for conveying the toxin to its site of action.

Endotoxins are part of the Gram-negative cell wall. They consist of polysaccharide surface c hains, which are virulence factors and somatic (O) antigens; a core polysaccharide; and **Lipid A, where the toxicity resides**. Endotoxins are taken up by host cells. They stimulate, particularly in macrophages, secretion o f mediator substances, s uch as **interleukin-1, tumour necrosis factor**, and **complement components**. These substances produce m anifestations o f e ndotoxaemia, i ncluding fever, headache, h ypotension, leukopaenia, thrombocytopaenia, i ntravascular coagulation, i nflammation, e ndothelial damage, h aemorrhage, fluid e xtravasation, and c irculatory collapse. Many of these result from: 1. **Activation of complement**, by either pathway, and 2. **Production of arachidonic acid metabolites, i.e., prostaglandins, leukotrienes, and thromboxanes**.

Immune-Mediated Damage

Tissue damage may occur from **immune reactions. C omplement-mediated responses** (such as inflammation) and reactions resembling immediate-type allergic phenomena can occur in response to endotoxins, or to peptidoglycans without preceding s ensitization.

Evasion of the Immune Response by Bacteria

Bacteria have d eveloped mechanisms b y w hich the i mmune r esponses can b e escaped. S ome bacteria, s uch as *B rucella a bortus*, *Mycobacterium tuberculosis, Listeria monocytogenes, Corynebacterium pseudotuberculosis, Campylobacter jejuni, Rhodococcus equi*, a nd t he salmonellae c an r eadily grow w ithin macrophages. I n addition, *L. monocytogenes*, c an travel from cell to cell without exposure to the extracellular fluid. **Bacteria employ several strategies for their survival within macrophages.** Some bacteria employ a **resistant coat** to protect themselves against lysosomal enzymes. For example, the cell wall waxes of *C. pseudotuberculosis* make this organism resistant to lysosomal enzymes. Other bacteria make sure that they are never exposed to these e nzymes. F or example, m ycobacteria a nd *B. abortus* c an p revent lysosomes f rom fusing w ith the p hagosome. The l ysosomes remain d istributed within the cytoplasm, and the bacteria continue to grow. A third mechanism to avoid destruction is to escape from the phagosome and remain free within the c ytoplasm. This method is e mployed by some mycobacteria a nd by *L. monocytogenes*.

Bacteria, such a s *Escherichia coli, M. tuberculosis*, a nd *P seudomonas aeruginosa* s ecrete molecules that depress phagocytosis by neutrophils. **Pseudomonas** bacteria also secrete a **leukotoxin** that kills neutrophils.

Staphylococcus aureus can inhibit chemotaxis and phagocytosis by producing toxins, such as streptolysin O, which lyse neutrophil cell membranes. The extreme form is seen in *Pasteurella haemolytica*, which secretes a toxin that kills ruminant alveolar macrophages and sheep lymphocytes.

Staphylococcus aureus also inhibits phagocytosis by means of **protein A** present on its surface. Protein A attaches to the Fc region of IgG molecules. **It prevents the immunoglobulin from binding to the receptors on the phagocytic cell and phagocytosing the bacteria.** Some bacteria avoid destruction by complement by using sialic acid in their capsules. The presence of this carbohydrate prevents activation of the alternate complement pathway. *P. aeruginosa* secretes a protease that causes destruction of cytokine interleukin-2. **Streptococci secrete proteases that destroy antibodies.** Some Gram-negative bacteria have long **polysaccharide O antigens**, which bind host antibody and activate complement at such a distance that the bacteria fail to be destroyed

This chapter is divided into three main sections (Table 15). The first includes diseases caused by various Gram-positive and Gram-negative cocci and rods. The **second section** includes members of the order Spirochaetales (spirochaetes). The **final section** covers the higher bacteria, mainly actinomycetes and mycobacteria, of the order Actinomycetales. **They are referred to as higher bacteria because they often produce lesions which resemble those caused by fungi.**

Table 15. Diseases caused by bacteria

1. Diseases caused by various Gram-positive and Gram-negative cocci and rods

Gram-positive Genera	Gram-negative Genera
Bacillus	Actinobacillus
Clostridium	Bordetella
Erysipelothrix	Brucella
Listeria	Campylobacter (Vibrio)
Staphylococcus	Escherichia
Streptococcus	Francisella
	Fusobacterium
	Haemophilus
	Klebsiella
	Moraxella
	Pasteurella
	Pseudomonas
	Salmonella
	Yersinia

2. Members of the order Spirochaetales
   (spirochaetes)

Family I.	Spirochaetaceae
	Genera
	Borrelia
	Treponema
Family II.	Leptospiraceae
	Genus
	Leptospira

3. The higher bacteria of the order Actinomycetales

Genera
Actinomyces
Corynebacterium
Dermatophilus
Mycobacterium
Nocardia
Rhodococcus

Diseases caused by Gram-positive Genera

Genus: Bacillus

Bacillus anthracis is the only pathogenic member of the genus **"Bacillus"**.

Anthrax

Anthrax is a peracute disease caused by *Bacillus anthracis*. It is characterized by septicaemia and sudden death accompanied by the exudation of tarry blood from the body orifices of the carcass. Anthrax is worldwide in distribution. **In India,** anthrax is mostly **seasonal**, occurring usually in rainy season. The disease takes a heavy toll of **cattle** life every year.

Anthrax is mainly a disease of herbivorous animals, but may affect a wide variety of species, including **humans. Cattle, sheep** and **goats** are most susceptible; **horses** and **mules** are slightly more resistant. **Pigs** are even more resistant, as are **dogs, cats,** and other species. However, anthrax does occur in these animals. In the more susceptible species (cattle, sheep, goat, horse), the disease is usually seen as a fulminant (sudden and severe) septicaemia. In the more resistant animals (pigs), the disease may be **localized** and confined to the regional lymph nodes, particularly those of the cervical region. **In wildlife**, anthrax has been reported in wild pigs, wild dogs, antelopes, elephant, lion, cheetah, leopard, giraffe, zebra, hippopotamus and hyena.

Cause

Bacillus anthracis is a **Gram-positive**, relatively large, encapsulated, **rod-shaped bacillus, which produces spores**. It grows well under aerobic conditions. In smears from tissues, it appears as short chains of square-ended rods. **Spores are not formed until it has been exposed to air.** Methylene blue and Giemsa's stain reveal purple to red capsules in some of the organisms.

Spread

Infection can follow **ingestion or inhalation of spores** or vegetative forms of the organism, or entry of the organism through the broken skin. **Highly resistant spores** released from infected animals can cause contamination of the area in which infection has occurred, **making it potentially dangerous for many years**. Spores are unharmed even by the gastric juice and pass on to the intestine, where they may set up infection. Infected animal products are also an important source of virulent organisms. In addition to carcasses, animal wastes and products such as bone-meal, wool, bristles, and hides from slaughterhouses have been involved in many infections.

Pathogenesis

Upon ingestion of the spores, infection may occur through the intact mucous membrane, through defects in the epithelium around erupting teeth, or through scratches from tough, fibrous food materials. Spores then germinate, and after localized multiplication, spread by means of lymphatics to lymph nodes and further to the bloodstream, leading to **massive septicaemia**. *B. anthracis* possesses both a **capsule** and an **exotoxin**. Antitoxic immunity is protective, but develops slowly. Moreover, toxin production continues for a long time, because the organism is encapsulated, and phagocytic cells are unable to eliminate its source. There is little cellular reaction of the host to the organisms, **whose capsules make them resistant to phagocytosis, as well as to neutralizing antibodies**. The severity of the disease is due to the production of a **lethal exotoxin** which causes oedema and tissue damage. Death results from shock and acute renal failure, and terminal anoxia mediated by the central nervous system. **The exotoxin has three components: 1. Oedema factor (EF), 2. Protective antigen (PA), and 3. Lethal factor (LF)**; also known as **factors I, II, and III**. The **oedema factor** is **adenylate cyclase**, which causes an increase in **cellular cAMP levels**, causing electrolyte and fluid loss. This factor is shared by the enterotoxins of *Escherichia coli* and *Vibrio cholerae*. The **protective antigen**, which is equivalent to the B fragment of other exotoxins (see 'direct damage'), is required for the activity of the other factors. It also has anti-phagocytic activity. The **lethal factor** stimulates macrophages to produce oxidizing radicals and cytokines, such as **interleukin-1-beta and tumour necrosis factor-alpha** which induce systemic shock and death.

Signs

In **cattle** and **sheep**, the disease occurs either in the **peracute or the acute form**. **Death** is the first indication of the presence of disease. In those animals in which symptoms are observed, anthrax is recognized as a febrile disease (fever up to 107° F), with signs of depression, weakness, bloody discharges from body orifices, cyanosis, dyspnoea, and occasional subcutaneous swellings. Most animals so affected die within a few hours, or a day. **In pigs**, anthrax may be acute or subacute. **Pigs** and **dogs** are usually infected by ingestion of infected meat from diseased sheep or cattle. Infection is usually **localized to the pharynx**, with enlargement of the cervical lymph nodes, **or** appears **as an acute haemorrhagic gastroenteritis**. Pharyngeal, or enteric disease, is also the usual picture in **horses**.

Lesions

The **gross lesions** in fatal cases of the **disseminated form** include oedematous and haemorrhagic changes in any part of the body, particularly in serous membranes. **The spleen is greatly enlarged, and engorged with dark, unclotted blood. Lymph nodes** are usually swollen, oedematous, and sometimes haemorrhagic. Lesions in other organs are inconstant. However, haemorrhages and swelling may occur in the intestinal tract, liver, and kidneys. **In localized infections in pigs**, oedema and haemorrhages are seen in the pharynx and cervical lymph nodes. In cases of longer duration, lymph nodes become enlarged and solid, with yellowish foci surrounded by fibrous connective tissue.

The **microscopic changes** in generalized cases are dominated by the presence of a large number of **anthrax bacilli in the blood, and most of the tissues**. The large rod-shaped organisms can be demonstrated in the smears or tissue sections. However, they cannot be distinguished from saprophytic bacilli without culturing them, and determining their pathogenicity in laboratory animals. In the **spleen**, the architecture is obscured by the presence of large numbers of erythrocytes. The lymphoid follicles are not noticeable; only the trabeculae remain as tiny islands in a sea of red cells and nuclear debris. These flood the splenic sinuses and the cords of Bilroth. Bacilli are readily demonstrated in sections of the spleen with Gram's stain. **Localized infection in lymph nodes of pigs** result in foci of necrosis surrounded by a layer of granulation tissue. Giant cells are usually not present.

Failure of the blood to clot, absence of rigor mortis, and the presence of splenomegaly are the most important necropsy findings.

Zoonotic Importance

Humans usually acquire anthrax from contact with infected animals, or animal products (hides, wool, shaving brushes made from infected pig bristles). The disease manifests as a **localized**, persistent **cutaneous pustule**, described as **"malignant pustule"** or **"malignant carbuncle"**; or as a **systemic**, often **fatal pulmonary disease**, known as **"woolsorter's disease"**.

Diagnosis

Presumptive diagnosis is made on the basis of history (few preceding signs, with sudden death of several animals in a herd), and the characteristic gross lesions found at necropsy. However, **a suspected anthrax carcass must not be opened, as it helps in the formation and dissemination of spores. Sporulation does not occur inside the body so long as the carcass is unopened**. Instead, blood smears may be made from one of the small ear veins and stained with methylene blue. The diagnosis is confirmed by demonstration of *Bacillus anthracis* in large numbers in **blood smears** (and also tissues, in case body is opened) of dead animals. It is important that the organisms be identified and differentiated from saprophytes on the basis of pathogenicity and morphological and cultural characteristics. Inoculation of organisms, intraperitoneally, kills a mouse in 12-24 hours, and a guinea-pig in 24-36 hours. Organisms are readily seen in tissues, and can be cultured from tissues of such inoculated animals.

Fluorescent techniques are available for use on blood smears and tissue sections. **Monoclonal antibodies** are also used to provide specific identification of anthrax organisms. *B. anthracis* antigens can be demonstrated in extracts of contaminated products by a precipitation test using high-titred antiserum (**Ascoli test**).

Genus: Clostridium

Organisms of the genus "**Clostridium**" are sporulating, **anaerobic** bacteria of rather larger size, about **0.8 μm** in width and **3-8 μm** in length. They occur singly, in pairs, or in chains. Most members of the genus are non-pathogenic, and are **commonly found in soil and in the intestinal tract of humans and animals**. Several members of the genus, however, are responsible for a number of diseases of humans and animals. These organisms can be divided into **two groups**: 1. Those which produce disease through **tissue invasion**, and 2. Those that owe their pathogenicity to the production of **toxins**. However, this division is not perfect, since all clostridia produce toxins which contribute to their pathogenicity.

Clostridium botulinum, which causes botulism, is completely **non-invasive**. Disease occurs from ingestion of toxins formed outside the body. *C. tetani*, cause of tetanus, is not particularly invasive. Disease results from circulating toxin produced by organisms, which after entry into the body, remain localized within sites of tissue damage with low oxygen tension. The **invasive clostridia**, such as *C. chauvoei, C. novyi,* and *C. haemolyticum* cause diseases characterized by extensive tissue invasion and necrosis. The invasion, however, requires tissue damage initiated through other mechanisms to produce an **anaerobic environment**. The pathogenesis of diseases caused by *C. perfringens* may involve both invasive and non-invasive mechanisms. It may be a pathogen in: **1.** Food poisoning by toxins produced outside the body, **2.** Various enterotoxaemias, resulting from toxins produced within the gastrointestinal tract, with or without significant tissue invasion, and **3.** Gas gangrene (also c aused b y o ther c lostridia), r esulting f rom proliferation i n areas of tissue damage with low oxygen tension. **Many of the clostridia (e.g., *C. septicum*) are normal inhabitants of the intestinal tract, and after death of the host, can invade and multiply.** They are easily seen, or cultured; and care must be taken so as not to consider them as the cause of death.

The pathogenic clostridia, and diseases caused by them, are listed in Table 16.

Table 16. Diseases caused by Pathogenic Clostridia

Clostridia	Disease	Animal species affected
C. chauvoei	Blackquarter (blackleg)	Cattle and sh eep
	Wound infections (gas g angrene)	Many species
C. septicum	Malignant oedema	Many species
	Braxy	Sheep
C. haemolyticum	Bovine b acillary haemoglobinuria	Cattle
C. novyi	Black disease, w ound infections (gas gangrene)	Many species
C. botulinum	Botulism	See Table 17
C. tetani	Tetanus	Many species
C. perfringens (Types - A-E)		See Table 18
C. difficile	Pseudomembranous colitis	Humans, monkeys, and pigs
Avian Diseases		
C. botulinum	Botulism (limberneck)	Chickens
C. colinum	Ulcerative e nteritis (quail disease)	Chickens, quail, p igeons, and other birds
C. perfringens	Necrotic e nteritis	Chickens, turkeys
	Gangrenous dermatitis (malignant oedema)	Chickens
C. septicum	Gangrenous dermatitis	Chickens

Blackquarter

Also known as "**blackleg**", blackquarter (BQ) is an acute, infectious, highly fatal disease of **mainly cattle**, and sometimes of other species, such as sheep, goats, pigs, and rarely horses. **In India, besides cattle, BQ is most common in sheep. In wildlife**, BQ has been reported in deer and antelope. BQ is caused by *Clostridium chauvoei*, and characterized by inflammation of skeletal and cardiac muscles, severe toxaemia, and a high mortality. *C. chauvoei* is also, along with other clostridia, a common secondary invader of traumatic or surgical wounds, resulting in gas gangrene, or clostridial sepsis. **BQ of cattle has a seasonal incidence with most cases occurring in the rainy season. The disease is enzootic in particular areas of India, and the mortality rate may approach 100%.** BQ is a cause of severe financial loss to cattle farmers. For the most part, major outbreaks can be prevented by vaccination, although outbreaks still occur, sometimes in vaccinated animals, but mostly in animals where vaccination has been neglected.

Cause

C. chauvoei is a **Gram-positive**, spore-forming, **rod-shaped bacterium**. The spores are highly resistant to environmental changes and disinfectants, and **persist in soil for many years**.

Spread

BQ is a soil-borne infection. **The portal of entry is through the alimentary mucosa after ingestion of spores** in contaminated feed. **In sheep**, the disease is almost always a **wound infection**, e.g., infection of skin wounds at shearing and docking, and of the navel at birth.

Pathogenesis

Following ingestion of the spores, the bacteria multiply in the intestine, cross the intestinal mucosa, and enter the general circulation. They are then deposited in a number of organs and tissues, **including the skeletal muscles**. Here, spores remain dormant until damage to the muscle sets up an **appropriate anaerobic environment** for germination and proliferation. The mechanisms which lead to this appropriate environment are not clear. It is also not known why damage to other tissues where the latent spores are present, such as the liver, does not initiate disease. Once the organisms begin to multiply, they release the **toxins** locally. *C. chauvoei* produces **four toxins**: 1. **Alpha toxin**, which is both necrotizing and haemolytic, 2. **Beta toxin**, which is a deoxyribonuclease (DNase), 3. **Gamma toxin**, a hyaluronidase, and 4. **Delta toxin**, a haemolysin. The alpha toxin is a phospholipase C. It degrades lecithin, a major component of cell membranes, and thus destroys red blood cells, platelets and muscle cells, causing **myonecrosis**. Thus, the release of toxins locally leads to **severe necrotizing myositis (myonecrosis)**, and systemic spread of toxins through the bloodstream **(systemic toxaemia) results in death.**

Signs

The disease is most common in young animals, **6 months to 2 years of age, on a good nutrition**, The disease runs an acute, usually fatal course, and **affected animals are often found dead before signs of illness are seen.** In some cases, there may be lameness, a high fever (106° F), and visible swelling of muscles. Any striated muscle may be affected, including the tongue, diaphragm, and myocardium; but the shoulder, pectoral, and **hindquarter (gluteal) muscles** are most commonly involved. In early stages, the **swelling is hot and painful to the touch but soon becomes cold and painless, and oedema and emphysema can be felt.**

Lesions

The lesions consist of **crepitant swelling** (i.e., making a crackling sound) in the muscles, particularly of the extremities. Clotting of the blood occurs rapidly. Incision of the affected muscles reveals the presence of a dark brown or dark red, swollen tissue, **streaked black**. Some areas appear moist, and on pressure, yield dark, gas-filled exudate. Other group of muscles are dry and sponge-like, **with numerous gas bubbles**. A peculiar **rancid or sweetish odour** may be noticed. The subcutaneous tissues overlying affected muscles are usually yellowish, gelatinous, blood-tinged, and **contain gas bubbles.** Similar lesions are usually seen in the heart, but rarely in the tongue (could be confused with **"woody tongue"**). Diffuse haemorrhagic lesions may occur even in the lungs

Microscopically, most important lesions are in the skeletal musculature. **Gas bubbles in tissue sections** are seen as spherical spaces, separating muscle bundles and fascia. There are irregular areas of necrosis, and collections of neutrophils and lymphocytes along the muscle septa. Oedema is uncommon. **Gram-positive organisms can be demonstrated in sections**, appearing singly or in small, irregular clumps.

Diagnosis

A presumptive diagnosis can be made by the characteristic gross lesions, and by demonstration of numerous single, or possibly paired, **bacilli** with rounded ends and occasional spores near, but not at the end of, the cell. The **spore** is somewhat greater in diameter than the bacillus in which it has formed. The lesions must be differentiated from other clostridial infections of muscle, particularly *C. septicum*, cause of malignant oedema (discussed next). Therefore, the diagnosis should be confirmed by culture, or use of specific immunological staining techniques.

Malignant Oedema (Gas Gangrene)

Malignant oedema is **an acute wound infection** caused by *Clostridium septicum*. There is an acute inflammation at the site of infection and a **profound systemic toxaemia**. It is most common in **horses, sheep**, and **cattle**, but most animal species and **humans** are susceptible. It is rare in dogs and cats. The disease is basically a form of gas gangrene, although **in malignant oedema gas production is minimal**. *C. septicum* is another ubiquitous organism (i.e., present everywhere) like *C. chauvoei*, which is found in soil and in the gastrointestinal tract of animals. It is similar in almost all characteristics to *C. chauvoei*.

Spread

The infection is usually soil-borne. Resistance of the spores to environmental influence leads to persistence of the infection for long periods. In most cases a wound is the portal of entry. Malignant oedema is seen as a sequel to wounds, such as those which occur during shearing or docking in sheep, or during parturition when aseptic precautions are ignored.

Pathogenesis

C. septicum owes its pathogenicity to various toxins like other clostridia. It produces the same four toxins: alpha, beta, gamma and delta as produced by *C. chauvoei* (see blackquarter). Of the several toxins produced, the haemolytic and necrotizing toxin, referred to as alpha toxin, is the most dangerous. Locally it causes extensive oedema and necrosis followed by gangrene, and when absorbed into the bloodstream, it causes death of the animal.

Signs

The disease is characterized by a febrile course of short duration with hot, painful swelling at sites of infection. A high fever (106⁰-107⁰ F) is always present. The swollen areas later become even more oedematous, but less painful and cooler.

Lesions

At necropsy, the involved tissues are oedematous and usually haemorrhagic, and they contain gas bubbles. Septicaemia often occurs, with haemorrhages distributed throughout the body. The lungs are congested and oedematous. Serous, blood-tinged effusion from the peritoneum may also be present. *C. septicum* can be easily demonstrated in the affected tissues.

Diagnosis

Association of profound toxaemia with local inflammation and emphysema is characteristic. The disease must be differentiated from blackquarter by the absence of typical muscle involvement, and the presence of wounds. A history of prior vaccination against blackquarter, and the age of the animal may be helpful in diagnosis. It is emphasized that clostridia are present in the alimentary tract of normal animals, and under favourable conditions postmortem invasion of the tissues may occur rapidly.

Braxy

Also known as "**bradsot**", braxy is **an acute infectious disease of sheep** characterized by haemorrhagic abomasitis, toxaemia, and a high mortality rate. It is caused by *Clostridium septicum*, the common cause of malignant oedema in animals. **The disease is mainly seen in Scotland and Scandinavia**, but also occurs in Canada and the northern United States. Its occurrence is associated with cold weather, and the ingestion of frost-covered foods. The disease affects mainly **young sheep**, and usually occurs during the **winter months**.

The **pathogenesis** is not understood, but it is presumed that a primary abomasitis, caused by the ingestion of frozen grass or other feed, permits invasion by *C. septicum* resulting in a fatal toxaemia. **Death is sudden, with few or no clinical signs**. At necropsy, the wall of the abomasum is thickened, oedematous, and haemorrhagic. Similar lesions may be seen in the small intestine. **Large bacilli can be seen in tissue section**, and are readily isolated from the lesions.

Clinically, **diagnosis** of braxy is most difficult. At necropsy, lesions of abomasitis are characteristic. Braxy may resemble black disease, but there are no liver lesions in braxy. The final diagnosis depends on isolation of *C. septicum* from typical alimentary tract lesions.

Bovine Bacillary Haemoglobinuria

Also known as "**red water disease**" and "**infectious icterohaemoglobinuria**", bovine bacillary haemoglobinuria is **an acute, highly fatal toxaemia of cattle and sheep**, characterized clinically by a high fever, haemoglobinuria and jaundice, and by the presence of necrotic infarcts in the liver. First described in California in 1916, **the disease occurs mainly in United States**, but has also been reported from other countries and also from Europe. The disease is caused by *Clostridium haemolyticum* (*C. haemolyticus bovis*), which is very similar, and identical in some respects, to *C. novyi* type B. The disease caused by the two organisms are also very similar.

Spread

Like certain other clostridia (*C. chauvoei, C. novyi*), infection occurs following **ingestion** of the organisms in the soil.

Pathogenesis

Following ingestion, organisms multiply in the intestinal tract, and finally enter into the systemic circulation. *C. haemolyticum* then localizes in the **liver**, and remains latent until an appropriate anaerobic environment allows its multiplication at this site. The migration of **liver flukes** is believed to be most effective method of causing the hepatic damage. This results in activation of the clostridia.

Exotoxins then c ontribute to further liver d\amage, with the production of a characteristic "**infarct**", haemolysis, and **death**. The main toxin is **beta toxin** (identical to that of *C. novyi*), a phospholipase C which hydrolyzes l ecithin and sphingomyelin and haemolyzes r ed blood cells.

Signs

The disease is characterized by sudden onset of **haemoglobinuria**, fever, anaemia, leukocytosis, collapse, and **death within a day or two**. The mortality rate is high.

Lesions

The typical lesion is a large area of necrosis in the liver, resembling an infarct. It is always a solitary (single) lesion, in contrast to black disease, where m ultiple areas o f h epatic n ecrosis can occur. **Microscopically,** the necrotic tissue contains t he G ram-positive bacilli and i s surrounded b y a polymorp honuclear infiltrate. The kidneys are mottled as a re sult of haemoglobinuria, and urine in the bladder is deep red.

Diagnosis

Diagnosis is b ased on t he pathological f indings of h epatic infarct and haemoglobinuria, and on isolation of *C. haemolyticum*. The disease must be differentiated f rom many o ther bovine d iseases which a re accompanied b y haemoglobinuria.

Black Disease

Also known as "**infectious necrotic hepatitis**", black disease is an **acute fatal infection of sheep**, and **rarely cattle**, caused by *Clostridium novyi* (*C. oedematiens*). Well-nourished adult sheep in the 2-4 year age group are particularly susceptible, l ambs being rarely affected. B lack disease w as first reported in Australia, but w as subsequently recognized in New Zealand and many other countries of the world, **including India**. There are similarities in the aetiology, p athogenesis, and lesions of this disease and bovine b acillary haemoglobinuria.

Cause

C. novyi is widely distributed in soil in the form of **three strains of A, B, and C**, and is a common inhabitant of the intestinal tract of sheep. T he strains are differentiated on the basis o f toxin production. **Type A** produces **alpha toxin**, a necrotizing and lethal toxin. **Type B** produces **both alpha toxin and beta toxin**, a necrotizing, haemolytic, and lethal toxin. **Type C** is **non-toxigenic** and non-pathogenic. *C. haemolyticum*, which produces **beta toxin**, is considered to be a toxigenic variant of *C. novyi*. The type B strain, which is almost similar to *C. haemolyticum*, is the strain which causes black disease.

Spread

Faecal contamination of the pasture by carrier animals is the most important source of infection. Spores of the causative clostridia are **ingested**, and are carried to the liver in the lymphatic system. A seasonal occurrence of the disease is noticed because of fluctuation in the liver fluke a nd h ost snail population. Many normal animals in flock in which the disease occurs carry *C. novyi* in their livers.

Pathogenesis

Following ingestion, *C. novyi* pass through the intestinal wall and lodge in the **liver**, where they remain as a **latent infection**. An **anaerobic environment** produced by the migration of the liver flukes (*Fasciola hepatica, Dicrocoelium dendriticum*) activates t he bacteria, w hich release e xotoxins. These f urther contribute to hepatic necrosis, and produce fatal toxaemia. The m ain toxin is **necrotizing** and called **alpha toxin**, or **lethal toxin**. A **beta toxin** is also produced, which is a necrotizing and haemolyzing lecithinase similar to the beta toxin of *C. haemolyticum*. **Death** of the animal may result without premonitory (preceding) s ymptoms.

Signs

Affected sheep u sually die d uring n ight without s howing any s igns of previous i llness. When o bservation is p ossible, there i s fever (105⁰-107⁰ F) which subsides to a subnormal level. The **course** from first illness to death is never more t han **a few hours**. C linical findings are t he same i n cattle as i n sheep, but the course is longer. **The disease lasts for 1-2 days**.

Lesions

Pathological changes include **characteristic multiple foci of necrosis in the liver**, petechiae on the epicardium and endocardium, and hydropericardium. Subcutaneous venous congestion causes a **dark discoloration of the skin (pelt)**, which is the reason for the name "**black disease**".

Diagnosis

Diagnosis is made on the basis of pathological findings and isolation of *C. novyi*. The organisms can be demonstrated with **fluorescent antibody technique** in smears, or sections of the liver. However, as the organisms are normal inhabitants of liver, and proliferate rapidly after death, the clinical manifestations and gross and microscopic lesions must also be considered in establishing a diagnosis.

Gas Gangrene (Clostridial Wound Infections)

Type A *Clostridium novyi* is a common contaminant of wounds and causes 'gas gangrene' in several species, including **humans**. The main toxin of the type A strain is **alpha toxin**.

Gas gangrene is the term applied to clostridial infections of **traumatic or surgical wounds**. Usually it is applied to such infections in humans. **Malignant oedema**, discussed earlier, is the term used for such conditions in animals, although in this disorder gas production is limited. Clostridia usually associated with gas gangrene are *C. perfringens, C. septicum, C. novyi, C. chauvoei,* and *C. histolyticum*. Gas gangrene is initiated by proliferation of clostridial organisms in areas of **tissue damage with low oxygen tension**, and is characterized by **extensive necrosis of muscle** with considerable oedema and cellulitis. The affected areas are swollen, exude sero-sanguineous fluid, and have a **putrid odour**. **Gas bubbles** of varying size are interspersed with necrotic tissue. The lesion is the result of **potent toxins**, released from the bacteria. They may enter the circulation, and lead to haemolytic anaemia and necrotizing lesions at other sites.

Botulism

Clostridium botulinum is responsible for an extremely serious **food intoxication, botulism**. Botulism is a rapidly fatal motor paralysis caused by ingestion of the toxin of *C. botulinum*. The bacterium was first called *Bacillus botulinus*. The name was taken from the Latin word "**botulus**" (sausage), because of the common association of the disease with ingestion of **sausage**.

Cause

C. botulinum is divided into **seven different toxigenic** (toxin producing) **strains**, namely, **A, B, C, D, E, F** and **G (Table 17)**. The strains are based on antigenically distinguishable toxins released on dissolution of the organism. On the basis of cultural characteristics, these **toxigenic strains are divided into four groups**. **Group I** consists of proteolytic organisms, including all strains of type A, and proteolytic strains of type B and F. **Group II** contains non-proteolytic strains of types B and F and all strains of type E. **Group III** contains types C and D, and **Group IV** consists of the type G strain.

Table 17. Botulism in Animals and Humans

Toxigenic type/strain	Species affected	Source of intoxication
A	Humans, birds	Canned vegetables, fruits, meat, and fish
B	Humans, horses, cattle, sheep, birds	Meat, usually pork; silage and forage
C-alpha	Cattle, sheep, horses, dogs, birds	Fly larvae, rotting vegetation, silage, carrion (i.e., dead and putrefying flesh)
D	Cattle, horses	Carrion

E	Humans, birds	Fish and marine animal foods
F	Humans	Liver paste (a food product)
G	Humans	Soil

Each toxigenic strain produces a single toxin of the same designation. However, certain strains produce more than one toxin, or more than one variant of the same toxin have been identified. Two strains of type C organisms exist: **type C-alpha and type C-beta. C-alpha** produces mainly classical **neurotoxin**, designated C1. **C-beta produces C2 toxin**, which is not a neurotoxin. But it is cytolytic through interference with adenosine diphosphate. **C2 toxin, however, is not involved in the disease botulism.** Another factor complicating the situation is that organisms different from *C. botulinum*, such as *C. barati* and *C. butyricum* also produce botulism toxin, and are involved in cases of botulism. Type A strains of *C. novyi* also are very similar to Group III type C organisms. **In general, all the botulinum neurotoxins behave in the same manner.** Molecularly, they are very similar to tetanospasmin toxin of *C. tetani*.

Spread

Botulism almost always results from the **ingestion of preformed toxin in a food source.** *C. botulinum*, a spore-forming anaerobe proliferates only in decaying animal or plant material. The **spores are extremely resistant**, and survive for long periods in most environmental circumstances. The **toxin** is also capable of surviving for long periods. In its vegetative form **the organism is a common inhabitant of the alimentary tract of herbivores.** The source of infection for animals is almost always **carrion** (i.e., dead and putrefying flesh), which includes domestic and wild animals, and birds.

Pathogenesis

As stated, botulism almost always results from the **ingestion of preformed toxin** in a food source. *C. botulinum* makes numerous extremely potent neurotoxins, which are released when the organisms die and autolyse. Botulinum toxins act at the peripheral nerve endings, where they get bound and cause nerve blockage. **These toxins cause death as a result of respiratory paralysis.** The dose of botulinum toxin required to block nervous activity is extremely small, only eight molecules are required to block transmission by a neuron. However, there are two other pathogenetic mechanisms which have been called "toxico-infectious". **The first is "wound botulism"** in which *C. botulinum* contaminates wound, grows, and produces toxin in them. This form of botulism is associated with proteolytic strains of **type A** and **type B**. It occurs in humans (type A and B) and horses (type B), but probably occurs in other species as well. Non-proteolytic strains do not grow and produce toxin at body temperature. **The second mechanism** in which the toxin is not ingested results from colonization of the gastrointestinal tract with *C. botulinum* (**type A** and **B**), with subsequent production of toxin and absorption by the host. **This is a true enterotoxaemia**. **In humans**, it has been referred to as **infant botulism**. It is seen mainly in infants less than 6 months of age. The condition results from ingestion of foods containing spores, not the toxin. The most often involved food in humans is **honey**. Enterotoxic botulism also occurs in **poultry** (see avian botulism).

Signs

The signs of botulism follow 1-5 day 'incubation period', and are characterized by a **descending and symmetrical paralysis**. After absorption into the bloodstream, the toxin enters peripheral nerves at their synaptic junctions, binds to nerve membranes, and prevents release of acetylcholine by synaptic vesicles. Only peripheral cholinergic nerves are affected. **The toxin does not enter the central nervous system**. Cranial nerves are first affected, but ultimately all muscles of the body may be affected. **Almost all animal species, including birds, are susceptible**.

In humans, botulism results from the consumption of inadequately sterilized canned food which is neutral in acidity. The organisms produce their powerful neurotoxins in these foods. Canned vegetables and some fish products are the most common sources. **In cattle**, botulism results from the ingestion of animal carcasses and their contaminated foodstuffs. Many small animals and birds carry type D organisms as part of their normal intestinal flora, and after death, the carcass can become extremely toxic. Botulism usually occurs in cattle with phosphorus deficiency who chew bones and remaining bits of decaying meat. This bone-chewing form of botulism is known as "lamsiekte" in South Africa, **"bulbar paralysis"** in Australia, and **"loin disease"** in the Unites States.

Forage poisoning is a form of botulism in **cattle**. It results from the **ingestion of silage or hay** that has become contaminated with a dead animal. **Type C is usually involved in this disease**. Poultry litter containing type C or type D toxin is also involved in botulism in cattle. Type B toxin in grains and silage, and drinking water contaminated with toxic animal carcasses, could also be important sources. Botulism in **sheep** is similar to that in cattle. **In horses**, botulism is seen sporadically. It is usually caused by ingestion of hay contaminated with dead cat, an excellent source of type C toxin. Wound botulism resulting from type B toxin occurs in humans and foals, and is known as "shaker foal syndrome". **Pigs** are relatively resistant to botulism. This is because the toxin is poorly absorbed. **In dogs**, botulism results from type C toxin, but is not common. **Botulism is seen in most species of birds, except, vultures**, which are resistant (see avian botulism).

Lesions

There are no specific gross or histopathological lesions.

Diagnosis

Although c ases of botulism are o ften suspected, i t is rarely possible t o establish t he diagnosis by demonstrating the presence o f toxin in the suspected food. The main evidence is provided by the feeding of suspect material to susceptible animals.

Tetanus

Also known as "**lockjaw**", tetanus occurs in **humans and animals**. It is a highly **fatal disease of all species of domestic animals** caused by the toxin of *Clostridium tetani*. Clinically, the disease is characterized by hyperaesthesia (unusual sensitivity to sensory stimuli, such as pain or touch), tetany (intermittent tonic spasms), and convulsions. Tetanus occurs in all parts of the world. It occurs in all farm animals mainly as individual, sporadic cases. **Horses are most susceptible and cattle the least**.

Cause

C. tetani is a **Gram-positive, sporulating, anaerobic, rod-shaped, bacillus**. It is **a normal inhabitant of the intestinal tract of herbivorous animals**, and is commonly present in the **faeces** of animals, especially **horses**, and in the **soil** contaminated by their faeces.

Spread

The **portal of entry is usually through puncture wounds**, often insignificant o nes, such a s nail-pricks, o r those p roduced by c astration, docking o r shearing, or t hose received during parturition. However, the **spores** may l ie dormant in the tissues for some time, and produce disease only when tissue conditions favour their proliferation. When t he wound is not visible, such a disease is called an "**idiopathic tetanus**" (occurs usually in very young cattle). It is possible that toxin is produced in the gut, or is ingested preformed in the feed.

Pathogenesis

The **tetanus bacilli remain localized at their site of introduction** and do not invade surrounding tissues. They start to proliferate and produce neurotoxin only if certain environmental conditions are attained, particularly a **lowering of the local tissue oxygen tension**. The **a naerobic environment** of certain wound allows germination of the spores, multiplication of the organism, and release of a **potent neurotoxin**. The neurotoxin prevents the function of inhibitory spinal i nterneurons by i nterfering with t he release o f transmitter substance at the presynaptic terminals. **Several biochemical events are initiated,** but the most important is the interference with release of **glycine**, the inhibitory transmitter at this site. The toxin known as **tetanospasmin**, reaches the interspinal site by entering the bloodstream, attacking the peripheral nerve endings, and travelling along nerves to the central nervous system. The secretion of inhibitory neuro-transmitters, which normally control muscle spasms, is blocked by tetanospasmin. As a result of this blockage, tetanic spasm of voluntary muscles, and ultimately, nerve block and paralysis occur. *C. tetani* also releases two other toxins: "tetanolysin (a haemolysin), and "non-spasmogenic toxin". The former may help *C. tetani* to establish itself in wounds, and the latter may interfere with motor nerve function. It is tetanospasmin, however, which is responsible for the clinical picture of tetanus. Death occurs from asphyxiation due to fixation of the muscles of respitation.

Signs

The clinical picture is similar in all animal species. The disease is characterized by prolonged spasmodic contractions of muscles, with extension of limbs, stiffness and immobilization. The muscles of mastication are often affected, immobilizing the jaws, hence the name "lockjaw". The entire musculature is eventually involved, and death follows from asphyxiation. The course of the disease varies both between and within species. The duration of a fatal disease in horses and cattle is usually 5-10 days, but the sheep usually die about the third or fourth day.

Lesions

No specific gross or microscopic lesions are produced; and have not been described.

Diagnosis

Diagnosis is based on clinical signs and a history of trauma. However, a wound is often not demonstrable, and if present, the bacilli are difficult to demonstrate.

Enterotoxaemia

A number of disorders, grouped under the heading "enterotoxaemia", result from the production of toxins by *Clostridium perfringens* (previously *C. welchii*) in the gastrointestinal tract. Some of the disorders are true enterotoxaemias, e.g., those caused by the type D organism. But others are characterized by a necrotizing enterocolitis more similar to the disease associated with *C. difficile* described as pseudomembranous colitis (discussed next).

There are five strains (or types) of *C. perfringens*: A, B, C, D, and E. Their pathogenicity is due to the production of one or more of four toxins, designated as alpha, beta, epsilon, and iota. There are others also, but these are the most important. The production of these four toxins by the five types of *C. perfringens*, and the diseases associated with them, are shown in Table 18.

Table 18. *Clostridium perfringens* types (strains), toxins, and diseases

Type (strain)	Toxins				Diseases
	Alpha	Beta	Epsilon	Iota	
A	+	-	-	-	Gas gangrene, food poisoning, infectious diarrhoea in humans; enterotoxaemia in lambs, cattle, goats, horses, dogs; colitis X in horses
B	+	+	+	-	Lamb dysentery, enterotoxaemia in calves, foals
C	+	+	-	-	Enterotoxaemia (necrotic enteritis) in lambs, goats, c attle, pigs; st ruck in adult s heep
D	+	-	+	-	Enterotoxaemia (overeating disease, pulpy kidney disease) in s heep, goats, cattle
E	+	-	-	+	Enterotoxaemia in calves, l ambs

+ = the strain contains this toxin
- = the strain does not contain the toxin

C. perfringens **secretes 12 toxins**, the most important of which is **alpha toxin**. **Alpha toxin**, produced by all five types, is a **phospholipase C** which causes tissue destruction (**necrosis**) and haemolysis. In this way it facilitates bacterial growth and invasion. This toxin is important in gas gangrene. **Beta toxin**, produced by types B and C has not been characterized. It is associated with increased vascular permeability and necrosis. **Epsilon toxin**, elaborated by types B and C, is first produced as a nontoxic compound, which is converted to a potent t oxin by p roteolytic enzymes s uch as trypsin. It causes increased vascular permeability and tissue necrosis. **Iota toxin**, produced by E, is a lso first p roduced as a protoxin a nd converted t o its a ctive form b y proteolytic enzymes. It increases vascular permeability markedly and causes necrosis.

All four types of *C. perfringens* are extremely common in the gastrointestinal tract of animals. Types B and E are considered obligate parasites. Type A is also found in soil.

Type A

C. perfringens type A is the m ost common c ause of **gas gangrene in humans and animals**. It also causes some forms of food poisoning in humans. Type A enterotoxaemia, known as **"yellow lamb disease"** has been described in lambs and calves in USA, but is a rare disease. It is **an acute syndrome** of short course and a high rate of mortality, characterized by intense jaundice, haemorrhagic anaemia, and haemoglobinuria. Lesions include jaundice, anaemia, excess pericardial fluid, dark kidneys, and an enlarged, friable liver. *C. perfringens* type A also causes a syndrome in **neonatal calves** characterized by rumen tympany and abomasitis. A disease of **horses** known as **"colitis X"** is associated with *C. perfringens* type A. Colitis X is characterized by foul-smelling, profuse diarrhoea, and dehydration. Besides haemorrhage in various organs, **lesions are restricted to the colon,** where there is haemorrhage and necrosis of mucosa. **Type A organisms** are also associated with enteric disease in goats, and dogs. In dogs, it often accompanies parvoviral enteritis.

Type B

C. perfringens type B causes **enterotoxaemia in lambs, calves, and foals**. It is a disease of very young animals. It affects lambs less than 2 weeks of age, calves up to 10 days of age, and foals in the first 2 days of life. The syndrome in lambs is known as **lamb dysentery**. It is **an extremely fatal condition**, deaths occurring without premonitory (preceding) signs. Or, lambs may show watery, often bloody, diarrhoea, lying down, refusing to suckle, and exhibiting signs of abdominal pain.

The **characteristic lesion is haemorrhagic enteritis**, usually with ulceration, and sometimes with perforation and peritonitis. Lesions are restricted to the small intestine, but may also affect the colon. Petechiae and ecchymoses are common on serous membranes of the epicardium and endocardium, and the pericardial cavity contains excess fluid. The **type B organism** is also associated with a wasting disease of older lambs in England, referred to as **"pine"**. **Microscopically**, the lesions are not pathognomonic, and are characterized by focal areas of necrosis involving the entire thickness of the mucosa and extending into the muscularis. The lesions in calves and foals are also characterized by haemorrhagic enteritis and ulceration.

Type C

Two different forms of type C enterotoxaemia have been described. **One** occurs in **adult sheep** and the **other in neonatal (newborn) lambs, calves,** and **piglets**. The **first form** is called **"struck",** a disease of **adult sheep** in Britain. **Clinical signs** are usually not observed. The disease is manifested by **sudden death**. Sometimes death is preceded by abdominal pain and convulsions. The **lesions** are **haemorrhagic enteritis** with ulceration of the mucosa, particularly of the jejunum and duodenum. A striking feature is peritonitis with a large volume of clear yellow fluid in the peritoneal cavity.

The **second form** of C enterotoxaemia, known as **"enterotoxic haemorrhagic enteritis"** occurs in the United States in calves, lambs, and foals in the first few days of life. **Clinically**, there is diarrhoea, but as with other forms of enterotoxaemia, death usually occurs without premonitory signs. **Lesions** include **haemorrhagic enteritis** with ulceration, particularly of the jejunum and ileum. H aemorrhages are common beneath the epicardium and thymus.

Type C enterotoxaemia also occurs in **suckling piglets**, usually during the first week of life. Most **affected pigs die within 12-48 hours** after onset of clinical signs, which include dehydration and diarrhoea, which is often bloody. The pathological changes are dominated by a **haemorrhagic or necrotizing enteritis**, mainly affecting the jejunum. There is haemorrhagic lymphadenitis of the draining lymph nodes; serosanguineous fluid in the peritoneal, pleural, and pericardial c avities; and h aemorrhage in t he epicardium, e ndocardium, and kidneys.

Type D

C. perfringens **type D** is responsible for enterotoxaemia of **sheep, goats, and cattle. It is an important killer disease of goats in India. In sheep**, the disease occurs in fatting (fattening) lambs, and less commonly, in adult sheep. The disease is known as **"pulpy kidney disease"**, or **"overeating disease"**. It occurs throughout t he world, i ncluding India, a nd is o ften associated w ith diets h igh in c oncentrated grains. D ecreasing the t otal amounts o f food, o r changing from a high concentration of grains with little roughage, to a ration consisting almost entirely of hay, appears to be an effective **preventive measure. Lambs are usually found dead**. However, a period of one-half to a few hours may be observed during which **opisthotonus** (an arched position of the body) progresses i nto coma. I n a f ew cases, c onvulsions take the place o f coma, and death is more quick. Sometimes, animals show a desire to push the forehead against a solid wall, such animals being referred to as **"blind staggers"**. Sometimes t hese acute s ymptoms are p receded by anorexia and d iarrhoea. There is usually **hyperglycaemia** and **glycosuria** (presence of glucose in the urine). **The disease in goats and calves is similar.**

The lesions result from absorption of epsilon toxin produced by *C. perfringens* **within the intestinal lumen**. Its injurious e ffect on vascular endothelium l eads to haemorrhage, oedema, and damage to parenchymal organs and the brain. There are petechial and ecchymotic h aemorrhages beneath the epicardial and endocardial surfaces, the serous surfaces of the intestines, in abdominal muscles, in the diaphragm, and in the thymus. Hydropericardium is usually present. There is **pronounced glycosuria**. Other findings include distension o f the r umen, reticulum, a bomasum, a nd l ower intestine by ingesta and gas. The intestinal mucosa is usually hyperaemic. The gallbladder is often distended. **The kidneys are soft and friable**, giving rise to the name "**pulpy kidney disease**". Usually, this i s the r esult of postmortem autolysis, which occurs rapidly.

Neurological signs are explained by lesions in the central nervous system, **which are the most specific and diagnostic for the disease**. These consist of bilaterally symmetrical focal malacia (softening) of the basal ganglia, substantia nigra, and thalamus, and bilaterally symmetrical demyelination in the internal capsule, subcortical white matter, and cerebellar peduncles. The harmful effect of the toxin on endothelium is particularly seen in the brain. Damaged endothelial cells develop pyknotic nuclei, and the vessels become surrounded by a zone of oedema.

Type E

Type E *C. perfringens* has been found in **calves** and **lambs**. However, the status of the disease is not known. Available information does not suggest that the disease is of importance.

Pseudomembranous Colitis (*C. difficile* Enterotoaxemia)

Clostridium difficile (so named because of the difficulty in its isolation) is an **inhabitant of the gastrointestinal tract of humans and animals**. In 1977 it was recognized as a cause of disease. Its association with disease results from the use of **antibiotics** to which *C. difficile* is resistant. This allows the organism to proliferate and secrete potent toxins. However, the organism has caused disease in the absence of antibiotic therapy in humans, monkeys, and pigs. **Two toxins** have been identified: 1. **Toxin A or enterotoxin**. This causes marked fluid accumulation in the intestines by unknown mechanisms, and 2. **Toxin B**, which is cytopathic.

The disease, which is characterized by severe colitis, and usually ileitis and caecitis, has been seen in **pigs, foals, monkeys**, and **humans**. The **lesions** begin in the superficial mucosa as focal areas of necrosis. This progresses to complete necrosis of the mucosa and its replacement by fibrin and debris. There is an intense neutrophilic inflammatory response. The organisms are not invasive, but remain within the lumen. These lesions are very similar to those induced by *C. perfringens* enteritis (enterotoxaemia).

Diagnosis

The early age at which enterotoxaemia occurs, the rapid course, and typical necropsy findings suggest the diagnosis, which can be confirmed by laboratory examination.

Avian Clostridial Infections

Clostridia are frequently found in low numbers in the normal bird's intestinal tract.

Botulism (Limberneck)

Botulism is an **intoxication** (a **toxaemia**) caused by exotoxin of rapidly multiplying *Clostridium botulinum*. The disease affects poultry worldwide. As indicated earlier (Table 17), there are **8 antigenically different toxigenic group-ings (A, B, C-alpha, C-beta, D, E, F and G). Almost all outbreaks in poultry are caused by type C-alpha.** Occasionally, however, **types A, B, and E** are involved. Botulism toxins are among the most potent toxins known. Type C toxin is produced under anaerobic conditions. **Type C-alpha cultures produce three toxins: C1, C2,** and small amounts of **type D toxin.**

Spread

C. botulinum **type C** is distributed worldwide. Type C organisms readily grow in the gastrointestinal tract of normal birds. Type C spores are com-monly found in and around poultry farms. **Presence of organisms in the gastrointestinal tract,** and resistance of spores to inactivation, favour spread of this organism. **Outbreaks occur in chickens when the toxin is consumed, usually in decaying poultry carcasses,** or toxin-containing maggots or bee-tles. Maggots are eaten up greedily by chickens, which can lead to botulism outbreaks. **Toxin** is produced by bacterial growth in rotting vegetation ex-posed during dry summers. The toxin may sometimes be both produced in, and absorbed from, the caeca of chickens, without any external source of toxin being available. Botulism is fairly rare in domestic poultry kept under good standards of management and hygiene in which carcasses are regularly and frequently removed.

Pathogenesis

Type C botulism can be caused by **ingestion of preformed toxin.** Because the organism is widely distributed in the gut, as indicated, dead birds provide conditions for *C. botulinum* growth and toxin production. Birds scavenging (i.e., searching for decaying flesh as food) such carcasses can readily obtain enough toxin to become affected. Botulism caused by A, B, and E occurs rarely, and generally has been associated with consumption of spoiled human food products fed to backyard chicken flocks.

The **pathogenesis** of botulism was once thought exclusively to be due to ingestion of preformed toxin. There is growing evidence that *C. botulinum* **type C produces toxin in the gut to cause disease.** The term "toxico-infec-tion" has been used to describe this form of the disease in broiler chickens. Experimental evidence suggests **caecum** as the site of toxin production.

Signs

Clinical signs appear within a few hours of ingestion of the toxin. In chickens, flaccid paralysis (i.e., lacking firmness of muscles) of legs, wings, neck, and eyelids are main features of the disease. Initially, affected birds are found sitting and reluctant to move. If forced to walk, they appear lame. Wings droop when paralysed. Affected birds have ruffled feathers. **Limberneck**, the original and common name for botulism, precisely describes the paralysis of the neck. Because of eyelid paralysis, birds appear comatose (in coma, unconscious), and may look dead. **Death results from cardiac and respiratory failure**.

Lesions

There are no gross or microscopic lesions. Sometimes, maggots or feathers may be found in the crop.

Diagnosis

The presumptive diagnosis of botulism is based on clinical signs and lack of gross or microscopic lesions. Definitive diagnosis requires detection of toxin in serum, crop, or gastrointestinal washings from sick birds. The presence of toxin is confirmed by the injection of serum, or extracts of crop, or gastrointestinal contents, into mice. Since toxin can be produced in decaying body tissues, material for examination should be from living birds, or fresh carcasses.

Ulcerative Enteritis (Quail Disease)

Ulcerative enteritis (UE) is an acute bacterial infection of **young chickens** and **turkeys** characterized by **sudden onset and rapidly increasing mortality**. The disease was **first seen in** enzootic proportions in **quail**, and was therefore called "**quail disease**". It has since been established that many avian species other than quail are susceptible. Therefore, the earlier name has been replaced by "**ulcerative enteritis**". UE is caused by *Clostridium colinum*, a new species of **Clostridium**. UE occurs worldwide. Predisposing factors appear to play an important role in the production of disease. They include coccidiosis, infectious bursal disease, and perhaps chicken infectious anaemia, stress conditions, and inadequate hygiene.

Signs

Birds dying from acute disease may show no premonitory signs. Or, they may be depressed, listless, huddled, anorexic, and show ruffled feathers. Mortality in chickens varies from 2% to as high as 12%.

Lesions

First, there are small, round, superficial **ulcers** with haemorrhagic borders in the mucosa of the **small intestines, caeca and upper large intestines**. These **later** coalesce and **penetrate deeper into the serosa** which may become **perforated and cause peritonitis**. In the **liver**, usually there are yellowish to grey **necrotic lesions** of varying size. The **spleen** is enlarged and haemorrhagic.

Diagnosis

The gross lesions are often sufficient, but the diagnosis should be confirmed by the demonstration of the organism in the intestine, liver, or spleen, by culture or immunofluorescence.

Necrotic Enteritis

Necrotic enteritis (NE) is a sporadic disease of chickens and turkeys. It occurs usually **in birds of 4 weeks of age or older**, and sometimes in **adults**. The disease is caused by the proliferation of *Clostridium perfringes* types **A or C** in the large intestine and caeca, and subsequent migration to small intestine where it produces toxins. **Alpha toxin** produced by *C. perfringens* **types A and C**, and **beta toxin** produced by **type C**, are believed responsible for intestinal mucosal necrosis, the characteristic lesion of the disease. **Both have been detected in faeces of chickens with NE**. Predisposing factors include outbreaks of coccidiosis, especially mild or subclinical, changes in diet, and inadequate cleaning of houses, utensils, and equipment.

Spread

C. perfringens can be found in faeces, soil, dust, contaminated feed and litter, or intestinal contents. **Contaminated feed or litter** are believed to be the **source of infection**.

Signs

Clinical signs include depression, decreased appetite, reluctance to move, diarrhoea, and ruffled feathers. **Clinical illness is very short**. Often there may be no clinical signs. **Birds are just found dead**.

Lesions

The **small intestine** is markedly thickened due to **extensive necrosis of the mucosa**, which is deeply fissured and often congested. In the lower part of the small intestine, lesions are quite dry. Acute cases have large amounts of necrotic epithelial debris in the lumen of the small intestine often with flecks of blood. **Microscopic changes** comprise severe necrosis of the intestinal mucosa with an abundance of fibrin mixed with cellular debris adherent to the necrotic mucosa.

Diagnosis

Diagnosis is based on typical gross and microscopic lesions and isolation of the causative agent. *C. perfringens* can be cultured **anaerobically** and identified.

Gangrenous Dermatitis (Malignant Oedema)

The two clostridia most commonly involved in this disease are *Clostridium septicum* and *C. perfringens* type A. However, in many outbreaks *Staphylococcus aureus* is also involved, and rarely, *C. novyi* (*C. oedematiens*) and other clostridial species. Gangrenous dermatitis (GD) is **mainly a disease of t he broilers over 4 weeks of age.** M ortality can r each up t o **60% in untreated cases**.

Predisposition

Clostridia are distributed in soil, faeces, dust, contaminated litter or feed, and i ntestinal contents. S taphylococci are u biquitous (present e verywhere), and **common inhabitant of skin and mucous membranes of poultry**, a nd areas where poultry are hatched, r eared, and processed. In many cases, GD occurs as a sequel t o disease produced by o ther infectious a gents, such a s infectious bursal d isease (IBD) v irus (due t o immunosuppression), c hicken infectious a naemia virus, r eticuloendotheliosis virus, a nd a vian adenovirus infections, including inclusion body hepatitis (IBH) virus. Both GD and IBH occur as a sequel to IBD. There are fewer cases of GD where protection against IBD in young s tock h as b een attained. S ome outbreaks o f G D h ave b een breeder flock-associated, i.e., progeny from a specific b reeder flock consistently develops GD. Another condition predisposing chickens to GD is "**blue wing disease (BWD)**". Characteristic lesions of BWD are **intracutaneous, subcutaneous, and intramuscular haemorrhages and oedema**, with atrophy of thymus, spleen, and bursa of F abricius. Numerous avian retroviruses and chicken infectious anaemia virus (CIAV) h ave been i solated from chickens affected with BWD. GD often occurs secondarily to the skin haemorrhages. **A compromised (damaged) immune system is the underlying predisposing factor which allows GD to occur.**

Signs

Clinical signs i nclude varying degrees of d epressicn, incoordination, inappetence (anorexia), leg weakness, a nd a taxia. **B ecause the period of illness is short, usually less than 24 hours, birds are often just found dead. Mortality ranges from 1-60%.**

Lesions

Gross lesions c onsist of **d ark, moist areas of skin**, u sually d evoid o f feathers, lying **under the wings, between the thighs and over the ribs and flanks** of birds. **Extensive blood-tinged oedema, with or without gas (emphysema)**, is present below the affected skin. Underlying musculature is discoloured grey or t an (yellowish-brown), a nd may contain oedematous f luid and gas between muscle bundles. In some cases, emphysema and serosanguineous fluid are present in subcutaneous tissue, but t here is no loss of integrity in the overlying skin. **In most cases there are no internal lesions**. However, discrete (separate) white foci (necrosis) in the liver, and small flaccid (not firm) bursa of Fabricius, presumably due to IBD virus infection, have been reported.

Diagnosis

Diagnosis can be made by the **typical gross and microscopic lesions,** and isolation of the causative agent(s). Clostridia and staphylococci can be isolated from exudates of skin and subcutaneous tissue, or underlying muscle. However, bacterial culture can be misleading **since both staphylococci and clostridial organisms are present on the skin of normal fowls.**

Genus: Erysipelothrix

This genus contains only one pathogenic member, *Erysipelothrix rhusiopathiae*, the cause of **swine erysipelas**.

Swine Erysipelas

Erysipelas is **an infectious disease of pigs** and appears in an **acute septicaemic form** usually accompanied by **diamond-shaped skin lesions,** and a **chronic form** manifested by a non-suppurative arthritis and a **vegetative endocarditis**. It is caused by *Erysipelothrix rhusiopathiae* (*E. insidiosa*). Erysipelas in pigs occurs throughout the world. The disease is important because it causes serious loss due to death of pigs and devaluation of pig carcasses due to arthritis. **Pigs of all ages are susceptible**. Besides pigs, *E. rhusiopathiae* also infects other species, including poultry, cattle, sheep, horse, and dogs. It causes **erysipeloid of humans**. The term **erysipelas, in humans**, is used to denote cutaneous infections with **beta-haemolytic streptococci.**

Cause

E. rhusiopathiae is a small, pleomorphic, and **rod-shaped**, either straight or curved organism. It is **Gram-positive**, and may have **beaded appearance**. The organism forms tiny colonies on ordinary agar media. At least 22 serotypes are known to exist. However, **serotypes 1 and 2 are the most common types** isolated from pigs affected with the disease. These are the only serotypes which cause the acute disease. The **other types are relatively unimportant**.

Spread

Soil contamination occurs through the faeces of affected or carrier pigs. Other sources of infection include infected animals of other species, and birds. **Thus, the clinically normal carrier animals are the most important source of infection**. The tonsils are the predilection site for the organism in such cases. Since **the organism can pass through the stomach without being destroyed,** carrier animals can reinfect the soil continuously, and this appears to be the main cause of environmental contamination. **The organism can survive in faeces for several months**. It survives for extremely long periods in alkaline soil, decaying flesh, and water. It is resistant to such preservative processes as salting, smoking, and pickling; and **many pigs carry the organism in their oropharynx**. Thus, sources of infection are easily provided. Once infection is established, a large number of bacteria are excreted. These provide the main source for spread within a herd. Although **infection** can occur through broken skin, **usually it occurs through the oral route**.

Pathogenesis

First, invasion of bloodstream occurs. Then, the development of either **an acute septicaemia**, or a bacteraemia with localization of organisms in organs **and joints (chronic form)**, depends on undetermined factors. **Type III (immune complex) reactions** may contribute to the development of arthritis. The **bacterial antigen** tends to **localize in joint tissues** where local immune complex formation then causes inflammation and **arthritis**. Virulence of the particular strain may be important. Concurrent viral infection, especially swine fever, may increase susceptibility. **Localization in the chronic form is usually in the skin, joints, and on heart valves**. Selective adherence of some strains may be important in the pathogenesis of endocarditis.

Signs

In pigs, the disease occurs in a **peracute, acute, or chronic form**. The **peracute or acute form** is a febrile disease with a **high rate of mortality. Death occurs before any specific signs can be detected**. The only outward sign may be discoloration of the skin. In severe cases, appearance of **rhomboid-shaped (diamond-shaped) areas of intense erythema in the skin are characteristic**, and therefore the common name **"diamond-skin disease"** is often applied to this disease. These erythematous lesions may progress to necrosis. Large patches of epidermis slough as healing occurs.

Chronic form is characterized by localization of the organism in the heart valves or joints. This leads to **vegetative endocarditis** or **arthritis**. Arthritis in one or more joints is manifested by a sudden painful hot swelling, particularly of the carpal or tarsal joints. **Vegetative endocarditis is a common sequel and may result in sudden death**. Hypersensitivity appears to play an important role in this disease, but is still inadequately understood.

Lesions

In acute septicaemic cases, non-specific lesions such as haemorrhages may occur in serous surfaces and elsewhere. Specific lesions of diagnostic importance develop as the disease progresses. The distinguishing lesions are found in the skin, synovial membranes, and endocardium. The **cutaneous lesions** are most common on the abdomen, but may occur elsewhere in the skin. They vary in size, but are almost always **of diamond, rhomboid, or rectangular** (with four sides and four right angles) **shape** and are sharply demarcated from the normal skin. At first, they are bright red, but later they become purplish, and eventually, dark blue. **Necrosis accounts for darkening of the skin**. The overlying epidermis dries and eventually peels off. Forcible removal of scabs from an incompletely healed lesion shows a raw, bleeding surface. The reason for the shape of the skin lesion is not adequately understood. However, the **lesions** themselves **result from** bacterially induced **arteriolitis** and **thrombosis**, which can be observed microscopically.

In the **subacute form** of the disease, microscopic evidence of synovitis may be seen, but in the **chronic form** damage to affected **joints** can be seen grossly. The joint capsule is visibly enlarged, thickened, and distended with excessive fluid, and the articular surfaces are roughened. Rugose thickening (i.e., full of wrinkles) of the joint capsule is particularly noticeable at the margins of the articular surfaces. **Microscopically**, the joint capsule is infiltrated with lymphoid cells, and the synovial lining is prominent and often thrown up into folds. Organisms can be identified in the synovial tissues early in the course of arthritis, but usually cannot be found in chronic arthritis. This has led to the belief that the lesions result from **immune mechanisms**.

Lesions in the **heart** are usually the result of **subacute bacterial endocarditis**. Most prominent are the large, irregular, coarse masses on the leaves of the **mitral (bicuspid) valve**, or less commonly, on the pulmonary valves. These nodular masses project into the lumen of the left ventricle, and at times, almost occlude it (**vegetative endocarditis**). The material adheres rather firmly to the valve leaflets, but it can be broken loose. Hypertrophy of the affected ventricle occurs in chronic cases. **Microcsopically**, the thickened valves are covered with fibrinous exudate made up of zones of organization, necrosis, leukocytes, and colonies of the organisms.

In sheep, *E. rhusiopathiae* is an important cause of **polyarthritis**. It is usually seen in **lambs**. The organism gains entry after docking or castration. Affected lambs are lame. The joints are swollen and contain fibrin and pus. The lesions progress to **degenerative osteoarthritis**. Valvular endocarditis, septicaemia, cutaneous lesions, or pneumonia can also develop in affected sheep.

Zoonotic Implications

Because of man's susceptibility, swine erysipelas has **some public health significance. Veterinarians** particularly are exposed to infection when vaccinating with virulent culture. It causes **erysipeloid (cellulitis) in humans**, particularly in **persons who work in slaughterhouses and fish markets.** The cutaneous lesions of erysipeloid are usually local but may become fulminant (severe), with widespread exanthematous or bullous lesions on the hands, face, or body.

Rarely, there may be endocarditis and encephalitis in humans who sustain an injury, such as a cut, while handling diseased carcasses.

Diagnosis

Typical symptoms and lesions are usually sufficient for diagnosis. However, recovery and identification of the organism are necessary in acute septicaemic cases and also in others. The organisms can be readily demonstrated by Gram's stain.

Avian Erysipelas

Erysipelas is **an acute, fulminating (sudden and severe) disease** caused by *Erysipelothix rhusiopathiae* (*E. insidiosa*). The disease is of great importance in **turkeys**, and of lesser significance in the **chicken. Chickens are less susceptible and have lower mortality**. In chickens there may be **depressed egg production**.

Spread

The source of infection may not be known, but often there is a history of **pigs** or **sheep** being previously housed on the same land. **The organism can survive for years in the soil, and it is shed for up to 40 days in the faeces of recovered birds. The organism enters the birds through breaks in the skin, or mucous membranes.**

Signs

The disease has a rapid onset. Birds in good condition may be found **suddenly dead,** after little or no prior signs of illness. A few birds may be drowsy, have diarrhoea, or show an unsteady gait prior to death. **T**urkeys often show cyanosis of the head. Mortality can range from 1-50%. **Most sick birds die.** Some recovered birds may show chronic lameness.

Lesions

There may be **dark, crusty lesions** over any part of the body, especially the head in **turkeys**. Lesions are of generalized bacteraemia and congestion, with small haemorrhages, usually in the skin, muscles, pericardial fat, gizzard serosa, mesentery, abdominal fat, liver, and under the pleura. **Liver, spleen, and kidneys** are usually enlarged, friable and mottled. There is usually marked **catarrhal enteritis. In very acute cases there may be no gross lesions.**

Diagnosis

Diagnosis is based upon the history and postmortem picture, together with the isolation and identification of the causative organism. Several sites, including the liver, spleen and bone marrow, should be cultured as *E. rhusiopathiae* **can be difficult to grow**. A tentative (provisional) diagnosis can be obtained by a Gram-stained smear of heart blood, especially in peracute cases.

Genus: Listeria

This genus too contains only one pathogenic member, *Listeria monocytogenes*, which causes **listeriosis.**

Listeriosis

Listeriosis is an infectious disease caused by *Listeria monocytogenes*. The disease is characterized by **encephalitis, systemic infection (septicaemia), or abortion.**

Cause

L. monocytogenes is a small, **rod-shaped, Gram-positive intracellular organism.** It causes disease in most species of animals (ruminants, pigs, dogs, cats), and **also in humans. In wildlife,** it has been reported in deer, fox and leopard. The organism is called '**monocytogenes**' since it causes **mononucleosis** (increased number of mononuclear leukocytes in the blood) **in rabbits,** in the systemic form of the disease. The organism is ubiquitous (present everywhere) in nature and can be recovered from soil, vegetation, dairy products, animal faeces, and **sometimes the oropharynx and tissues of healthy animals.**

Spread

With **septicaemic disease** and **abortion,** the organism is transmitted by **ingestion of contaminated material. Lambs** which develop septicaemic disease may acquire infection from contamination on the ewe's teat, from the ingestion of milk containing the organisms from ewes with subclinical bacteraemia, from the navel, and as a congenital infection. The **encephalitic form** of the disease results from infection of the terminals of the trigeminal nerve following injuries of the buccal mucosa from feed, from nibbling on plantations, or from infection of tooth cavities.

Pathogenesis

Listeria have the ability to penetrate epithelial cells, such as the conjunctiva, urinary bladder, and intestine. Recent studies have revealed that *L. monocytogenes* has on its surface **leucine-rich proteins called internalins. The internalins are required for penetration of the bacterium into epithelial cells. Internalins bind to E-cadherin on host epithelial cells, which acts as a receptor for internalin. Thus, the organisms enter into the cells.** Here, they multiply, destroy the cells, and are then released. Following release, they are phagocytized by macrophages. **To avoid destruction,** they escape from the phagosome and persist free within the cytoplasm and multiply here. Thus, they can survive and multiply inside normal macrophages. Moreover, *L. monocytogenes* can travel from cell to cell without exposure to the extracellular fluid. However, **activated**

macrophages which depend on cell-mediated immunity, phagocytose and kill bacteria. Transport by macrophages is thought to result in a septicaemic phase in some cases. Centripetal movement (i.e., toward the centre) of organisms within the branches of the trigeminal nerve eventually makes them to reach **medulla oblongata.** Bacteria appear to move along fibre tracts, but also within axons. In experimentally infected ewes in the latter half of gestation, organisms penetrated the placenta and reached the foetal liver. Here multiplication occurred, resulting in the death of the foetus. **Listeria organisms can be carried and excreted in the faeces of animals in the absence of disease.**

Signs and Lesions

Listeriosis occurs in **three different syndromes,** which usually do not occur together. These are: 1. **Encephalitis** in humans, cattle, sheep, goats, and pigs, 2. **Systemic infection (septicaemia)** in humans, cattle, sheep, pigs, dogs, and cats, and 3. **Abortion** in humans, cattle, and sheep. Less commonly, the organism causes endocarditis and purulent lesions in other organs and tissues.

Encephalitis

Involvement of the central nervous system is the most characteristic form of the disease **in ruminants.** It is manifested by the animal's abnormal posturing (position) of the head and neck, walking aimlessly in a circle ("**circling disease**"), nystagmus (constant involuntary movement of the eyeball), blindness, and paralysis. The **encephalitic form** can also occur in **horses, dogs, pigs,** and **humans.** The organism is thought to invade the central nervous system by ascending peripheral nerves, particularly the **trigeminal nerve.**

The **lesions** in the CNS can be recognized only by microscopic examination and are confined to the brain stem, particularly medulla oblongata and spinal cord. The primary lesion is a circumscribed collection of mononuclear cells, with or without neutrophils, adjacent to blood vessels. Diffuse cellular infiltration and frank abscesses may occur, but there is little tissue necrosis. Nerve cells are destroyed, but the lesions are not restricted to grey matter. **The organisms, being Gram-positive, can be demonstrated in tissue sections without difficulty with appropriate stains.** They are found in the centre of the lesions in the medulla oblongata or spinal cord. Intense meningeal infiltration by lymphoid cells is a charactertistic finding. Lesions in various organs, similar to those met with in septicaemic listeriosis (described below), occur in listeric encephalitis in both cattle and sheep.

Systemic Infection (Septicaemia)

Generalized listeriosis is the most common form in monogastric animals **(pigs, dogs, cats),** and in **human newborns** and **infants. The most characteristic lesion is focal necrosis of the liver.** Less commonly, lesions occur in the spleen, lymph nodes, lungs, adrenal glands, myocardium, gastrointestinal tract, and brain. **Microscopically**, lesions consist of focal areas of necrosis infiltrated with mononuclear cells and some neutrophils. The organisms are easily demonstrated in appropriately stained tissue sections.

Abortion

Abortion is important mainly in **cattle** and **sheep**. Abortion usually occurs in the **last quarter of gestation** without signs of infection in the dam (mother). The **foetus** dies in uterus and may be severely autolyzed when expelled. If not damaged by autolysis, **focal hepatic necrosis** containing stainable organisms in the foetal liver is the main lesion of diagnostic value.

Diagnosis

Diagnosis of encephalitis can be confirmed by demonstration of the typical microscopic lesions. These are: 1. Microabscesses, diffuse purulent inflammation, or glial nodules; 2. Perivascular accumulation of lymphocytes; and 3. Lymphocytic leptomeningitis along with the presence of Gram-positive organisms in these lesions. Although the lesions in listeric septicaemia and abortion are less specific than encephalitis, demonstration of the organisms within the necrotic lesions allows presumptive diagnosis. Confirmation can be made by isolation of the organisms in appropriate culture media inoculated with suspension of tissue.

Avian Listeriosis

Listeriosis in poultry is caused by *Listeria monocytogenes*, which is widespread in nature. It is found in the soil, sewage, water, and in faeces of domestic and wild birds. **The organism can be recoverd from the apparently normal domestic poultry. It can survive outside the body for several years.** In chickens, turkeys, and ducks, **spread** can occur through the **faeces**. However, it may be difficult to determine the source and spread of infection. **There is no evidence for egg transmission.**

In poultry, disease associated with this organism is very rare and sporadic. The signs are not pathognomonic, and may include depression, diarrhoea, and emaciation. In the less common encephalitic form, there may be ataxia (muscular incoordination) and torticollis (stiff neck). The **gross lesions** are those associated with septicaemia, and include myocarditis with pale necrotic foci, hydropericardium, focal hepatic necrosis, and less frequently, splenomegaly with necrotic foci, nephritis, oedema of the lungs, thickening of the airsac walls, enteritis and conjunctivitis.

Diagnosis

Diagnosis of the infection is made by isolation and identification of the organism. Isolation can be made from the blood, myocardium, liver, spleen, or brain. The organism can be identified by biochemical means. An ELISA has been developed for the recognition of listeria.

Genus: Staphylococcus
Staphylococcal Infections

There are more than two dozen different species of staphylococci. However, only a few are pathogenic. Staphylococci cause pyogenic infections of various organs and tissues, particularly of the skin, mammary glands, lungs, joints, and uterus, in almost all species of animals. The important pathogenic staphylococci are: *S. aureus*, *S. epidermidis*, *S. intermedius*, and *S. hyicus*.

S. aureus is a haemolytic, coagulase-positive organism which can cause a variety of purulent inflammatory diseases. In humans, it is associated with septicaemia, severely necrotizing and purulent pneumonia, endocarditis, upper respiratory infections, subcutaneous abscesses (furuncles and boils), cellulitis, enterocolitis, and toxic shock syndrome. *S. aureus* is also a cause of food poisoning, which occurs from the ingestion of preformed heat-stable enterotoxins produced by its growth in contaminated foods. In animals, *S. aureus* is associated with purulent lesions of the skin, such as pyoderma, furunculosis (condition in which inflamed hair follicles rupture spilling exudate and causative agent), and impetigo (a superficial, pustular, bacterial epidermitis). At times these lesions may become disseminated. One such example is "tick pyaemia" in sheep. There is a generalized staphylococcal infection which is introduced into young lambs by bites of the sheep tick, *Ixodes ricinus*, and is characterized by multiple disseminated abscesses and polyarthritis. The pathogenesis of these types of disorders is not entirely understood. The most important diseases of *S. aureus* in animals are: 1. Botryomycosis, 2. Staphylococcal bovine mastitis, and 3. Exudative epidermitis of swine (greasy pig disease).

Pathogenesis

S. aureus and other virulent staphylococci possess a large number of "virulence factors". These include surface proteins involved in adherence, enzymes that degrade proteins, and toxins which damage host cells. *S. aureus* has, on its surface, receptors for fibrinogen, fibronectin, and vitronectin. It uses these receptors as a bridge to bind to host endothelial cells. *S. aureus* also has a laminin receptor which is similar to that of metastatic tumour cells. The receptor allows bacteria to bind to host extracellular matrix proteins and invade host tissues.

Staphylococci produce a variety of toxins which include coagulases, fibrinolysins, hyaluronidase, haemolysins (alpha, beta, gamma, delta), and enterotoxins. The lipase of *S. aureus* destroys lipids on the skin surface, and thus gives bacteria the ability to produce skin abscesses. Alpha toxin, a pore-forming toxin, penetrates into the plasma membrane of host cells and depolarizes them (i.e., destroys their polarity). Gamma-haemolysin and leukocidin lyse (destroy) erythrocytes and leukocytes, respectively. *S. aureus* can inhibit chemotaxis and phagocytosis by producing toxins, such as streptolysin O, which lyse neutrophil cell membranes. *S. aureus* also prevents phagocytosis by means of **protein A** present on its surface. Protein A binds to the Fc portion of IgG molecules, and prevents the immunoglobulin from binding to the receptors on the phagocytic cell and phagocytosing the bacteria.

Botryomycosis

Botryomycosis is **a chronic pyogranulomatous inflammation** caused by *S. aureus*. It is so named because the pyogranulomatous **lesions resemble a bunch of grapes** (G. botrys = bunch of grapes). The condition occurs in **cattle, sheep, horses, dogs, cats,** and **pigs,** and probably in other species as well.

Lesions

The lesions are usually in the subcutaneous tissues, but may occur in any organ. **In cattle,** the mammary gland may be affected, causing **granulomatous staphylococcal mastitis. In horses,** the stub (short piece left) in geldings (castrated horses) is a common site.

Grossly, the lesions are composed of **multiple firm nodules with purulent centres** containing white granules referred to as **grains.** These are similar to the "**sulphur granules**" seen in some other bacterial and mycotic granulomas. However, the grains are rarely sufficiently firm to be felt with fingers, like the granules of actinomycosis. **Microscopically,** a core (centre) of neutrophils is surrounded by granulation tissue, containing epithelioid cells, some lymphocytes, plasma cells, and rarely multinucleated giant cells. This granulation tissue is surrounded by fibrous connective tissue. Within the cores are brilliantly eosinophilic "**rosettes**" (**Splendore-Hoeppli material**), which closely resemble the rosettes of actinomycosis and actinobacillosis, but these show less tendency to form "**clubs**" at the periphery. **These are the grains seen grossly. Gram's stain** shows these rosettes as surrounding the colonies of cocci. However, the organisms usually die out in the centre, the oldest part of the colony.

Staphylococcal Bovine Mastitis

This may occur as a **chronic infection** which results in **botryomycosis (as** an acute gangrenous inflammation), or as an acute to clinically not noticeable purulent lesion. Variations in the virulence of the infecting organisms, which gain entry through the teat, probably account for the differing severities of the infection. *S. aureus* also **causes mastitis in sheep, goats, pigs and horses.**

Exudative Epidermitis of Swine (Greasy Pig Disease)

Exudative epidermitis of **suckling pigs** is caused by *Staphylococcus hyicus*. **Clinically,** it is characterized by the appearance of an acute, generalized,

seborrhoeic dermatitis (i.e., by increased sebum production). The source of the organism is unkown, but the **gilts** or **sows** are probably inapparent **carriers. The organism is a common inhabitant of the skin of normal pigs.** Although the main lesion is an inflammatory-exudative reaction in the dermis and upper layers of the epidermis, the disease is probably a systemic rather than local one.

Signs

In the **peracute form** which occurs usually in the **piglet,** there is a sudden onset of marked **cutaneous erythema,** with severe pain on palpation. Anaemia and severe dehydration are present, and **death occurs within 24-48 hours.** The entire **skin coat** is wrinkled and reddened, and is covered with a **greasy, grey-brown exudate** which accumulates around the eyes, behind the ears, and over the abdominal wall. Hence the name **greasy pig disease.** In the **less acute form,** seen in **older pigs,** the greasy exudate becomes thickened, and peels off in scabs, leaving a pink-coloured to normal skin surface. There is **no** irritation or pruritus. In the **subacute form,** the exudate dries into brown scabs. In the **chronic form,** there is thickening with wrinkling of the skin and thick scabs, which crack and form deep fissures. **Most peracute cases die, while piglets with the less severe forms survive if treated.**

Avian Staphylococcosis

Staphylococcus aureus **infections are common in poultry;** the most common sites being bones, tendon sheaths, and joints of the leg. A wide variety of diseased conditions of the chicken and turkey are associated with *S. aureus*. They include **arthritis and tenosynovitis (inflammation of a tendon sheath), gangrenous dermatitis, yolk sac infection, subdermal abscesses (bumble foot), spondylitis and osteomyelitis,** and **staphylococcal septicaemia.**

S. aureus **is often found in the skin, in the nares, on the beak and on the foot of apparently normal chickens.** The organism can survive away from the host for many months, particularly under dry conditions and in pus. All species of domestic poultry and other birds are susceptible to staphylococcosis. **Injury to the skin or mucous membrane** (as in pecking, toe-clipping and debeaking), and in fowl-pox, may predispose to tissue infection. The **unhealed navel in chicks** may also be route for infection.

Diseases

Arthritis and Tenosynovitis

The **affected joints,** usually the **hocks,** are swollen and painful, and affected birds are usually depressed, lame and reluctant to walk. When the phalangeal joints are affected, subdermal staphylococcal, plantar abscesses ("**bumble foot**") may occur. The synovial membranes of joints and tendon sheaths (usually in the region of hock and feet) become thickened and oedematous. There is some necrosis and the exudate may later become **caseous**. If the bird survives, the condition becomes chronic with the formation of fibrous tissue.

Gangrenous Dermatitis (GD)

This is usually seen in **broiler chickens**. The wing tips and the dorsal pelvic region are the sites usually affected. Lesions are dark, moist, and gangrenous in appearance with crepitation. Staphylococci are usually associated with *Clostridium perfringens* **type A**, which may be the primary pathogen. Immunosuppression resulting from damage to the bursa of Fabricius may predispose to gangrenous dermatitis in growing chickens.

Yolk Sac Infection

See "yolk sac infection" under "colibacillosis".

Subdermal Abscesses

Subdermal abscesses usually affect the feet ("**bumble foot**") and sternal bursa. There is abscess formation with swelling, heat, and some pain. In bumble foot the undersurface of the foot is first affected. The lesion may then spread to involve the whole foot. There is caseous and necrotic tissue and some haemorrhage.

Spondylitis and Osteomyelitis

S. aureus can cause abscesses in the bodies of the **5th to 7th thoracic vertebrae** with periostitis and osteomyelitis. These abscesses may press on the spinal cord resulting in paresis and paralysis. The head of the femur, tibiotarsus and sometimes other bones may also be affected with osteomyelitis.

Staphylococcal Septicaemia, Endocarditis and Granuloma

Septicaemia usually follows a primary staphylococcal focus. It is rare and may result in sudden death. The lesions include haemorrhages and **necrotic foci in the liver**, lungs, spleen, kidneys, and myocardium. In **chronic cases**, these may develop into **granulomas**. **Endocarditis** may also be a sequel, and vegetations, particularly affecting the left atrio-ventricular valves, are seen at necropsy.

Diagnosis

The clinical history, signs, and lesions are helpful, but other organisms, such as *Escherichia coli*, Salmonella, *Pasteurella multocida*, *Mycoplasma synoviae* and **reoviruses**, may cause some of these conditions. It is therefore necessary to isolate and identify *S. aureus* to confirm diagnosis.

Genus: Streptococcus

Streptococcal Infections

Streptococci are spherical, **Gram-positive** organisms which grow in pairs or chains. They are **pathogenic for humans and animals**. The importance of these infections has increased greatly during the past few years because of the widespread use of antibiotics. Several different systems of classification for streptococci have been proposed. However, usually the various species are **classified according to their Lancefield Group** (a system based on antigens known as **group-specific antigens**. These antigens are polysaccharides or teichoic acids), and the type of haemolysis induced in the culture. **Important streptococci classified in this way, along with their associated diseases, are listed in Table 19.** In addition to these specific diseases, sreptococci are common invaders of wounds, leading to local purulent inflammation which can spread to distant organs. They are often recovered from purulent otitis media, arthritis, pneumonia, lymphadenitis, and other diseases.

Table 19. Streptococcal Infections

Species	Lancefield group	Diseases
S. pyogenes	A	Scarlet fever in **humans**; pyogenic infections in monkeys; rarely **affects animals**
S. agalactiae	B	Bovine mastitis; mastitis in sheep and goats; pyogenic infections in **humans**
S. dysgalactiae	C	Bovine mastitis
S. equi	C	Equine strangles
S. equisimilis	C	Cervical abscesses in horses; various pyogenic infections in pigs, dogs
S. zooepidemicus	C	Pyogenic infections, including pneumonia, in horses; mastitis in cattle; **streptococcosis in poultry**
S. bovis	D	Gastrointestinal commensal in cattle, sheep; rare cause of endocarditis in **humans**
S. equinus	D	Gastrointestinal commensal in horses
S. faecalis (genus **Enterococcus**)	D	Pyogenic infections in various animals
S. uberis	Mixed	Bovine mastitis

S. porcinus	E	Cervical abscesses in pigs
S. canis	G	Genital infections in dogs and cats; abscesses in cats
S. suis	D	Septicaemia, meningitis, arthritis in pigs
S. pneumoniae	None	Lobar pneumonia in **humans**, monkeys; **rare cause of disease in domestic animals**

Pathogenesis

Streptococci possess a **protein** on their surface, **M protein**, that prevents bacteria from being phagocytosed. They also possess a **complement C5a peptidase**, which destroys this chemotactic peptide. The M protein of *Streptococcus equi* can reduce opsonization by interfering with the deposition of equine complement on the bacterial surface. *Streptococcus pyogenes* M protein can bind fibrinogen, thus masking (hiding) C3b binding sites. Streptococci also have surface molecules, including **lipoteichoic acid**, which enable bacteria to bind to the host extracellular matrix protein **laminin and invade host tissues**. Streptococci secrete a **pyrogenic exotoxin** that causes fever.

Strangles

Also known as "**adenitis equorum**" and "**distemper**", strangles is an upper respiratory infection accompanied by purulent adenitis of horses caused by *Streptococcus equi*. This organism is an obligate parasite of **horses** which rarely affects other animals. **The disease is most common in young horses living in crowded conditions. It is usually introduced by carrier horses.**

Spread

Inhalation is the most important route of infection. **Ingestion** is possible.

Pathogenesis

Infection of the pharyngeal and nasal mucosa causes an acute pharyngitis and rhinitis. Drainage to lymph nodes results in **abscessation**. The infection may then spread to other organs causing suppurative processes in the kidney, brain, liver, spleen, tendon sheaths, and joints. After an attack of strangles has subsided, **purpura haemorrhagica** (a syndrome characterized by many petechial or ecchymotic haemorrhages) may occur **due to the development of sensitivity to streptococcal protein.**

Signs

There is fever, a mucopurulent nasal discharge, often conjunctivitis, and oedematous swelling of the pharyngeal region. This may produce inspiratory dyspnoea. The submaxillary lymph nodes become enlarged and hot, and soon form abscesses. **These abscesses yield large quantities of creamy yellowish pus when they rupture** spontaneously, or are incised. Recovery usually follows drainage of the abscess, but in some cases, the infection spreads to other lymph nodes, or reaches the general circulation. In such cases, abscesses may form in any organ, but are most common in the lungs, kidneys, liver, and spleen, and less common in the brain.

Lesions

Organisms which penetrate the upper respiratory mucosa cause acute inflammation in the neighbouring structures, particularly **lymph nodes**, where they form **abscesses**. Such abscesses may become encapsulated, or more commonly, rupture into the oral or pharyngeal cavities, or through skin of the inter-mandibular region. There is catarrhal or purulent rhinitis and pharyngitis, often with small abscesses in the pharynx and on the soft palate. **Metastatic abscesses occur in the lungs, liver, kidneys, spleen, and sometimes, brain**. Septicaemia is sometimes observed, with few or no abscesses. Abscesses in the retropharyngeal lymph nodes may drain into the **guttural pouches**, leading to **empyema** (accumulation of pus).

Purpura haemorrhagica may be a complication of strangles. In such cases, large subcutaneous areas of oedema and haemorrhage are associated with septic emboli in blood vessels of the tissues involved.

Diagnosis

Clinical history, presence of characteristic gross lesions, and the demonstration of *S. equi* in abscesses are sufficient to establish the diagnosis at postmortem. Demonstration and identification of the organisms in submaxillary, or other abscesses, confirms the clinical diagnosis in living animals.

Streptococcal Mastitis

Streptococcus agalactiae is the most important streptococcus as a cause of **bovine mastitis**. It is an obligate parasite of the bovine mammary gland, i.e., it requires the mammary gland for its survival. It is a specific contagious disease of **cattle** which is transmitted from cow to cow by means of a milker's hands, or contaminated milking equipment. **The bacteria enter through the teat canal, and colonize within the ducts, ductules, and acini**. The infection is thought to be permanent. Although the streptococci do not invade deep into the interstitium of the gland, the living epithelium is disrupted and an intense polymorphonuclear inflammatory reaction occurs. This is followed by replacement of polymorphonuclears by macrophages, **proliferative fibroblastic connective tissue**, and nodules of lymphocytes. Ducts may become obstructed, resulting in cysts lined by villous epithelial projections, and sometimes, metastatic squamous epithelium. Multiple foci of acute inflammation result in chronic inflammation and scarring. This ultimately leads to a **fibrotic gland**, which is firm to the touch. During the acute stages of the disease, **the milk may contain fibrin and pus**, but later the gland becomes dry.

Other streptococci, which do not require the mammary gland for survival, are also important as causes of mastitis. However, the associated diseases do not depend solely on the presence of the organism, as is the case with *S. agalactiae*. These streptococci include *S. uberis*, *S. dysgalactiae*, *S. faecalis*, and *S. zooepidemicus*. In a few cases, **streptococci of human origin** (*S. pyogenes*) may be involved in the outbreaks of bovine mastitis. They then contribute to epidemics of "**septic sore throat**" in persons who drink the milk from infected cows. With the exception of *S. uberis*, these other streptococci cause acute purulent mastitis. *S. uberis* is associated with less severe and more chronic disease.

Urogenital Infections

Streptococci are often associated with vaginitis, cervicitis, and endometritis. Sometimes they also cause placentitis and abortion. *S. zooepidemicus* is the most common in horses, and *S. canis* in dogs. Streptococci also sometimes cause inflammatory lesions of the testes and male accessory sex glands, as well as urethritis and pyelonephritis.

Cervical Lymphadenitis of Pigs

Abscesses known as "**swine strangles**" and "**jowl abscess**" sometimes occur in the cervical lymph nodes of pigs. **Streptococci of Lancefield group E** are the most commonly isolated organisms. These have been termed *Sreptococcus porcinus*. Group C streptococci, *Corynebacterium pyogenes*, *Pasteurella multocida*, and *Staphylococcus aureus* have also been recovered from abscesses of cervical lymph nodes. **Haematogenous spread** of the organisms occurs sometimes, causing abscesses in other parts of the body, or streptococcal endocarditis or meningitis.

Sreptococcal Meningitis and Arthritis in Pigs

A specific streptococcal infection of **young pigs** is caused by *S. suis*. The organism enters through the oral or respiratory routes. Infections may be subclinical or result in pharyngitis and cervical lymphadenitis. In some young pigs, septicaemia may develop with localization of the organism in the meninges and joints. This leads to **fibrinopurulent meningitis** and **polyarthritis**.

Neonatal Streptococcal Infections

Streptococcal infections occur in neonates (newborns) of **humans** and **most domestic animals**, particularly **foals, calves, lambs**, and **pigs**. Infection is thought to occur through the umbilicus ("**navel-ill**"). The infection usually results in suppurative polyarthritis ("**joint-ill**") and meningitis. However, localization in the valvular endocardium, kidneys, and choroid of the eye is not uncommon, especially in **lambs**.

Avian Streptococcosis

Among the streptococci, *Streptococcus zooepidemicus* of **Lancefield group C** has usually been **associated with diseases in poultry**. However, **diseases associated w ith streptococci i n poultry a re r elatively u ncommon**. *S. zooepidemicus* is intestinal inhabitant o f birds, and spread is direct through the egg, or indirect by t he oral route or respiratory routes, and perhaps skin wounds. **The organism affects mainly adult chickens.**

The **disease** caused may occur as **acute** or **chronic**. In the **acute form** of the disease, **death may occur without prodromal (preceding) signs**. Signs include cyanosis of the face and comb, blood-stained nasal exudate, and rapid loss of weight. **Mortality may be as high as 50% of the flock**. T he **gross lesions** include serosanguineous fluid su bcutaneously and i n the pericardial sac, p eritonitis, and e nlargement of t he liver, s pleen, and k idneys. **Small necrotic foci** from pinpoint to 1cm in diameter may be seen **in the liver**. In the **chronic form**, the clinical signs include progressive loss of condition, diarrhoea, lameness, and f ever (110^0 F). G ross lesions include emaciation, a rthritis, misshapen ova, peritonitis, endocarditis with vegetations on the heart valves, pericarditis, p erihepatitis, and pneumonia.

Clinical signs and gross lesions are an indication of possible steptococcal infection, but other pathogens such as staphylococci, **Erysipelothrix**, **Pasteurella**, and some strains of *E. coli* produce similar conditions. **Diagnosis** depends on the demonstration o f Gram-positive c occi i n s mears f rom the blood, l iver, spleen, or any of t he lesions. Culture and identification of the organism are necessary to c onfirm the diagnosis.

Diseases caused by Gram-negative Genera

Genus: Actinobacillus

Five members of the genus **Actinobacillus** cause disease **actinobacillosis** in animals. *A. equuli* and *A. suis* cause septicaemia in **foals** and **piglets**, respectively. *A. l ignieresii* i s the cause o f "**wooden tongue**", also known a s "**woody tongue**", of **cattle**. The fourth organism *A. seminis* causes epididymitis and polyarthritis in sheep. The fifth organism *A. capsulatus* is the cause o f arthritis in rabbits.

Actinobacillosis (Wooden Tongue)

Also known as "**woody tongue**", actinobacillosis **is a specific infectious disease of cattle and sheep** caused by *Actinobacillus lignieresii*. The disease is most common in cattle and worldwide in distribution. It is usually of sporadic occurrence on individual farms.

Spread

A. lignieresii (named after **J. Lignieres**) **is present normally in the oral cavity of cattle and sheep. Infection occurs from traumatic injury** to the oral mucosa. In cattle infection usually occurs through ulcerating or penetrating lesions of the tongue, and ulcerations to the side of the tongue caused by the teeth.

Signs

In cattle, the disease may produce signs and lesions which resemble those of actinomycosis, **but differ in several respects**. This organism may infect the jaw of cattle, but usually it invades the tongue, lymph nodes of the head, neck, and thorax. Tongue is replaced by fibrous tissue. It becomes hard, shrunken and immobile (**"wooden tongue"**). Less often the organism invades the lung, and rarely, other organs. In cattle, this infection is therefore much more common in soft tissues **than in bones, a point of differentiation from actinomycosis. Actinobacillosis is rare in sheep.** It usually affects soft tissues and lymph nodes of the mouth and pharynx. Lesions in the internal organs are rare. **Actinobacillosis does not occur in other species, including dogs and humans.**

Lesions

Microscopically, lesions closely resemble those of actinomycosis. There are discrete (separate) colonies of organisms surrounded by radiating clubs, suspended in pus, and encapsulated by dense connective tissue. **The colonies are much smaller, radiating clubs longer and more slender, and the purulent exudate is more abundant than in actinomycosis.** Gram's staining of smears or sections reveals **Gram-negative**, rod-shaped organisms in the centre of the colonies. However, they are difficult to detect because of the acidophilic staining of the background.

In the tongue, the abscesses are usually small. Diffuse proliferation of connective tissue sometimes causes such great enlargement that the stiff, partially mobile tongue protrudes from the mouth. This is the so-called "**wooden tongue**" **of cattle.** In **lymph nodes**, there is formation of an abscess, filled with thick, smooth, shiny pus. In the lungs and other tissues, the abscesses are usually much smaller.

Diagnosis

In tissue sections, Gram-negative material in the centre of the colonies is sufficient to differentiate actinobacillosis from actinomycosis, nocardiosis, and staphylococcal infections (**"botryomycosis"**). Demonstration of rosettes and the absence of Gram-positive organisms in fresh preparations also establish the diagnosis in bovine material. Culture and identification of the organisms may be used to confirm the diagnosis.

Actinobacillus equuli

A. equuli causes a specific infection of **young foals**. The organism, a tiny **rod-shaped**, **Gram-negative** and non-sporulating bacterium, is usually carried in the **gastrointestinal tract of normal horses**. It is present in the aneurysms caused by *Strongylus vulgaris*. Foals are infected in the uterus, or soon after birth. Migrating strongyles may serve to infect the foetus. **Most infected foals die within the first 3 days of life**, but others may survive longer. Sometimes, adult horses are affected. *A. equuli* is the most common cause of "**joint-ill**", "**navel-ill**", and "**septicaemia of foals**".

Signs

The disease must be suspected in newborn foals which are weak; are unable to stand to nurse; have swollen, hot, and painful joints; have fever and depression; or which die suddenly within a few days of birth.

Lesions

It is difficult to find lesions in foals which die soon after birth from an acute, septicaemic infection. However, if the foal survives a few days, **gross lesions** may become noticeable. **Infected joints are enlarged**, and contain excessive amounts of synovial fluid mixed with sanguineous or purulent exudate. The most characteristic lesions are observed in the **kidneys**. These contain tiny grey foci in the centre. The medulla is remarkably free from the grey foci which are microscopically tiny abscesses. These abscesses result from bacterial emboli which lodge in the capillaries, particularly in the glomerular tufts. Similar abscesses occur in other organs, but are much less common than in the kidneys.

A. equuli and *A. suis* sometimes cause infection in **pigs**. The infection resembles *A. equuli* in **foals**. It is usually a septicaemia of piglets, although pneumonia and arthritis are described in older animals. Both organisms have been associated with endocarditis in piglets.

Diagnosis

Diagnosis can be confirmed by isolation of the organisms, or by demonstration of typical gross and microscopic lesions in which bacteria are present.

Actinobacillus seminis

A. seminis causes epididymitis in rams. The organism, which is present in semen, localizes in the epididymis and testis. It produces a **chronic pyo-granulomatous inflammation** similar to that caused by *Brucella ovis*. The infection may be inapparent, or cause gross distortion of the epididymis and testis with ulceration and draining a bscesses.

Genus: Bordetella

The genus **B ordetella**, w hich are **G ram-negative rods**, c ontains t hree pathogenic species: *B. pertussis*, *B. parapertussis*, and *B. bronchiseptica*. *B. pertussis* is an obligate parasite of **humans**, and causes the respiratory infection known as "whooping cough". *B. parapertussis* is also an obligate parasite of **humans** and causes respiratory disease. It is also pathogenic for **sheep**, and is associated with chronic non-progressive pneumonia.

B. bronchiseptica is also an obligate parasite, but has a **broad host range** which include **dogs, cats, pigs, horses,** guinea-pigs, rabbits, non-human primates(monkeys, apes), and sometimes, humans. In contrast to *B. pertussis*, it can be carried in the absence of disease. The organism is readily spread between individuals by contact and aerosols. It readily establishes itself in the ciliated respiratory mucosa, where it proliferates in the cilia without invading further. A mucopurulent l aryngotracheitis d evelops. Upper r espiratory disease c aused by *B. bronchiseptica* occurs in most of the species listed above, but is most important in dogs and pigs. **In dogs,** it is an important bacterial pathogen in **infectious tracheo-bronchitis ("kennel cough"),** and usually **contributes to the pneumonia in canine distemper. I n** pigs, *B. bronchiseptica* is usually found in cases of **atrophic rhinitis.** It is considered by some to be the primary pathogen in this disease. However, its role remains controversial.

Bordetellosis (Turkey Coryza)

Bordetella avium causes an acute upper re spiratory infe ction **(rhinotracheitis) in turkeys.** T he syndrome w as first described i n 1967 i n Canada. *B. avium* is a small, **Gram-negative,** rod-shaped bacterium. Turkeys appear t o be the natural h ost. T he onset of t he d isease is usually s udden, morbidity reaching 100% within 24-48 hours. **Clinical signs** include conjunctivitis, sneezing and coughing. Mortality may vary, but can be extremely high.

Genus : Brucella

Brucellosis

The discovery a nd identification o f brucella o rganisms were i mportant steps in t he development o f knowledge c oncerning the complex disease o f humans and animals, n ow k nown as "brucellosis". *Brucella melitensis,* t he first member of t he genus to be r ecognized, was i solated in 1 887 from the spleen of patients who died from **"Mediterranean fever", "gastric fever",** or **"Bruce's septicaemia",** later called **"Malta fever"** by **Sir David Bruce,** a Brit-ish a rmy surgeon. T he genus **"Brucella"** and t he d isease **"brucellosis"** a re named after him. In 1905, the infection was traced to **goat's milk.** Even today milk of goat is the most common source of the organism, although it has been isolated from the milk of infected cattle and from aborted foetuses of sheep.

A **second step forward** ten years later, in 1897, was isolation and identification of *Brucella abortus* from aborted bovine foetuses and foetal membranes by the Danish veterinarian **Frederick Bang**. The infection of cattle caused by *B. abortus* has since been known as **"Bang's disease"** or **"Bang's abortion disease"**. Later on it became known that the causative organism was ubiquitous (present everywhere), and that natural infections occur not only in **cattle**, but also in **humans, horses, sheep, dogs,** and **fowl. One important source of infection for human is cow's milk**. However, contact with aborted bovine foetuses or slaughtered cattle has also produced the disease. The characteristic undulating or recurrent fever usually seen in the human disease has given rise to the name **"undulant fever"** (undulant = rising and falling like waves; L. unda = wave). **Brucellosis is widely prevalent in cattle in our country**.

The third organism was identified in 1914 by Traum **in aborted pig foetuses**. This organism, *Brucella suis*, also infects **humans**, and has been isolated from naturally infected **horses, cattle, pigs, dogs,** and **fowls**. The disease in humans, usually acquired from contact with pigs, does not differ much from brucellosis caused by *B. abortus*, except that it tends to be more severe and persistent.

The remaining two pathogenic **Brucella** species were more recently identified: *Brucella ovis*, as the cause of **epididymitis in rams** in the 1950s; and *Brucella canis*, as the cause of **abortion in dogs** in the 1960s.

Brucella are small, **Gram-negative**, bacillary (rod-like) organisms, varying from 0.4-3.0 μm in length and 0.4-0.8 μm in width. Coccoid (spherical) forms outnumber rod forms under some culture conditions. The three species, *B. melitensis*, *B. abortus* and *B. suis*, are similar in morphological and other characteristics, but can be differentiated by bacteriological methods. Some bacteriologists, however, think that each of these is only a strain of the same species.

Pathogenesis

After entry, organisms first localize in regional lymph nodes, where they proliferate within reticulo-endothelial cells. **Most infections are acquired by ingestion**. The organisms enter and travel through the intestinal epithelial cells overlying Peyer's patches by endocytosis. Then they enter into the lymphatics. Development of **bacteraemia** allows localization of the bacteria in a variety of tissues. Bacteria have a particular affinity for male and female reproductive organs, placenta, foetus, and mammary glands. The organisms may also localize in other organs, such as lymph nodes, spleen, liver, joints, and bones, resulting in different clinical signs. **At all sites, brucella organ-**

isms proliferate intracellularly. The affinity of brucella for placenta and foetus, particularly for chorio-allantoic trophoblasts, is due to the presence of erythritol in these tissues. This sugar also promotes growth of brucella organisms *in vitro*. It is the striking proliferation of brucella in trophoblasts which causes placentitis, infection of the foetus, and abortion, which characterize brucellosis in animals. Usually, infections with brucella are chronic, or persistent, often without clinical signs.

Although readily phagocytosed by macrophages, *B. abortus* is resistant to intracellular destruction. It can survive and multiply inside normal macrophages. This is because *B. abortus* has a resistant cell wall, and can prevent lysosomes from fusing with the phagosome. That is, it blocks phagosome-lysosome fusion. Thus, the bacteria are never exposed to lysosomal enzymes. The lysosomes remain distributed in the cytoplasm and bacteria continue to grow within phagosome inside the macrophages. As a result, antibodies are ineffective against these organisms, and the bacteria are distributed throughout the body inside macrophages. The macrophages ultimately rupture as a result of the expanding physical bulk of the growing bacteria. Protection against this type of infection develops as a result of macrophage activation following stimulation of Th1 helper cells. This activation is caused by the Th1 cytokines - interferon-gamma and interleukin-2. Interferon-gamma is the most potent macrophage-activating agent.

Signs

Brucellosis in cattle is usually caused by *B. abortus*. However, cattle can be infected with *B. melitensis* and *B. suis*. *B. abortus* may also infect sheep, dogs, horses, and humans. The infection in cattle is of worldwide distribution. It is usually spread by contact, and ingestion of infective uterine discharge, aborted foetus, or placenta. The organism is also excreted in milk. Transmission through coitus is rare. Bulls are relatively resistant to infection. Prepubertal animals (i.e., before puberty) are susceptible, but most eliminate the organism, and only a few become persistently infected. In cows exposed after puberty, a persistent infection and disease is the usual outcome. The main clinical sign is abortion between the seventh and eighth months of gestation.

Brucellosis in pigs is usually caused by *B. suis*. However, pigs can be infected with *B. abortus* and *B. melitensis*. *B. suis* may also infect dogs, horses, and humans. Transmission is typically through coitus. Infected sows abort between the second and third months of gestation. Orchitis occurs in infected boars. Localization in other tissues, particularly the skeleton, is much more common in pigs than in other species.

Brucellosis in sheep and goats is caused by *B. melitensis*, and is widely prevalent in India. It is characterized by late abortion, and sometimes, orchitis in male goats. Transmission is similar to that of *B. abortus* in cattle. Sheep and goats are also susceptible to *B. abortus*, and *B. melitensis* can infect pigs, dogs, and humans. *B. ovis* naturally infects only sheep. Infection leads to epididymitis in rams and abortion in ewes.

Canine brucellosis is caused by *B. canis*. It is transmitted both by exposure to uterine discharges or aborted foetuses, or by coitus. The infection in bitches leads to abortion, usually after 50 days of gestation; and in male dogs to orchitis and epididymitis. *B. abortus*, *B. melitensis*, and *B. suis* can infect dogs. Infection of **humans** with *B. canis* has been reported.

Brucellosis in horses is caused by *B. abortus* along with *Actinomyces bovis*. It is associated with **"poll-evil"** and **"fistulous withers"**, disorders initiated by *Onchocerca cervicalis*.

Lesions

Lesions of brucellosis in animals are as varied as the clinical manifestations. As mentioned, after the onset of bacteraemia, organisms localize in a variety of tissues. These differ somewhat according to animal species, and species of brucella. In the tissues, particularly the lymphoreticular system, the organisms attract macrophages and proliferate within them, producing **small granulomas**. Macrophages may take on the appearance of epithelioid cells, and become surrounded by lymphocytes. **As the granuloma grows, caseous necrosis occurs in the centre**, and a large number of organisms enter the lesions. Fibrous connective tissue is then laid down at the periphery. Usually, multinucleated giant cells are not part of the lesion. These granulomas are visible grossly, or may be of microscopic size. **This process is the classical lesion of brucellosis.** However, it is not always present, except **in B. suis infection**, where **granulomas are the rule in all tissues**. Also, granuloma formation is usually not the lesion in the placenta associated with abortion, except again for *B. suis*. **Abortion is the most serious outcome of brucellosis in most domestic animals.**

In the bovine placenta, there is extensive proliferation of B. abortus in the chorionic epithelium and trophoblasts. This leads to necrosis of cotyledons. The inter-cotyledonary chorion is oedematous and becomes filled with an odourless, sticky, brownish exudate. As the disease advances, yellowish granular necrotic areas become clearly visible in the cotyledons. Rest of the chorion is opaque and thickened, with a leathery consistency. **Microscopically**, many organisms can be demonstrated in the chorionic epithelial cells. There is necrosis and inflammatory exudate, containing both macrophages and neutrophils. Granulomas are not seen in placenta, although small collections of epithelioid cells may be present in the endometrium. Similar lesions are seen in sheep and goats affected with *B. melitensis*. Similar lesions may also be caused by *B. ovis*, but this organism is mostly associated with epididymitis. **In contrast, lesions caused by B. suis in pigs are typical granulomas.** The aborted bovine foetus is oedematous, with serosanguineous fluid in the body cavities. The most characteristic lesion is bronchopneumonia, which is mainly characterized by a mononuclear infiltrate, with less number of neutrophils. Foetal lymph nodes are hyperplastic, and thymus smaller than normal.

The bovine mammary gland and the supramammary lymph nodes are common sites of localization of *B. abortus*. This results in **induration** (hardening). **Microscopically,** there is diffuse inflammation. Lymphocytes and neutrophils predominate. Collections of epithelioid cells and occasional Langhans' giant cells are present in some areas. As the disease progresses, there is atrophy of the glandular tissue and fibrosis. The epididymis and testicle of the bull sometimes show lesions caused by localization of *B. abortus*. The scrotum becomes enlarged and indurated. This can be detected in the living animal. In some cases, necrosis of the contents of the sac formed by the tunica may result in suppuration, rupture, and discharge of the contents. *B. abortus* can usually be recovered in pure culture, from the affected scrotal contents.

In pigs, *B. suis* usually produces lesions in the **uterus**. However, the infection is also often generalized with localization in many organs, including bone, mammary glands, testicles, epididymis, seminal vesicles, lymph nodes, spleen, liver, kidneys, and brain. **Grossly,** the affected organs show tiny white to yellowish nodules. **Microscopically, these are typical brucella granulomas with necrosis,** containing some neutrophils in their centres.

In rams, *B. ovis* infection typically **involves tail of the epididymis**. The lesions begin as perivascular oedema and lymphocytic infiltration. This is followed by hyperplasia and degeneration of the tubular epithelium and intertubular fibrosis. Escape of spermatozoa from damaged tubules produces a granulomatous response. This is responsible for the major changes in the epididymis. Primary changes do not occur in the testicle. However, stasis results in secondary testicular degeneration. The disease closely resembles infection caused by *Actinobacillus seminis* in rams. Lesions caused by *B. melitensis* infection of sheep and goats resemble those of *B. abortus* infection in cows.

B.canis infection **in the bitch** is accompanied by **uterine and placental lesions** similar to bovine brucellosis. Bronchopneumonia is seen in aborted pups. Lesions include hyperplasia and plasmacytosis (increased number of plasma cells) of lymph nodes, orchitis, epididymitis, prostatitis, and hyaline thickening of glomerular tufts. *B. canis* is also associated with osteomyelitis in dogs, as are *B. suis* and *B. abortus*. **Dogs** have been suspected **as sources of human infection** with both *B. canis* and *B. suis*.

In horses, *B. abortus* has been isolated from necrotizing and purulent lesions involving **ligamentum nuchae**. These lesions occur near the occipital attachment of the ligamentum nuchae. The name **"poll-evil"** indicates some of its c linical c haracteristics. I n the r egion of t he t horacic attachment of the ligametum nuchae, s imilar necrotizing a nd purulent l esions are called as "**fistulous withers**".

B. abortus infection is sometimes reported in **dogs**. Lesions include arthritis, orchitis, epididymitis, and abortion.

Diagnosis

Precise diagnosis of brucellosis is often difficult, both in humans and animals. Isolation of the organism is the most reliable method. An agglutination test can be used to detect antibodies. Immunological staining, or the use of molecular probes, are precise techniques w hich can be used to detect the presence of organisms in tissues.

Genus : Campylobacter (Vibrio)

The genus C ampylobacter contains s everal pathogenic b acteria, w hich were previously classified in the genus **Vibrio**. The name "**Campylobacter**" is derived f rom the **Greek word for "curved rod",** because of the c urved, spiral, or S-shaped morphology of these bacteria. Campylobacter are slender, **spirally curved, motile, Gram-negative rods**. They cause i nfections of t he genital tract, resulting in abortion and infections of the gastrointestinal tract (**Table 20**). T he o rganisms invade a nd p roliferate **within epithelial cells,** chorionic epithelium , or g astrointestinal tract e pithelium. **They cause cell death, or by some unknown mechanism, proliferation.** O rganisms can b e seen with s pecial staining t echniques, immunofluorescence a nd by electron microscopy, as slightly curved (comma-shaped) organisms **within epithelial cells** of affected tissues. Campylobacter also produce an **enterotoxin** similar in a ction to t hat o f **V ibrio cholerae**, w hich causes increased s ecretion and profuse d iarrhoea.

Table 20. Diseases caused by Campylobacter species

Species	Hosts and diseases
C. foetus subsp. *venerealis*	Endometritis, sterility, abortion in cattle
C. foetus subsp. *foetus*	Abortion in sheep (sometimes in cattle); possible cause of enteritis in sheep, cattle, pigs
C. jejuni (*C. foetus* subsp. *jejuni*)	Abortion i n sheep; e nteritis in h umans, monkeys, cattle, foals, dogs, c ats, and **fowl**
C. coli	Enteritis i n humans, m onkeys, and o ther animals. Also **fowl**
C. sputorum subsp. *bubulus*	Commensal of female genital tract of cattle and sheep

C. sputorum subsp. *mucosalis*	Swine proliferative ileitis; adenomatosis in pigs
C. upsaliensis	Probable cause of enteritis in dogs, cats, and humans
C. pylori (Helicobacter pylori)	Gastritis in children and monkeys

Campylobacter foetus subsp. venerealis

This organism (previously known as *Vibrio foetus* var. *venerealis*) causes a **specific venereal disease in cattle**. It is spread either by coitus, or through artificial insemination. **Infection of bulls is not associated with any lesion or disease.** In bulls the infection is eliminated spontaneously, but some bulls carry the organism for long periods. **Infection in cows is characterized mainly by temporary infertility and prolonged oestrus cycles.** The cow is infected during breeding, and although fertilizatin and implantation are normal, *C. foetus* subsp. *venerealis*, which has a marked tropism for chorionic epithelium, soon kills the embryo and produces endometritis. **Neither death of the embryo nor endometritis are manifested by clinical signs.** Endometritis may prevent conception at succeeding oestrus periods. Recovered cows are usually resistant to reinfection. Sometimes, the organisms may also cause **abortions,** usually between 4 and 7 months of gestation.

Pathogenesis

The main immunoglobulin in cervico-vaginal mucus is IgA, and within uterus it is IgG. When *C. foetus* subsp. **venerealis** infects the genital tract, vaginal IgA antibodies immobilize and agglutinate the organisms. If the mucous membrane becomes inflamed, IgG antibodies derived by transudation from serum also help in protection. However, *C. foetus* subsp. venerealis shows **cyclical antigenic variation.** As a result, destruction of most of this bacterial population by the local immune response leaves a **residual population of bacteria that possess new and different epitopes.** This residual population multiplies and is largely eliminated by a second immune response, **leaving a residual population of a third antigenic type.** This process may be repeated over a long period, **resulting in a persistent infection.**

Lesions

Lesions in cattle are usually not clearly noticeable. Lesions have been described as a **subacute, diffuse mucopurulent endometritis.** The uterine mucosa is infiltrated with lymphocytes, often in the form of small nodules. Similar infiltrates are found in the cervix and vagina. When abortion occurs, the foetus and placenta are autolyzed as a result of intrauterine death.

Diagnosis

Diagnosis m ay be p ossible from h erd h istory, b ut the d isease must be differentiated from **trichomoniasis**. Campylobacter species are visible in tissue sections of the placenta, and can be identified with immunological staining t echniques.

Campylobacter foetus **subsp.** *foetus*

Also known as *Vibrio foetus* var. *intestinalis*, this organism infects **sheep**. However, i n contrast t he subspecies *v enerealis* infection i n cattle, **is not a venereal disease** and is **characterized by abortion**. Infection is acquired by the **oral route**. The ram does not play a role in transmission. **Birds** are capable of carrying t he organism, c ontributing to its spread. **I n ewes**, t he o rganism localizes in the pregnant uterus, and after a brief bacteraemia, results in late abortion, stillbirth, o r birth o f weak l ambs. T hese u sually die a fter birth. Immunity follows abortion.

Cattle a re also s usceptible to *C. foetus* subsp. *f oetus* and l ate a bortion may occur, b ut incidence i s far l ess than it is i n sheep. T he organism a lso causes abortion in horses, and enteritis in cattle, sheep, pigs and horses, similar to that caused by *C. jejuni*. In sheep, *C. jejuni* also causes abortion with lesions similar to those caused by *C. foetus* subsp. *foetus*.

Lesions

Lesions are usually found in the placenta, but may also occur in the foetus. **The bacteria first localize in the placentomes**. This results in vascular change and thrombosis of small vessels, causing separation of the chorion with formation of h aematomas. S ubsequent invasion o f the c horion and c horionic capillaries leads to necrosis at this site, and invasion of the foetus. **Both hypoxia from placental damage and foetal invasion contribute to foetal death**. The placenta, p articularly the c otyledons, are oedematous and i nfiltrated with neutrophils and mononuclear cells and contain foci of necrosis. The foetus is oedematous a nd often macerated. In s ome, s pecific l esions i n t he f orm of focal, diffuse, n ecrotizing hepatitis a re seen g rossly as m ultiple grey foci. Diagnosis can be made by finding and identifying the organisms in the placenta or foetus.

Campylobacter jejuni

Also known as *C. foetus* subsp. *jejuni* or *Vibrio jejuni*, **this organism is a normal inhabitant of the intestinal tract of cattle, sheep, goats, dogs, cats, and many species of birds.** *C. jejuni* and other campylobacters (*C. laridis*, *C. upsaliensis*, a nd others) have emerged recently as an important cause o f **enteritis and diarrhoea in humans, dogs, cats, cattle, foals, and monkeys**, either as a primary pathogen, or in association with enteric viruses.

Lesions

Usually, **the lesions are not specific**. They consist of stunting and fusion of villi, dilation of crypts and crypt abscesses, mild cellular infiltration of the mucosa, and sometimes ulceration and haemorrhage. **Lesions tend to be most severe in the proximal small intestine**, but can affect the entire small intestine and colon. With silver stains, comma-shaped organisms can be seen on the surface of epithelial cells and within the lamina propria. *C. jejuni* **can grow readily within macrophages**.

C. jejuni also causes late abortion and stillbirths in **sheep** and **goats**. This must be differentiated from that caused by *C. foetus* subsp. *foetus*. *C. jejuni* may also cause mastitis in cattle.

Campylobacter sputorum subsp. *mucosalis,* and *Campylobacter hyointestinalis*

These organisms cause **"swine proliferative ileitis syndrome"** in pigs. Campylobacters are found within the cytoplasm of crypt and glandular epithelial cells. The proliferative lesions begin in, and mainly involve the epithelium of crypts and glands. Hyperplasia results in crowding of cells and development of a pseudostratified appearance. Villi overlying such areas become shortened (atrophic) and fused. Crypts contain neutrophils and mononuclear cells, and there is extensive mononuclear inflammation in the mucosa and submucosa.

Campylobacter coli

This organism may cause **enteritis** in **humans** and **animals**, but it does not appear to be an important pathogen.

Campylobacter pylori

Also known as *Helicobacter pylori*, this organism is now recognized as a cause of **gastritis** in **humans**. It is also important in the pathogenesis of **peptic ulcer**, and has a strong association with an increased risk for **gastric carcinoma**.

Zoonotic Importance

In humans, infection with *C. jejuni*, *C. laridis*, and *C. upsaliensis* can be a **zoonosis**. It may be acquired from dogs, cats, sheep, birds, and other infected animals. *C. jejuni* has emerged in recent years as a major cause of **enterocolitis** (inflammation of intestines and colon) **in humans**.

Avian Campylobacteriosis

The **three main pathogenic species** of campylobacters in poultry are *C. jejuni*, *C. coli*, and *C. laridis*. All three species can be isolated from poultry, **but the main pathogenic species is** *C. jejuni*. Campylobacters are found in the intestinal tracts of a wide variety of animals and birds often without causing disease. Except *C. foetus*, they are not major pathogens. Their main significance lies in the ability of infected animals and birds **to serve as reservoirs of infection for human disease.**

Infection occurs mainly **in broiler breeder flocks**, and has been found to be as high as 80%. *C. jejuni* is the most frequently isolated species from poultry. Sometimes *C. coli* and *C. laridis* are found. Flocks may be infected with more than one species of campylobacter.

Spread

Vertical transmission, by either transovarian infection or by penetration of the eggshell after oviposition (egg laying), appears unlikely, as eggs and newly hatched chicks from infected breeder flocks are found free of campylobacters, although large numbers of campylobacters (*C. jejuni*) are normally present in the avian intestinal tract. There is **horizontal spread** of infection to broilers by contact with infected birds, or indirect transmission by vectors or other vehicles. **Contaminated feed can introduce infection to young chicks. Drinking water** may also act as a vehicle of infection for growing broiler chicks. Campylobacters survive well in cold water. Insects have been shown to be carriers of *C. jejuni*. House flies can spread *C. jejuni* to chicks. Rodent droppings can be an important source of infection for flocks, especially if there are **rodents** around the poultry houses or food stores. Infection can also be spread by **movement of personnel** between broiler houses or farms. Campylobacters have been recovered from the **shoes of poultry farm workers** and surface water near poultry houses.

Pathogenesis

The mechanisms by which these bacteria cause disease are unknown. However, **virulence** has been associated with **cytotoxin** or **enterotoxin production, adhesion and invasion, flagella and motility.**

Signs

There is no recognized clinical syndrome in poultry flocks attributed to infection with these bacteria. The clinical signs are usually confined to depression and diarrhoea. The severity of these signs depends on infective dose, strain of *C. jejuni* or *C. coli*, and age of the host. The purpose of controlling infection in poultry **is to reduce the potential for food-borne spread of the bacteria to humans.**

Gross Lesions

The main change with *C. jejuni* in chicks is **distension of the intestinal tract**. There is accumulation of mucus and watery fluid, and depending on the cytotoxic properties of the campylobacter involved, haemorrhages may be present. Newly hatched chicks may show the presence of red or yellow mottling of liver parenchyma.

Microscopic Lesions

Microscopic changes caused by *C. jejuni* include congestion and mononuclear cell infiltration of the lamina propria, and **destruction of mucosal cells in the entire intestinal tract**. Oedema of the mucosa is seen in the ileum and caeca.

Poultry Processing

Campylobacters are commonly found in birds at slaughter. Caeca and intestines of infected birds have been shown to contain very large numbers of bacteria. The organism appears to survive the processing operation and procedures such as scalding, plucking and evisceration, and immersion chilling. **Surveys have shown that more than 50% of chicken carcasses are contaminated.**

Public Health Significance

Human campylobacteriosis is a food-borne condition of emerging significance. In UK, campylobacters have become the most frequently involved cause of **human gastroenteritis.** All species are involved, but *C. jejuni* is by far the most important and is isolated from 98% of cases. There is no evidence that campylobacteriosis in humans is due to the consumption of eggs. **Consumption or handling of table chicken,** on the other hand, **has been identified as a major source of campylobacter infection for humans.** Highest rates of infection are in **children and young adults,** particularly **males.** The staff of poultry processing plants are exposed to campylobacteriosis by handling contaminated material, and the condition can be regarded as an **occupational disease**.

Most human cases are sporadic, and large outbreaks are relatively rare. Illness occurs 2-10 days after exposure, and the **symptoms** are watery diarrhoea accompanied by nausea, abdominal pain, and sometimes fever. The enteritis does not usually require antibiotic therapy as the **disease is self-limiting,** lasting about 5 days. Complications are uncommon, but can be serious and even fatal. It is mainly in the form of a post-infectious neurological disorder. **In developing countries,** although human infection is hyper-endemic, clinical illness in adults (unlike developed countries) is rare. **This is due to the early development of immunity by children persistently exposed to multiple strains of infection.**

The exact role which the infected animals and birds play in the human disease is not clearly defined. **However, the majority of infections are food-borne and that poultry are the major source of infection.** *C. jejuni* isolation rates in broiler farms and poultry processing plants have been found high. Case-control studies in the human population have blamed at least half of all cases **to the consumption, or handling of chicken.** Despite various control measures, incidence of human enteritis continues to be high. This is due to a combination of factors, and include the high numbers of organisms present on raw chicken, the **low infective dose**, and cross-contamination during food preparation to utensils or foods, which are afterwards not cooked. **It has been shown that a small drop of raw chicken juice can be sufficient to provide an infective dose for humans.**

However, there are also less important sources of human infection. These include red meats (beef, mutton, lamb), unpasteurized milk, or contamination of milk delivered to the doorstep by wild birds pecking through the bottle tops, contaminated water, and direct contact with infected animals, especially domestic pets.

Diagnosis

Campylobacters can be isolated from faeces, and caecal and jejunal contents. Since the main site of colonization in the bird is the caeca, the caecal contents are the diagnostic sample of choice. However, **faecal samples are also suitable as infected birds shed large numbers of campylobacters in their faeces.** Isolation requires incubation of cultures for 48-72 hours at 43^0 C in a microaerobic atmosphere. Selective media are required to suppress the growth of faecal and other samples. A solid selective medium, containing antibiotics to inhibit unwanted organisms, is used routinely for isolation.

Direct examination in smears is not used routinely because it lacks sensitivity. However, molecular techniques such as **polymerase chain reaction-based restriction fragment length polymorphism (PCR-RFLP) analysis of flagellar genes** are currently in development, and may prove useful for rapid detection and typing purposes in future. Latex agglutination kits are also available but are only to be used for confirmation purposes.

Genus : Escherichia

Genus **Escherichia** is composed of several species, but only *Escherichia coli* is an important pathogen of animals, causing **colibacillosis**. Members of the genus **Escherichia** are **Gram-negative, flagellated rods** 2-3 μm in length and 0.6 μm wide.

Colibacillosis

Colibacillosis is caused by *E. coli*. **The species is the normal inhabitant of the digestive tract of mammals and birds,** and most strains are not pathogenic. There are **hundreds of serotypes of *E. coli*.** These are classified on the basis of various surface antigens (see **Fig. 9, page 233**), which are: 1. **O (somatic) antigen.** The O antigen is the **endotoxin** liberated following lysis of smooth cells. 2. **K (capsular) antigen.** These are polymeric acids. They are associated with virulence, and are present on the surface of the cell. 3. **H** (flagellar) antigen. These are not associated with pathogenicity. 4. F (fimbrial or pilus) antigen. F antigens are involved in attachment to cells.

Only a few *E. coli*, however, are true pathogens. These are mainly associated with enteric disease, and are referred to as "enteropathogenic", "enterotoxigenic" or "enterotoxic" *E. coli*. They are important causes of diarrhoea in humans, pigs, cattle, sheep, horses, and probably other species. *E. coli* also causes oedema disease of swine, which results from production of a toxin which is absorbed into the bloodstream (enterotoxaemic *E. coli*). Other strains are responsible for septicaemia, especially in calves. *E. coli* are also usually associated with septic infections, such as inflammation of the lower urinary tract, pyelonephritis, infected wounds, pneumonia, peritonitis, mastitis, and meningitis. In these conditions, *E. coli* is considered to be an opportunistic pathogen, rather than a primary pathogen.

Pathogenesis

The walls of *E. coli* (i.e., of Gram-negative bacteria) consist of lipopolysaccharide (endotoxin). Most of the biological activity of lipopolysaccharide, including the production of fever, come from lipid A and the core sugars, and are mediated through the production of host cytokines, including tumour necrosis factor (TNF) and interleukin-1 (IL-1) (see 'bacterial endotoxins' under General Considerations). *E. coli* also secretes molecules that depress phagocytosis by neutrophils.

E coli also secretes an enterotoxin, which is an ADP-ribosyltransferase. The enzyme generates excess cyclic adenosine monophosphate (cAMP), which causes intestinal epithelial cells to secrete isosmotic fluid, resulting in diarrhoea and loss of water and electrolytes.

Fimbriae or pili present on the surface of *E. coli* are non-flagellar filamentous structures (see Fig. 9, page 233). At the tips of the pili are minor protein components that determine to which host cells the bacteria will attach ("bacterial tropism"). In *E. coli*, these minor proteins are antigenically different and are associated with particular infections. For example, type I proteins bind mannose and cause urinary tract infections, type P proteins bind galactose and cause pyelonephritis, and type S proteins bind sialic acid and cause meningitis. A single bacterium can express more than one type of pili as well as non-pilar adhesins.

Enteric Colibacillosis

Three distinct pathogenetic mechanisms have been identified with the enteropathogenic *E. coli*: 1. Enterotoxic (enterotoxigenic) colibacillosis, 2. Enteroinvasive colibacillosis, and 3. Enteroadherent colibacillosis.

Enterotoxic (Enterotoxigenic) Colibacillosis

Also k nown as "**enterotoxigenic diarrhoea**", t his i s the m ost c ommon form of colibacillosis in domestic animals. This disease results from: 1. Colonization of *E. coli* on t he surface o f e nterocytes (intestinal cells) , and 2. Production of toxins. **The ability to adhere to mucosal cells is a special quality of these pathogens**, and is due to the characteristic antigens present on the surface of these *E. Coli*, known as "**fimbrial or pilus" antigens. These antigens bind to ganglioside receptors on enterocytes.**

Two classes of toxins are produced by enterotoxigenic strains of *E. coli*: 1. **Heat-labile e nterotoxin** or **labile t oxin (LT)**, and 2. **Heat-stable enterotoxin** or **stable toxin (ST)**. The heat-labile enterotoxin acts in a manner similar to cholera toxin (of *Vibrio cholerae*) by activating enzyme **adenylate cyclase (Fig. 10)**. Activation of a denylate c yclase l eads to **a n increase in intracellular cyclic-AMP**, which causes a marked increase in cellular secretion from intestinal cells.

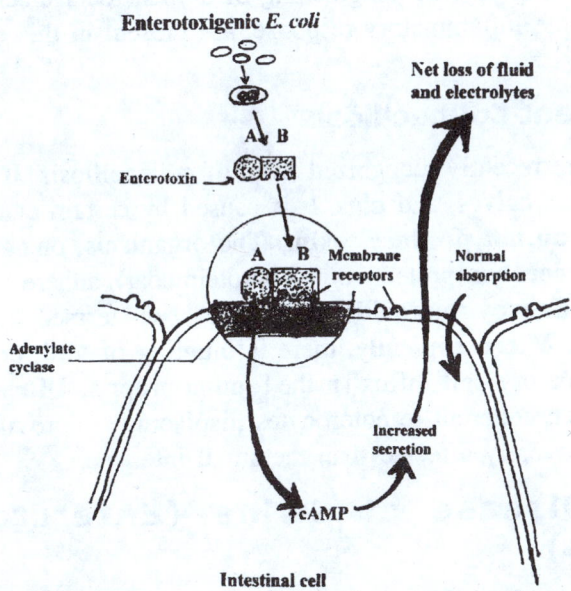

Fig. 10. Mechanism of action of **heat-labile enterotoxin of *E. coli*** in its induction of increased secretory activity.

This results in **diarrhoea**. The **action of LT** is of relatively **slow onset and long duration**. On the other hand, **action of ST** is **more rapid and of shorter duration than that of LT**. ST specifically activates particulate **enzyme guanylate cyclase**. It also induces fluid loss and diarrhoea. **Two types of ST** have been identified: **STa** and **STb**. A lthough there m ay be villous atrophy, lesions i n both forms of enterotoxic colibacillosis are minimal to absent. This is helpful in differentiating the disease from several enteric viral diseases, such as those caused by rotaviruses and coronaviruses. **This form of colibacillosis is most common in young piglets, calves, and lambs during the first week of life**. A condition known as post-weaning enteritis ("**post-weaning diarrhoea**") of **piglets** is also caused by toxigenic *E. coli*. This condition is usually seen in association with oedema disease.

Enteroinvasive Colibacillosis

This is mainly a disease of **humans**. However, there are a few examples of enteroinvasive colibacillosis in **pigs** and **cattle**. This form of colibacillosis is similar to **shigellosis** or **salmonellosis**. The organisms penetrate enterocytes, penetrate the lamina propria, and may extend to mesenteric lymph nodes and further. The enteropathogenic (enterotoxic) *E. coli* responsible also produce a **toxin** which **inhibits protein synthesis**. This leads to **necrosis of enterocytes**, usually in the **colon**. The toxin has been called "**shiga-like toxin or SLT**" (**Vero toxin**). In contrast to enterotoxic colibacillosis, microscopic lesions consisting of blunting of villi, lengthening of crypts, focal ulceration, and an accompanying acute inflammatory response, are present in this enteroinvasive form.

Enteroadherent Colibacillosis

This is a more recently recognized form of colibacillosis. It has been described in **humans, calves**, and **pigs**. It is caused by certain enteropathogenic serotypes **which do not produce toxins**. The organisms, on the other hand, **penetrate the glycocalyx** (protective glycoprotein coat), adhere to the mucosal cell surface, and **destroy microvilli**. They have been termed "**attaching and effacing**" *E. coli*. Microscopically, there is blunting of villi, crypt hypertrophy, and inflammatory cell influx in the lamina propria. **Ultrastructurally**, organisms are seen adherent to enterocytes displacing microvilli. The colon is usually more severely affected than the small intestine.

Oedema Disease of Swine (Enterotoxaemic Colibacillosis)

The disease attacks previously healthy pigs without warning. The course is short, and characterized by incoordination and paralysis of limbs, coma, and often diarrhoea, causing death within a number of hours, or a day or two. The disease is not contagious, but morbidity may approach 35%, **and mortality may reach 100%**.

The **pathogenesis** is not entirely clear. However, the disease appears to result from production of a toxin by certain strains of *E. coli*, which adhere to and colonize in the intestinal mucosa. The mechanism by which organisms adhere is not established. However, **it is not dependent on fimbrial antigens**.

The toxin, referred to as "**oedema disease toxin**" (Shiga-like toxin II), **is absorbed into the circulation** and acts on small arteries and arterioles. It causes a **necrotizing arteritis**, characterized by swelling and proliferation of endothelium, and necrosis and hyalinization of the media, resulting in non-inflammatory oedema. Necrotizing arteritis can be found in almost all organs of the body, including the brain.

The oedema is usually found in the wall of the stomach. The thickness of the stomach wall may be increased to 3 cm. The **coiled portion of the colon is another common site of oedema.** The body cavities usually contain varying amounts of fluid. The organs of the abdomen usually appear normal.

Septicaemic Colibacillosis (Colisepticaemic Form)

In this form of colibacillosis, the organisms invade host through the oral cavity, respiratory system, pharynx, or umbilicus. They produce an **endotoxin** which causes the lesions. Unless the enterotoxic form occurs simultaneously, the **bacteria do not reach the small intestine. Thus, diarrhoea or intestinal lesions do not occur.** This form has been best described in young calves. Calves which are **deficient in immunoglobulin** (as a result of failure to receive colostrum) are **most susceptible.**

The **signs** and **lesions** are those of bacterial arthritis, polyserositis (pericarditis, pleuritis, and peritonitis are collectively referred to as "**polyserositis**"), meningitis, ophthalmitis, and pyelonephritis, with bacterial emboli and necrotizing, purulent, or fibrinous exudate.

Summary

Thus, different strains of *E. coli* have the ability, under certain conditions of the host, to produce pathological manifestations **involving at least five pathogenetic mechanisms, discussed above.** It is possible that future research may change these concepts, or strengthen them by elucidating certain hitherto unknown mechanisms.

Avian Colibacillosis

As described, *Escherichia coli* **is a normal inhabitant of the digestive tract of mammals and birds, and most strains are non-pathogenic. Certain serotypes, however, can cause disease in poultry.** Colisepticaemia, egg peritonitis, yolk sac infection, and coligranuloma (**Hjarre's disease**) are the well-recognized results of *E. coli* infection. These conditions are collectively grouped under the heading "**colibacillosis**".

Colisepticaemia

The disease is usually seen in **young chickens. It is the most serious form of colibacillosis.** Coccidiosis, viral infections, Ranikhet disease or infectious bronchitis **even in live vaccine form**, infectious bursal disease (IBD), *Mycoplasma gallisepticum* infection, and nutritional deficiencies, all predispose the bird to the disease.

Spread

E.coli **persist for long periods outside the bird's body in dry, dusty conditions. Faecal contamination of the eggs** may result in the penetration of *E. coli* through the shell, and is considered to be **the most important source of infection.** Other sources may be **ovarian infection or salpingitis. It has been estimated that between 0.5-6% of eggs from normal hens may contain the organism.** *E. coli* may spread to other chickens during hatch, and is often associated with high mortality rates, or it may give rise to **yolk sac infections.**

Coliform bacteria can be found in the **litter, dust,** and **faecal matter. Feed is often contaminated. Rodent droppings** usually contain pathogenic coliforms. Pathogenic serotypes can also be introduced into the poultry flocks through **contaminated well water.**

Pathogenesis

E. coli **are always found in the digestive tracts of poultry,** particularly in large numbers in the lower part of the small intestine and caeca. The serotypes which cause septicaemia are also likely to be found in the throat and upper trachea. However, healthy birds with intact defences are remarkably resistant to naturally occurring *E. coli*. **The infection occurs when pathogenic *E. coli* invade the bird's body from the respiratory tract when mucosal barriers are compromised** (i.e., damaged from viral, bacterial, or parasitic infections; toxins; ammonia fumes; poor ventilation, nutritional deficiencies, immunosuppression, contaminated water, overcrowding, dry dusty conditions, feed/water restriction, poor litter condition, temperature extremes). **Mycoplasmal infection increases susceptibility to *E. coli*.** Exposure to dust and ammonia results in **deciliation** (removal of cilia) of the upper respiratory tract, permitting inhaled *E. coli* to colonize and and cause respiratory infection. The resulting disease is commonly called **"airsac disease"** or **"chronic respiratory disease (CRD)".**

Signs

Birds between 4 and 12 weeks of age are usually affected, and the first sign is **a drop in food consumption.** The birds then appear listless, stand dejectedly with ruffled feathers, develop **laboured breathing,** and **a characteristic "snicking"** (i.e., making short sharp sound). Morbidity and mortality vary. Losses are usually less than 5%, **but morbidity can be over 50%.**

Lesions

The gross lesions are characteristic, and include **airsacculitis, peritoni-**

tis, p erihepatitis, and p ericarditis. B esides these l esions, p neumonia and **pleuropneumonia** are also usually present. Less commonly, **salpingitis** may occur following sepsis. When the **left abdominal airsac** is infected by *E. coli*, females may d evelop **chronic salpingitis** characterized b y a l arge c aseous **mass** in a dilated, thin-walled oviduct. Size of the caseous mass may increase with time. Infection of the peritoneal cavity (**peritonitis**) is characterized by acute mortality, fibrin, and free yolk. Infection occurs when bacteria ascending through the oviduct grow rapidly in yolk material that has been deposited in the peritoneal cavity. Salpingitis can also occur from an **ascending infection from the cloaca**. The carcass is septicaemic. Liver, spleen, lungs and kidneys are d ark and c ongested. The **a irsacs** are t hickened, o paque and w hite w ith **caseous deposits**. A **fibrinous pericarditis**, with the pericardial sac thickened, **white and adhering** to the surface of the heart, is **a characteristic finding**. The **surface of the liver is usually covered by a thin layer of fibrinous material**.

Microscopically, the pseudostratified, columnar epithelium of the trachea is replaced by immature non-ciliated cells. Changes in airsacs consist of oedema and heterophil infiltration. Later, there is fi broblast proliferation and **accumulation of vast numbers of necrotic heterophils in caseous exudate**.

Diagnosis

Colisepticaemia can be diagnosed after a gross postmortem examination. However, diagnosis can be confirmed by isolation of a profuse pure growth of *E. coli* on direct culture from the heart, liver, lungs, and airsacs.

Egg Peritonitis

The term "egg peritonitis"covers a number o f reproductive disorders o f poultry. These include **peritonitis, salpingitis** (inflammation of oviduct), and **impaction of the oviduct**. Postmortem examination may reveal **egg debris, inspissated yolk, caseous material or milky fluid in the abdominal cavity**, along with i nflammation and d istortion of t he ovaries, a nd salpingitis. T he oviduct may be obstructed b y i nspissated inflammatory d ebris which m ay sometimes result in rupture of the oviduct wall. A whole or partly formed egg may b e impacted i n the o viduct. A profuse pure g rowth of *E. coli* c an b e isolated from the oviduct and caseous inspissated material.

In any flock of laying birds there will be a small number of deaths from egg peritonitis, **o ften about 1% a month**. This is usually c onsidered to be unavoidable. **However, egg peritonitis can occur as a flock problem.** Flock peritonitis outbreaks a re usually linked t o **cannibalism,** or **vent pecking. Overcrowding** and huddling lead to vent pecking and egg peritonitis.

Yolk Sac Infection

Also known as "mushy chick disease" and "omphalitis", yolk sac infection is probably the commonest cause of mortality in chicks during the first week after hatching. *E. coli* can be involved either as the primary and sole causal agent, or as a secondary opportunist. **Yolk sac infection can be associated with an inflamed navel, or bacteria can multiply in the hatching egg following faecal contamination of the shell.** Yolk sac infection can cause **100% mortality** in the first week of life, but deaths are usually between 5% and 10%. Other bacteria, such as *Bacillus cereus*, staphylococci, **Pseudomonas, Proteus,** and clostridia can also cause yolk sac infection, either on their own, or more commonly, along with *E. coli*. *E. coli* multiplies rapidly in the intestines of newly hatched chicks. Infection spreads rapidly from chick to chick in the hatchery and brooders.

Signs and Lesions

Affected chicks have **distended abdomens**, and a tendency to huddle. **Navel** may be visibly thickened, prominent, and necrotic. Postmortem examination reveals subcutaneus and yolk sac blood vessels engorged and dilated. Lungs are congested, and liver and kidneys dark and swollen. **The main finding is an inflamed unabsorbed yolk sac, yolk being abnormal in colour and consistency.** The yolk may be yellow and inspissated, or brown green and watery, and is **usually fetid (foul-smelling).** There is peritonitis with haemorrhages on the serosal surfaces of the intestines. A pure growth of non-haemolytic *E. coli* can be recovered from the abdominal viscera, and particularly from the yolk sac, on direct culture.

Coligranuloma (Hjarre's Disease)

This condition usually causes sporadic death in adult hens. **The clinical signs are non-specific.** Affected birds are usually found dead, or die after depression and loss of condition. **Postmortem examination** shows hard, yellow, **nodular granulomas in the mesentery and wall of the intestine**, particularly the **caeca.** Sometimes, the liver is similarly affected, and is hard, discoloured and swollen.

Other Clinical Conditions

E. coli is also involved in a number of other clinical conditions. These include **synovitis, arthritis, tracheitis, airsacculitis, panophthalmitis,** and **localized abscesses. This organism is a great opportunist.** However, it rarely causes disease in the field **unless there is a precipitating managemental fault, or some underlying pathogen.**

Genus: Francisella

The genus **Francisella** has been established recently to include *Francisella* *tularensis*, the cause of **tularaemia**. *F. tularensis* is a **Gram-negative** organism.

Tularaemia

Tularaemia is **a highly contagious disease mainly of wild animals**. However, it is transmissible to **farm animals**, causing a severe septicaemia and a high mortality.

The history of tularaemia began in 1910, when a bacterial organism was isolated from **"plague-like disease" of squirrels** in the Tulare County of California, USA. The organism was named *Bacterium talarense* after the Tulare County. The organism was later designated *Pasteurella tularensis*, and more recently *Francisella tularensis* . Then, there occurred an accidental infection of **laboratory workers** with this organism, and finally the natural occurrence of the **human disease** was established. A human disease in USA, known as **"deer fly fever"** was later identified as tularaemia. **Localized cutaneous ulceration and lymphadenitis** occurred after the bite of a blood-sucking fly, *Chrysops discalis*, which is responsible for spread of the disease among wild animals. Later on a more important source of **human infection** was established in **wild rabbits**. **"Rabbit fever"** of rabbits proved to be tularaemia, livers containing the organisms.

Tularaemia is most important as a disease of humans, wild rabbits and rodents. However, it may occur in **sheep, pigs, horses, dogs, monkeys,** and **in wild animals** in rhesus monkey, deer, wild boar and fox. Most mammals are susceptible. Guinea-pigs are also readily infected. **In humans,** the disease is described as **"ulcero-glandular"** when the site of entry is skin and initial lesion cutaneous; **"oculo-glandular"** when the initial entry is through the conjunctiva; or **"glandular"** when the site of entry is not clear.

Spread

The major reservoirs and transmitters of infection are rabbits, hares, wild rodents, ticks, and flies. **In sheep,** spread occurs mainly through the **bites of certain ticks.** The ticks become infected in the early part of their life cycle, when they feed on rodents. Sheep are relatively resistant to tularaemia, but become clinically affected when the infection is massive and continuous. Spread to **pigs** and **horses** is thought to occur mainly by **tick bites.**

Pathogenesis

Tularaemia is an acute septicaemia. However, localization occurs, mainly in the parenchymatous organs, with the production of **granulomatous lesions.**

Signs

In sheep, heavy tick infestation is usually present. The signs include stiffness of gait, hunching of the hindquarters, fever up to 107° F, and cough.

There is diarrhoea, the faeces being dark and fetid. Death occurs usually within a few days, but may be as long as 2 weeks. Animals which recover are solidly immune for long periods. The disease is latent in **adult pigs**, but **young piglets** show fever up to 107° F, accompanied by profuse sweating and dyspnoea. The course of the disease is about 7-10 days. **In horses,** fever up to 107° F and stiffness and oedema of the limbs occur. **Foals** are seriously affected and may also show dyspnoea and incoordination.

Lesions

In humans, the **ulcero-glandular form** is the most common. The first sign is a small, indurated, **cutaneous swelling** at the site of an insect bite, or on the fingers, or hands **after dressing wild rabbits**. The lesion becomes hot and painful, eventually filled with pus, and ulcerating. This is followed by extension to **regional lymph nodes**. These become enlarged and painful, and may also ulcerate through the skin. **General lymphadenopathy** occurs with involvement of other viscera, such as the spleen, liver, lungs, heart, and bones. This **widespread involvement usually results in death.**

In **rabbits** and **squirrels**, the disease is usually recognized by the presence of multiple, chalky, focal lesions scattered in the liver, spleen, and lymph nodes.

Microscopically, a central mass of caseous necrosis is surrounded by a zone of lymphocytes, mixed with a few neutrophils, macrophages, and sometimes, multinucleated giant cells. Thrombosis of small blood vessels is common and areas of necrosis may coalesce. **The causative organisms, being Gram-negative, are difficult to demonstrate in tissue sections.** However, they are present in large numbers, particularly in macrophages at the margin of lesions.

Zoonotic Implications

F. tularensis has remarkable invasive powers, and **infection in humans can occur through the unbroken skin.** The most common source of **infection is from the handling of infected rabbits and other wildlife.** Infections can also occur from bites of ticks and the deer fly (**Chrysops discalis**). The disease is **an occupational hazard to workers in the sheep industry** in areas where the disease occurs. Spread of the disease to humans may also occur in **abattoir workers who handle infected sheep carcasses.** The inhalation or intradermal injection of as few as 10 organisms can establish infection in humans. Proper precautions should be taken in clinical and postmortem examination of suspect cases.

Diagnosis

Diagnosis can be made on the basis of gross and microscopic lesions, isolation o f the c ausative organisms, or specific identification with f luores-cence antibody techniques. Increased agglutination antibody titre i s of diag-nostic value in non-fatal human cases.

Genus: Fusobacterium

Infection by **Fusobacterium** sp., especially *Fusobacterium necrophorum* (previously *Sphaerophorus necrophorus*) is common in **all species of farm animals**, and is referred to as **"necrobacillosis"**. In many instances the organ-ism is p resent **as a secondary invader**, rather than a s a primary c ause of disease.

Necrobacillosis

Necrobacillosis is a wide-ranging term applied to a number of lesions and disorders associated w ith *Fusobacterium necrophorum*. T his organism, a **filamentous, Gram-negative strict anaerobe**, is a commensal in the diges-tive tracts of animals and humans. Although *F. necrophorum* can be recov-ered from various l esions of a nimals, including d eer and a ntelope, there i s some doubt as to whether it is a primary pathogen. However, it does produce a v ariety of e xotoxins and e ndotoxins, w hich o nce established i n n ecrotic tissue, a llow them to cause m ore s evere n ecrosis. These i nclude **a potent endotoxin, a polysaccharide capsule, a n exotoxin (a leukocidin), and a haemolysin**.

In cattle, necrophorus organisms are found in the necrotic plaques of the larynx, pharynx, a nd trachea; t he disease c aused by t hem is r eferred to a s **"calf diphtheria"**. They h ave also been d emonstrated i n c attle which d ied from **pneumonia**. Large **foci of necrosis** also occur in the **liver** and **spleen of adult cattle**, particularly those which are heavily fed. The hepatic lesions are associated with ulcerations of the rumen.

Foot rot ("infectious pododermatitis") (G podo=foot) in **cattle** and **sheep** is always associated with *F. necrophorum*, but the exact causes of the disease are not entirely understood. I t appears t hat the disease develops only in the presence of an obligate G ram-negative anaerobe (a bacterium) of the h oof, *Bacteroides nodosus*. Progression of the disease is due to *B. nodosus*, and not due to *F. necrophorum*. The disease can be produced by experimentally in-fecting the inter-digital skin of normal animals with both organisms. *Actinomyces pyogenes* has been recovered from foot rot in cattle and sheep, and *Spirochaeta penortha* (a bacterium) from sheep foot rot.

In sheep, f oot abscesses and **"lip-and-leg ulceration"** h ave been a ttrib-uted to necrophorus infection. However, it is doubtful that this organism is the cause of these diseases in sheep.

In horses, *F. necrophorum* is associated with a necrotizing disease of the feet in animals which are forced to remain for long periods in deep manure and urine-soaked mud. This "**gangrenous dermatitis**" begins at the heel, or in the frog, and results in large, irregular areas of sharply demarcated necrosis. It usually produces serious disability.

In pigs, ulcerative, necrotizing stomatitis and enteritis have been suspected to be due to *F. necrophorum*, as also a disfiguring type of rhinitis ('**bull-nose**').

Of the various conditions caused by *F. necrophorum*, "calf diphtheria" being important, will be described further.

Calf Diphtheria

Calf diphtheria is a disease **characterized by necrotic stomatitis, laryngitis, and pharyngitis**. It is caused by *F. necrophorum*.

Spread

F. necrophorum is a common inhabitant of the environment of cattle. Under unsanitary conditions the infection can spread to dirty milk buckets and feeding troughs. **Entry in the mucosa is probably through the injuries** caused by rough feed and erupting teeth.

Pathogenesis

F. necrophorum is a **normal inhabitant of the oral cavity**, and causes inflammation and necrosis following injury of the mucosa of the oral cavity, pharynx, and larynx. *F. necrophorum* **produces a variety of endotoxins and exotoxins**. These cause extensive **coagulative necrosis** of the tissues. Oedema and inflammation of the mucosa of the larynx result in closure of the rima glottidis (elongated slit between the vocal cords) and inspiratory dyspnoea and stridor (harsh sound during respiration). **The presence of the lesion causes discomfort, painful swallowing, and toxaemia.**

Signs

A most painful cough, accompanied by **severe inspiratory dyspnoea**, salivation, **painful swallowing movements**, and complete anorexia are the characteristic signs. The temperature is high (106° F), pharyngeal region may be swollen and is painful on palpation, and there is salivation and nasal discharge. The breath has a most foul rancid smell. **Death is likely to occur from toxaemia, or obstruction to the respiratory passages**, between 2nd to 7th day. Most affected calves die without treatment. Spread to the lungs may cause a severe, supportive bronchopneumonia.

Lesions

Grossly, the lesions appear as large, raised, well-defined, plaques of yellow-grey, adherent necrotic tissue (**diphtheritic membrane**), surrounded by a zone of hyperaemia. Once the necrotic tissue sloughs, large ulcers over the granulation tissue become visible. **Microscopically,** the lesion consists of a **superficial pseudomembrane** composed of a homogeneous mass of eosinophilic, coagulated protein, surrounded by a zone of hyperaemic granulation tissue containing neutrophils, macrophages, lymphocytes, and plasma cells. The **long, filamentous organisms are found** at the interface between necrotic and viable tissue. Calves may also develop necrotic lesions in other portions of the alimentary tract.

Diagnosis

Calf diphtheria is characterized by dyspnoea and stridor (harsh sound), toxaemia and fever; and oedema, inflammation and necrotic lesions of the laryngeal mucosa. Bacteriological examination of swabs from lesions may help in confirming the diagnosis.

An enzyme-linked immunosorbent assay (ELISA) for the detection of *F. necrophorum* antibodies in the serum of cattle and sheep has been developed.

Genus: Haemophilus

Haemophilus organisms are short, **Gram-negative** bacteria. **They reside in the oropharynx or genital tract of humans and many species of animals.** Most of them are non-pathogenic, or of very limited pathogenic potential. Some of them, under appropriate conditions, are capable of causing specific and serious disease. **These are listed in Table 21.**

Pathogenesis

More is known about *H. influenzae* which causes life-threatening acute lower respiratory tract infections and meningitis in **young children.** Pili on the surface of *H. influenzae* mediate adherence of the organisms to the respiratory epithelium. In addition, *H. influenzae* secretes a factor that disorganizes ciliary beating and a protease that destroys IgA, the major class of antibody secreted into the airways. Survival of *H. influenzae* in the bloodstream is due to the capsule which prevents opsonization by complement and phagocytosis by host cells. *H. pleuropneumoniae* secretes a toxin that kills porcine macrophages. *H. somnus* is capable of inhibiting the respiratory burst in the macrophages, and thus prevents the bactericidal activities of these cells.

Table 21. Diseases caused by Haemophilus species

Haemophilus species	Diseases and the animal species affected
H. pleuropneumoniae (*Actinobacillus pleuropneumoniae*)	Contagious pleuropneumonia, meningitis, and arthritis in pigs
H. parasuis (*H. suis*)	Polyserositis, meningitis, and arthritis (Glasser's disease) in pigs; pneumonia in pigs

H. somnus	Infectious thrombo-embolic meningo-encephalitis, pneumonia, and arthritis in cattle
H. paragallinarum	Infectious coryza (fowl coryza)
H. influenzae	Upper respiratory tract infections and pneumonia in **humans**
H. equigenitalis	Contagious equine metritis

Contagious Pleuropneumonia of Swine

Contagious pleuropneumonia of **pigs** is caused by *Haemophilus pleuropneumoniae*. It is not carried by healthy animals, like *H. parasuis*. Infection is spread through the respiratory route by infected animals, and pigs with subclinical disease. **Young animals, up to 6 months of age, are most susceptible. Infection can be very acute and cause death in a day or two.** However, infection usually causes a pneumonia of several days duration. Mortality may be more than 50%. **Clinical signs** include fever, respiratory distress, and nasal discharge, which is often tinged with blood.

Lesions

Lesions are those of an acute **fibrino-purulent pneumonia** with extensive necrosis and haemorrhage. There is also **fibrinous pleuritis.** Large areas of lungs may become sequestered and walled off by granulation tissue. These are usually discovered as incidental findings in slaughtered pigs. Meningitis and arthritis may accompany pneumonia. **Haemophilus endotoxins** are the main contributors to the pathogenesis of the lesions. These include alveolar and interlobular oedema, dilation of lymphatics, congestion, haemorrhage, and intravascular fibrinous thrombus.

Diagnosis is confirmed by isolation of the organism from affected lung.

Glasser's Disease

Haemophilus parasuis (*H. suis*), **a normal resident of the oropharynx of pigs, causes Glasser's disease.** The disease occurs in **young pigs** after some form of stress, such as weaning or transport. **Clinically,** it is characterized by sudden onset of fever, lameness, respiratory distress, and neurological signs. Affected pigs develop convulsions and paresis (partial or incomplete paralysis).

Lesions

The lesions have been described as **polyserositis** (pericarditis, pleuritis, and peritonitis are collectively referred to as "**polyserositis**"). Polyserositis is characterized by serofibrinous inflammation of the meninges, pleura, pericardium, and synovia (synovial membranes) of joints. **Meningitis** is most severe in the basal meninges, but may also involve the spinal meninges. Extensive deposits of fibrin cover the serosa of the body cavities. **Joints are swollen,** contain excessive cloudy fluid, and the lining is covered with accumulated fibrin. Usually, the limb joints and the atlanto-occipital joints are the most severely affected. **Microscopically,** the main lesion is **fibrinous inflammation.** The lesions resemble mycoplasmal polyserositis of pigs (see Chapter 7), and must be differentiated from it. Mycoplasmal polyserositis usually lasts longer, and is microscopically characterized by significant lymphocytic infiltration.

Diagnosis of Glasser's disease can be confirmed by isolation of the organism.

H. parasuis also causes **pneumonia in pigs**, usually in association with swine influenza virus.

Infectious Thrombo-Embolic Meningo-Encephalitis of Cattle

This disease of cattle is caused by *Haemophilus somnus*. It has been reported mainly from the United States, Canada, and Europe. *H. somnus* is carried in the nasal cavities, prepuce, and female genital tract of healthy cattle, and is easily **spread**. Sometimes, it has been associated with bovine abortion.

Signs

The course is rapid, and clinical signs usually go unnoticed. When observed, signs include fever, weakness, staggering, somnolence (sleepiness), ataxia (muscular incoordination), blindness, and paralysis. Signs of pneumonia (dyspnoea), and arthritis are also common. Mortality rates are high.

Lesions

Grossly, the most characteristic lesions are multiple foci of necrosis and haemorrhage in the brain. Any part of the brain may be affected. **Microscopically,** the basic lesion is **vasculitis** with **thrombosis** and **septic infarction**. Vasculitis is most common in the brain, but may be generalized. Necrotic foci contain bacterial colonies, and become infiltrated with neutrophils. The thrombi are mainly fibrinous. **Meningitis is characterized by fibrino-purulent exudate.**

Diagnosis is made on the basis of lesions, and recovery and identification of *H. somnus*.

Haemophilus somnus is also associated with diseases of other systems, in the absence of central nervous system involvement. These include polyarthritis, endometritis and abortion, orchitis, septicaemia, and especially, bronchopneumonia. *H. somnus* pneumonia is more prevalent in **calves**, and is characterized by fibrino-purulent bronchopneumonia and pleuritis.

Haemophilus Septicaemia of Lambs

This is an acute septicaemia of lambs caused by *Haemophilus agni*. Clinical signs include fever, depression, and reluctance to move. However, as the course is less then 12 hours, animals are usually found dead without premonitory (preceding) signs.

Gross lesions include multiple haemorrhages throughout the body, including skeletal muscles, where they are of diagnostic value. Other important lesions are focal necrosis of the liver and splenomegaly. Microscopically, generalized bacterial embolism and vasculitis account for the gross findings.

Definitive diagnosis requires isolation and identification of H. agni.

Contagious Equine Metritis

Contagious equine metritis in horses is caused by *Haemophilus equigenitalis*. The organism is spread mainly by coitus. It persists in the genital tract of infected horses (both mares and stallions) indefinitely. Infected mares tend to return to oestrus after a reduced dioestrus and usually develop a mucopurulent vaginal discharge. Microscopically, the organism causes severe, purulent, necrotizing endometritis. Culture is the only definitive means of diagnosis. No lesions have been reported in infected stallions.

Infectious Coryza (Fowl Coryza)

Infectious coryza (IC) is an acute, highly contagious disease of the upper respiratory tract of chickens caused by *Haemophilus paragallinarum*. The disease is limited to chickens. Chickens of all ages are susceptible, but older birds react more severely. Not much is known about virulence factors, but it is established that presence of the capsule and the specific haemagglutination antigen are necessary for the pathogenicity of H. paragallinarum. The disease occurs worldwide and causes economic losses due to increased culling in growing chickens, and reduced egg production in layers. Infectious coryza can turn into a chronic respiratory disease.

Spread

The main source of infection are diseased and carrier birds. Because only a few organisms are necessary for the infection, it can be spread by drinking water contaminated by nasal discharge, as well as by airborne means over a short distance. Lateral transmission occurs readily by direct contact.

Pathogenesis

After entry, organisms first adhere to the ciliated mucosa of the upper respiratory tract. The capsule and the haemagglutination antigen (HA) play an important role in the colonization. Toxic substances released from the organism during proliferation are associated with the production of lesions in the mucosa, and appearance of the clinical signs. **The capsule acts as a natural defence substance against the bactericidal power of complement** through the alternate pathway.

H. paragallinarum **is a non-invasive organism with a strong tropism for ciliated cells**. It migrates into the lower respiratory tract (lungs, airsacs) **only after synergistic interaction with other infectious agents, or when encouraged by immunosuppression**. Factors which predispose to more severe and prolonged disease (chronic respiratory disease) include intercurrent infections with infectious bronchitis virus, laryngotracheitis virus, *Mycoplasma gallisepticum*, or *Escherichia coli*, and unfavourable environmental conditions.

Signs

The disease is characterized by rapid spread, high morbidity, and low mortality. The period of incubation is 1-3 days after contact infection, and susceptible birds in the flock show signs within 7-10 days. If not complicated by other infections, the **course** of the disease is **not more than 10 days in the mild form, and about 3 weeks in the more severe form**. The first characteristic signs include **sero-mucoid nasal and ocular discharge and facial oedema**. In severe cases marked conjunctivitis with closed eyes, swollen wattles, and dificult breathing can be seen. **Feed and water consumption is decreased**. This results in **a drop in egg production**, or an increase in the rate of culling. A reduction of egg production of more than 20% indicates multifactorial disease. If complicated with other infectious agents, a more severe and prolonged disease may develop with the clinical picture of a **chronic respiratory disease**.

Lesions

Chickens have **catarrhal to fibrino-purulent inflammation of the nasal passages**, and **infraorbital sinus** and **conjunctiva**. Subcutaneous oedema of the face and wattles is prominent. The upper trachea may be involved, **but the lungs and airsacs are affected only in chronic complicated cases. Microscopically**, lesions include loss of cilia and microvilli, cell oedema, degeneration and desquamation of mucosal and glandular epithelium, infiltration of leukocytes, and deposition of mucopurulent substances, followed by infiltration of mast cells into the lamina propria of the mucous membrane.

Diagnosis

The history of a rapidly spreading disease, its clinical signs and lesions may allow a tentative diagnosis. The diagnosis has to be confirmed by cultural isolation and identification of the causal agent. **Swabs from an infraorbital sinus** (the nasal exudate is usually contaminated) of 2 or 3 diseased chickens should be cultured on blood agar plates cross-streaked with a feeder organism such as *Staphylococcus epidermidis*. Swabs from the trachea and airsacs may be taken, a lthough *H. paragallinarum* is l ess frequently i solated from these areas. T he organism sh ould be identified by m orphology, biochemistry a nd immunofluorescence. A number of serological tests are used for the examination of sera for specific antibodies against *H. paragallinarum*. These include **agglutination, haemagglutination inhibition,** and **fluorescent antibody tests.**

Genus: Klebsiella

Klebsiella pneumoniae (**Friedlander's bacillus**) is the only m ember of this genus which is of pathological importance. **It is a normal inhabitant of the gastrointestinal tract.** Under conditions which are poorly understood, *K. pneumoniae* may be a causative factor in a variety of inflammatory processes. **In humans and monkeys,** it is an important cause of severe pneumonia and upper respiratory and middle ear infections. **In domestic animals, pneumonia caused by *K. pneumoniae* is seen only rarely.** Other conditions associated with *K. pneumoniae* include meningitis in monkeys, mastitis in cattle and pigs, genitourinary infections in mares and bitches, and wound infections in many species.

Genus: Moraxella

Infectious Bovine Kerato-Conjunctivitis

Also known a s "**pink eye**", *M oraxella bovis* is t he cause o f i nfectious **bovine kerato-conjunctivitis in cattle.** T he frequent r ecovery of *M. bovis* from healthy conjunctiva caused a lot of confusion regarding the importance of this organism as a pathogen. However, it is now recognized that only certain strains (piliated) are c apable of a dhering to corneal epithelial cells and are associated with the disease. Other environmental factors, however, are necessary in the development of t he disease. These include exposure to su nlight, dust, insects, and other infections. *M. bovis* can be carried by recovered animals in the ocular and nasal tissues, **providing a constant source for new infections.**

The **clinical signs** include photophobia (unusual intolerance of light), excessive lachrymation, purulent blepharitis (inflammation of the e dges of t he eyelids), and u lceration with v ascularization of t he cornea. L esions usually heal, but often with a corneal scar. **In severe cases, the cornea may rupture, leading to loss of an eye. M icroscopically,** the lesions a re not specific. However, organisms can be found within and on the surface of corneal and conjunctival epithelial cells, and also within the necrotic tissue lying on the ulcers.

Generalized and localized infections of **piglets** with a **Moraxella** species have been d escribed. Other species of **Moraxella** have a lso been associated with kerato-conjunctivitis i n several animal species, b ut their e xact role a s pathogen has not been determined.

Moraxella anatipestifer (previously known as *Pasteurella anatipestifer*), has now been placed in the genus **Riemerella**, and is now known as *Riemerella anatipestifer*. It causes "infectious serositis" of ducks, which is also known as "new duck disease" or "duck septicaemia". It is an important septicaemic disease of growing ducklings throughout the world.

Genus: Pasteurella

Pasteurella are **Gram-negative**, facultatively **anaerobic, rod-shaped bacteria**. They are named after **Louis Pasteur**, who described the type species, *Pasteurella multocida*, and demonstrated it to be the cause of **fowl cholera**. Two species of **Pasteurella**, *P. multocida* and *P. haemolytica*, are important pathogens for cattle, sheep, and pigs. Although both *P. multocida* and *P. haemolytica* are obligate parasites, **they exist as normal commensals in the oropharynx of cattle, sheep, and other mammals.** On the basis of capsular (most pathogenic strains produce capsules) and somatic antigens and other characteristics, there are multiple serotypes of each species. They often have well-defined geographical distributions, and some are more highly pathogenic than others. **The events which allow the organisms to produce disease are not entirely clear,** but during various stressful situations, such as inclement weather, shipping (hence the name "**shipping fever**"), or dipping, the most pathogenic strains outgrow others that are present. Initiation of disease by other organisms, such as viruses or mycoplasmas, also creates a situation for **Pasteurella** to become **important secondary invaders in pneumonia.**

The serotypes of *P. multocida* have been classified as **type 1 (or B), 2 (or A), 3 (or C), and 4 (or D),** and there is a relationship between the serotype and the host species. There is also a relationship between the serotype and the disease produced. With *P. haemolytica* also a number of serotypes occur. **Haemorrhagic septicaemia of cattle is caused by *P. multocida* serotype 1 (or biotype B), and occasionally serotype 4 (D) and serotype E. It is the classical disease of southern Asia.** Pneumonic pasteurellosis of cattle is caused by *P. haemolytica* serotype 1 or biotype A and *P. multocida* serotype 2 or biotype A. It is a common disease in Europe and the western hemisphere. *P. haemolytica* also causes a fulminating fibrinous lobar pneumonia, and *P. multocida* causes a fibrinous bronchopneumonia. **Pasteurellosis of sheep and goats is usually associated with infection by *P. haemolytica*.** It is usually pneumonic in form, but a septicaemic form of the disease is not unusual in lambs. **Pasteurellosis in pigs is usually associated with infection by *P. multocida*,** and is mainly pneumonic in form.

Haemorrhagic Septicaemia

Also known as "**septicaemic pasteurellosis**" and "**barbone**", haemorrhagic septicaemia (HS) is **an acute infection of cattle, buffaloes, sheep and goats,** caused by *P. multocida* serotype B, and occasionally **D and E.** To a much smaller extent, HS also occurs in **camels, pigs, and horses**. The disease occurs mainly in Southeast Asian countries, and also in Africa, where it causes very heavy death losses. **HS is one of the most important bacterial diseases of cattle and buffaloes in India. The disease occurs mainly during the rainy season**. It sp reads rapidly among groups o f animals, causing morbidity a nd mortality between 50 and 100%. **The overall mortality in buffaloes is nearly three times more than in cattle**. In **wildlife**, the disease has been reported in deer, antelope, wild pigs, bison, elephant, kangaroo and sea lion.

Spread

Spread occurs by the ingestion of contaminated foodstuffs, the i nfection originating from clinically normal carriers or clinical cases, or possibly by ticks and biting i nsects. **The saliva of affected animals contains large numbers of organisms during the early stages of the disease**. Although infection occurs b y i ngestion, t he organism d oes not s urvive on pasture for more than 24 hours. HS occurs in outbreaks during periods of environmental stress, the causative organism in the intervening periods persists on the tonsillar and nasopharyngeal m ucosa of carrier animals. About 45% of healthy cattle in herds associated with the disease harbour the organism compared to 3-5% in cattle from herds unassociated with the disease.

Signs

The disease is an acute septicaemia. Clinically, it is characterized by an acute onset of fever (106^0-107^0 F), profuse salivation, submucosal petechiation, severe depression, **a nd death within 24 hours**. Localization m ay occur i n subcutaneous tissue resulting in the development of **warm, painful swellings about the throat, dewlap, brisket or perineum. Severe dyspnoea** occurs if the respiration is obstructed. In the later stages of an outbreak, some affected animals develop signs of pulmonary or alimentary involvement. Pasteurellae can be isolated from the saliva or bloodstream. **The disease in pigs is similar to that in cattle.**

Lesions

Widespread petechiae and ecchymoses on mucous and serous membranes are the main pathological findings, along with **oedema of the lungs and lymph nodes**. There m ay b e o edema of the subcutaneous t issue with gelatinous fluid, and in a few animals there are lesions of early **pneumonia** and **haemorrhagic gastroenteritis**.

Diagnosis

Apart from its regional distribution, clinical and necropsy findings of the disease are not much helpful in diagnosis. HS can only be differentiated from anthrax, blackquarter and acute leptospirosis by bacterial examination. Isolation i s best a ttempted from h eart blood a nd spleen. A rapid e nzyme-linked immunoassay is now available for the identification of specific serotypes of *P. multocida* responsible for HS.

Pneumonic Pasteurellosis of Cattle

Also known as "**shipping fever pneumonia**" or simply as "**shipping fever**", pneumonic pasteurellosis of cattle is caused by *Pasteurella haemolytica* **biotype A (serotype 1)**. [There are **two biotypes** of *P. haemolytica*: biotype A (serotype 1) and biotype T. Different disease syndromes are associated with the two biotypes. Pneumonic pasteurellosis of cattle, sheep and goats is associated with biotype A (serotype 1), whereas biotype T is associated with systemic pasteurellosis in sheep and goats.] *P. multocida* is isolated or ly occasionally. However, the mechanisms by which bacteria get into the lungs and produce the lesions have not been determined. Other pathogens like viruses or mycoplasma may act synergistically to allow the bacteria to be pathogenic.

Spread

Spread of pasteurella occurs by the **inhalation of infected droplets** coughed up or exhaled by infected animals which may be clinical cases, or recovered carriers in which the infection persists in the upper respiratory tract.

Pathogenesis

The **pathogenesis** of pneumonic pasteurellosis **is complex and still not clearly understood**. Lot of research has focussed on finding out how pasteurella, **which are part of the normal flora of the upper respiratory tract**, get down into the terminal bronchioles and alveoli, and when they reach these locations how the lesions develop. Under normal conditions, bovine lungs are free of pasteurella due to an effective **lung clearance mechanism**. The **current hypothesis** is that a combination of viral infection of the respiratory tract and/ or devitalizing influences from transportation, temporary starvation, weaning, rapid fluctuations in ambient (surrounding) temperature, and mixing of cattle from different origins can all collectively promote an increase in the total numbers and virulence of pasteurella in the nasopharynx which are then inhaled into the alveoli and not effectively cleared. Under normal conditions, alveolar macrophages effectively clear pasteurella from alveoli by phagocytic mechanisms. Bovine pulmonary macrophages release '**superoxide anion**' (**free radical**) when exposed to *P. haemolytica*. The response depends on the presence of opsonizing antibody and the quantity of organisms presented to the phagocyte. This is an important mechanism by which the pulmonary macrophage/phagocyte can initiate microbicidal activity. **It is believed that viral-bacterial synergism is an important part of the pathogenesis.** The virus interferes with the lung clearance of *P. haemolytica*.

Four virulence factors have been associated with *P. haemolytica*: fimbriae, a polysaccharide capsule, endotoxin (lipopolysaccharide), **and**

leukotoxin. The interactions of these virulence factors contribute to the pathogenesis of the disease. **Fimbriae** enhance the colonization of the upper respiratory tract. The **capsule** of the organism inhibits complement-mediated serum killing as well as phagocytosis and intracellular killing of the organism. The capsule also increases neutrophil-directed migration and adhesion of the organism to alveolar epithelium. The **endotoxin** can alter bovine leukocyte functions, and is directly toxic to bovine endothelium. It also raises circulating **prostanoids, 5-hydroxytryptamine (serotonin), cAMP, and cGMP. Leukotoxin** is produced by all known serotypes, and is **a pore-forming cytolysin which affects bovine leukocytes and platelets.**

P. haemolytica produces a soluble, bovine leukocyte-specific cytotoxin **(leukotoxin)**, which is **highly toxic to bovine neutrophils and macrophages.** Following inhalation of *P. haemolytica* into the lung there is an accumulation of neutrophils, which when destroyed by the **leukotoxin**, results in the release of proteolytic enzymes, oxidant products, and basic proteins **which degrade cellular membranes, increasing capillary permeability**. This results in fluid accumulation in the interstitium of the alveolar wall, alveolar wall necrosis, and pulmonary oedema. The **endotoxin** of *P. haemolytica* is capable of causing **direct injury to bovine pulmonary arterial endothelial cells**, which may be a contributing pathogenetic mechanism. **Death occurs as a result of hypoxaemia and toxaemia.**

Signs

The close examination of the typical case of pneumonic pasteurellosis reveals a fever of 104°-106° F, and evidence of **bronchopneumonia**. In severe cases, the **dyspnoea is marked**. The course of the disease is usually short, 2-4 days. If treated early, affected cattle recover in 24-48 hours, but severe cases and those which have been ill for a few days before being treated, may die or become chronically affected in spite of prolonged therapy. On an affected farm, **calves** may be affected with pneumonia, but very young calves may die of septicaemia without having shown previous signs of illness.

Lesions

The pneumonia is a **classical fibrinous or lobar pneumonia**, mainly affecting the cranio-ventral portions of the lungs. Interlobular septa are thickened, the pleura is covered with fibrin, and alveoli are filled with neutrophils and mononuclear inflammatory cells. Numerous bacteria are present as are areas of necrosis.

Diagnosis

Nasal swabs taken from clinical cases often yield an almost pure culture of pasteurella, but *P. haemolytica* serotype 1 or biotype A is the most common isolate obtained from cattle with acute pneumonic pasteurellosis. The levels of **plasma fibrinogen** are raised, and parallel the increase in body temperature. They are a more reliable indication of the presence of the lesion than clinical assessment. Young cattle with clinical signs of acute respiratory disease and a fibrinogen concentration greater than 0.7 g/dl, and a temperature greater than 104⁰ F are likely t o have pneumonic p asteurellosis. Haematological examinations are of little value.

Pasteurellosis of Sheep and Goats

Pasteurella haemolytica is the cause of pasteurellosis in sheep and goats. The most common manifestation is **pneumonic pasteurellosis**, which occurs in all ages. Other manifestations of *P. haemolytica* infections in **sheep** include **septicaemic pasteurellosis** in **very young lambs,** w hich usually occurs i n association with pneumonic pasteurellosis in the same flock, systemic pasteurellosis in weaned lambs, and mastitis in ewes. There are **two biotypes** of *P. h aemolytica*: **biotype A (serotype 1)** and **biotype T**. **Pneumonic pasteurellosis is associated with biotype A.** Biotype A is also associated with septicaemic pasteurellosis o f young lambs a nd mastitis i n e wes. S ystemic **pasteurellosis is associated with infections by biotype T.** *P. haemolytica* **is a normal inhabitant of the upper respiratory tract of sheep.**

Pneumonic Pasteurellosis

Pneumonic pasteurellosis causes losses in **sheep** in most parts of the world, through both deaths and reduction of body weight gains. **The disease affects sheep of all ages.** Outbreaks usually start with sudden death in **lambs** from the **septicaemic pasteurellosis,** and progress to **pneumonic pasteurellosis in the ewes** and also in the **lambs** as they get older. **The pathogenesis in sheep and goats** is in g eneral the same a s in p neumonic pasteurellosis of cattle. *P. haemolytica* **is a primary pathogen in very young lambs,** but older lambs are more resistant and predisposing factors are required for the production of disease. Infection with **parainfluenza-3 (PI-3) virus** impairs the bactericidal activity of ovine neutrophils and the clearance of *P. haemolytica* by the ovine lung.

Clinically, outbreaks of the disease commence with **sudden deaths in the absence of preceding signs.** As the outbreak progresses, signs of respiratory involvement include dyspnoea, slight frothing of the mouth, cough, and nasal discharge. Affected s heep have f ever from 1 05⁰-107⁰ F, a nd are depressed and anorectic. **Death may occur within 12 hours,** but in most cases the course is about 3 days. S heep that r ecover have evidence of c hronic p neumonia. **Lesions** include petechial and ecchymotic haemorrhages throughout the body. There is a greenish gelatinous exudate over the pericardium, and large quantities of straw-coloured pleural exudate. The lungs are enlarged, oedematous, and haemorrhagic. **Microscopically,** there is diffuse alveolar necrosis, oedema of the i nterlobular septa, a nd sloughing o f bronchial m ucosa. In d **iagnosis,** nasal swabs for culture are of little value due to the high carrier rate of healthy sheep for the organism in the nasopharynx.

Septicaemic Pasteurellosis

Also known as a "septicaemic disease", septicaemic pasteurellosis is caused by *P. haemolytica* biotype A and also T. The condition mainly affects **lambs, but sheep of all ages are susceptible.** Affected animals die suddenly without any specific clinical signs. **Pathologically,** there are widespread haemorrhages on serosal surfaces, congestion and oedema in lungs and lymph nodes, and necrotizing pharyngitis. **Microscopically,** bacterial emboli are widespread throughout most organs.

Systemic Pasteurellosis

This is associated with *P. haemolytica* **biotype T and also B.** Clinical disease in systemic pasteurellosis is seldom seen as the clinical course is usually less than 6 hours, and **affected sheep are found dead.**

Both *P. multocida* and *P. haemolytica* are sporadic causes of various inflammatory disorders of most species of animals. These include **mastitis, arthritis, otitis, sinusitis, meningitis, and encephalitis.** *P. multocida* type D along with *Bordetella bronchiseptica* are associated with **atrophic rhinitis.**

Pasteurellosis of Pigs

Pasteurella multocida is an important pathogen of pigs. **It causes pneumonic pasteurellosis and septicaemic pasteurellosis. Pneumonic pasteurellosis** is characterized by chronic pneumonia, purulent bronchopneumonia, and pleurisy. Isolates are mainly capsular **serotype A strains** with some **serotypes D strains.** Affected pigs have fever of up to 106⁰ F, are anorectic and disinclined to move. They show significant **respiratory distress,** often breathing through the mouth. Death is common after a clinical course of 4-7 days. There is a marked tendency for the disease to become chronic, resulting in reduced weight gains, and frequent relapses. **On postmortem examination** there is a chronic bronchopneumonia with abscessation. Pleuritis is common and there may also be pericarditis. Peracute cases show an acute necrotizing fibrinous bronchopneumonia.

Septicaemic Pasteurellosis

Septicaemic disease with death occurring within 12 hours and without signs of pneumonia is sometimes observed in **baby pigs. In India,** it is associated with infection by capsular **serotype B.** The disease occurs in all ages of pigs including adults, and is manifested by fever, dyspnoea, and oedema of the throat and lower jaw. **Lesions** include haemorrhage and congestion on serosal surfaces. **Microscopically,** there is widespread vascular damage with thrombus formation, and the presence of colonies of bacteria in the blood vessels of internal organs.

Fowl Cholera

Also known as "**avian pasteurellosis**", "**avian cholera**" and "**avian haemorrhagic septicaemia**", fowl cholera (FC) is a contagious disease affecting domestic and wild birds. It is caused by *Pasteurella multocida*. **In the peracute form, fowl cholera is one of the most virulent and highly infectious diseases of poultry**. The disease is worldwide in distribution. **All species of birds are susceptible**, although turkeys are more so than fowl. Ducks and geese are also highly susceptible. **Adult birds,** or those in the late growing stage, are more frequently affected than younger stock. The **immune status** of the bird may be associated with protection against the strain of organism with which they have previously had contact. But they are often susceptible to other strains.

Spread

Sources of infection include carrier birds (survivors of a natural outbreak), clinically diseased poultry and their excretions, and carcasses of birds which have died of the infection. **Rats are also a reservoir for** *P. multocida*. However, the organism is not usually found in normal poultry or wild birds. Airborne spread of infection does occur between pens, **but spread through water and feed troughs is more important**. The infection does not appear to be egg-transmitted. Disease tends to recur on the same site. **Poultry may be infected by oral, nasal, and conjunctival routes, and through wounds.**

Pathogenesis

Virulence (pathogenicity) of *P. multocida* **in relation to fowl cholera is complex**. It varies depending on the strain, host species, and variations within the strain or host, and conditions of contact between the two. The ability of the organism to invade and reproduce in the host is increased by the presence of a **capsule**, which surrounds it. **Virulence is related to some chemical substance associated with the capsule**, rather than with its physical presence.

P. multocida usually enters tissues through mucous membranes of the pharynx or upper air passages, but it can also enter through the conjunctiva or cutaneous wounds. **Endotoxins are produced by all** *P. multocida*, both virulent and non-virulent. **They contribute to virulence.** However, invasion and multiplication of a strain are necessary for production of sufficient quantities of **endotoxin** to contribute to pathological processes. Signs of acute fowl cholera can be induced in chickens by injection of fractional (very small) amounts of endotoxin. Free endotoxin induces active immunity.

Signs

Fowl cholera occurs in **several forms: peracute, acute, chronic, and localized disease**. In the **peracute form**, there are **no warning signs and large**

numbers of birds are found dead, but in good bodily condition. In the **acute form** marked depression, anorexia, mucus discharge from the orifices, cyanosis and fetid (foul-smelling) diarrhoea may be seen. The **chronic form** occurs in birds which survive the more acute disease, or it may result from infection with an organism of relatively low virulence. The clinical signs include depression, conjunctivitis, dyspnoea, and in a few cases lameness, torticollis, and swelling of the wattles.

Lesions

Gross lesions in the peracute and acute forms include marked congestion of the carcass, multiple petechiation throughout the viscera, and **multiple pinpoint necrotic foci in the liver**. In laying hens, free yolk may be present in the body cavity. In the **subacute disease**, oedema of the lungs (especially in turkeys), pneumonia and perihepatitis are seen. **Chronic lesions** include caseous arthritis of the hock and foot joints, swelling with induration of one or both wattles (chickens), and caseous exudate in the middle ear.

Diagnosis

A presumptive diagnosis can be made from clinical observations, necropsy findings, or isolation of *P. multocida*. A conclusive diagnosis is based on all three. Demonstration of the causal organisms confirms the diagnosis. In the peracute form, **impression smears of the liver or smears of the heart will show bipolar organisms when stained with methylene blue**. In the pneumonic form, similar smears from the lungs may be helpful. Isolation and identification of the organism depends on cultural and biochemical procedures. Isolation can be readily achieved by injection of Pasteurella-free mice (or rabbits) with an inoculum of ground tissue from an affected animal. *P. multocida* kills the experimental animal in 24-48 hours.

Genus: Pseudomonas

Of the numerous species of **Pseudomonas**, only **three** are responsible for diseases of animals: *P. mallei* (glanders), *P. pseudomallei* (melioidosis), and *P. aeruginosa* (purulent infections).

Glanders

Glanders is **a contagious disease** of horses, mules and donkeys (solipeds), occurring in either acute or chronic form, and characterized by **nodules or ulcers** in the respiratory tract and on the skin. It is caused by *Pseudomonas mallei* (previously known as *Malleomyces mallei, Pfeifferella mallei, Actinobacillus mallei, Bacillus mallei*). The disease is **highly fatal**, and of major importance in any affected horse population. The disease is still common in some parts of Asia, **including India**.

P. mallei is a short, **rod-shaped** organism with rounded ends. It is **Gram-**

negative, non-sporulating, aerobic, and an obligate parasite. **Horses tend to develop the chronic form, mules and donkeys the acute form. Humans** are susceptible and the **infection is usually fatal. Dogs** and **cats** are also susceptible. The disease has been seen in large cats in zoos. Guinea-pigs are readily infected. Intra-peritoneal injection of infected material into male **guinea-pigs** ("Straus test") results in **acute purulent orchitis** in 3-4 days. The organisms can be isolated in pure culture from the testicular lesions.

Spread

Infected animals, or carriers which have made an apparent recovery from the disease, are the important sources of infection. **Spread to other animals occurs mostly by ingestion.** The infection spreads on fodder and utensils, particularly watering troughs, contaminated by nasal discharge or sputum. Rarely the cutaneous form appears to arise from **contamination of skin abrasions** by direct contact, or from harness or grooming tools. Spread by **inhalation** can also occur but this mode of infection is probably rare under natural conditions. Dogs and cats acquire the infection from ingestion of contaminated horse meat.

Pathogenesis

Invasion occurs mostly through the intestinal wall, and a **septicaemia (acute form),** or a **bacteraemia (chronic form)** develops. The respiratory mucosa and lungs are most commonly affected, but disseminated lesions may occur. Localization always occurs in the lungs, but the skin and nasal mucosa are also common sites. Other viscera may become the site of the typical nodules. Terminal signs are mainly those of bronchopneumonia. **Death is caused by anoxic anoxia.**

Nasal involvement is indicated by a copious and persistent nasal discharge. It is first catarrhal, later purulent. **Ulceration usually occurs in the nasal mucosa,** and **chronic cough** may indicate pulmonary infection. **Cutaneous involvement** ("farcy") produces indolent (not painful) ulcers in the skin, with thickening of the superficial lymphatics. This sometimes leads to abscesses in superficial lymph nodes.

Signs

In the **acute form**, there is a high fever, cough and nasal discharge with ulcers on the nasal mucosa, and nodules on the skin of the lower limbs or abdomen. **Death from septicaemia occurs in a few days.** In the **chronic form**, signs are related to the lesions. When the localization is mainly pulmonary, there is a chronic cough, frequent epistaxis, and laboured respiration. The chronic nasal and skin forms usually occur together. **Nasal lesions** appear on the lower parts of the turbinates, and the cartilaginous nasal septum. They commence as **nodules** (1 cm in diameter) which **ulcerate** and become conflu-

ent. In the early stages, there is a **serous nasal discharge** which may be unilateral. **Later it becomes purulent and blood-tinged**. Enlargement of the
submaxillary lymph nodes is common. On healing, the ulcers are replaced by
a characteristic stellate (star-shaped) scar. The **skin form** is characterized by
the appearance of **subcutaneous nodules** (1-2 cm in diameter) which so on
ulcerate and discharge pus. In some cases, the lesions are more deeply situated and discharge through fistulous tracts. Thickened fistulous lymphatics
radiate from the lesions, and connect one to the other. **Lymph nodes** draining
the area become involved and discharge to the exterior. The cutaneous lesions
are more common in the medial aspect of the hock, but they can occur on any
part of the body.

Lesions

The **nasal lesions** appear as erosive, **deep ulcerations of the mucosa**,
particularly over the septum. With time, ulcers heal, leaving star-shaped scars.
The **pulmonary lesions** are usually discrete (separate) **granulomatous nodules** resembling tubercles, but sometimes they coalesce. In a few cases, the
disease is manifested as acute purulent bronchopneumonia. **The granulomas
usually have a caseous necrotic centre surrounded by epithelioid cells, a
few giant cells, and some lymphocytes**. Granulomas sometimes occur in the
liver, spleen, or other viscera.

The **skin lesions** are most common on the legs. They appear as persistent
ulcers connected by tortuous, indurated, thick-walled lymphatics. **Superficial
lymph nodes** usually get involved, suppurate and **discharge thick tenacious
pus**. Healing occurs slowly with scarring. Healed ares may break down, leaving
persistent indolent ulcers.

Zoonotic Importance

Humans are susceptible, where the disease may occur as **an acute, often
fatal pyaemia** or a chronic granulomatous disease, as is usually seen in horses.
Cases usually occur in persons working with the organism in the laboratory, **or in
close contact with affected animals**.

Diagnosis

Clinical diagnosis is usually confirmed by the intradermal **mallein test**. This
test has been an effective means for detecting asymptomatic infections, and
making control of the disease possible. Other tests used are complement fixation
test on serum, an indirect haemagglutination test using mallein as antigen, conglutinin
complement absorption test, and the injection of pus from lesions into guinea-pigs.
Diagnosis at necropsy is based on the presence of *P. mallei* by culture methods,
or guinea-pig inoculation. **A dot ELISA test has been developed in India in
recent years which is suitable for use in all soliped species**. It is reported to
have high sensitivity, and can be used as a field test without specialized

equipment.

Melioidosis

Melioidosis is a disease which resembles glanders, and is therefore often called "**pseudoglanders**". It is caused by *Pseudomonas pseudomallei* (previously called *Malleomyces pseudomallei*). Melioidosis is primarily a disease of **rodents** with an occasional case occurring in **humans**. Although infection may be latent, **melioidosis is usually a fatal disease of humans, monkeys, horses, cattle, goats, pigs, dogs,** rabbits, guinea-pigs, and wild rodents. Most mammals appear to be susceptible. **In horses, clinical and necropsy findings are similar to those of glanders.**

Spread

The source of infection is an infected animal which passes the organism in its faeces. The disease in rodents runs a very long course, making these animals important reservoirs of infection for man, and possibly other species. **Infection is spread by ingestion of contaminated food or water,** by insect bites, cutaneous abrasions, and possibly inhalation.

Pathogenesis

Pathogenesis is believed to be the **same as in glanders** with an initial septicaemia or bacteraemia, and subsequent localization in various organs.

Signs

In humans the disease is **a highly fatal acute septicaemia,** terminating after an illness of about 10 days. Melioidosis in **rodents** is also highly fatal. Signs in **sheep** consist mainly of weakness and recumbency (lying down) with death occurring in 1-7 days. In **goats,** the syndrome may resemble the acute form as seen in sheep, but usually runs a chronic course. The disease in **pigs** is usually chronic and is manifested by cervical lymphadenitis. In **horses,** the syndrome is that of an acute metastatic pneumonia with high fever and a short course. Cough and nasal discharge are minimal. Other signs include colic, diarrhoea, and lymphangitis of the legs. Affected horses may survive for several months.

Lesions

The **lesions are characterized by the formation of granulomatous nodules** with a **caseous centre,** which in some cases may become **purulent.** The solid, granulomatous nature of the nodule distinguishes them from frank abscesses. The organisms are found in colonies in the nodule's caseous centre, surrounded by layers of granulation tissue. Giant cells are seldom seen. In **young pigs,** the lungs are often affected by bronchopneumonia. The intrathoracic lymph nodes are oedematous or contain granulomas. In **adult pigs** usually nodules involve the lungs, thoracic lymph nodes, liver, spleen, and lymph nodes. In **goats**, lesions are usually more widely distributed than in pigs, and the nodules are smaller. Ulcers may be found in the mucosa of the nasal septum and trachea; nodules and consolidated areas occur in the lungs; and multiple nodules are seen in the respiratory lymph nodes, spleen, and liver. In **horses**, nodules of 2-3 mm diameter occur in the lungs with a yellowish caseous centre. The lungs may be oedematous and consolidated.

Diagnosis

Diagnosis depends on demonstration, isolation, and identification of the causative organism, *P. pseudomallei*. Intraperitoneal inoculation of guinea-pigs may lead to orchitis ("**Straus reaction**"), as with *P. mallei*.

Pseudomonas aeruginosa Infection

Pseudomonas aeruginosa (previously known as *Pseudomonas pyocyanea*, *Bacterium pyocyaneum*, and *Bacillus aeruginosus*) is a **normal inhabitant of skin and mucous membranes**. It is associated with **sporadic infections of animals and humans,** usually in association with other bacteria or fungi. *P. aeruginosa* is a small, **Gram-negative, rod-shaped** organism. It is actively motile, with 1-3 polar flagellae, and does not produce spores. Most strains produce characteristic **blue-green pigment** in tissues and in cultures. The pigments are complex, and include **pyocyanin** and **pyoverdin**. Other substances with antibiotic and bactericidal properties have been recovered from the organisms. *P. aeruginosa* produces **exotoxins**, including **protease** and **elastase**, which appear to be responsible for their pathogenic properties.

Pathogenesis

P. aeruginosa has **pili** and **adherence proteins** which mediate adherence to epithelial cells and lung mucin. It has an **endotoxin** that causes the symptoms and signs of Gram-negative **sepsis. Pseudomonas** also has a number of "**virulence factors**", such as **alginate, exotoxin A, exoenzyme S, phospholipase C** and **an elastase. A**lginate covers the bacteria and protects them from antibacterial antibodies, complement, and phagocytes. **Exotoxin A** inhibits protein synthesis and **exoenzyme S** may interfere with host cell growth. **Phospholipase C** lyses red blood cells and degrades pulmonary surfactant, and **elastase** degrades IgGs and extracellular proteins, and are both therefore important in tissue invasion. Finally, *P. aeruginosa* also produces **iron-containing compounds** that are **extremely toxic to endothelial cells** and therefore **cause the vascular lesions** characteristic of this infection.

Lesions

The lesions are not characteristic, and consist of necrotizing, purulent and haemorrhagic inflammatory reactions of affected tissues. The more common situations include pneumonia, otitis media, traumatic reticulitis, mastitis, metritis, enteritis, dermatitis, and keratitis. In acute pneumonia, the lesions are described a s vasculitis w ith infiltration b y large number of b acteria in the walls, but not the lumen, of arteries and veins. More prolonged infection of any organ or tissue results in the formation of abscesses or granulomas with purulent cores, called "**botryomycosis**" (see staphylococcal infections).

Pseudomonas Infection in Poultry

Pseudomonas aeruginosa (*P. pyocyanea*) is a **Gram-negative** motile rod and a strict a erobe. It is ubiquitous i n nature, b eing found i n soil, s ewage, lakes, and t he intestinal c ontents of a nimals and birds. It causes disease i n chickens, ducks, t urkeys a nd pheasants. A lthough all ages are s usceptible, young birds a re m ore susceptible t han older stock. I nfection in e ggs kills embryos.

The organism is an opportunist pathogen. Infection occurs through the contamination o f egg dips, or c ontaminated inoculum i n vaccination. T hese result in high mortality in embryos or young chicks. It can also spread from infected flocks to susceptible ones under conditions of poor hygiene.

Factors which cause stress and pathogens, particularly those causing immunodeficiency, aggravate the effect of the organism. Signs may v ary greatly a nd include depression, incoordination, ataxia, swelling of the h ead, wattles and j oints (especially o f the l eg), diarrhoea, and conjunctivitis. T he **duration** of the disease is **very short** - from a few hours to few days. **Lesions are similar to those seen in colisepticaemia, with pericarditis, perihepatitis, and airsacculitis**. There may be subcutaneous oedema especially of the head and neck, excess fluid in affected joints, and necrotic focal lesions in the liver and s pleen. **Diagnosis** depends. on t he isolation and identification o f the organism which can be grown on common bacteriological media.

Genus: Salmonella

Salmonellosis (Paratyphoid)

Genus "Salmonella" is named after an eminent veterinary bacteriologist, **Daniel E. Salmon, an American**. It contains **hundreds of serovars (i.e., species)**, which are· subdivided into **five subgenera** on the basis of biochemical characteristics. The **pathogenic members** primarily **belong to subgenera I and III**, and are mainly associated with **enteric diseases. In humans, typhoid fever** is the classical form o f salmonellosis. **In animals, the infections are often referred to as "paratyphoid"**. S almonella a re **rod-shaped, Gram-negative**, non-sporulating **motile** (by peritrichous f lagella, i.e., covering the entire surface) organisms. Some of the salmonella are host-specific, whereas others may infect a wide variety of animal species. *S. typhi*, the cause of typhoid fever in h umans and *S . choleraesuis* of p igs, are e xamples of h ost-specific salmonella. In contrast, *S. typhimurium* produces gastroenteritis, sometimes leading to septicaemia, in cattle, horses, pigs, humans, and other species. The more important pathogenic members of the genus are listed in Table 22. **Salmonellosis occurs in all animals but is most common in cattle (*S. dublin*, *S. typhimurium*), horses (*S. typhimurium*), and pigs (*S. choleraesuis*, *S. typhimurium*).** It is rare in dogs and cats. Birds are affected by their own species of salmonella as well as *S. typhimurium*.

Table 22. More important Pathogenic Salmonellae

Host	Organisms
Cattle	*S. dublin, S. typhimurium, S. anatum, S. newport, S. montevideo*
Horses	*S. typhimurium, S. newport, S. heidelberg, S. anatum, S. copenhagen, S. agona, S. abortus equi*
Sheep and goats	*S. abortus ovis, S. montevideo, S. typhimurium, S. dublin, S. arizonae*
Pigs	*S. choleraesuis, S. typhimurium, S. dublin, S. heidelberg*
Dogs and cats	*S. typhimurium, S. panama, S. anatum*
Poultry	*S. pullorum, S. gallinarum, S. typhimurium, S. enterica, S. enteritidis, S. agona, S. anatum*
Humans	*S. typhi, S. paratyphi-A, S. typhimurium, S. enteritidis*

Spread

Salmonellae are spread by direct or indirect means. Infected animals are the source of organisms which they excrete and infect other animals directly, or indirectly by contamination of the environment, mainly feed and water supplies. **Infection is acquired by ingestion** of material contaminated with infected faeces from either clinically ill animals, or carrier animals. The carrier state is particularly important in the maintenance and transmission of the disease. Because salmonellae are facultative intracellular **organisms which survive in the phagolysosome of macrophages,** they can **dodge the bactericidal effects of antibody and complement. Thus, persistence of infection in animals (the carrier state)** and in the environment are important features of salmonellosis.

Pathogenesis

The bacteria adhere to enterocytes (intestinal cells) **through fimbriae or pili, and colonize** (settle and proliferate in) the **small intestine.** They then **penetrate enterocytes,** where **further multiplication occurs** before they cross the lamina propria. They continue to proliferate, both free and within macrophages. Many salmonella infections do not progress further. However, with some of the more pathogenic species, especially in **young animals**, the organisms are transported by macrophages to mesenteric lymph nodes. Further multiplication ultimately leads to **septicaemia**, with localization of bacteria in many organs and tissues. This includes the spleen, liver, meninges, brain, and joints. Thus, the **infection may range from a mild enteritis to serious and often fatal enteritis with septicaemia.**

Recent studies have revealed that invasion of intestinal epithelial cells is controlled by **invasion genes** in these bacteria that are induced by the low oxygen tension found in the intestine. These genes produce **proteins** that are involved in **adhesion**. Similarly, growth inside macrophages is important in pathogenicity. This is achieved through **bacterial genes** that are induced by the acid pH within the macrophage phagolysosome.

In humans, the mildest form of salmonellosis is **food poisoning**, resulting from ingestion of contaminated foods. **Fluid loss from diarrhoea** is important in the development of clinical signs and the outcome of the infection. The mechanism appears to involve both an **e**nterotoxin which causes increased secretion by enterocytes (as in cholera and *E. coli* infections), and **exsorption** (opposite of absorption) resulting from the inflammatory process. **Abortion** may occur during the acute enteritic or septicaemic form of salmonellosis, especially **in cattle**. Certain salmonella species, however, cause abortion in the absence of visible enteritis, such is the case with *S. abortus ovis* in sheep and *S. abortus equi* in horses.

Signs

The disease can be described as **three syndromes: 1. Septicaemia, 2. Acute enteritis**, and 3. **chronic enteritis. Septicaemia:** This is the characteristic form in newborn foals and calves and guinea-pigs. Affected animals show profound depression, dullness, prostration, high fever (105°-107° F), and **death within 24-48 hours. Acute enteritis:** This is the common form **in adult animals of all species.** There is a high fever (104°-106° F) with **severe fluid diarrhoea**, sometimes dysentery, and with tenesmus (spasmodic contraction of anal sphincter) occasionally. Other signs include anorexia, and faeces having a putrid smell, containing mucus, and sometimes blood and fibrinous casts. **Pregnant animals usually abort.** Mortality may reach 75%. In all species, severe dehydration and toxaemia occur; the animal becomes recumbent **and dies in 2-5 days. Chronic enteritis (subacute enteritis):** This is a common syndrome in **pigs** and occurs sometimes in **cattle** and **adult horses.** In **calves**, there is persistent diarrhoea, with the occasional passage of spots of blood, mucus, and firm fibrinous casts, moderate fever (102° F), loss of weight and emaciation.

Lesions

The lesions of salmonellosis, or "paratyphoid fever" in animals are those of enterocolitis and septicaemia. The stomach and small intestine are usually spared. Enteritis commences in the ileum and through the colon. The mucosa is hyperaemic, frankly haemorrhagic, thickened, and usually covered with a red, yellow, or grey exudate. It contains distinct ulcers. Microscopically, in the mucosa there is haemorrhage, oedema, necrosis, and leukocytic infiltration, mainly composed of macrophages. Lesions in other organs are less consistent. Although not pathognomonic, lesions found in the liver are more specific. These include small foci of necrosis, and the so-called "paratyphoid nodules" ("typhoid nodules" in typhoid fever of humans). "Paratyphoid nodules" consist of small aggregations of reticulo-endothelial cells (histiocytes, macrophages). These nodules may occur in association with or independent of hepatic necrosis.

Reticulo-endothelial hyperplasia is present in lymph nodes and spleen, which may cause enlargement of these tissues. Haemorrhage and necrosis are common in mesenteric lymph nodes. In septicaemic cases, petechiae or ecchymoses on the pleura, peritoneum, endocardium, kidney, and meninges always develop. Microscopic examination, in the septicaemic form, reveals fibrinoid necrosis of vessel walls and hyaline material deposited in glomerular capillaries and minor vessels of the dermis. This material is the result of thrombosis with fibrin and densely packed erythrocytes. This situation has been compared to the generalized Shwartzman reaction, and has been reproduced in pigs by the intravenous injection of killed *Salmonella choleraesuis*, which was repeated 24 and 48 hours later. This procedure resulted in disseminated vascular thrombosis and bilateral cortical necrosis of the kidneys, characteristic of the generalized Shwartzman reaction.

Prolonged ulcerative proctitis (inflammation of the rectum and anus) associated with infection caused by *S. typhimurium* leads to rectal stricture (narrowing). The stricture results from annular (ring-shaped, circular) fibrous thickening of the submucosa and muscularis. Partial or complete obstruction of the rectum occurs with subsequent distension of the rectum, colon, and abdomen.

Abortion

S. abortus equi is a cause of abortion in mares. *S. abortus ovis* and *S. montevideo* are causes of abortion in sheep. Either abortion characteristically occurs late in gestation, or infected foals or lambs are born at term and die within a few days. There are no specific lesions in the placenta or foetus. The placenta is oedematous and contains focal haemorrhage and necrosis. There is usually oedema of the foetus.

Diagnosis

Salmonellosis can be suspected on the basis of gross and histopathological findings. However, the lesions are not specific, and isolation and identification of the causative agent in association with lesions is necessary for confirmation. Serum ELISA is available for the detection of *S. dublin* mammary gland infection in carrier cows. The DNA probe is a sensitive method for screening large numbers of samples to detect potentially virulent **Salmonella** sp.

Salmonella Infections in Poultry

Infections with bacteria of the genus Salmonella are responsible for a variety of acute and chronic diseases in poultry. Infected poultry also comprise one of the most important reservoirs of salmonellae **which can be transmitted through the food chain to humans.** Isolations of salmonella are reported more often from poultry and poultry products than from any other animal species. This reflects the high prevalence of **Salmonella** infections in poultry. The genus **Salmonella** consists of **more than 2300 serologically distinguishable variants (serotypes/serovars.).** These serotypes are usually named after the place of initial isolation.

Infections of poultry with salmonellae can be grouped into **three categories.** The **first group** includes infections with **two non-motile serotypes,** *S. pullorum* and *S. gallinarum*, which are generally host-specific for avian species. **Pullorum disease**, caused by *S. pullorum*, is an acute systemic disease of chicks and poults (young turkeys). **Fowl typhoid**, caused by *S. gallinarum*, is an acute or chronic septicaemic disease which usually affects mature birds. Both of these diseases have been responsible for serious economic losses to poultry farmers in the past. The **second group** includes infections with a group of **motile Salmonella serotypes**, referred to collectively as "**paratyphoid salmonellae**". The disease produced by them is called "**salmonellosis**" or "**paratyphoid infections**". **Paratyphoid infections are important mainly as a cause of food-borne disease in humans.** Although paratyphoid infections of poultry are very common, they rarely cause acute systemic disease, except in highly susceptible young birds subjected to stressful conditions. The **third group** includes infections with the **various motile serotypes of the sub-genus Arizona**, the most important species being *S. arizonae*, which was formerly designated as *Arizona hinshawii*. The disease caused by this group of organisms is known as "**arizonosis**", which is of particular economic significance in **turkeys.**

Pullorum Disease

Pullorum disease (PD) is caused by the bacterium *Salmonella pullorum*. The disease was previously known as "**bacillary white diarrhoea or BWD**", but a s white diarrhoea is n ot always a clinical f eature, it b ecame known as "pullorum disease". It is **septicaemic disease affecting mainly chickens** and turkeys, but other birds are susceptible.

Spread

The most important method by which pullorum disease spreads is from an infected h en t hrough the ovary t o t he n ewly hatched chick (**transovarian transmission**). A proportion of infected birds become **adult carriers**, with *S. pullorum* **persisting in the ovaries and being excreted in the ova**. Such infected hens become poor egg layers, but only a small percentage of the eggs laid are likely to be infected. The fertility and hatchability of infected eggs is also below average. However, viable chicks do hatch from such infected eggs and become a source of infection. Fluff (soft fur/fibres) from such chicks is heavily contaminated with *S. pullorum*, and as it dries, the bacteria are rapidly disseminated through t he incubator o r b rooder. T hus, pullorum disease i s passed from hen to chick **by vertical transmission**, and then there is **rapid lateral spread** from chick to chick in hatcheries and rearing units.

Signs

Pullorum disease is seen m ainly **in chicks under 3 weeks of age**. First indication is usually excessive numbers of **dead-in-shell chicks**, and **deaths soon after hatching**. S igns include depression with a t endency to h uddle, respiratory distress, lack of appetite, and w hite v iscous (thick a nd sticky) droppings which adhere to the feathers around the vent. **The mortality varies considerably, and in extreme cases can be 100%.**

A **subacute form** with lameness and swollen hock joints may be seen **in growing birds**, a nd result i n poor g rowth r ates. Older b irds appear l istless (depressed, dull), and have pale and shrunken combs. **Reduced egg production may be the only sign of the disease in adult birds.**

Lesions

Chicks which die soon after hatching have **peritonitis** with an **inflamed, unabsorbed yolk sac. Lungs** may be congested and **liver** dark and swollen with haemorrhages visible on the surface. Sometimes, in chicks which die in the acute phase, there are no specific lesions, or only those of **a septicaemia** with the liver congested and the subcutaneous blood vessels dilated and prominent. **In chicks which die after showing signs of disease for 1 or 2 days**, there may be typhlitis (inflammation of the caecum). The caeca are enlarged and distended with casts of hard, d ry necrotic m aterial. Discrete (separate), **small, w hite, necrotic f oci** are also usually found in the liver, lungs, myocardium, and g izzard wall. **In growers** affected with arthritis, the h ock joints are usually enlarged due to the presence of excess orange-coloured gelatinous material around the joints. **In general, the lesions in chicks are**

neither characteristic nor constant.

In adult birds, the characteristic lesion is **an abnormal ovary** with the **ova being irregular, cystic, mis-shapen, discoloured and pedunculated with prominent thickened stalks.** There m ay also be **peritonitis, arthritis, and pericarditis.** In some infected hens, the **ovary is inactive** with the ova small, **pale, and undeveloped.**

Diagnosis

The clinical s igns a nd l esions in p ullorum disease a re variable (inconstant) a nd are n ot sufficiently characteristic to m ake a f irm diagnosis. **The disease is diagnosed in the chick by isolating the causal organism** after cultural examination o f the v iscera. Infected o lder birds c an be d etected by demonstrating. *S. pullorum* antibodies in blood samples by **agglutination tests.** Antibodies t ake several d ays to appear and m aximum antibody p roduction may not occur until 100 days after infection. **They may not be detectable, therefore, until the bird has reached immunological maturiry at 16 weeks of age.** A number of tests are available to detect the antibodies, but the **two** which have been most commonly used are the **rapid slide agglutination test** on whole blood using a stained antigen, and a **tube agglutination test** carried out on serum. More recently, enzyme-linked immunosorbent assay (**ELISA**) for detecting *S. pullorum* antibodies has been developed by using lipopolysaccharide (endotoxin) from this s almonella as a ntigen. This t echnique can be used for screening large numbers of blood samples.

Fowl Typhoid

Fowl typhoid (FT) is caused by *Salmonella gallinarum*. It is **a septicaemic disease** affecting mainly chickens and turkeys, but other birds are susceptible. The disease constitutes a serious poultry health problem. Unlike other avian salmonella infections, **the disease is usually seen in growers or adult birds, although chicks can be infected.**

Spread

S. gallinarum is passed out by infected birds in the **droppings. Lateral spread is by the ingestion of such material in contaminated food or water.** *S. gallinarum* persists in faeces for at least a month, and in infected carcasses for much longer periods. **Recovered birds usually remain carriers for long periods,** a nd the m ovement o f s uch b irds could be a means b y w hich the disease spreads rapidly. **Egg transmission also occurs.** It may then spread the infection to contact birds in the hatchery or rearing u nits. Likewise **attendants, visitors etc**. may carry infection from one farm to another, or house to house, unless appropriate disinfection procedures are followed.

Signs

In acute outbreaks, the first sign is **an increase in mortality** followed by a **drop in food consumption**. If the birds are in lay, there is a **drop in egg production**. Depression, with affected birds standing still with ruffled feathers and their eyes closed, is a common feature. Respiratory distress with rapid breathing can occur, but the most characteristic clinical sign is a **watery to mucoid yellow diarrhoea**. In birds which do not die within 2-3 days, **a chronic phase** follows. There is progressive loss of condition. An **intense anaemia** develops which produces shrunken, pale combs and wattles. The disease spreads rapidly through the flock, and can result in **losses of 50% or more**.

Subacute outbreaks may result in a **sporadic mortality over a long period**. Egg transmission is not a regular feature of the disease, but can occur, and leads to an increase in **dead-in-shell embryos**, and small, weak, moribund or dead chicks on the hatching trays. When **young chicks** are affected, the signs are non-specific, and similar to those seen in pullorum disease or salmonellosis. Weakness, reluctance to move, a tendency to huddle, and a drop in food consumption all occur. Yellow, pasty droppings, which adhere to the feathers around the vent, are also seen. Sometimes there is respiratory distress with rapid breathing and gasping.

Lesions

The carcass of the bird died in **acute phase** has a septicaemic, jaundiced appearance. The subcutaneous blood vessels are hyperaemic and prominent, and the skeletal muscles congested and dark in colour. A consistent finding is a **swollen friable liver** which is dark red or almost black, and the **surface has a characteristic coppery bronze sheen** (glistening brightness on the surface). **Spleen** may be **enlarged**, and a **catarrhal enteritis**, particularly involving the small intestine, is usually present. The intestines contain viscous, slimy, bile-tinged material. A characteristic feature is a dark brown bone marrow. Lesions in birds dying in the **chronic phase** include emaciated and an intensely anaemic carcass with focal necrosis in the heart, intestines, pancreas and liver. Greyish-white necrotic foci are also seen in the myocardium, the first part of the intestine, and in the pancreas. A **pericarditis**, with turbid yellow fluid in the pericardial sac and fibrin attached to the surface of the heart, is a feature of chronic fowl typhoid. In **young chicks**, additional findings are discrete necrotic foci in the lungs and gizzard. Well-defined necrotic foci in the testicles have been reported in cockerels in FT. **In laying birds, there may be retained yolks which may later rupture**.

Diagnosis

A definite diagnosis of FT requires isolation and identification of *S. gallinarum*. A tentative diagnosis, however, can be made based on flock history, clinical signs, mortality, and lesions. **Serological tests include** the macroscopic tube agglutination (TA) test, rapid serum (RS) test, stained antigen whole blood (WB) test, and microagglutination (MA) test using tetrazolium-stained antigens. ELISA test for detecting *S. gallinarum* antibodies has been developed by using lipopolysaccharide (endotoxin) from this salmonella as antigen. This technique has been used for screening a large number of blood samples.

S. gallinarum has the same antigenic structure as *S. pullorum*. The rapid plate agglutination test or whole blood, using **the stained *S. pullorum* antigen, can therefore be used to detect carriers of *S. gallinarum*.** Positive birds can then be removed from the flock. This is the main reason why fowl typhoid has been virtually eradicated from most countries with a progressive poultry industry.

Salmonellosis (Paratyphoid Infections)

Motile Salmonella serotypes, other than those in the *S. arizonae* subgenus are often referred to as "**paratyphoid (PT) salmonellae**". These organisms can infect a wide variety of hosts, **including humans**. In some cases they result in asymptomatic intestinal carriage (transport), and in other cases produce clinical disease. More recently, PT salmonellae have been the subject of great interest **as agents of food-borne disease transmission to humans**. Commercial poultry constitute one of the largest and most important reservoirs of salmonellae **that can be introduced into the human food supply. Contaminated poultry meat and eggs** have consistently been among the most frequently implicated sources of human **Salmonella** outbreaks.

Cause

Although **more than 2300 serotypes of Salmonella have been identified**, only about 10% of these have been isolated from poultry. The most commonly isolated serotypes from chickens (i.e., PT salmonellae) in USA include *S. heidelberg*, *S. enteritidis*, *S. hadar*, *S. montevideo*, *S. kentucky*, and *S. typhimurium*. The serotypes most commonly isolated **from humans** include *S. typhimurium*, *S. enteritidis*, *S. heidelberg*, *S. hadar*, *S. newport*, and *S. agona*.

Spread

Paratyphoid salmonellae can be introduced into poultry flocks from many different sources. Among the most common sources of infection are **contaminated feed**, and various animal and insect vectors. PT salmonellae can be **spread vertically** to the progeny of infected breeder flocks, and **horizontally** within and between flocks.

Contaminated feeds, particularly those **containing animal proteins**, are the likely sources of introduction of PT salmonellae to poultry flocks, e.g., fish meal, meat and bone meal, and poultry offal and feathermeal. **Vegetable protein** may also become contaminated with salmonellae either before or during processing. **Biological vectors** can both disseminate and amplify salmonellae in poultry flocks. **Insects,** including cockroaches and mealworms (larvae of various beetles), can carry salmonellae internally and externally, and spread them throughout poultry houses. **Rats and mice** have been identified as particularly important vectors for *S. enteritidis* in laying flocks.

Vertical transmission of PT salmonellae to the progeny of infected breeder flocks can result from the production of **eggs contaminated by salmonellae** in the contents, or on the surface. Some PT serotypes, particularly *S. enteritidis*, can be deposited in the contents of eggs before oviposition (egg laying). **The resulting transovarian transmission of infection to progeny is an important aspect of the epidemiology of** *S. enteritidis* **in chickens. Transmission through shell penetration occurs from faecal contamination of the egg during egg laying.** As the egg passes through the cloaca, salmonellae in faeces attach themselves to the warm wet surface of the shell **and are drawn inside as it cools.** This can result in direct transmission of infection in the developing embryo, or can also lead to exposure of the chick to salmonellae when the shell is broken during hatching.

After introduction into poultry, **PT salmonellae can spread horizontally within and between flocks. Horizontal transmission** can be brought about by direct bird-to-bird contact, through ingestion of contaminated faeces or litter, contaminated water or feed, personnel and equipment, and a variety of other means. Salmonellae can spread from one poultry farm to another through movement of vehicles, equipment and utensils, including hatchery egg trays and trolleys contaminated with the organisms. Also, **staff on a poultry farm** can carry salmonellae mechanically from one unit to another on contaminated footwear, clothing and hands. **Humans may also be salmonella excretors and infect poultry in their charge. Control of salmonellosis from all such sources can be achieved only by maintaining a high standard of farm management, farm hygiene, and biosecurity.**

Pathogenesis

Three general categories of toxins have been reported to play roles in the pathogenicity of PT salmonellae. **Endotoxin** is associated with the lipid A portion of **Salmonella** cell wall lipopolysaccharide (LPS). If released into the bloodstream when bacterial cells are lysed, endotoxin can produce fever. *S. enteritidis* endotoxin causes liver and spleen lesions. LPS also contributes to the resistance of the bacterial cell wall to attack and digestion by host phagocytes. Loss of the ability to synthesize complete LPS is associated with a loss of virulence for *S. enteritidis*, and an impaired ability of *S. typhimurium* to colonize the caeca and invade to the spleen. **Two proteinaceous toxins**

have also been identified in salmonella. **Enterotoxin** (heat-labile) of salmonella induces a secretory response in epithelial cells which results in fluid accumulation i n the i ntestinal lumen. **C ytotoxin** (heat-stable) o f salmonella c auses structural damage to intestinal epithelial cells, by inhibiting protein synthesis.

The **adherence** of P T salmonella to intestinal epithelial cells is the first step in the sequence of events which produces disease. Adherence is associated with **type 1 fimbriae** and with a **mannose-resistant haemagglutinin**. Although adherence does not require metabolically active salmonella, the subsequent b acterial invasion o f host c ells r equires p rotein synthesis b y l ive salmonella. **The overall virulence of salmonella depends mainly on the initial degree of mucosal (of mucosa) invasiveness.** Mechanisms for salmonella invasion into intestinal cells include **type 1 fimbriae** and **various bacterial proteins** induced by c ontact with e pithelial cell surfaces. T he replication (multiplication) of salmonella within host cells has b een found to be necessary for the full expression of pathogenicity.

Serotype specific plasmids of characteristic molecular weight have been **directly linked with virulence for a number of salmonella**. Plasmids are extra-chromosal DNA elements which have been usually associated with bacterial pathogenicity. H owever, **pathogenicity of salmonella does not always require the presence of the serotype-specific plasmids**.

Paratyphoid salmonellae strains are usually found to differ in their ability to cause disease, or death in young poulrty. However, the bacterial characteristics r esponsible for the pathogenicity d ifferences between S almonella strains are still incompletely understood.

Signs

Disease caused by paratyphoid salmonellae is uncommon, and is usually seen in chicks, poults (young turkeys) or ducklings and **rarely in birds over 4 weeks of age**. The morbidity and mortality vary greatly. **Deaths are usually less than 20%, but in exceptional cases can approach 100%. The clinical signs are not specific** and are similar whichever serotype of salmonella is involved. Affected birds are depressed, reluctant to move, and stand with t heir eyes closed and w ith ruffled feathers and d rooping wings. **D iarrhoea with pasting of the feathers around the vent is commonly seen**. In some o utbreaks visual i mpairment, due t o t he c orneal o pacity o r caseous plaques in the eyeball, has been reported.

Lesions

These vary considerably, f rom the c omplete absence t o a s epticaemic carcass with the lungs, liver, spleen and kidneys swollen and congested. When **baby chicks** are affected, **an inflamed, unabsorbed yolk sac** is a common feature. Discrete (separate) **necrotic lesions in the lungs, liver and heart,** peritonitis and **haemorrhagic enteritis** may be seen in birds which do not die, in the acute septicaemic phase. The most characteristic lesion is **typhlitis**, with the caeca distended by hard white necrotic cores.

Diagnosis

Confirmation of the diagnosis requires the isolation and identification of the causal agent. **Salmonella** are readily isolated from infected tissues by direct culture. In chicks dying of septicaemia, direct isolations can be made from the liver, gallbladder, or yolk sac. **In older birds salmonella are often confined to the intestine; the caeca being the most likely site for isolation.** The value of serological tests depends to some extent on the salmonella serovar. involved. *S. pullorum* and *S. gallinarum* **do not colonize the digestive tract**, but readily infect the rest of the bird's body. This stimulates the production of antibodies which c an be d etected by serological tests. O ther salmonella colonize the alimentary tract, but do not readily invade the tissues and thus may not stimulate the production of antibodies.

A number of serological tests have been developed for the diagnosis of salmonella infections in poultry. As discussed, the whole blood test (WBT), which u ses a stained antigen, and the serum agglutination test (SAT) h ave been used successfully for more than 50 years for the identification of flocks infected with *S. pullorum* and *S. gallinarum*. **Because *S. enteritidis* possesses the same group D somatic antigen as *S. pullorum*, the WBT and related tests can be used for the diagnosis of this infection.** In recent years other tests, such as the ELISA, have been developed for the identification of *S. enteritidis*-**infected flocks** and are now in use in many countries.

Rapid Detection Technologies

Specific antibodies to Salmonella antigens have been used to develop a variety of ELISA methods. These tests, using **polyclonal antibodies to Salmonella** LPS or flagella, have been reported to detect salmonellae in eggs, tissues, cloacal swabs, litter, and feed. **Monoclonal antibodies** to outer membrane proteins or flagella have been used as the basis for ELISA tests to specifically detect *S. enteritidis* in eggs, tissues, and environmental samples. Another application of antibodies for detecting **salmonellae** involves coating **small magnetic beads** with specific antibodies. When mixed with the sample to be tested, the **antibody-coated beads** will bind to any Salmonella target antigens present, and a magnetic field can then be applied to recover the bead-antibody-antigen complex. Another approach to rapid testing for salmonellae in poultry, which has received considerable attention in recent years, involves **using probes for particular DNA sequences unique to salmonellae.** Hybridization of the probe with DNA extracted from the sample indicates a positive result.

Public Health Significance

Salmonellae remain among the leading sources of food-borne illness throughout much of the world. In a developed country like United States, salmonellosis m ay a ffect a s m any a s 1-5 m illion people e ach year. **A bout 20,000 hospitalizations and 500 deaths associated with Salmonella are reported annually.** P oultry products are c onsistently i dentified as i mportant sources of salmonellae **which cause illness in humans.** More than one-third of f ood-borne s almonellosis o utbreaks i n t he United S tates between 1 983-1987 were associated with **poultry meat or eggs. Thus, paratyphoid infections in birds (salmonellosis) acquire great importance because of the human illnesses caused from the consumption of contaminated poulty products.**

Arizonosis

Arizonosis is **an acute septicaemic disease, mainly of young turkey poults,** caused by the bacterium, *Salmonella arizonae*.

Spread

If an **adult turkey** is infected, the organism localizes in the intestine **and such a bird then becomes a carrier and excreter of arizonas for long periods.** Also, after a female has recovered from infection, **the organism can localize in the ovary,** a nd from t here be **transmitted to progeny through the egg.** However, transmission through the egg occurs usually after contamination of the shell with i nfected faeces. **A rizona bacillus can readily penetrate the shell and shell membranes at 37⁰ C.** Once an embryo or poult (young turkey) is infected, **lateral transmission,** in the hatcher or hatchery by aerosol and in the brooder by direct contact and through contaminated food and water, can readily occur.

Signs

The signs shown by poults are similar to those shown by chicks with salmonellosis. However, eye abnormalities are seen more often, and nervous signs a re regular additional feature. Affected birds t end to huddle, look dejected, and have pasty faeces which sticks to the ventral feathers. Morbidity and mortality vary, but losses of up to 90% in a group of pullets have been reported. Adult chicks usually show no clinical signs of disease, but can be carriers and excrete the organisms for long periods.

Lesions

The carcass is septicaemic with generalized **peritonitis. Yolk sacs are inflamed** and the **airsacs** thickened with opaque white to yellow, cheesy, caseous deposits. **Liver** may be swollen, and discrete necrotic foci are sometimes found throughout t he liver. There is e nteritis, and a characteristic f inding as w ith salmonellosis, is **typhlitis** with white caseous casts filling the caecal lumen. **Eye lesions are a characteristic feature**.

Diagnosis

The c linical signs a nd lesions i n birds a ffected with a rizonosis are n ot specific, and c annot be d ifferentiated from o ther forms o f salmonellosis. However, if t here are any poults with incoordination and eye abnormalities, arizonosis should be strongly suspected. Confirmation of the diagnosis is by isolation and identification of the causal agent.

Genus: Shigella
Shigellosis
Bacillary Dysentery

Monkeys, apes, and humans are the only hosts which are naturally susceptible to infection with dysentery bacilli. The disease is well known in **humans**, and has been described in a variety of non-human primate species. *Shigella flexneri* is the most common pathogen, but *S. sonnei* and *S. dysenteriae* also commonly occur. These strains are infectious to humans, but they are not the strains which produce severe dysentery in humans, and **fortunately transmission from monkeys to humans is rare**.

Clinically, dysentery varies from mild **diarrhoea** to severe watery or mucoid diarrhoea m ixed w ith b lood. Animals b ecome dehydrated and rapidly l ose condition. **Lesions** are non-specific, and confined to the **colon**. T he colonic mucosa is s wollen, with p atchy or diffuse haemorrhage. U lceration may o r may not be present. The intestinal lumen contains varied quantities of mucus and blood. **Microscopically, colitis** is characterized by hyperaemia, oedema, haemorrhage, necrosis, and desquamation o f the mucosal epithelium. L arge numbers o f neutrophils a nd macrophages i nfiltrate the m ucosa. It i s due to their ability to p enetrate epithelial c ells that S higella organisms exert t heir pathogenic e ffects.

Genus: Yersinia
Yersiniosis

Genus Yersinia contains three important pathogens. These are: *Y. pestis*, *Y. pseudotuberculosis*, and *Y. enterocolitica*. *Y. pestis* is the cause of **bubonic plague ("black death") in humans**. It is mainly an infection of rats, squirre!s, and other rodents. It is transmitted between rodents, and to humans by the rat flea, *Xenopsylla cheopis*. T he bacteria i nfect the f lea, causing o esophageal obstruction and regurgitation of the deadly bacteria when they take their blood meal. **The disease in humans is an extremely acute septicaemia. Plague is not a disease of domestic animals**, although there have been isolated reports, **particularly in cats**.

Y. pseudotuberculosis and *Y. enterocolitica* have **a variety of molecules on their surface** which are involved in attachment to and phagocytosis by host epithelial cells. They include a protein called **"invasin"** which binds to host cell **integrins**. (Integrins are a family of adhesion proteins found on cell membranes). Multiplication of *Y. enterocolitica* and *Y. pestis* within host cells depends on the presence of a virulence plasmid.

Y. pseudotuberculosis and *Y. enterocolitica* produce **enteric** and **systemic diseases** which are similar but not identical. Unfortunately, both diseases have been described as **"pseudotuberculosis"**, mainly because of the gross appearance of the visceral lesions. Use of the term **"yersiniosis"** has been suggested for these two infections.

Y. pseudotuberculosis infection causes disease mainly in **guinea-pigs, rats,** other **rodents** and **poultry** ("see avian pseudotuberculosis"). Infection, however, has also been reported in many other species, including **humans**, cats, pigs, sheep, goats, horses, rabbits, and mice. The infection may occur as a fatal, acute septicaemia with few specific gross lesions. Usually it occurs as a **chronic infection** which results in discrete, **white or grey nodules in the liver**, spleen, lymph nodes, and lung. **Abortion** has been described in cattle, sheep, and goats, with typical lesions in the placenta and foetus. **Microscopically**, lesions consist of a necrotic core of pus and bacteria surrounded by a zone of macrophages. Epithelioid cells may be present in the lesions of prolonged duration, and a fibrous capsule may be formed. **Giant cells are absent.** In the small intestine, the necrotic lesions containing colonies of organisms usually include the mucosa to the level of muscularis mucosa.

Y. enterocolitica, a similar organism, but distinguishable from *Y. pseudotuberclulosis*, has a similar host range. It produces an enteric infection, usually limited to intestines and mesenteric lymph nodes. It may, however, become generalized and result in visceral lesions. There are ulcers in the lower ileum and necrosis in liver, spleen, and lymph nodes. Colonies of organisms can be seen under the light microscope in the necrotic zones, which are surrounded by neutrophils and macrophages.

Avian Pseudotuberculosis (Yersiniosis)

Avian pseudotuberculosis (AP) is a contagious disease of domesticated and wild birds. It is characterized by an **acute septicaemia** of short duration, followed by **chronic focal infections** which result in **caseous nodules** resembling the tubercles of tuberculosis. *Yersinia pseudotuberculosis* is widespread in almost all domestic poultry and rodents throughout the world. **It has been reported in humans, but is not an important zoonosis. Among domestic poultry, the turkey is most frequently affected**, and mortality of up to 80% has been recorded. Young birds of 4-10 weeks are most susceptible. Infection is spread by contamination of food by an infected host. **The organism gains entry through the intestinal mucosa,** or sometimes through breaks in the skin.

Signs and Lesions

Clinical signs are sometimes similar to those of fowl cholera. Birds may show no premonitory (warning) symptoms and **are found dead.** In the **more chronic cases** there is usually persistent diarrhoea, weakness, ruffled feathers, lameness, and progressive emaciation. Gross lesions include **enlargement of the liver and spleen in acute cases,** while in the more **chronic form** there are **multiple caseous tubercle-like lesions** of varying size in the liver, spleen, and sometimes lungs. Severe enteritis may be present.

Diagnosis

Clinical signs and gross lesions are helpful in diagnosis, but confirmation of the disease depends upon isolation and identification of the organism from the blood in acute cases, and from lesions in chronic cases.

Diseases caused by Spirochaetales Organisms

These bacterial organisms are commonly called "spirochaetes". They are currently grouped in one order, Spirochaetales, which contains **two families: Spirochaetaceae** and **Leptospiraceae. The family Spirochaetaceae contains six genera,** of which **Borrelia, Serpulina,** and **Treponema** contain species pathogenic for animals, birds, and humans. **The family Leptospiraceae contains two genera,** only one of which, **Leptospira,** contains pathogens **(Table 23).**

Table 23.　Classification of Order Spirochaetales

Family	Spirochaetaceae
Genus I	**Borrelia**
	Many species of varying pathogenicity. Diseases include spirochaetosis in **poultry,** Lyme disease (Lyme borreliosis), borreliosis of cattle, sheep, and horses
Genus II	**Serpulina**
	S. hyodysenteriae. Causes **avian** intestinal spirochaetosis
Genus III	**Treponema**
	Only four pathogenic species. Disease includes swine dysentery (porcine ulcerative spirochaetosis)
Family	**Leptospiraceae**
Genus	**Leptospira**
	One pathogenic species (*Leptospira interrogans*), subdivided into several serogroups. They cause leptospirosis in **humans** and animals

In general, spirochaetes are slender, helically coiled, single-celled bacteria measuring 5-30 μm in length. They **are motile** due to periplasmic **flagella**, which are encased within the outer sheath of the organisms. They **multiply by binary fission**, and are best observed by phase-contrast or dark-field microscopy and silver staining techniques. **Specific species cause important diseases in humans** (syphilis, yaws, pinta, relapsing fever, Lyme disease, leptospirosis) **and animals** (spirochaetosis, leptospirosis, and borreliosis).

Genus: Borrelia

Avian Spirochaetosis

Also known as "**borreliosis**", spirochaetosis is caused by the spirochaete, *Borrelia anserina* (*Spirochaeta anserina*, *Treponema anserinum*). It is usually **an acute, septicaemic disease** characterized by marked illness, variable morbidity, and high mortality. Spirochaetosis occurs worldwide. The disease is transmitted by the soft tick, *Argas persicus*. It is therefore limited in distribution to areas where the tick is common. **Spirochaetosis is endemic in certain parts of India**, and causes significant economic losses. The spirochaete can infect a wide variety of birds, **but disease mainly occurs in young fowl.**

Spread

Soft ticks of the genus Argas are the main reservoirs of the organism. *B. anserina* is capable of surviving in either the bird or environment **for long periods**. The organism must rely on the tick for its continued existence. Not all species of **Argas** function as biological vector of spirochaete. *A. persicus* **is the important vector**. After it feeds an infected chicken, spirochaetes **are** numerous in the gut lumen. Within 2 hours, spirochaetes penetrate the gut wall and are present in haemolymph, where they increase in number during the next seven days. By the 7th day, organisms can be found in the tick's tissues, particularly the central nervous mass, **salivary glands**, and gonads, where they remain at least 60 days. *B. anserina* is transmitted transovarially from one generation to the next. Infection rates in larvae from infected female ticks may be as high as 100%.

Ticks become infective 6-7 days after biting a host **and can remain infective up to 488 days**. Although spirochaete **outbreaks** can occur throughout the year, they are **most common during warm, humid seasons. Birds can become infected from saliva introduced by the tick when bitten,** or by ingesting infected ticks or ova. **Recovered birds are not carriers.** Organisms disappear from tissues shortly after they disappear from the circulation.

Signs

Birds are visibly sick with cyanosis or pallor, especially of comb and wattles. Other signs include ruffled feathers, huddled-up appearance, **greenish**

diarrhoea, and birds are inactive and anorectic (anorexic). Characteristically, there is **an abrupt, marked elevation in body temperature,** and a rapid loss of body weight. Body temperature is elevated when spirochaetes are in the circulation, even if their numbers are too low. Affected birds pass fluid, **green droppings** containing excess of bile and urates, probably resulting from anorexia, and have increased water consumption. **Late in the disease,** birds develop paresis (partial paralysis) or paralysis, and become anaemic and are comatose (in coma). **Body temperature is subnormal just prior to death.** Recovered birds are often emaciated and may have paralysis of one or both wings or legs.

Lesions

Grossly, marked enlargement and mottling of the spleen is the most characteristic lesion. Splenomegaly, however, may not be as noticeable when birds are infected with low virulent strains, or early in the disease. The liver may be enlarged and contain small haemorrhages and pale foci. **Kidneys are swollen and pale with urates visible in ureters.** Intestinal contents are usually green and mucoid and there is often variable degree of **haemorrhage,** especially at the **proventriculus-ventriculus junction.** Sometimes, there is mild fibrinous pericarditis, but other serous membranes are not involved.

Microscopically, splenic lesions result from an inflamatory reaction characterized by increased macrophage response, mononuclear-phagocyte system (MPS) hyperplasia, erythrophagocytosis, and haemosiderin deposits. Massive areas of haemorrhage may be present in some birds. The **liver** is congested with increased periportal infiltrates of mixed lymphocytes, haemocytoblasts, and phagocytic cells with vacuolated cytoplasm. **Erythrophagocytosis** and **haemosiderin** are seen in Kupffer cells. Extramedullary haematopoiesis may be present. Silver stains reveal spirochaetes in intercellular spaces and bile canaliculi. Organisms within hepatocytes are usually fragmented or coiled, forming small rings. Lymphoplasmacytic (lymphocytes and plasma cells) infiltrations may be found in **kidneys** and **intestinal lamina propria.** A mild to moderate meningo-encephalitis is sometimes present.

Diagnosis

A clinical diagnosis of spirochaetosis can be made on finding characteristic lesions in birds with signs consistent with the disease. Confirmation requires demonstration of *B. anserina*, or its antigen. During clinical disease, spirochaetes can be found in **stained blood, or organ smears, wet mounts stained by dark-field or phase microscopy, or by immunofluorescence.** Stained blood smears are best used when only a small quantity of blood is available. **Giemsa stain** is usually used, but the organism stains readily with most aniline and Romanowsky dyes. For demonstrating spirochaetes in **tissue sections, silver**

impregnation procedures are used.

Dark-field microscopy is the diagnostic method of choice because of its ease, rapidity and accuracy. Early in the disease, spirochaetaemia may be so low that detection of the organsim is difficult. *B. anserina* can be concentrated in the buffy coat. Spirochaetes undergo agglomeration (formation of a jumbled mass or collection) followed by lysis in the termial stages of the disease, and may no longer be seen in blood or tissues. In some cases, spirochaetal antigens can usually be identified in liver or spleen **by serological tests, or immunofluorescence**.

Spirochaetes can be cultured by inoculating embryos or chicks with infective blood, or organ suspensions. Six-day-old embryonated eggs from spirochaete-free hens inoculated through the yolksac are preferred for embryo culture. Serological tests to identify antibodies in immnue birds include serum plate agglutination test, slide agglutination and immobilization tests, agar gel precipitation test, and indirect fluorescent antibody test.

Lyme Disease

Also known as **"Lyme borreliosis"**, Lyme disease is **most important in humans**, where in many respects it resembles syphilis. Lyme disease was first reported in humans in 1977 as a peculiar form of **arthritis** occurring in Lyme, Connecticut, USA. The disease is now recognized as **a complicated multi-system syndrome** caused by *Borrelia burgdorferi*, so named after **Burgdorfer** who first isolated the spirochaete and associated it with the disease, in 1982. Serological evidence of infection with *Borrelia burgdorferi* has been recorded in several domestic animals - **dogs, cats, horses, cattle, and sheep**.

Spread

The spirochaete is **transmitted to humans by the bite of *Ixodes ticks***. The organism is maintained in the white-footed mouse. **The mice serve as the reservoir hosts for *B. burgdorferi*,** carrying the spirochaete without developing any disease.

Lyme Disease in Humans

Typically, the infection begins with an expanding, **ring-like, pruritic skin rash** known as **"localized erythema migrans" at the site of the tick bite**. Sometimes, it is accompanied by fever, chills, malaise, and meningeal symptoms (**stage I or localized stage**). This is followed weeks to months later by cardiac or neurological involvement, usually accompanied by migratory joint pain (**stage II or disseminated stage**). Months to years later this is followed by oligoarthritis, i.e., chronic arthritis usually of one to a few large joints, particularly the knee (**stage III, late infection, or persistent infection**). Chronic cardiac and central nervous system manifestations are also features of this stage.

At a ll stages, various affected t issues are infiltrated with l ymphoblasts **and plasma cells.**There m ay be n ecrosis, as well as c ellular infiltration, in lymph nodes and spleen. **Arthritis** is characterized by proliferative synovitis, fibrinaceous deposits, and aggregates of lymphoblasts, plasma cells and mast cells. Late in its course, there are erosions of cartilage and bone. Organisms are e asily demonstrable (using silver s taining or i mmunological staining methods) in the early skin lesions. **In stage 2 or 3 lesions, it is difficult to find the organisms. Pathogenesis** of the lesions still remains to be determined, but **immune mechanisms** are thought to play an important role both in the initial and chronic lesions.

Lyme Disease in Animals

None of the domestic species (dogs, cats, horses, cattle or sheep) are considered reservoirs for **Borrelia** species. **A variety of clinico-pathological findings have been described as caused by the spirochaete B. burgdorferi in animals.** These i nclude **arthritis** (one of the m ost c onsistent lesions), encephalitis, uveitis, myocarditis, heart b lock, h epatitis, p neumonia, lymphadenopathy, lymphoblastic/plasmacytic infiltration of various tissues, and immune complex glomerulonephritis. **This list is similar to many of the manifestations of the disease found in humans.** In several of these lesions, *B. burgdorferi* has been isolated or specifically demonstrated, but in many cases the organism cannot be demonstrated or isolated. **The true significance of Lyme disease in domestic animals remains to be clarified.**

Public Health Significance

Birds may be important in the spread of Lyme disease, a borreliosis of humans c aused by *B . b urgdorferi*. This s pirochaete appears to be unique among borrelia i n its a bility to infect by n atural means b oth mammals a nd birds.

Bovine Borreliosis

Bovine borreliosis was first described by **Theiler** in South Africa in 1904. The causative organism *Borrelia theileri*, found in the blood of **cattle**, in South Africa and Australia, is transmitted by several species of ticks. *B. theileri* **is relatively non-pathogenic**, but it has been associated with fever, haemoglobinuria, a nd anaemia. S heep and horses are su sceptible, a nd m ay develop v ery mild d isease.

Genus: Serpulina

Avian Intestinal Spirochaetosis

Avian intestinal spirochaetosis is **a subacute to chronic, non-septicaemic intestinal disease** c haracterized by spirochaetes in the **caecum and/or rectum,**and variable clinical illness, morbidity, and mortality. It is caused by

Serpulina hyodysenteriae. **It is different from** *Treponema hyodysenteriae* **of swine dysentery.** *S. hyodysenteriae* is mildly pathogenic for **young chicks** and **adult hens**. In fact, intestinal spirochaetes are a heterogeneous group of **spiral bacteria** which colonize the large intestine of a variety of avian hosts.

Spread

Intestinal spirochaetes are **transmitted by the faecal-oral route. Ticks and biting insects are not transmission vectors**. Rats, mice, flies, or other animal species can serve as mechanical vectors.

Pathobiology

Avian intestinal spirochaetes can be divided into **three pathotypes:** 1. **Subclinical** or **apathogenic**, 2. **Mildly to moderately pathogenic**, and 3. **Severely pathogenic. They are usually found in the caeca**, but sometimes can be found in the **rectum** and **ileum**. Duodenum and jejunum are not sites of colonization. Naturally occurring infections can result in : 1. Subclinical infection, 2. Mild-to-moderate clinical disease, or 3. Severe clinical disease.

Subclinical disease is characterized by mild transient diarrhoea **in chicks** and yellowish green, frothy caecal contents. **Mild-to-moderate disease is seen in layer chickens**. Clinical signs include wet faeces, diarrhoea, pasty vents, retarded growth rates, delayed onset of laying, production of dirty, faecal-stained eggshells, and reduced mean egg weights. Infected chickens have slimy to frothy, yellowish to brown, fluid-filled caeca, and either lack inflammation or have mild lymphocytic typhlitis. **Severe disease** is characterized by **necrotizing typhlitis** with mortality rates which can vary from 25-80%. The disease usually occurs in **young rheas** (rhea is South American three-toed ostrich). **Clinically**, birds have reduced body weights and pass watery faeces. However, **rheas usually die suddenly without clinical signs**. Caeca are dilated and have thickened walls with ulcerations, and lumina contain thick pseudomembranes.

Diagnosis

Diagnosis can be made on clinical signs, absence of gross lesions at necropsy, and finding of the causal organisms by immunofluorescence in scrapings of the caecal mucosa, or in droppings.

Genus: Treponema

Treponemal Infections

Treponema organisms are most important as pathogens of humans. *T. pallidum*, the cause of **syphilis**, is the most important. Only one **Treponema** species is of importance as a cause of disease in animals, *T. hyodysenteriae*, the cause of **swine dysentery**. There are several non-pathogenic species, which are commensals of humans and animals. The **Treponema** species are **Gram-negative**, but c an be b est seen i n tissue s ections with **silver impregnation staining** methods. In wet smears or cultures, **dark field illumination** is best. They are helical in shape, 5-20 μm in length, motile by means of periplasmic flagella, and a naerobic.

Swine Dysentery

Also known a s **"porcine ulcerative spirochaetosis"**, swine dysentery i s caused by *Treponema hyodysenteriae*. T he disease i s s pread by recovered pigs, which may carry the organism for several months after recovery; and by wild rodents, which can carry the organism without c linical disease.On **ingestion**, the organism establishes itself in colonic epithelium and goblet cells, but d oes not invade deeper. **Infection leads to diarrhoea** containing mucus and blood. Within a herd, morbidity up to 90% and mortality up to 50% result from dehydration and electrolyte imbalance. **Piglets 8-14 weeks of age are the most susceptible.**

Lesions

Lesions are restricted to the colon, caecum, and rectum. However, they are most constant and severe in the spiral colon. The affected mucosa is folded and rugose (corrugated, wrinkled), covered with a fibrinous mucinous exudate with foci of haemorrhage, and eventually, **ulcers. Microscopically**, the mucosa is initially thickened, but later the superficial cells become necrotic and are sloughed. Crypts and epithelial cells contain many spirochaetes.

Diagnosis

The diagnosis is made from the nature of the lesions, and by demonstrating the spirochaetes in the colonic mucosa, using silver stains, immunofluorescent techniques, or electron microscopy.

Genus: Leptospira

Leptospirosis

Genus Leptospira has only one pathogenic species, *Leptospira interrogans*. T his p athogenic s pecies is s ubdivided into **many serogroups** (23) which contain **numerous serovars** (over 212). **These cause leptospirosis in humans and animals (Table 24)**. In other words, the one pathogenic species *L. interrogans* is composed of more than 200 different, but related, organisms. On the basis of serological relatedness, as determined by cross-agglutination and agglutination-absorption tests, these species (serovars) are divided into s erogroups (serotypes), su ch as *L. pomona*, *L. canicola*, a nd *L. icterohaemorrhagiae*. Within each serogroup, there are multiple antigenically distinct organisms, which a re referred t o as s erovars. Thus, d ifferentiation between serovars, belonging to a particular serogroup is done by cross-agglutination tests. Two strains are considered different if, after c ross-absorption with adequate amounts of heterologous antigen, 10% or more of the heterologous titre regularly remains in either of the two antisera. Because this system is considered subjective (i.e., based on personal assessment), the **restriction endonuclease analysis (REA) of leptospiral DNA has been used as a genotyping taxonomic tool**. This method is much less time and labour consuming than cross-agglutination-absorption and gives highly reproducing results.

The **pathogenic serotypes and serovars are not limited to a single host species**. The various serovars cause leptospirosis. **Leptospirosis is a disease of humans and animals with varying clinical and pathological manifestations**. The disease appears to be **worldwide in distribution, including India. In wildlife,** leptospirosis has been reported mainly in deer.

Leptospira are thin (G. leptos = thin) spiral organisms, single and helical, with bent, hooked or curved ends. They are 6-20 μm or more in length by 0.1 μm in diameter. They are motile by means of periplasmic flagella, and are best seen by darkfield microscopy as well as the electron microscope.

Table 24. Host/organism relationship for some of the Leptospira

Serogroup	Serovar	Reservoir (maintenance host)	Other susceptible (accidental) hosts
L. icterohaemorrhagiae	icterohaemorrhagiae	Rats, other wild mammals	Dogs, cattle, pigs, humans
L. canicola	canicola	Dogs, wild mammals	Cattle, pigs, humans
L. pomona	pomona	Pigs, skunk	Cattle, sheep, horses, humans
L. grippotyphosa	grippotyphosa	Raccoon, skunk	Cattle, pigs, dogs
L. sejroe	hardjo balcanica	Cattle	Sheep, humans, cattle
L. australis	bratislava	Horses	-
L. hebdomadis	szwajizak	-	Cattle

Spread

L. pomona is the commonest infection in all animals. **The source of infection is an infected animal** which contaminates pasture, drinking water and feed by infected urine, aborted foetuses, and infected uterine discharges. All the leptospiral species are transmitted in this way a nd can pass between the animal species. **Urine is the chief source of contamination** because animals, particularly **pigs**, even after recovery, may **pass leptospira in the urine for log periods**. They are considered to be a common source of infection to calves on a composite farm. Cattle pass leptospira in the urine for a mean period of 36 days (10-118 days), with the highest excretion rate in the first half of this period. The **semen** of an infected **bull** may carry leptospira, and transmission from such a bull to heifers by coitus and artificial insemination has been reported.

Pathogenesis

Organism enters into the body through cutaneous or mucosal abrasions. Transplacental transmission is not common, but neonatal infection, probably contracted *in utero*, has been recorded. **In all species**, after an interval of bacteraemia, **the organisms localize in the kidney** where they multiply in the lumen of the proximal convoluted tubule and are **excreted in the urine**. This provides the principal mode of transmission and leads to acute or chronic nephritis. **Leptospirosis manifests itself as a disease in a number of ways.** There are **acute** and **subacute forms, a chronic or abortion form**, and an **occult form** in which there is no clinical illness. Which form of the disease occurs depends largely on the species of the host.

Certain serovars are well adapted to their hosts (**reservoir hosts**) and remain in the kidney for long periods. They serve as a constant source of infection to other members of the same species, or accidently infect a species in which the organism is less well adapted (**accidental host**), **but in which more serious disease may result**. For example, rats infected with serovar *icterohaemorrhagiae* shed the organism in the urine for life with little or no ill effect to the host. Ordinarily disease, if present in the reservoir host, is limited to chronic nephritis. When **dogs** (and other susceptible species) are exposed to infectious rat urine, the same organism can cause serious disease. Infection in these "accidently" infected hosts can vary from subclinical to peracute.

Clinical Signs and Lesions

Clinical signs and lesions, which may be **acute and severe**, may develop during the bacteraemic phase of infection, before localization in the kidneys. **The signs and lesions vary somewhat. This depends on the species affected and the serogroup of leptospira**. However, they include extensive haemorrhage, haemolytic anaemia, hepatocellular damage leading to jaundice, and abortion. In addition to the kidneys, leptospira may localize for long periods in other tissues, including uterus, where reproductive disorders follow, and the aqueous humour, where they have been associated with chronic or recurrent iridocyclitis (inflammation of iris and ciliary bidy).

Canine Leptospirosis

Leptospirosis in dogs results from infection with several different serogroups of **Leptospira. Serogroup** *canicola* **is the most common leptospira which infects dogs.** Dog is the reservoir host for this serogroup, with transmission occurring mainly from dog to dog. Serogroup *icterohaemorrhagiae*, acquired from clinically infected rats, is also a common cause of leptospirosis in dogs. O ther s erogroups, s uch a s *g rippotyphosa* occur sporadically. The incidence of infection, especially with serogroup *canicola*, is much more than the incidence of clinical disease.

Leptospirosis in dogs presents itself clinically and pathologically as either an **acute to peracute infection**, with haemorrhage, hepatic dysfunction, and jaundice as the major signs, or **as a subacute nephritis**. The acute infection is usually a ssociated with serogroup *icterohaemorrhagiae*, and the subacute infection with serogroup *canicola*. The two are, however, not separate conditions. Both leptospira c an be associated with e ither condition, a nd dogs recovered from the acute hepatic disease may succumb to uraemia from nephritis. The **acute disease** is characterized by fever, haemorrhages, bloody diarrhoea, vomiting, jaundice, increased erythrocyte sedimentation rate, albuminuria, se vere debilitation, a nd often d eath. The p eracute form, w ith few signs other than haemorrhage, is most common in **puppies**. The **subacute or nephritic form** of the disease, also known as "**Stuttgart disease**", is characterized by typical signs of uraemia, and include "**uraemic**" **breath**, ulcerative stomatitis, vomiting (often bloody), weight loss, dehydration, coma, and death.

Lesions

For c onvenience, lesions f or the " **acute**" and " **subacute**" p hases of t he disease are described separately.

Acute Phase Lesions

In dogs which die during the "**acute**" or "**septicaemic stage**" of the disease, the m ain lesions are **severe dehydration and j aundice**, with many petechiae o n the p leura, peritoneum, a nd nasal a nd oral m ucosa. The l iver usually shows characteristic microscopic changes, although there are no significant gross changes. **The most striking lesion is in the liver cells.** Liver cells sh rink and b ecome dissociated from one another, breaking up the normal columns of liver cells into individually separate cells. This **individualization of liver cells** is not limited solely to leptospirosis, **but is particularly striking in this disease**. The a ffected liver cells have c oarsely granular, eosinophilic cytoplasm and small hyperchromic nuclei. Regeneration of liver parenchyma is a ccompanied by binucleate cells, large hyperchromic n uclei, and mitotic figures. Foci of necrosis of liver parenchyma may be found. Bile retention is indicated by plugging of bile canaliculi, but larger bile ducts are usually e mpty. Kupffer c ells contain large amounts o f haemosiderin. P ortal veins are usually congested. **Leptospira** can be demonstrated with appropriate silver impregnation technique. These organisms are seen in the sinusoids and within liver cells as thin, tightly coiled, spiral organisms with hook-shaped ends.

Changes in the **kidney** during the acute stage are only grossly visible petechiae, but significant changes can be seen on microscopic examination.**The glomeruli do not show much change, but convoluted tubules are usually severely affected**. The epithelial cells of the covoluted tubules are swollen, coarsely granular, and deeply eosinophilic, or vacuolated and partially or completely desquamated into the lumen. In some tubules, only the basement membrane of the tubule is left. In others, the lumen is filled with eosinophilic epithelial cytoplasmic debris, containing some nuclei and occasional erythrocytes. Some tubules may show regenerating epithelium, as indicated by mitosis, hyperchromatic nuclei, and cells which coalesce to appear as multinucleated giant cells. Leptospira are demonstrable singly or in small groups in affected tubules by **silver impregnation techniques**. Affected tubules are surrounded by lymphocytes, plasma cells, and occasional erythrocytes. These diffusely infiltrate the interstitial stroma.

Lymph nodes and **spleen** are usually enlarged, and may contain areas of oedema and haemorrhage. **Microscopically**, there is a lack of mature lymphocytes and an increase in reticular cells. Erythrocytes are present in the medullary sinuses, either free or in macrophages. **Gastric mucosa** usually shows diffuse haemorrhages in the fundic portion, which may be associated with necrosis, neutrophilic infiltration, and desquamation of the mucosa. Haemorrhages may also be present in the submucosa and the muscularis. The intestine may contain small petechiae in the serosa and mucosa.

Haemorrhages and areas of oedema may be seen in other organs, such as myocardium, submucosa, and muscularis of the urinary bladder, adrenal gland, pancreas, gallbladder, and lung. In the **lung**, gross haemorrhages on the pleural surface may be striking, the entire surface being covered with tiny spherical haemorrhages, or larger ones a few millimetres in diameter.

Subacute Phase Lesions

Animals which survive, or escape the "acute septicaemic form" of the disease, die from **uraemia** caused by renal involvement. These animals then show **a subacute course**. At postmortem of such animals, dehydration, emaciation, and **a strong "uraemic" smell** are observed, but **jaundice and haemorrhages are rare. The renal lesions are most significant**. Lesions in other organs are not constant. **The kidneys** are enlarged, surface is usually smooth, capsule is tense and white or greyish, sometimes with haemorrhages. The cut renal parenchyma shows petechiae, **but the most striking changes are at the cortico-medullary junction**. Here, grey masses of firm, swollen tissue replace the normal renal parenchyma. This grey tissue forms a wide band on the inner margin of the cortex. In animals during recovery, these lesions may be focal in pattern. **The microscopic appearance of these lesions is characteristic.** Covoluted tubules undergoing degenerative changes are surrounded, or replaced by large dense masses of cells. These include lymphocytes, plasma cells, macrophages, occasional neutrophils, and sometimes small nests of erythrocytes. A lthough c onvoluted t ubules are s everely affected, **g lomeruli are usually spared**. S ilver preparations d emonstrate leptospira i n the lumen o f tubules, or in the cytoplasm of the tubular epithelium. **The organisms occur singly or in tangled nests**.

Lesions resulting from uraemia are found elsewhere in the body. They include severe gastric h aemorrhage with microscopic deposits of calcium in the gastric mucosa, and calcareous deposits in the wali of the aorta and large arteries.

Bovine Leptospirosis

Leptospirosis in cattle is associated with a wide range of clinical signs and syndromes. T hese include h aemolytic a naemia, hemoglobinuria, jaundice, mastitis, abortion, and nephritis. Several serovars cause disease in cattle. These include *hardjo*, for which **cattle** are the reservoir hosts; *pomona*, which is usually maintained by **pigs**, but is also well adapted to cattle; *icterohaemorrhagiae*, *grippotyphosa*, c *anicola*, s *zwajizak*, a nd b *alcanica*.

Acute disease is most severe in calves, and is characterized by **haemolytic anaemia**. In animals which survive this phase, or in which the bacteraemic phase is subclinical, leptospira localize in the kidneys and produce **interstitial nephritis**. Abortion may occur during the acute or chronic phase of the disease. Abortion usually occurs in the latter half of pregnancy, and is associated with specific lesions in t he placenta o r foetus. Mastitis is usually associated with serovar *hardjo*.

Lesions

The disease in cattle is very similar to that in dogs. It may occur as an "acute septicaemic form" or as a "chronic nephritic type". The latter is rarely fatal. The lesions in these two types are similar to those observed in dogs.

In the **acute form**, jaundice, swollen yellowish liver, and petechiae are the main gross findings, as in dogs. **Haemolytic anaemia**, which is not a feature of the canine disease, a ccounts for h aemoglobinuria in c alves and p artially contributes to the jaundice and hepatic lesions. **Microscopic changes** include portal h epatic lymphocytic infiltration, s plenic h aemosiderosis, and severe centrilobular necrosis of the liver caused by anaemic anoxia. In the kidneys, swelling and disorganization of convoluted tubular epithelium are associated with bile pigment and haemoglobin in the lumen.

Animals which survive the acute septicaemic disease have focal lesions in the kidney parenchyma (**chronic nephritic type**). These foci are usually separate and scattered throughout the cortex, **not concentrated at the cortico-medullary junction, as is the case in dogs. Microscopically**, the epithelial cells and affected tubules have granular, swollen, or vacuolated cytoplasm. These affected tubules are surrounded by dense masses of leukocytes, mainly lymphocytes and plasma cells. In some cases, syncytial giant cells of the Langhans' type have been observed. Leptospira are usually but not constantly, demonstrated in sections impregnated with silver. They are located within affected tubular epithelium or in the lumen of the tubule.

Porcine Leptospirosis

Pigs, like most other species, are susceptible to several serogroups of **Leptospira**. The most common pathogen is the serovar *pomona*, for which pigs are the reservoir host. Most infections with this serovar are subclinical. Urinary excretion spreads the organism in the pigs, and serves as a source of infection for other species, which are more severely affected. These include **cattle** and **humans**, in whom the disease has been termed "**swineherd's disease**". Serovar *pomona* infection is mainly associated with chronic lymphocytic interstitial nephritis. This serovar along with others, such as *icterohaemorrhagiae* and *canicola*, are an important cause of abortion, still-births, and deaths of neonatal pigs. In young pigs, the latter two serovars can cause acute leptospirosis similar to that seen in cattle, with haemolytic anaemia, haemoglobinuria, hepatitis, and icterus.

Stillborn pigs and aborted foetuses are expelled mainly in the last third of gestation. The most characteristic lesion in aborted foetusus and stillborns is **focal necrosis of the liver**, without significant cellular infiltration. Organisms can usually be isolated, but are difficult to demonstrate in tissues.

Leptospirosis in Other Species

Serological evidence indicates that leptospirosis is a relatively common infection in **horses**, but clinical disease is rare. Serovars *icterohaemorrhagiae*, *pomona*, and *hardjo* are associated with febrile illnesses, abortion, periodic ophthalmia, and rarely jaundice. **Leptospirosis in sheep and goats resembles the disease in cattle.** The most common serovars are *pomona* and *hardjo*. Acute haemolytic disease, abortion and interstitial nephritis are the main conditions associated with leptospirosis in these species. **Cats** are susceptible to several leptospiral serovars, but the infection is not associated with clinical or pathological changes.

The Higher Bacteria

Order Actinomycetales

The order **Actinomycetales** is composed of several families, some of which contain pathogenic o rganisms. **These organisms are referred to as higher bacteria since they usually induce lesions which resemble those produced by fungi.** Some of the o rganisms even have morphological and biochemical characteristics which are shared by fungi. **They are, however, bacteria lacking eukaryotic nuclei and mitochondria.** The classification used is over-simplified, but the i mportant animal pathogens are i n the f ollowing genera: **Actinomyces, Corynebacterium, Dermatophilus, Mycobacterium, Nocardia, and R hodococcus.**

Genus: Actinomyces

Actinomycosis

Actinomycosis occurs fro m infection by org anisms of the genus **Actinomyces. Although not fungi, the lesions produced by these bacteria closely r esemble the t rue mycotic d iseases.** The currently recognized Actinomyces, t heir hosts, and the d iseases they p roduce are listed in **Table 25.** Other species also exist, but are not pathogenic. All the actinomyces are of **low pathogenicity, and are mostly commensals in the oral cavity and intestinal tract. They gain entry into tissues through injuries.** The classical disease, caused by *Actinomyces bovis*, occurs in **cattle,** but many sp ecies can be infected by *A. bovis* under natural conditions. The most important manifestation of **actinomycosis in cattle** is the hard, irregular enlargement which o ccurs from i nfection of t he mandible (lower jawbone), a nd less often the maxilla (upper jawbone), which gives the disease its common name **"lumpy jaw". In wildlife,** actinomycosis has been reported in deer and antelope.

Table 25. Actinomycosis

Actinomyces	Host(s)	Tissues affected/diseases caused
Actinomyces bovis	Cattle, pigs, horses	Mandible, maxilla, soft tissues, or generalized
A. israeli	Humans, cattle, pigs	Soft tissues, may be generalized
A. naeslundii	Pigs Humans	Foetus (abortion) Bony and soft tissues, eye
A. pyogenes	Humans, cattle, sheep, horses	Skin abscesses, mastitis, peritonitis, lymphadenitis
A. hordeovulneris	Dogs	Pleuritis, peritonitis, visceral abscesses, arthritis
A. suis	Pigs	Mammary gland, foetus (abortion)

A. viscosus	Humans, pigs, cats, dogs	Bony and soft tissues, periodontal disease
A. denticolens	Cattle	Oral cavity commensal
A. howellii	Cattle	Oral cavity commensal

In dogs actinomycosis is usually caused by *A. hordeovulneris*. It affects soft tissues and may become generalized. **In humans,** *A. israeli* is the usual infecting organism; the cheek, mouth, skin of the chest, appendix, and intestine are the usual sites of involvement. Infection of the mammary glands **in pigs** by *A. suis* is not uncommon. *A. suis* and *A. naeslundii* also have been associated with abortion in pigs, causing typical lesions in the uterus and foetus, particularly in the lungs. **Actinomyces** have also been identified in association with *Brucella abortus* in equine "**fistulous withers**".

Actinomycosis in Cattle (Lumpy Jaw)

Actinomycosis in cattle is caused by *Actinomyces bovis*. However, other bacteria may be present in extensive lesions. The most common manifestation of actinomycosis is **a rarefying osteomyelitis** of the bones of the head, particularly the **mandible** and **maxilla.** At times it involves soft tissues, particularly the alimentary tract. It is reported from most countries of the world. Occasional cases occur in **pigs** and **horses.**

Spread

A. bovis **is a common inhabitant of the bovine mouth,** and infection occurs through wounds in the buccal mucosa caused by sharp pieces of feed or foreign material. Infection may also occur through dental alveoli. This may account for the more common occurrence of the disease in **young cattle** when teeth are erupting. Infection of the alimentary tract is related to laceration by sharp foreign bodies.

Signs

Actinomycosis of the jaw begins as a **painless, bony swelling** which appears on the **mandible** or **maxilla,** usually at the level of the central molar teeth. The enlargement may be diffuse or localized. In the case of **mandible,** it may appear only as a thickening of the lower edge of the bone with most of the enlargement in the intermandibular space. Some lesions enlarge rapidly within a few weeks, others slowly over a period of months. **The swellings are very hard,** are immovable, and in the later stages, painful to the touch. They usually break through the skin and discharge through one or more openings. The **discharge of pus** is small in amount and consists of sticky, honey-like fluid containing minute, hard, yellow white granules. In severe cases, **spread to contiguous (neighbouring) soft tissues** may be extensive and involve the muscles and fascia of the throat. Excessive swelling of the **maxilla** may cause dyspnoea. Involvement of the local lymph nodes does not occur.

The most common form of **actinomycosis of soft tissues** is involvement of the oesophageal groove region. It then spreads to the lower oesophagus and the anterior wall of the reticulum The syndrome is one of impaired digestion. There is periodical diarrhoea with the passage of undigested food material, chronic bloat, a nd a llotriophagia (perverted appetite f or injurious, u nusual and nonedible s ubstances).

Lesions

The organisms grow in colonies of microscopic size. They are located in purulent centres surrounded by dense granulation tissue, which displaces the normal tissues. W hen organisms p enetrate the b one, t he bone b ecomes enlarged and honeycombed as a result of **rarefaction** (process of making the bone more porous) and regenerative proliferation. The cut surface of the lesion is usually white and glistening from the dense connective tissue in which the **small abscesses** are embedded. Occasional sinus tract may drain through the skin, or into the oral cavity. The squeezing of yellowish pus **from the abscesses** yields tiny hard masses called "**sulphur granules**". They are so called because of their gross consistency and yellowish colour. **Microscopically**, these masses may a ppear as r osettes (something that resembles r ose) w hich a re s imply separate colonies of actinomyces organisms growing in characteristic fashion. In H & E stained sections, a colony apperas as a basophilic mass, 20 microns or more in diameter, surrounded by a zone of radially arranged ((i.e., arranged like rays) eosinophilic projections.

The central part of the colony can be demonstrated by Gram's stain. It is made up of a mass of **Gram-positive, rod-shaped, or long filamentous organisms**, which are sometimes b ranched. The m ass of o rganisms is s urrounded by zones of r adiating (spreading out like r ays) club-shaped s tructures. Beyond t he radiating c lubs, there i s usually a zone o f neutrophils, surrounded b y an o uter area o f large m ononuclear (epithelioid) cells w ith abundant, often foamy c ytoplasm. Giant cells of t he Langhans' t ype and lymphocytes are sometimes found. The dense vascular connective tissue which separates the many abscesses from one another usually encapsulates the entire lesion.

The colonies of actinomyces may become **calcified** in cases of long standing. They then assume a **gritty texture** as blue-staining **granules of calcium salts** replace the organisms. Actinomycosis of other tissues, and in other species, may h ave a s imilar microscopic a ppearance. In so me situations, h owever, as in actinomycotic pleuritis and peritonitis (usually in dogs), the lesions are a more diffuse purulent inflammation, **without distinct g ranuloma formation**.

Diagnosis

The characteristic lesions can be identified by using **Gram's stain on tissue sections**. This will differentiate the Gram-positive organisms at the centre of the colonies. Organisms can also be demonstrated in smears of fresh, unfixed material stained by Gram's method. The rosettes with the radiating clubs can be demonstrated in **wet preparations of fresh pus** compressed under a coverslip and examined under low illumination.

Differential diagnosis must include other granulomatous infections, particularly actinobacillosis, nocardiosis, and staphylococcosis (botryomycosis). The morphology of the bacterial colonies and individual organisms and their staining reactions differ in each of these infections. This allows ready differentiation.

Genus: Corynebacterium

Corynebacteria are involved in a wide variety of lesions in many domestic animals, as well as in humans. The best known organism in this genus is *Corynebacterium diphtheriae*, cause of **human diphtheria**. Other members of this group are referred to as **"diphtheroid bacteria"**. Many of these are of low pathogenicity, and exist as commensals in otherwise normal animals. Predisposing factors play an important role in the induction of disease. The lesions produced by various corynebacteria show much variety. The tissue reaction to some is mainly **necrotizing**, to most it is **suppurative**, and to others **granulomatous**.

Corynebacteria are **Gram-positive**, non acid-fast, and sometimes "beaded" in stained tissue sections. They share features with **Mycobacteria** and **Nocardia**, but can be easily differentiated. The pathogenic corynebacteria are listed in **Table 26**.

Table 26.   Pathogenic Corynebacteria

Corynebacterium	Disease
C. diphtheriae	Diphtheria in humans
C. renale C. cystitidis	Pyelonephritis, ureteritis, cystitis in cows Haemorrhagic cystitis and pyelonephritis in cows
C. pilosum	Cystitis and pyelonephritis in cows
C. pseudotuberculosis (C. ovis)	Caseous lymphadenitis in sheep and goats; ulcerative lymphagitis and pectoral abscesses in horses
C. bovis C. suis (Eubacterium suis)	Rare cause of mastitis in cattle Pyelonephritis and cystitis in pigs

C. pyogenes *(Actinomyces pyogenes)*	Suppurative infections in cattle, sheep, goats, and pigs
C. ulcerans	Wound infections and abscesses in many species
C. equi (Rhodococcus equi)	Pneumonia in horses

C.pyogenes, now called *Actinomyces pyogenes*, is a common and important organism in **pyogenic processes** in cattle, pigs, sheep, and goats. **In cattle**, the organisms are found in abscesses, many of which are encapsulated, and in necrotic and suppurative pneumonias. They have also been isolated from suppurative arthritis and umbilical infections in calves, and from purulent metritis and mastitis in cows. **In pigs**, the "**diphtheroid**" organisms produce diseases resembling those of cattle. Arthritis is a common manifestation. **In sheep** and **goats**, purulent pneumonias and abscesses in the upper respiratory tract have been described.

C. renale is commonly associated with "**bacillary pyelonephritis**" of cattle, in which chronic purulent cystitis and urethritis accompany the inflammatory changes in the ureters and renal pelvis. **Horses** and **sheep** may become infected, but dogs are rarely infected. **In cattle**, the disease is mainly confined to **cows**; it is **rare in bulls**. In affected herds, *C. renale* can be recovered from healthy individuals. The lesions may affect the entire urinary tract. The bladder, ureters, and renal pelvis are dilated with thickened walls and necrosis and haemorrhage of the mucosa. The mucosa becomes covered with a fibrino-necrotic membrane. Abscesses may be present throughout the kidneys.

Two other corynebacteria also cause cystitis and pyelonephritis in cows. *C. pilosum* causes a disease similar to that produced by *C. renale*, and *C. cystitidis* is associated with a severe haemorrhagic cystitis and also pyelonephritis in cows. **In pigs**, an organism which has been called *C. suis*, but is now classified as *Eubacterium suis*, causes cystitis, pyelonephritis, and metritis in sows.

C. pseudotuberculosis (*C. ovis*) is the cause of caseous lymphadenitis or pseudotuberculosis of sheep and goats. *C. pseudotuberculosis* also causes ulcerative lymphangitis, pectoral abscesses and folliculitis (inflammation of hair follicle) in **horses**.

A bacterium which has been called *Corynebacterium equi*, but is more correctly classified as *Rhodococcus equi*, is the cause of a specific **pneumonia in foals**, and sometimes, pneumonia in cattle, sheep, humans, and other species. This is discussed under **Rhodococcus**.

Ovine Caseous Lymphadenitis (Pseudotuberculosis of Sheep and Goats)

Caseous lymphadenitis is **a chronic disease of sheep and goats characterized by the formation of abscesses in lymph nodes**. The disease is caused by *C. pseudotuberculosis* (*C. ovis*), a *Gram-positive* diphtheroid bacillus.

Spread

The organism gains entry by **way of abrasions** in the skin or oral mucous membranes, and less commonly, through **inhalation**. Infection is seen rarely in cattle.

Pathogenesis

Spread of infection from infected skin sites leads to involvement of local lymph nodes, and the **develoment of abscesses**. *C. pseudotuberculosis* **is an intracellular organism and lives inside cells**. Although readily phagocytosed by macrophages, these bacteria are resistant to intracellular destruction. *C. pseudotuberculosis* **produces an exotoxin (a phospholipase D) and possesses toxic surface lipid, which allows the organism to survive within macrophages**. The high lipid content of the bacterial cell wall gives resistance to the lysosomal enzymes of the phagocyte, **and the organism persists as an intracellular parasite**. The disease is **characterized by abscesses of lymph nodes**, usually the prescapular and prefemoral, but may become generalized from haematogenous spread of the organism from these local lesions with abscess formation in many organs, including lungs, liver, kidney, brain, and spinal cord.

Signs

There is palpable **enlargement** of one or more of the **superficial lymph nodes**. Those most commonly affected are the submaxillary, prescapular, prefemoral, supramammary, and popliteal nodes. **The abscesses usually rupture and thick, green pus is discharged**. In cases in which systemic involvement occurs, chronic pneumonia, pyelonephritis, ataxia (incoordination) and paraplegia (paralysis of hind portion of the body and of both legs) may be present.

Lesions

Lesions are usually restricted to lymph nodes, particularly prescapular, prefemoral, and mediastinal nodes, and less often, lungs, kidneys, and other viscera. **Microscopically**, the lesion starts as a small nidus (focus) of epithelioid cells but is soon transformed into **caseous necrosis**, which becomes the main feature. The central caseous mass is soon surrounded by a thin layer of epithelioid cells mixed with lymphocytes, to which an external layer of fibrous connective tissue is added. **As the lesion grows**, the epithelioid and fibrous reactive layers undergo necrosis; the epithelioid layer dies first. While the fibrous layer still remains visible, new reactive layers form outside it, one after another become necrotic. **The result is a spherical, onion-like, concentrically laminated mass.** Calcification may occur, **but giant cells are not seen**.

The **gross appearance of lymph nodes is characteristic**. The entire node is greatly enlarged and almost replaced by a single spherical lesion. In cross section, it is concentrically laminated. Layers of fibrous capsule alternate with caseous, friable material which is greenish, and sometimes gritty. In the **lungs**, the lesions may resemble an abscess, with a central, semifluid mass of yellowish or greenish pus.

Zoonotic Implications

Human infection has been reported on rare occasions and is **an occupational disease of shearers** (persons who cut sheep's wool). Infection occurs through cuts. *C. pseudotuberculosis* may be present in the milk of goats from udders where the mammary lymph node is affected.

Diagnosis

The **gross and microscopic features, if typical, are practically diagnostic**. Examination of pus taken by needle biopsy for the presence of *C. pseudotuberculosis* is the usual laboratory technique. Isolation of the causative organism depends on demonstrating its diphtheroid morphology and cultural characteristics. The serological tests which have been examined detect antibodies to the exotoxin of *C. pseudotuberculosis* and include indirect haemagglutination, haemolysis inhibition, and immunodiffusion. ELISA tests have also been developed to detect antibody to cell wall antigens as well as to exotoxin. None of these tests has good specificity and sensitivity.

Ulcerative Lymphangitis of Horses and Cattle

Ulcerative lymphangitis is a mildly contagious disease mainly of **horses** and sometimes **cattle characterized by lymphangitis of the lower limbs**. It is caused by *C. pseudotuberculosis*. Infection occurs through abrasions on the lower limbs and is more likely when horses are crowded together in dirty, unhygienic quarters. Infection of skin wounds is followed by invasion of lymphatics and the **development of abscesses** along their course. Lymph node involvement is unusual.

Signs and Lesions

In horses the initial wound infection is followed by swelling and pain of the pastern, sufficient to cause severe lameness. **Nodules** develop in the subcutaneous tissue **around the fetlock**, but can spread to subcutaneous sites on all parts of the body. These may enlarge 5-7 cm in diameter and rupture to discharge a **creamy green pus**. The **resulting ulcer** has irregular edges and a necrotic base. Lymphatics draining the area become enlarged and hard, and secondary ulcers m ay develop along them. Lesions heal i n 1 -2 weeks but fresh crops may occur, and cause persistence of the disease for up to 12 months. The lesions in **cattle** are similar to those in **horses**, except that there may be lymph node enlargement and the ulcers discharge a gelatinous clear exudate.

Isolation of *C. pseudotuberculosis* from discharging lesions is necessary to confirm the **diagnosis**.

Genus: Dermatophilus

Dermatophilus Infection (Cutaneous Streptothricosis)

Infection by the bacterium *Dermatophilus congolensis* has also been termed mycotic dermatitis, proliferative dermatitis, cutaneous streptothricosis, strawberry foot-rot (sheep), lumpy wool, and cutaneous actinomycosis. **Dermatophilus infection** has been described in cattle, sheep, goats, horses, pigs, cats, m onkeys, fowl, and **humans. I n each of these species, with the exception of humans, the gross and histopathological changes are similar.**

Pathogenesis

The organism invades and multiplies within the epidermis as branching filaments. These filaments divide i n a c haracteristic fashion, g iving rise to multiple rows of coccoid organisms. They do not invade the dermis, but **produce an extensive purulent exudate beneath the epidermis**, separating it from the dermis. The invaded epidermis c ornifies, and a new e pidermis forms u nder the exudate, which i n turn i s invaded by hyphae at the p eriphery. A second inflammatory exudate separates the n ew epidermis f rom the d ermis, and a third epithelium is generated. **The process is repeated**, a nd results in thick scab composed o f alternate l ayers of c ornified epidermis a nd exudate. T he organisms can be seen in H & E stained tissue sections, **and are clearly visible as Gram-positive filaments, or chains of cocci in sections with Gram's technique.**

The disease is spread by the coccoid forms, which result from division of the hyphae. This stage is known as "**zoospore**". It is motile and released when the scabs a re exposed t o moisture. Spread can be direct or indirect through contaminated water o r g rasses. F lies and ticks are the principal m eans o f spreading zoospores.

Dermatophilus infection rarely affects tissues other than the skin. It can produce granulomatous lesions containing colonies of organisms in the subcutis, lymph nodes, tongue, tonsils, and u rinary bladder in c ats, c attle, goats, pigs, and humans. In the **granulomas in cattle**, colonies of *D. congolensis* are surrounded by r adiating c lubs resembling actinomycosis. The granulomas consist of a central core of neutrophils containing organisms, surrounded by a zone of macrophages, multinucleated giant cells, and fibrous connective t issue.

Lesions

The infection is usually limited to the skin. It produces raised, alopecic, and sometimes p apillomatous lesions caused by t hick keratinaceous c rusts. The lesions may be well-circumscribed or confluent (fused), a nd may affect the sk in of a ny portion of the b ody. At t imes, organisms m ay reach lymph nodes r esulting in a granulomatous r esponse.

Diagnosis

Diagnosis usually can be made from the morphology of the exudate, and demonstration of the organisms. If necessary, the organism can be cultured.

Genus: Mycobacterium

Tuberculosis

Tuberculosis is a disease caused by certain organisms of the genus **Mycobacterium**. Mycobacteria are **curved o r r od-shaped**, sometimes filamentous, **acid-fast bacteria**. They a re r elated t o the genera **Nocardia, Corynebacterium**, and **Rhodococcus**. Many species of **Mycobacterium**, other than those causing tuberculosis, are pathogenic for humans and animals. These are listed in **Table 27**.

Table 27. Mycobacterial Infections

Organism	Host(s)	Disease
M. tuberculosis	Humans, monkeys, dogs, rarely other domestic animals	Tuberculosis
M. bovis	Humans, cattle, dogs, cats, sheep, goats, pigs, horses, monkeys	Tuberculosis
M. avium	Domestic and wild fowl, pigs, humans, monkeys, rarely other domestic animals	Tuberculosis
M. ulcerans	Humans	Indolent (without pain) skin ulcers
M. intracellulare	Humans, monkeys, cattle, pigs	Pulmonary disease (tuberculosis)
M. kansasii	Humans, cattle	Pulmonary disease, lymphadenitis
M. farcinogenes, and	Cattle	"Bovine farcy"

M. senegalense		
M. lepraemurium	Cats?	Feline leprosy
M. paratuberculosis	Cattle, sheep	Paratuberculosis (Johne's disease)
M. leprae	Humans	Leprosy
M. fortuitum	Humans, dogs, cats, cattle, pigs	Soft tissue infections
M. smegmatis	Cattle	Mastitis (usually a commensal)

Apart from cattle, pigs, monkeys, and domestic fowl, tuberculosis is not a common disease of animals. In wildlife, it has been recorded in camels, deer, antelope and llamas.Throughout most of the world, **the bovine disease is widespread, including India.** In most countries, contol of bovine tuberculosis has significantly reduced the prevalence of infection of the bovine type in both humans and animals. **Three species of Mycobacterium cause tuberculosis.**

Mycobacterium tuberculosis is the type species and the main cause of tuberculosis in humans and monkeys. It occasionally causes tuberculosis in dogs, but other domestic animals, such as cattle and cats, are relatively resistant. Among laboratory animals, **guinea-pigs** are highly susceptible, but rabbits and birds are resistant. **Spread** of infection is **mainly by aerosol** (fine particles/droplets s uspended in a ir) from i nfected humans. The organism i s rarely maintained in other species.

Mycobacterium bovis is closely related to *M. tuberculosis*. It is the **cause of tuberculosis in cattle** and in o ther domestic a nimals. **Humans are also susceptible,** usually acquiring the **infection from ingestion of infected milk.** It is a lso pathogenic for **sheep, goats, dogs, cats, horses, pigs,** and s ome species of birds, such as **parrots.** Rabbits, guinea-pigs, and monkeys are easily infected, whereas mice are more resistant. The organism is only slightly pathogenic for rats. D omestic fowls are not s usceptible. The o rganism is maintained in cattle, and is spread in cattle mainly by aerosol, **but calves can be infected by ingestion of milk or *in utero*.**

Mycobacterium avium is the main cause of tuberculosis in domestic fowl and wild birds. It is also an important p athogen for **pigs,** but rarely causes tuberculosis in other animals, although it may infect dogs, cats, horses, sheep, goats, monkeys, and **humans.** It is clearly re lated to *Mycobacterium intracellulare* and isolates are usually named *M. avium-intracellulare*. At times these cause tuberculosis in animals as well a s in **humans,** especially in immunocompromised (immunologically d amaged) individuals. *M. avium* is not pathogenic for guinea-pigs and rats, but can infect rabbits and mice. *M. avium* is maintained in birds, and **spreads mainly by ingestion**. The source of infection for other species is not always related to contact with infected birds. For example, **both healthy pigs and monkeys carry the organism in their digestive tracts**, the most common site of lesions. Immuno-suppression allows its presence to progress to disease in monkeys, where lesions may be present in a high percentage of certain herds.

Pathogenesis of Tuberculosis

Recent studies on *M. tuberculosis* have given a new insight into the pathogenesis of tuberculosis. **Pathogenicity of *M. tuberculosis* is due to its ability to escape killing by macrophages and induce delayed type hypersensitivity. This is on account of several components in its wall. First is cord factor**, a surface glycolipid. Virulent strains of *M. tuberculosis* have cord factor on their surface, whereas avirulent strains do not. It causes formation of characteristic granuloma. **Second is lipoarabinomannan (LAM)**, a heteropolysaccharide similar in structure to the endotoxin of Gram-negative bacteria. It inhibits macrophage activation by interferon-gamma. LAM also induces macrophage to secrete tumour necrosis factor-alpha, which causes fever, weight loss, and tissue damage; and interleukin-10 that suppresses mycobacteria-induced T cell proliferation. **Third, is complement**. When activated on the surface of mycobacteria, it opsonizes the organism and facilitates its uptake by the macrophage complement receptor (CR3). However, this occurs without triggering the respiratory burst necessary to kill the organisms. **Fourth**, a highly immunogenic *M. tuberculosis* **heat-shock protein**. This has a role in autoimmune reactions induced by *M. tuberculosis*.

The primary phase of *M. tuberculosis* begins with inhalation of the mycobacteria and ends with a T cell-mediated immune response which produces hypersensitivity to the organisms. Inhaled *M. tuberculosis* is first phagocytosed by alveolar macrophages and transported by these cells to lymph nodes. Normal macrophages are unable to kill the mycobacteria, which multiply, destroy the host cell, infect other macrophages, and sometimes spread through the blood to other parts of the lung and elsewhere in the body. **After a few weeks, T cell-mediated immunity develops**. Mycobacteria-activated T cells interact with macrophages in **three ways. First**, CD4+ helper T cells secrete **interferon-gamma**, which activates macrophages to kill intracellular mycobacteria through nitrogen intermediates, such as **NO (nitric oxide), NO2, and HNO3 (nitric acid)**. This is associated with the formation of epithelioid cell granulomas and clearance of mycobacteria. **Second**, CD8+ suppressor T cells lyse macrophages infected with mycobacteria. **Third**, CD4- CD8- **(double-negative) T cells** lyse macrophages, without killing mycobacteria. Lysis of macrophages results in the formation of **caseating granulomas** (delayed type hypersensitivity reactions). Direct toxicity of the mycobacteria to the macrophages may contribute to the **necrotic caseous centres. To conclude**, development of cell-mediated or type IV hypersensitivity to the tubercle bacillus, is probably due to the organism's destructiveness in tissues and also to the emergence of resistance to the organisms.

Tuberculosis caused by *Mycobacterium bovis*

M. bovis is the specific cause of tuberculosis in **cattle**. The disease is characterized by the progressive development of tuberculosis in different organs. **All species, including humans, and all age groups are susceptible to *M. bovis*. Cattle, goats and pigs are most susceptible**, sheep and horses showing high natural resistance.

Spread

Infected cattle are the main source of infection for other cattle. Organisms are excreted in the expired air, in sputum, faeces (both from intestinal lesions and swallowed sputum from pulmonary lesions), milk, urine, and vaginal and uterine discharges. Usually, entry occurs through **inhalation** or **ingestion**. **Inhalation is the most common portal of entry** in housed cattle, and even those at pasture it is considered to be the main method of transmission. Infection by **ingestion** is more likely at pasture when faeces contaminate the feed, and common drinking water and feed troughs.

Pathogenesis

Tuberculosis **spreads** in the body **in two stages**, the **primary complex** and **post-primary dissemination**. The **primary complex** consists of the lesion at the point of entry, and in the local lymph node. A lesion at the point of entry is common when infection is by **inhalation**. When infection occurs through the alimentary tract, a lesion at the site of entry is uncommon, although tonsillar and intestinal ulcers may occur. Usually the only visible lesion is in the pharyngeal or mesenteric lymph nodes. **Post-primary dissemination** from the primary complex may take the form of acute miliary (small tubercles like a millet seed) tuberculosis, discrete nodular lesions in various organs, or chronic organ tuberculosis caused by endogenous or exogenous reinfection of tissues rendered allergic to tuberculoprotein. In cattle, horses, sheep, and goats, the disease is a progressive one. Although generalized tuberculosis is uncommon in pigs, the disease is usually characterized by localized abscesses in the lymph nodes of the head and neck.

Signs

Cattle

Some cows with extensive miliary tuberculous lesions are **clinically normal**, but in most cases **progressive emaciation** unassociated with other signs occurs. This should arouse suspicion of tuberculosis. An erratic appetite and fluctuating temperature are also usually associated with the disease. The hair coat may be r ough. Pulmonary i nvolvement is c haracterized by a chronic cough due to bronchopneumonia. Rarely tuberculous ulcers of the small intestine cause diarrhoea. **Tuberculous mastitis is of great importance because of the danger to public health,** and spread of the disease to calves.

Pigs

Tuberculous lesions in cervical lymph nodes u sually c ause no clinical abnormality, u nless they r upture to the exterior. G eneralized cases p resent signs similar to those seen in cattle. However, tuberculous involvement of the meninges and joints is more common in pigs.

Horses

The commonest signs in horses are caused by the involvement of the **cervical vertebrae** in which a painful osteomyelitis causes stiffness of the neck, and inability to eat from the ground.

Sheep and Goats

Bronchopneumonia is the commonest form of the d isease i n these species, and is manifested by cough and terminal (fatal) dyspnoea. In some goats, intestinal ulceration with diarrhoea, and enlargement of the lymph nodes of the alimentary tract occur. In both species, the disease is only slowly progressive.

Lesions

The characteristic lesion of tuberculosis is the tubercle. It is **a classical granuloma** composed of a collection of **epithelioid cells** surrounded by a rim of fibroblasts w ith s cattered l ymphocytes. The c entre of the g ranuloma i s usually necrotic and calcified. The **tubercle** is the host's reaction to the invading organism. Its p athogenesis depends on a n immunological r esponse, k nown as **hypersensitivity.** The initial lesion consists of a small group of neutrophils surrounding invading bacilli. This is replaced in few hours by a rim of macrophages. The mycobacteria are ingested, **but multiply intracellularly, due in part to mycobacterial glycolipids which prevent fusion of phagosomes with lysosomes.** W ith unchecked intracellular multiplication, the organisms gain entry into lymphatics and are carried to regional lymph nodes and distant sites.

With the onset of **an immune response,** t he lesion d evelops the typical features of **a granuloma.** The rim of macrophages takes a different a ppearance. The cells acquire an abundant e osinophilic cytoplasm a nd are t ermed **epithelioid cells,** si nce they are su ggestive of epithelial c ells. Although derived from circulating monocytes and phagocytes, epithelioid cells contain abundant e ndoplasmic reticulum s uggestive of a n adaptation t o a s ecretory cell. Fusion of epithelioid cells leads to the formation of multinucleated giant cells up to 50 microns in diameter. These are called **Langhans' giant cells**, in which the nuclei are arranged in a wreath (ring) or crescent (sickle-shaped) at the periphery of the cell. As the granuloma increases in size, the central cells undergo **caseous necrosis. Calcification** may occur in the caseous centre of the tubercle, **except in avian tuberculosis in birds**, where it is almost unknown. Tubercle bacilli can be demonstrated with **acid-fast stains** in the cytoplasm of Langhans' giant c ells, epithelioid c ells, and i n the c aseous necrotic d ebris. Their number m ay be v ery few, a nd finding t hem may r equire a laborious search.

As the lesion progresses, collagenous connective tissue surrounding the lesion increases in amount and maturity. If the bacteria in the lesion are eventually overcome, the tubercle is reduced to a mass of fibrous or hyaline scar tissue. There is some evidence, however, that even with healing, the organisms may n ot be c ompletely eliminated, b ut persist a s a latent infection. **I f the immune responses are not effective, the lesions continue to grow**, develop large cavitary centres (i.e., containing cavities), and c ontinue to disseminate to other organs. Most tubercles are between 1mm to 2cm in diameter, but big tubercles m ay be formed by the growth a nd fusion of one or more adjacent single t ubercles.

Infection with tubercle bacilli does not always result in the formation of typical tubercles. This occurs particularly in meningeal tuberculosis, a rapidly fatal infection. In this, the pathological changes consist of a scanty fibrinous or fibrino-purulent exudate on the surface of pia mater, and only a small number of epithelioid cells in meninges. Tissue reaction of a similar diffuse type may occur in very severe infections in sensitized animals.

Grossly, a tubercle is a firm or hard, white, grey, or yellow nodule, whether it is deep i n soft t issue like l iver and l ungs, or b ulging from a mucous o r serous surface. **On cut section**, its yellowish, caseous, necrotic centre is dry and solid **in contrast to the pus in an abscess. Calcification** is common in many animals. O n cutting a tubercle, **a gritty sensation** and g rating s ound indicate the presence of calcareous material.

Sometimes a tubercle breaks into a blood vessel, or by other means the blood is se eded with l arge numbers of tubercle bacilli. The bacilli lodge in capillaries of the parenchyma of visceral organs, where they give rise to innumerable tubercles, 2-3 mm in diameter, and all of the same age and size. To early o bservers, these lesions appeared a s if m illet seeds were sprinkled o n the organ su rfaces. They t herefore gave t he name m iliary tuberculosis (L. miliaris = like a millet seed) to infection of this rapidly fatal type.

Lesions in Different Species

Although the general features of tuberculous lesions are similar in most species, **certain differences in tissue reaction are specific for each species. In cattle, c alcification** is usually p rominent, particularly i n **lymph nodes**. Disseminated tubercles over the pleural and peritoneal surfaces are also common. The appearance of these individual tubercles, usually from 0.5-1.0 cm in diameter, gives the disease its common descriptive name "**pearl disease**". **Certain bovine skin lesions** are of particular i nterest. Although t hey are histologically indistinguishable from those of tuberculosis, they are not caused by infection with tubercle bacilli. Acid-fast bacilli which do not cause systemic disease, produce these **tuberculoid lesions**. Certain bovine skin lesions occur most frequently on the legs and are usually associated with lymphangitis. This disease has been termed "**skin tuberculosis**". As stated, although the disease is histologically indistinguishable from those of typical tuberculosis, it is not caused by infection with tubercle bacilli. In most cases, organisms cannot be cultured. However, a species termed *M. vaccae* has been recovered from some lesions and from lacteal glands of cattle. The disease produces sensitivity to bovine tuberculin, **a point of considerable practical importance**.

In the horse, lesions of tuberculosis are usually of chronic proliferative character, and **rarely show caseation or calcification. Alimentary infection is the usual form**, with possible extension elsewhere. In **birds** also, calcification is seldom observed. In contrast, lesions of tuberculosis of the **avian type in pigs** appear as multiple caseo-calcareous, encapsulated foci, usually affecting lymph nodes of the head and neck, mesenteric lymph nodes, and intestinal mucosa.

In dogs and cats, lesions may be discrete **granulomas with caseous centres**, or t hey may be characterized by a m ore diffuse mixture of e pithelioid cells, L anghans' giant c ells, and connective tissue l acking organizational structure, c aseation, a nd calcification. In m onkeys, the d isease is u sually **pulmonary** and may run a very severe course. Miliary lesions are common, caseation is usually prominent, but calcification is rare.

Infection by *M. avium-intracellulare* usually results in lesions of a very different nature from those already described. Although *M. **avium*** infection leads to the formation of classical t ubercles, there are a number of circumstances in which lesions are characterized by infiltration of tissues with diffuse sheets of epithelioid cells containing countless o rganisms. The number of organisms in a cell can be s o numerous t hat, with acid-fast stains, i ndividual b acteria cannot be seen nor cellular morphology recognized. **E verything is reduced to a red mass. Giant cells, necrosis, calcification, and fibroplasia are completely absent**. A vian tuberculosis is f urther d iscussed, next, in detail.

Zoonotic Importance

Tuberculosis can occur in all species, including humans, and is of importance for public health reasons. The case and frequency of the spread of tuberculosis from animals to humans in an uncontrolled environment makes this **an important zoonosis. Infection in humans occurs largely through consumption of infected cow's milk by children,** but spread can also occur by **inhalation.** Spread to humans can be almost completely eliminated by pasteurisation of milk, but only complete eradication can protect the dairy farmer and his family. The widespread occurrence of tuberculosis in **wild animals** maintained in captivity adds to the public health importance of these infections.

Diagnosis

The diagnosis of tuberculosis **in living animal** is based on the **tuberculin test,** X-ray findings, and demonstration of the organisms in exudates, or excretions.

In tissues obtained surgically (biopsy) or at necropsy, demonstration of acid-fast organisms within typical tubercles is sufficient to establish the diagnosis. However, bacterial isolation is necessary to establish its type. Acid-fast bacteria (mycobacteria) appear to infect many different species. Therefore, it is important that in each case organisms be recovered in culture for careful identification.

Avian Tuberculosis

Tuberculosis of poultry is a contagious disease caused by *Mycobacterium avium.* **It is characterized by chronicity,** persistence in a flock when once established, and tendency to induce unthriftiness, decreased egg production, and finally death. **Avian tuberculosis (AT)** in chickens is worldwide in distribution, and also occurs in a variety of avian and some other species. The condition is of importance because **pigs** and **rabbits** may be readily infected. Although avian tuberculous bacillus has been isolated in a few cases from human beings, **cases of this infection in humans are extremely rare** and poultry are not of much importance in the epidemiology of human tuberculosis. However, recent information indicates that *M. avium* infection is common **in patients with acquired immune deficiency syndrome (AIDS).** *M. avium* **serovar 1,** the organism usually isolated from wild birds, has been isolated from patients with AIDS. *M. avium* **serovar 2,** the organism usually isolated from chickens, is not commonly isolated from humans.

M. avium is **acid-fast** when stained by the Ziehl-Neelsen method and usually appears **beaded.** There are a large number of serotypes of this organism, **but types 1, 2, and 3 are most virulent and mainly responsible for the disease.** *M. avium* is relatively resistant compared with other mycobacteria to antimicrobials and disinfectants. **Outside the body it can survive for many years**. The organism does not show tropism for any particular tissue, but **gross lesions** of the **liver, spleen, intestine**, and **bone marrow** are usually seen. All species o f birds c an be i nfected, but s usceptibility among domestic b irds appears in this order - **chickens, ducks, geese**, and **turkeys**. AT in turkeys is relatively uncommon. Cage birds may also succumb to AT, but **tuberculosis in parrots and canaries may usually be caused by the human species of organism**. The disease is observed usually in older poultry. It is less prevalent in young fowl not because the younger birds are more resistant to infection, but because i n older b irds the d isease has a greater o pportunity to b ecome established through a longer period of exposure. Among mammals, *M. avium* can cause a progressive disease in **pigs** and **rabbits**, and **can cause sensitivity in cattle to the tuberculin test**. Taken together, reasons for the control and elimination of avian tuberculosis are: **1**. Affected birds are unthrifty, **2**. Tuberculous chickens are u ndesirable for h uman food, **3**. Diseased b irds produce fewer eggs, **4**. Tuberculous c hickens are t he source o f tuberculosis of pigs, and rarely sheep, **5**. Avian tubercle bacilli are capable of sensitizing cattle to mammalian tuberculin, and **6**. Avian tubercle bacilli have been isolated from lesions in humans.

Spread

In the spread of infection **the most important source of the organism is the infected bird;** and secondarily, because of the prolonged survival of *M. avium* outside the body of the host, **items contaminated with the droppings of such birds**. These usually include l itter, contaminated pens and pasture, equipment and implements which come into contact with infected fowls, and the hands, feet and clothing of attendants. **Tubercle bacilli may be carried by persons whose shoes have become soiled with faecal matter.**The t remendous number of tubercle bacilli e xcreted from u lcerated tuberculous lesions of t he intestine i n poultry c reates a c onstant s ource o f v irulent b acterium. Although other sources of infection exist, **infective faeces is the most important material in spread of AT**. Faecal discharges may contain tubercle bacilli from lesions of the liver and mucosa of the gallbladder expelled through the common duct. The **respiratory tract** is also a potential source of infection, especially if the lesions occur in the tracheal mucosa.

The **egg** a ppears to be only of minor importance i n the sp read of a vian tuberculosis. Other sources of spread are **carcasses of tuberculous fowl** which die of the disease and offal from chickens dressed for food. **Pigs** may h ave **ulcerative intestinal lesions** from avian tubercle bacilli, and thus constitute a source of infection for other animals and birds.

Pathogenesis

The capacity of *M. avium* to produce disease appears to be related to **cell** wall constituents, which are certain complex lipids such as cord factor, sulphur-containing glycolipids (sulphatides), or strongly acidic lipids. However, the effect of these components alone or together on phagosome-lysosome fusion cannot account for virulence. Delayed-type hypersensitivity (DTH) develops following exposure to mycobacteria. Once activated, macrophages demonstrate an increased capacity to kill intracellular *M. avium*. The DTH responses are mediated by lymphocytes, which release lymphokines that act to attract, immobilize, and activate blood-borne mononuclear cells at the site where virulent bacilli or their products exist. Tumour necrosis factor, alone or in combination with interleukin-2, but not gamma-interferon, is associated with macrophage killing of *M. avium* serovar 1. The DTH which develops contributes to accelerated tubercle formation, and is partly responsible for cell-mediated immunity in tuberculosis.

Activated macrophages that lack sufficient microbicidal components to kill virulent tubercle bacilli are destroyed by the intracellular growth of the organism, and a lesion develops. Recent information indicates that a combination of toxic lipids and factors released by virulent *M. avium* may 1. Cause disruption of the phagosome, 2. inhibit phagolysosome formation, 3. Interfere with release of hydrolytic enzymes from the affected lysosomes and/ or 4. Inactivate lysosomal enzymes released into the cytoplasmic vacuole. Recent information further suggests that toxic oxygen metabolites are not responsible for killing activated macrophages. However, the significance of hydrogen peroxide, activated oxygen radicals, and nitric oxide in resistant macrophages of birds exposed to virulent *M. avium* remains to be clarified.

Signs

The condition is usually chronic and symptoms may continue over a period of weeks or months before death. There is usually progressive but slow loss of condition, loss of energy, and increasing lethargy (a lazy state). Although appetite remains good, there is eventually gross emaciation with marked atrophy of the sternal muscles. The "keel" becomes prominent or even "knife edged". The face and comb become pale. Persistent diarrhoea with soiling of the tail feathers is usually seen. An occasional bird may show a hopping, jerkey type of locomotion caused by tubercular lesions of the bone marrow of the leg bones, or joints, and this is usually unilateral. Sometimes birds may die suddenly in good body condition, and yet show advanced lesions of tuberculosis. In such cases rupture of the affected liver or spleen with resultant internal haemorrhage is the precipitating cause of death.

Gross Lesions

Gross lesions are usually seen in the liver, spleen, intestines and bone marrow, but they may be found in any organ or tissues. Regardless of the organ involved, the lesions are typical tubercular granulomas. They are ir-

regular, **grey-white nodules**, varying in size from pinpoint to large masses of
fused tubercles. **When cut, the nodules are firm and caseous.** The centres
may be of pale yellow colour, particularly in those from the bone marrow. The
liver and spleen are usually **grossly enlarged** and sometimes **rupture**, with
resultant blood in the body cavity. The smaller tubercles in these organs can
be easily enucleated (removed entirely) from the surrounding tissue, particularly when they protrude from the surface. This is in contrast to leukosis, in
which somewhat similar lesions cannot be enucleated from the surrounding
tissue. Protrusion of tubercles from surface of the spleen, **gives spleen an
irregular, "knobbly"** (having many small hard lumps) **appearance**. The wall
of the **intestine** is always studded with similar irregular **lesions**, varying in size
from a millimetre to several centimetres in diameter. They usually involve the
whole thickness of the intestinal wall. They **eventually ulcerate** into the lumen
of the intestine, with discharge of bacilli and **constituting the major source of
infection in the droppings**. The **bone marrow** of the long bones of the legs
usually contains **tubercular nodules**. These can be best seen grossly if the
bones are split longitudinally, particularly in the region of femoro-tibiotarsal
and tibiotarsal-tarsometatarsal joints. They are pale yellow in colour, and vary
in size and number. **This is one of the characteristic features of tuberculosis
in the chicken. Lungs** are less frequently affected in the domestic chicken,
but in waterfowl (**mainly ducks**) they are commonly affected. Tubercle bacilli
have been isolated from some cases of arthritis affecting the phalangeal joints
in the fowl. This is known as "**bumble foot**". It is also caused by staphylococcal
infection (see avian staphyococcosis).

Histopathology

Microscopically, the **tubercle** is a closely packed collection of pale-staining cells with vesiculated nuclei. These **epithelioid cells** are derived from fixed
tissue elements known as histiocytes. The histiocytes phagocytose tubercle
bacilli early in the process. The cellular mass or "**primary tubercle**" gradually
expands as histiocytes proliferate at the periphery. **Within 3-4 weeks, signs of
degeneration can be seen in epithelioid cells in the central zone**. The degeneration is partly due to the avascularity of the cellular mass, and partly to the
toxic substances of the tubercle bacilli. As the cellular mass becomes larger,
epithelioid cells have tendency to fuse and form syncytia. Outlines of the
individual cells become less distinct, or disappear. This is followed by a
necrobiotic change resembling coagulative necrosis. Nuclei of epithelioid cells
become pyknotic and may disappear. The cellular mass, **except the peripheral portion**, becomes fused and stains deeply with eosin. The necrotic bacilli
multiply and appear singly or in clumps throughout the necrotic tissue.

While the **epithelioid cells in the central zone** under necrobiotic changes,
an outer zone of epithelioid syncytia persists as a rim around the entire periphery. From these, giant cells are developed. Their nuclei are situated **away**

from the central zone of necrosis. The cells are arranged usually in palisade formation, i.e., like a fence of stakes. Immediately peripheral to the zone of giant cells, there is a diffuse collection of epithelioid cells and histiocytes, from which they are derived. Fibrocytes and minute blood vascular channels also occur near the outer portion of the peripheral area. **Bacilli are more numerous in the central or necrotic zone of the tubercle.** However, they are also found in large numbers in the epithelioid zone next to giant cells.

The final phase in the formation of tubercle is development of a zone of encapsulation. It consists of fibrous connective tissue, histiocytes, some lymphocytes, and an occasional eosinophil. **New tubercles** develop in the epithelioid zone immediately external to giant cells. As a result, a tubercle as seen grossly, consists of the original or parent tubercle and several smaller ones.

The degenerative process in the central zone of the tubercle is somewhat unusual, in that the integrity of the cells is maintained for a long period before disintegration. **Caseous necrosis eventually occurs, and may affect all or part of the central zone. Calcification of the tubercle occurs only rarely in fowl. Amyloid-like degeneration** is sometimes seen in portions of the parenchymal elements surrounding the tubercle in liver, spleen, and kidney.

Acid-fast bacilli occur in great numbers in smears of lesions, and in appropriately stained tissue sections.

Diagnosis

A **presumptive diagnosis** of tuberculosis in fowl can usually be made **on the basis of gross lesions.** Demonstration of acid-fast organisms in smears of infected livers, spleen, or other organs is very helpful in diagnosis. **There is rarely any difficulty in demonstrating the organisms. They are present in very large numbers,** particularly in young lesions and those from the bone marrow. However, cultural examination for isolation and identification of the causal agent is necessary for definitive diagnosis.

Immunological tests are also of value in finding out the infected birds during life. They include the **tuberculin test**, a rapid agglutination test, and ELISA. The tuberculin test consists of injection of avian tuberculin into one wattle, the other uninjected serves as the control. The test is read 48 hours after the injection of tuberculin. A positive reaction shows a hot, soft, oedematous swelling in the injected wattle. When administered properly, the tuberculin test provides a satisfactory procedure for determining presence of avian tuberculosis in a flock. The **agglutination test** is a rapid whole blood test. It is also helpful in the diagnosis of AT in fowl. The **ELISA** has been developed and has been used for detecting antibodies in sera of tuberculous chickens.

Johne's Disease (Paratuberculosis)

Johne's disease (JD) is a chronic, infectious, granulomatous enteritis of ruminants characterized clinically by **chronic diarrhoea** and **progressive emaciation**. JD is caused by **an acid-fast organism**, *Mycobacterium paratuberculosis*, which is known to affect **cattle, sheep, goats**, and **other ruminants. In India**, besides **cattle**, JD is also widely prevalent in the **sheep** and **goat** population. **In wildlife**, it has been reported in deer. The disease remains virtually undetectable clinically until the onset of diarrhoea. **Pigs** and **horses** can be infected, but lesions are minimal or absent. Most laboratory animals are resistant to infection. However, a model of the disease has been reproduced in athymic (without thymus) mice. **Three strains** of *M. paratuberculosis* **are capable of causing the disease in cattle**, the usual **bovine strain**, and **two sheep strains**. The disease is of worldwide distribution and constitutes an important economic problem in cattle. It is less frequently encountered in **sheep** and **goats**. In **cattle**, it causes a wasting illness with a prolonged course, during which intractable (not easily controlled/cured) diarrhoea, emaciation, and eventually death occur. **Young calves are most susceptible to infection**, which is usually acquired during the first year of life.

Spread

Faeces containing the organisms serve as the primary source of infection, which is acquired by **ingestion** of feed and water contaminated by the faeces of infected animals which are excreting the organism. Because of the long incubation period, infected animals may excrete organisms in the faeces for 15-18 months before clinical signs appear. The organism has been isolated from the genitalia and the **semen of infected bulls**. Foetal infection occurs in cows with and without clinical signs of the disease. *M. paratuberculosis* persists without multiplication in pasture for long periods, **and such pastures are infective for up to one year**. Infection occurs in animals at a very early age, usually under 30 days of age. **However, clinical disease does not occur until 3-5 years of age.**

Pathogenesis

Following ingestion, the organisms localize in the mucosa of the small intestine, its associated lymph nodes, and to a lesser extent, in the tonsils and supra-pharyngeal lymph nodes. The organisms then penetrate the intestinal mucosa, and set up residence within macrophages. **Here, they multiply intracellularly without killing the host cell**, and like other mycobacteria, **are resistant to cellular digestion**. *M. paratuberculosis* is an intracellular organism and lives inside the cells. Although readily phagocytosed by macrophages, **these bacteria are resistant to intracellular destruction**. They grow within macrophages and are distributed throughout the body inside these cells. The primary site of bacterial multiplication is the **terminal ileum** and also the **large**

intestine. Recent evidence indicates that **intestinal M cells** play a key role in the transport of bacteria across the mucosa. This would explain the primary localization of lesions in the terminal ileum.

Three different groups of animals can occur depending on the host-bacteria relationship. In the **first group**, animals quickly develop resistance, contol the infection, a nd **do not become shedders**. These a nimals are c alled "**infected-resistant**". In the **second group**, infection is not completely controlled. Some animals control the infection only partially and **shed the organisms intermittently**, while o thers become i ntermediate cases. That is, they are incubating the disease and **will later be heavy shedders of the organism**. In the **third group**, the organism persists in the intestinal mucosa, and it is from these animals the **clinical cases develop**. The organism is phagocytosed by macrophages. They then proliferate in large numbers and infiltrate the submucosa, which results in **decreased absorption, chronic diarrhoea, and malabsorption**. There is a reduction in protein absorption, and also leakage of protein into the lumen of jejunum. **In cattle**, loss of protein results in much wasting, hypoproteinaemia, and oedema. **In sheep**, a compensatory increase in protein production in the liver makes for the protein loss, and clinical signs appear only when this compensatory mechanism fails. **Within the macrophages, the bacteria remain viable and protected from humoral factors.** *In vitro* studies indicate that blood-derived macrophages from clinically normal c ows, o r cows i nfected with *M. paratuberculosis* are incapable of destroying the organism.

The **immunological response** following infection is variable, and depends on the stage of the infection. That is, whether or not the clinical disease develops. In general, infected animals initially develop **a cell-mediated response**. This is followed by a **humoral response** initiated by the release of bacteria by **dying macrophages** as the disease progresses. Type III (immune complex) reactions may c ontribute to the development of intestinal lesions in Johne's disease. Type I or t ype III r eactions occurring i n the intestinal mucosa may result i n an i ncreased outflow of fluid and diarrhoea. In the late stages of clinical disease **anergy** (irreversible functional inactivation of lymphocytes, i.e., failure of a sensitized animal to respond to an antigen) occurs, and neither cell-mediated nor humoral immunity is detectable. These immunological features occur independent of the st ages of c linical disease. They can appear at any time during the clinical course.

The bacteria are carried by macrophages to other sites, particularly uterus, foetus, and the mammary gland, and the testes and semen of bulls. **In cows**, infection may penetrate to the foetus and cause **prenatal (before birth) infection**.

The important features of the disease are the long incubation period of

2 years or more, and the development of **sensitization to johnin and to mammalian and avian tuberculin**. This sensitivity develops in the preclinical stage. It u sually disappears by the t ime c linical s igns become n oticeable. On t he other hand, complement fixing antibodies appear late in the disease and usually rise with increasing severity of the lesions. This suggests that two independent antibodies are involved in the two reactions.

Signs

Clinical signs are seen only after several months. Infection in **cattle** and **sheep** does not always lead to clinical disease. However, even in the absence of clinical infection, **the organism is shed in the faeces**, providing a source of infection for young animals. A lthough lesions a re usually r estricted to the intestinal tract and lymph nodes, the organism can infect other tissues, including the uterus, which can lead to **congenital infection and abortion**.

In cattle, c linical signs do not appear before 2 years of age, and a re commonest in t he 2-6 y ear a ge group. **Emaciation** is the m ost noticeable abnormality, and i s usually a ccompanied by s ubmandibular oedema. T he oedema has a tendency t o disappear a s d iarrhoea d evelops. A f all in milk yield and a bsence of f ever a nd toxaemia a re present. T he a nimal eats w ell throughout, but thirst is excessive. **The faeces are soft and thin, and without foul smell**. There is absence of blood, epithelial debris, and mucus. Diarrhoea may be continuous or intermittent. The course of the disease varies from weeks to months, but it always terminates in **severe dehydration, emaciation, and weakness**, necessitating d estruction/disposal. Cases occur sporadically (i.e., isolated cases), because of the slow rate of spread of the disease.

In sheep and goats, the disease is manifested mainly by **emaciation**, although shedding of wool may occur in sheep. Diarrhoea is not severe. However, faeces are sufficiently soft to lose their usual pelleted form in both species. Affected **sheep** may lose weight, be partially anorexic, and their faeces may appear normal until t he t erminal s tages, when the faeces may b e s oft a nd pasty. Depression and dysponea are noticeable in **goats**, but are less obvious in **sheep**.

Lesions

The terminal part of the ileum is the most common site of the specific lesions. Lesions also occur in the remaining small intestine and large intestine, and the mesenteric lymph nodes. **Microscopic lesions** reveal the lamina propria of the mucosa to be closely packed with large, discrete epithelioid cells which have a dundant foamy c ytoplasm, and a re often m ultinucleated. These c ells also infiltrate and thicken the submucosa, but leave the muscularis mucosae and the m uscular layer i ntact. N ests o f these e pithelioid cells m ay a lso b e found in mesenteric lymph nodes, but rarely elsewhere. In impression **smears** or sections of these lesions, Ziehl-Neelsen's stain demonstrates a large number of **acid-fast, rod-shaped organisms in the cytoplasm of the epithelioid cells** where they multiply. **As with the mycobacteria which cause tuberculosis, *M. paratuberculosis* is resistant to cellular digestion.**

Secondary changes in the intestinal mucosa include oedema, which results from local interference with circulation; nests of neutrophils; and increased numbers of eosinophils. The eosinophils may perhaps be due to helminthic parasitism. **Of importance is the absence of caseous necrosis, nodule formation, and calcification.** In contrast to cattle, nodule formation with necrosis and calcification has been described is **sheep, goats, and wild ruminants**.

The **gross appearance** is directly related to the microscopic changes. **The affected intestinal wall is thickened**, sometimes oedematous, and its mucosal surface has many broad, closely placed, transverse folds, or **rugae** (i.e., **corrugations**; wrinkled, rough, irregular folds). These rugae result from thickening of villi and give the surface **a corrugated appearance,** which does not disappear when the intestinal wall is stretched.

Although the lesions are usually confined to the intestines and lymph nodes, generalized infection has been reported in cattle, sheep, and goats. Lesions then occur in the liver, spleen, lungs, kidneys, uterus, placenta, and non-mesenteric lymph nodes.

Zoonotic Implications

The disease in ruminants is **not a zoonosis**, but injury and illness from accidental inoculation of the **bacterin** used for the vaccination of cattle is a potential veterinary occupational hazard. The most common injury is a **needle-stick exposure to the bacterin**. The likelihood of exposure is directly related to the number of doses administered.

Diagnosis

The **gross lesions** in the intestine are highly suggestive, but confirmation of the diagnosis depends on the **demonstration of the epithelioid cells containing acid-fast bacilli** in huge numbers in smears or sections of mucosa or submucosa. In about 60% of affected cattle, lesions containing organisms extend into the colon and rectum. This makes it possible to diagnose the disease in the living animal by microscopic examination of mucosal scrapings collected from the **rectum**.

The diffuse nature of the lesions, their confinement to the intestinal mucosa and mesenteric lymph nodes, and the presence of **innumerable acid-fast bacilli** serve to differentiate Johne's disease from tuberculosis. In tuberculosis nodule formation, fibrosis, necrosis, calcification, and only a few acid-fast bacilli are characteristic. In s heep and goats, lesions with c aseation and c alcification require greater care in differentiating tuberculosis. However, the diffuse distribution of the lesions in Johne's disease usually allows this differentiation.

Bacteriological examination of the faeces is a valuable diagnostic aid for detecting infection in clinically diseased animals. **Faecal culture is at present recognized as the most reliable index of infection in live cattle**. It is both 100% specific and 100% sensitive on herd basis. A major advantage of faecal culture is it can identify cattle 1-3 years **prior to the appearance of clinical signs**. But current procedures are laborious and fail to detect animals shedding low numbers o f organisms. **M olecular genetics** can p rovide a n ew way to identify organisms through the u se of **D NA probes**. C ompared with faecal culturing, a **DNA hybridization** probe identifies 34% more mycobacterium-containing faecal samples, and testing takes only 72 hours to complete.

Various serological tests and the **i ntradermal johnin test** are c heaper and much more rapid than faecal culture, and several are available. However, neither a pproach is c ompletely satisfactory. T he serological t ests include complement fixation test (CFT), agar gel immunodiffusion test (AGID), and ELISA. The l ipoarabinomannan antigen e nzyme-linked immunosorbent as-say (**LAM-ELISA**) i s c onsidered s uperior t o b oth C FT a nd the protein D antigen agar g el immunodiffusion (D-AGID).

Feline Leprosy

Leprosy of the **domestic cat** was first described in New Zealand in 1962, as a non-tuberculous granulomatous lesion involving the dermis and subcutis. Since t hen t he disease h as been reported from m any other c ountries. The causative a gent h as not been s pecifically i dentified, b ut i s v ery similar to *Mycobacterium lepraemurium*. The **lesions** usually appear as **single or multiple nodules** involving the skin and subcutis in almost any part of the body, but particularly the head and limbs. **Microscopically**, the lesions resemble leprosy of humans, taking the form of either tuberculoid or lepromatous leprosy.

Leprosy of Buffaloes

Leprosy of buffaloes is a disease characterized by **persistent cutaneous and subcutaneous nodules** on the legs, and lower parts of the abdomen and thorax. It has been reported from Indonesia and other East Asian countries. It is of particular interest because of the similarity of its histological features to those of human leprosy. The disease is uncommon, and usually does not result in death, or serious disability. **The causative organism, although demonstrable in tissue, has not been cultured successfully.**

The c utaneous lesions occur from accumulation of large n umbers of epithelioid cells in the dermis. **Microscopically**, these cells have greatly distended, foamy, u sually v acuolated c ytoplasm in w hich numerous acid-fast bacilli are demonstrable. The large vacuoles are the result of lipid production by the bacilli, and are similar to those in the large "**lepra cells**" of human leprosy. Giant cells of Langhans' type may be seen, but caseation, necrosis and calcification do not occur.

Bovine Farcy

Bovine farcy is believed to result from infection with *Mycobacterium farcinogenes* or *Mycobacterium senegalense*. The disease occurs as a chronic suppurative granulomatous inflammation of the skin, lymphatics and draining lymph nodes, usually confined to the limbs.

Genus: Nocardia

Nocardia are aerobic, **Gram-positive**, mycelial (filamentous) organisms. These, under some conditions, have "**acid-fast**" staining properties. These organisms infect **humans and animals**, particularly **dogs and cats**. They cause purulent, necrotizing, and at times, granulomatous disease. The genus **Rhodococcus** has similar morphology and staining characteristics, and is easily confused with Nocardia.

Nocardiosis

Nocardiosis is mostly caused by *Nocardia asteroides*, but *N. brasiliensis* and *N. caviae* are also pathogenic, and sometimes identified.

Lesions

In dogs, infection of the lungs and pleura is most common. However, systemic infection can occur, and the organisms can localize in peritoneal and pleural cavities, in the brain, or in any visceral organ. **Microscopically**, the lesions are tangled colonies of organisms, surrounded by cellular necrotic debris, purulent exudate, and granulation tissue. **Distinct granulomas are usually not a feature.** However, chronic lesions are characterized by a surrounding zone of macrophages, lymphocytes, plasma cells, and sometimes multinucleated giant cells along with fibrovascular connective tissue. Usually, eosinophilic clubs (**Splendore-Hoeppli material**) are not present surrounding the colonies of organisms, but they have been reported. **This makes the differentiation from actinomycosis very difficult.** The colonies are not surrounded by radiating clubs. The organisms can usually be demonstrated in the tissues as G ram-**positive, branching filaments**. These are acid-fast when appropriately stained. Culture identification of the organism is necessary to establish diagnosis, although presumptive diagnosis can be made from tissue sections.

Nocardiosis is less common in other species. It may be a sporadic cause of **mastitis or pneumonia in cattle**, and pneumonia in monkeys. The lesions in these or other species are similar to those described in the dog. Infection of the bovine foetus and placenta, resulting in abortion, has been associated with nocardiosis.

Genus: Rhodococcus

Bacteria of Rhodococcus genus closely resemble those of Nocardia genus. They are Gram-positive, usually mycelial (filamentous), and **partially acid-fast**. Of the several species, only *Rhodococcus equi* is an important pathogen for animals. This species, previously classified as *Corynebacterium equi*, is a variably acid-fast coccobacillus. It is an important cause of a **specific granulomatous pneumonia of horses**, and sometimes of **cattle, sheep, pigs**, and other species. *R. equi* has also been associated with pyogranulomatous inflammation of submandibular and cervical lymph nodes of **pigs**, and arthritis in **lambs**. It has been reported as a cause of pneumonia and pleuritis in a **monkey**. It has also emerged as an important cause of **pneumonia in immunosuppressed human patients**, usually in individuals **with a history of exposure to horses**.

The organism is believed to enter through the respiratory route. *R. equi* is an intracellular organism and lives inside the cells. Although it is readily phagocytosed by macrophages, **these bacteria are resistant to intracellular destruction**. They grow within macrophages and are distributed throughout the body inside these cells. **Foals** between 2-4 months of age are most susceptible. Infection in horses over 6 months of age is rare, unless they are **immunocompromised** (immunologically damaged). Morbidity can approach 20% and mortality may be up to 80%. **The pneumonia is a severe bronchopneumonia** characterized by filling of alveoli with neutrophils, macrophages, and multinucleated giant cells. Enlarging foci of necrosis, surrounded by this mixed cellular infiltrate and fibrosis, lead to multiple, often coalescing pyogranulomas.

Microscopically, these pyogranulomas have a central area of caseous necrosis containing neutrophils surrounded by macrophages and multinucleated giant cells. **The infection can be systemic with** pyogranulomatous inflammtion in many organs and joints. Enteritis, metritis, abortion, and lymphangitis may result from *R. equi* infection in foals, independently of pneumonia. The most common lesion is purulent and mononuclear **enterocolitis**, often with ulcers and associated pyogranulomatous lymphadenitis. **In all forms of the infection, the organisms can be found within macrophages**.

Zoonotic Implications

R. equi is an occasional pathogen for humans. Infection is more common in immunocompromised people, but there is not a particular association of contact with farm animals.

4

Fungal Diseases

Fungi are the most plant-like of animal pathogens. Fungal cells are relatively l arge (5-300 µm) and t heir thick c ell walls c ontain **ergosterol** and **polysaccharides rather than the peptidoglycans of bacteria.** Some species have antiphagocytic capsules; others have wall components resistant to phagolysosomal attack. **F ungi therefore can produce the whole range of bacterial pathology from acute pyogenic to chronic granulomatous infection,** a nd they may not r eveal their presence until i dentified by.l aboratory methods. F ortunately, their s turdy cell w alls make f ungi d etectable m icroscopically in t issues, even i n the m idst of n ecrosis. However, s ome are s o tightly bound that they are rarely visible in body fluids or exudates, and tissue samples are required to find them. **Fungal morphology can be characteristic enough for tentative microscopic species identification,** but often culture is required. Fungi grow well, but slowly, on appropriate media. But contaminating spores of free-living or commensal fungi also grow well on media. **Therefore, culture and tissue diagnosis together provide the most useful information.**

In tissues, fungi reproduce by simple division of round, yeast-like forms, or of slender, tubular **hyphae** that form a **mycelium** (a mycelium is a collection of hyphae). Rarely, fruiting bodies called '**conidia**' (asexual reproductive units) or '**sporangia**' (sacs enclosing spores) are also formed, but the free-living and sexual reproductive stages are missing. Thus, **fungi may have more than one form in tissue or in culture,** and usually grow by extension and branching of filamentous structures. Some species form infective spores only in nature or in culture **and these differ markedly from their tissue forms,** which are noncommunicable (**dimorphic fungi**).

Pathogenic fungi produce mycotoxins and enzymes, b ut with f ew exceptions, their role in disease is still unclear. Their antigens, rich in polysaccharides, a re sometimes d iagnostically detectable. S ome can i nduce strong **hypersensitivity responses of types III and IV.** P hagocytic competence plays an important role in antifungal defence, and leukopaenic patients are as vulnerable to fungi as to bacteria. **Corticosteroids and**

immunosuppressive drugs favour fungal infections of all varieties and species.

Majority of the fungi are saprophytes and do not cause disease in animals, even when they enter into the body through inhalation or other means. Depending on their capability to set up infection, **fungi and fungal diseases can be classified into five groups:**

1. The only obligate parasites are the **dermatophytes**. These live in keratin layers of the skin and cause **ringworm**. Such infections are called **"superficial mycoses"**. Dermatophytes do not live as saprophytes, and **spread is direct**. However, they **are not invasive**. Transmission is direct. All other disease-producing fungi live as saprophytes, and cause disease only when the host is unable to restrict their growth in tissues. Usually, the organisms are destroyed after entry into the host and do not lead to disease.

2. **Some fungi, however, are capable of establishing themselves in normal individuals.** These fungi cause "systemic or deep mycoses." Examples include histoplasmosis, coccidioidomycosis, blastomycosis, and sporotrichosis. They generally live in **mycelial forms** in the soil or on plants, and in **yeast forms** in tissue (**dimorphic fungi**). Even these fungi are usually checked after entering into an animal host. **Debilitated and immunocompromised** (immunologically damaged) **animals are the most susceptible.**

3. The third group of mycosis is the **"subcutaneous mycoses"** or "**mycetomas**". Infection with these saprophytic fungi occurs following their **entry into the skin** through wounds where they grow **in mycelial form, producing localized lesions which usually do not spread.**

4. The fourth group of fungi are capable of **causing both localized and disseminated disease**, growing as mycelia in tissue. This group includes aspergillosis and the zygomycoses. These are most common in debilitated animals.

5. The **yeasts** comprise a fifth group. Yeasts grow as single-celled fungi. Some form pseudomycelia. **They are not highly pathogenic and rarely cause disease in the normal animal. Candidiasis is the most common yeast infection.** It is usually a superficial infection of mucous membranes, but may cause serious systemic disease. **Cryptococcosis is the other yeast infection of importance in animals.**

Many bacteria (so-called **higher bacteria**) **produce diseases that closely resemble mycoses**, and are usually included in discussions of diseases caused by fungi. These include **Actinomyces, Nocardia, Dermatophilus, and**

Mycobacteria. These have been discussed under bacterial diseases.

Lesions

In almost all cases fungi can be easily seen in tissue sections stained with either **haematoxylin** and **eosin**, or with special stains such as **Gomori methenamine silver (GMS), periodic acid-Schiff (PAS) reaction, or Gridley stain**. A characteristic morphological feature of some of these diseases is the presence of a homogeneous, brightly eosinophilic material known as "**Splendore-Hoeppli material**", surrounding individual organism or colonies of organisms. It exists as a rim, usually more than 100 μm, or as a surrounding collar of radially arranged clubs or baseball bats (radially arranged = arranged like rays). The **clubs** are coarse, 3-10 μm in diameter and 10-30 μm in length. It is believed that they are product of the host, **most likely an antigen-antibody complex**. Splendore-Hoeppli material is a feature of coccidioidomycosis and sporotrichosis. But it may also be a feature of many other mycoses, and also of certain diseases caused by higher bacteria, such as **actinomycosis**.

The lesions produced by deep (systemic) fungi are usually "classical granulomas". There is **a central core of necrotic debris, usually containing pus**. It is surrounded by a zone of epithelioid cells, macrophages, and multinucleated giant cells. Variable number of lymphocytes, plasma cells, and sometimes eosinophils may be present. The entire lesion is surrounded by fibrovascular connective tissue of varying maturity.

The superficial mycoses (dermatophytoses) do not produce granulomas, because the organisms are restricted to the superficial layers of the skin and are not invasive.

Defence Against Fungal Infections

The first line of defence against invasive fungi, such as **A spergillus** or **Candida**, is activation of the alternate pathway of the **complement system**. This results in attraction of neutrophils which attempt to ingest the invading **hyphae** or **pseudohyphae**. Because of their size, neutrophils cannot totally ingest the invading fungi. Nevertheless, by releasing their enzymes into the tissue fluid, **neutrophils can severely damage fungal hyphae**. Very small fungal fragments or spores may be ingested and destroyed by **macrophages**, or by **natural killer (NK) cells**.

Immunity to Fungal Infections

Once established, fungal infections can only be destroyed by **T cell-mediated mechanisms**. Thus, some species of **Aspergillus** are facultative intracellular parasites, and chronic or progressive fungal diseases are usually associated with defects in the T cell system. **T cells in fungal infections act mainly by activating macrophages**, and by promoting epidermal growth and keratinization. Some

T a nd NK c ells cause a direct c ytotoxic effect on yeasts, s uch as *Candida.
albicans* and *Cryptococcus neoformans*. It is not uncommon for r ecovered
animals to develop a type IV hypersensitivity to fungal antigens.

Superficial Mycoses or Dermatomycoses

Also known by several other names, such as "**ringworm**" "**trichophytosis**",
"**favus**", "**tinea**", and "**dermatophytosis**", **dermatomycoses are those infections of the skin and its adnexae** (hair follicles, sebaceous and sweat glands)
that are caused by the dermatophytic fungi (dermatophytes). These fungi
comprise many species which inhabit the skin of **humans** and **animals**, and
produce lesions under certain conditions. **Forty-two species of dematophytes
are recognized**. The most important of these are listed in **Table 28**. Members
of the genus **M icrosporum** and **Trichophyton** infect a nimals a nd h umans.
Humans are a lso infected b y the t hird genus **E pidermophyton** (Table 2 8).
**Infection is acquired by contact with infected animals, or contaminated
fomites. (A fomite is any s ubstance that absorbs and t ransmits i nfectious**
material). **Animals may serve as reservoirs for human infection, and humans
may transmit infection to animals.** Those fungi which primarily infect humans
are called "**anthropophilic**", while those primarily affecting animals are termed
"**zoophilic**". A third g roup, "**geophilic**", are m ainly soil s aprophytes, and
sometimes infect both humans and animals. The dermatomycoses are usually
classified as "**ringworm**", or in human infections, as "**tinea**" (from Latin for
gnawing worm, i.e., biting or chewing worm).

**Table 28. Important dermatophytes which cause ringworm in man and
animals**

Genus: Microsporum

M. canis (zoophilic)	Dogs, cats; sheep, calves, monkeys, apes; tinea capitis in humans
M. audouinii (anthropophilic)	Tinea capitis in humans; infects dogs, monkeys
M. gypseum (geophilic)	Ringworm of scalp in humans; also infects dogs, cats, horses, pigs
M. nanum (zoophilic)	Pigs
M. distortum (zoophilic)	Dogs, cats, m onkeys

Genus: Trichophyton

T. mentagrophytes (zoophilic)	Tinea capitis in humans (tinea cruris, tinea

	barbae, tinea pedis); ringworm in dogs, cats, cattle, sheep, goats, horses, monkeys
T. rubrum (anthropophilic)	Tinea corporis, tinea pedis, tinea cruris, and tinea barbae in humans; ringworm in dogs and monkeys (rare)
T. tonsurans (anthropophilic)	Tinea capitis and tinea corporis of man
T. schoenleinii (anthropophilic)	Cats, tinea favosa (favus) of man
T. concentricum (anthropophilic)	Tinea imbricata of man (rare)
T. violaceum (anthropophilic)	Tinea imbricata and tinea barbae of man
T. verrucosum (zoophilic)	Cattle; also horses, sheep, dogs; tinea favosa and tinea barbae of man
T. megninii (anthropophilic)	Tinea favosa of man
T. equinum (zoophilic)	Horses; also cattle; tinea barbae of man
T. gallinae (zoophilic)	Chickens, turkeys, man
Genus: Epidermophyton *E. floccosum* (anthropophilic)	Tinea cruris, tinea pedis, tinea unguium, tinea corporis of man

In humans, these superficial mycoses are classified on the basis of anatomical site of the lesion, as well as on their clinical appearance. Superficial mycoses in humans include: **tinea pedis**, **"athlete's foot"** or **ringworm**; **tinea cruris**, a ringworm of the groin or **"jock itch"**; **tinea capitis**, ringworm of the scalp; **tinea favus**, a form of tinea capitis with a honeycomb appearance; **tinea unguium**, a ringworm of the nails (onchomycosis); **tinea glabrosa**, also called **tinea circinata** or **tinea corporis** (**tinea imbricata** when particularly severe), ringworm of the glabrous (hairless) skin; **tinea barbae**, **"barber's itch"**, ringworm of the bearded area; and others.

In animals, the dermatomycoses are characterized by growth of organisms upon or within the hairs, in the stratum corneum of the epidermis in the hair follicles, or in the nails. **The infection does not spread to deeper structures.** The organisms appear as **septate** (dividing, branching) **hyphae** (filaments of mycelium), or as individual or chains of **arthrospores**, derived from the mycelial form. *In vitro*, fungi produce both microconidia and macroconidia.

(**Conidia** are asexual spores of fungi). **The conidia are useful in identification, but are not produced in tissue**. It is easy to see the organisms in or on
hair, where two main types of growth are seen: 1. **Ectothrix dermatophytes**.
This type of growth is characterized by mycelial invasion within the hair with
arthrospores on the outside of the hair shaft (G. thrix=hair), and 2. **Endothrix
mycelia and arthrospores**, found within the hair. **All animal pathogens are
of the ectothrix type**.

Lesions

**Lesions of dermatomycosis are limited to the hairs, nails, epidermis,
and dermis**. The fungi grow within or upon the surface of stratum corneum, or
the hairs. Growth of the fungi usually binds hairs together, or causes them to
fall, depending upon the fungus and host. Dry, scaly, or powdery crusts may
form, or the hair may be bound together in a scutulum (thin crust). This leaves
a red, sometimes raw and bleeding surface, when it is removed. The lesions
are often circumscribed and may involve any part of the skin surface. The
name "ringworm" is given because of the circinate (circular) nature of the
lesions that sometimes result from the outward growth of the organisms from
the healing areas in the centre.

Microscopically, lesions are not very noticeable and can be easily over-
looked in routine sections. Thickening of the stratum corneum may be the
only change seen in sections stained with H & E. However, special methods,
such as **PAS reaction, Gridley fungus stain and Bauer stain**, usually make it
possible to recognize the fungi in tissue sections. Hypertrophy of the epidermis occurs in severe cases, accompanied by congestion and infiltration of the
underlying dermis. In deeper infections in which hair follicles are involved,
severe destruction of the follicle with resultant inflammation in the dermis
may be seen. Organisms also can be identified in hairs and skin scrapings
cleared with a concentrated aqueous solution of sodium or potassium
hydroxide and examined under the microscope, using decreased illumination.

Diagnosis

Diagnosis is facilitated by clinical findings. **Ringworm** is most commonly
seen in **dogs** and **cats** with *Microsporum canis* as the most frequent agent, and
in **cattle**, where *Trichophyton verrucosum* is the usual cause. **Horses** housed in
groups are usually affected with *T. equinum*. The disease in **pigs** is rare, and
sheep are seldom affected. The clinical diagnosis of some of the superficial
mycoses is helped by the use of filtered ultraviolet light (Wood's light) to examine the lesions in a darkened room. Some species, particularly of **Microsporum**,
exhibit fluorescence under ultraviolet light, making it possible to recognize mild
infections.

Systemic or Deep Mycoses

Aspergillosis

Aspergillus sp. are saprophytic moulds. They are extremely common in nature, occurring on foodstuffs as a white, fluffy, sporulating mould. **Ordinarily they are not pathogens, but rather opportunists**. However, once established in susceptible host, aspergillosis can be a serious disease. Debilitated and immunocompromised animals and those on prolonged antibiotic therapy are at particular risk. **Most infections are established through inhalation of spores leading to pneumonia. Haematogenous spread is common** due to the tendency of Aspergillus to **invade blood vessels** and establish mycelial emboli. Certain **Aspergillus** sp. also produce **toxins**, known as **aflatoxins**, which cause **mycotoxicosis (aflatoxicosis)**. Mycotoxicosis is discussed later in this chapter. Of more than 100 species in the genus **Aspergillus**, *A. fumigatus*, *A. flavus*, *A. niger*, *A. nidulans*, and *A. terreus* are the species most commonly associated with disease in animals.

Aspergillosis is most common and severe in poultry. This is discussed in detail later in this chapter, under avian fungal diseases. **Young chicks** and turkey poults are especially prone and become infected from contaminated bedding, usually while they are in the brooder stage of growth. Hence the term "**brooder pneumonia**" (see avian aspergillosis). The infection may occur as an epizootic with high mortality. **In mammals**, aspergillosis is seen in most species, **but usually as an isolated event**. The infection is not communicable. In most species, superficial infections of the skin and cornea occur as well as pneumonia. Sometimes infection spreads to other organs, such as kidneys, gastrointestinal tract, liver, spleen, and central nervous system. **In cattle**, mastitis, placentitis and abortion, rumenitis, and gastritis may result from aspergillosis, usually in association with other fungi. Infection of the guttural pouch **in horses** results in a clinical syndrome characterized by recurrent epistaxis and visceral and locomotor disturbances. The infectious granulomas may spread from the guttural pouch to the nasal cavity, and through the optic nerves, to the cerebrum.

Lesions

Acute or invasive aspergillosis is characterized by extensive necrosis and haemorrhage with a purulent and mononuclear inflammatory response. Colonies of organisms are large and invade adjacent tissues. **Invasion into the walls of arteries leads to thrombosis and infarction**. This further enlarges the necrotizing lesion. Lesions of larger standing take the form of **granulomas** with a central core of **caseous necrosis**, in which the organisms are surrounded by a wide zone of epithelioid cells. Multinucleated giant cells of the foreign body type may be present, also lymphocytes and a collar of fibroblasts in chronic lesions.

In tissue, organisms may be present as large colonies of radiating hyphae. This is typical of the invasive disease. Or, they may be present as small colonies of irregularly scattered hyphae. This is more common in granulomas or superficial infections. The **hyphae** are slender, 3-6 μm wide, of uniform diameter but of variable length. They are septate and branching. The branches form at acute angles. **The hyphae are usually basophilic.** Despite this, they often do not stain well with H & E stain. Stains for glycogen (**PAS, Gridley fungus, Bauer**) differentiate the mycelia by colouring the cell wall intensely. Spores are usually not formed in tissues, but on surfaces exposed to air, such as those on airsacs (in birds) and the lining of external orifices and trachea. The organisms may produce long mycelia-bearing **conidiophores**, which project into the lumen. The mycelial growth in these sites is like that in cultures on artificial media. Sometimes, mycelia are surrounded by eosinophilic, radiating clubs (**Splendore-Hoeppli material**) similar to that seen in actinomycosis and certain other mycotic infections.

Diagnosis

Diagnosis can be confirmed by demonstrating the characteristic fungi with their slender, branching septate hyphae, **in tissue sections**. Or, they can be recovered in cultures from typical lesions.

Blastomycosis

Blastomycosis is an infectious disease of **humans** and **animals** caused by the **dimorphic** (i.e., occurring in two different forms - yeast form in tissue, mycelial in culture) **fungus** *Blastomyces dermatitidis*. Among animals, blastomycosis is **most common in dogs**, but has been reported in **cats** (particularly Siamese), **horses** (mammary gland), and an African lion. **Blastomycosis usually occurs in dogs and humans of the same household** (i.e., living together in a house). The fungus has been recovered from soil, and **infection** is acquired by **inhalation**. **It is not a communicable disease.**

In **dogs** and **cats**, **pulmonary infection is the most common**, but organisms may spread to any system. Lungs, skin, bones, lymph nodes, testicle, and eyes are the most commonly affected organs. In **humans**, infection usually presents as cutaneous blastomycosis, but the primary site is the lung, with secondary spread to the skin.

Lesions

Blastomycosis is characterized by a **mixed cellular reaction**. A **purulent reaction** is characteristic of the **early lesions**, whereas a **typical granulomatous reaction** characterizes the **chronic lesions**. The typical lesion in **dogs** consists of a central core of neutrophils and caseous necrosis, surrounded by an intense infiltration of epithelioid cells, also containing foci of neutrophils and lymphocytes. **Multinucleated giant cells** may be present. There is little tendency towards encapsulation of the lesions.

In the **lungs of dogs, grey nodules of consolidation** may be seen in some cases. In others, **consolidation** may be diffuse with the cut surfaces yielding purulent exudate. **Microscopically**, the pulmonary lesion is characterized by an intense infiltration of epithelioid cells, in which foci of neutrophils and lymphocytes may be found. **Caseous necrosis** may occur, but there is little tendency towards encapsulation. **Multinucleated giant cells** of the foreign body type may be seen. **Calcification is rare**. The lesions are usually limited to the lungs. However, spread with abscess formation has been described in the subcutis, spleen, kidneys, lymph nodes, liver, brain, bones, adrenal glands, eyes, and intestines.

Fungi, which vary in number from a few to countless, are found in the lesions free, or in macrophages as spherical, yeast-like cells, 8-20 μm in diameter, with double-contoured walls. In H & E stained sections, organisms are seen as a central granular mass, surrounded by a refractile, double-contoured, unstained zone, bounded by a thin outer wall. An occasional cell may be seen extruding a daughter cell (**budding**). The **buds** are always single with a broad base. This is helpful in differential diagnosis. Stains for bound glycogen (**PAS, Gomori methenamine silver, Gridley fungus, Bauer**) stain the outer wall of the fungi selectively. This differentiates them more clearly from the surrounding tissue.

Diagnosis

Microscopic examination of the affected tissues is necessary to establish diagnosis. The organisms are readily demonstrable in typical lesions, and can be stained differentially with glycogen stains. They are larger than *Histoplasma capsulatum*, smaller than *Coccidioides immitis*, and do not have the wide, mucicarmine-staining capsule of *Cryptococcus neoformans*. The tissue reactions in histoplasmosis and cryptococcosis are also different from that of blastomycosis. Cultural identification of the fungus is important, but it is more important that any fungus recovered in culture also be demonstrated in characteristic lesions.

Candidiasis (Moniliasis, Thrush)

Candidiasis is caused by the spores of the fungus **Candida**, usually *Candida albicans*, and is **mainly a superficial mycosis of mucous membranes. It is mostly seen in avian species**, affecting the mouth, oesophagus, crop, and proventriculus. In mammals also, superficial infection of oral mucous membranes is the most common form, and is seen in **humans, dogs, cats, pigs, and monkeys**. Superficial infection of the skin is another form. **Systemic infection** is less common, but has been described in **humans, calves, and pigs. In cattle**, systemic disease may affect the gastrointestinal tract, lungs, liver, kidneys, or brain. Mastitis a nd abortion have also b een attributed t o **Candida**. In p igs, especially piglets, i nfection of t he stomach i s most c ommon, usually a long with oral and oesophageal infection. **In general, candidiasis is most common in young animals**, debilitated patients, and also as a complication of antibiotic therapy.

Lesions

Gross lesions in the superficial form are characterized by white pseudomembrane lying o ver the s kin, or m ucous membranes. **Microscopically**, the membrane is composed of masses of entangled pseudohyphae, septate hyphae, and budding yeast-like organisms 3-4 μm in diameter. The fungi are difficult to be seen clearly in H & E stained sections, but are clearly demonstrated with the **periodic acid-Schiff, Gridley, and Gomori methenamine silver techniques. Pseudohyphae** are chains of yeast-like cells, called **blastoconidia** or **blastospores**, which have remained attached after division. A leukocytic infiltration, composed mainly of neutrophils and lymphocytes, accumulates beneath the epidermis. Lesions in systemic candidiasis, which involve particularly kidneys, are characterized by necrosis and suppuration. **Only rarely is a granulomatous reaction present.**

Diagnosis

Diagnosis depends upon d emonstration of t he fungi i n characteristic le-sions. **The presence of blastoconidia and pseudohyphae is diagnostic.** When only yeast-like forms are p resent, other m ycoses, such a s histoplasmosis or blastomycosis, must be c onsidered.

Coccidioidomycosis (Coccidioidal Granuloma)

Coccidioidomycosis occurs both in humans and a wide variety of do-mestic and wild animals. T hese include **dogs, sheep, cattle, horses, mon-keys, wild deer and Bengal tigers. In humans**, infection is usually subclinical, or may occur as an acute, febrile, respiratory disease with a short course. In a few cases, the infection progresses to a serious disease with disseminated lesions and fatal outcome. **In animals**, the disease usually acquires the chronic pro-gressive form with primary lesions in the lungs, and spread first to regional lymph nodes a nd then t o most o rgans. Inapparent p ulmonary infection h as been seen in cattle. **Among domestic animals, disseminated disease is most common in dogs.**

The causative organism, *Coccidioides immitis*, is a dimorphic fungus which lives in soil. **Inhalation of spores (arthroconidia) produced by the mycelia causes the disease in humans and animals.** Direct transmission from one ani-mal to another does not appear to occur. The organism grows well in cultures, producing mycelia which form a small, spherical colony. **In tissues mycelial structures are not observed.** The fungus takes the form of spherules 5-50 μm in diameter with double-contoured walls. **Reproduction i n tissues i s by endosporulation**. Therefore, **endospores** may be found in some of the larger spherules.

Clinical signs are usually absent, particularly in cattle. The first indication of the infection is the presence of lesions in the pulmonary lymph nodes in apparently healthy animals at slaughter. Generalized infections run a slow course; the signs are non-specific a nd may include emaciation, inappetence, low-grade f ever and cough.

Lesions

Gross lesions resemble those of tuberculosis in many respects. They may be present as discrete (separate) or **confluent granulomas**, with or without suppuration o r calcification. **I n cattle**, lesions usually a ppear as s mall nodules in the lungs, and as diffuse enlargements of bronchial or mediastinal lymph nodes. Purulent foci may be surrounded by a band of granulation tissue and a fibrous capsule. On incision of an affected lymph node, thick, yellowish pus comes out. In this disseminated form of the disease, as in the **dog**, greyish nodules of various sizes may be found in the lungs, lymph nodes, liver, spleen, meninges, eye, bone marrow, and other organs.

Microscopically, the characteristic **appearance of the lesion varies with the developmental stage of the fungus**. T he largest s pherules, filled w ith endospores, are surrounded by a zone of epithelioid cells, admixed with a few neutrophils and so me lymphocytes. **I n cattle** these large s pherules are su r-rounded b y a c orona (ring) o f radiating c lub-shaped structures (**Splendore-Hoeppli material**). This somewhat resembles the "**rosette**" around a colony of *Actinomyces bovis*. When the large spherule ruptures, releasing its **endospores**, the tissue reaction becomes rich in neutrophils and lymphocytes, with fewer e pithelioid cells. A s these e ndospores mature, l eukocytes and epithelioid cells predominate i n the inflammatory exudate. Fungi within the cytoplasm of Langhans' giant cells are clearly seen in sections stained with H & E. However, stains for the bound glycogen (**PAS, Gridley fungus, Bauer**) demonstrate the double-contoured wall selectively.

Diagnosis

Microscopic demonstration of the fungi in the lesions usually establishes the diagnosis. When organisms are few, special stains (PAS, Gridley fungus, Bauer) are helpful in revealing them. The size of the largest spherules (50 µm), p resence o f e ndospores, a nd the a bsence o f b udding all s erve to differentiate *C. i mmitis* f rom *B lastomyces d ermatitidis* or *Cryptococcus neoformans*. The spherules of *Rhinosporidium seeberi* are similar to those of **Coccidioides**, but may be much larger, have a thicker wall, and contain larger endospores.

Cryptococcosis

Also known as "torulosis", **cryptococcosis is a disease of many animal species**. It is caused by a yeast-like fungus, *Cryptococcus neoformans*. Two varieties exist: *C. neoformans* var. *gratti* and *C. neoformans* var. *neoformans*. Most i nfections in a nimals are d ue to v ar. *neoformans*. In nature, *C. neoformans* var. *n eoformans* is f ound in m anure, e specially t hat of b irds, mainly **pigeons. C ryptococcosis is usually acquired by inhalation**, is non-communicable, and is often an opportunistic infection in immunocompromised animals. The disease occurs in most domestic animals, which include **cattle, sheep, pigs, horses, cats** and **dogs**, and also in a variety of wild species.

Cryptococcosis may i nvolve many d ifferent systems, b ut it u sually af-fects the respiratory and central nervous systems. Any portion of the respi-ratory system may be invaded, from the external nares to the lungs. The or-ganism has a strong affinity for the cerebrospinal meninges and brain. It may gain entry through haematogenous spread, or by direct extension through the turbinates.

Lesions

Gross lesions are not diagnostic, but usually quite characteristic. Although they may appear as **nodules** typical of other granulomatous diseases, usually the lesions consist of expanding masses of a mucinous or gelatinous translucent material. The **tumour-like masses** project fro m the org ans and displace them. **Microscopically, the findings are diagnostic. Lesions contain masses of pro-liferating organisms**. The fungi in tissues occur as ovoid or spherical, thick-walled, yeast-like b odies that s ometimes show s ingle budding a nd are s ur-rounded by a wide capsule. The cell inside the capsule is 5-20 μm in diameter; the capsule increases the diameter to 30 μm. In sections stained with H & E, the cell w all and so metimes its c ontent are v isible, but the capsule remains unstained. **The capsule stains selectively by the PAS method and mucicarmine technique for glycogen.**

In m ost places, o rganisms grow a nd multiply r apidly, producing **c ystic lesions**. This is a prominent feature in **brain**. Organisms grow in the pia mater over t he surface, a nd deep i nto the c erebral convolutions w here they f orm cystic areas and displace brain parenchyma. Cystic lesions may occur in lungs, adrenal glands, l ymph nodes, and mammary glands.

Diagnosis

Diagnosis can be made from the characteristic microscopic lesions in which organisms can be demonstrated, and identified culturally or morphologically. The wide capsules, which selectively stains with mucicarmine stain, differenti-ates *C. neoformans* in tissue from *Blastomyces dermatitidis*. The budding of *C. neoformans*, and its smaller size and capsule, differentiate it from *Coccidioides immitis*, which produces endospores and is not encapsulated.

Epizootic Lymphangitis

This is a disease of the **skin and superficial lymphatics of horses, mules and donkeys,** but **rarely humans.** Epizootic lymphangitis is caused by a fungus currently known as *Histoplasma farciminosum.* The organism is yeast shaped in tissue and cannot be differentiated from *Histoplasma capsulatum.* **The disease remains endemic in India.** The **clinical features are those of chronic indurative (hardened) ulceration of the skin,** especially in the **limbs,** with thickening of the superficial lymphatics, enlargement of regional lymph nodes, formation of abscesses, and **discharge of purulent material.** This is followed by the development of new **indolent (painless) ulcers.** Sometimes infection may occur as conjunctivitis, or naso-lachrymal infection. Only rarely it becomes generalized, involving internal organs. **The disease runs a chronic course over a period of months,** but eventually resolves.

The mode of transmission is unknown. Direct contact does not appear important unless infective material is conveyed to previously injured skin.

Lesions

Cutaneous lesions reveal **granulomatous tissue reactions** with a large number of macrophages, and sometimes **multinucleated giant cells.** Their cytoplasm is distended with oval organisms, each about 2.0 by 3.0 μm and enveloped by a thin, clear capsule. The central mass of the fungus in sections can be demonstrated with H & E. The capsule, however, remains unstained. Stains for bound glycogen **(PAS, Gridley, Bauer)** identify the capsule selectively, staining it red and leaving the central body unstained. Lymphocytes, plasma cells and some neutrophils are present within the granulomatous tissue reaction. Secondary infection leads to the formation of abscesses which may drain to the surface.

Diagnosis

Diagnosis can be confirmed by the demonstration of typical fungi in characteristic lesions (tissue sections), cultures, or stained smears of exudate. The fungi cannot be differentiated from *H. capsulatum*, but the nature of the two diseases is different. *Sporothrix schenckii* (of sporotrichosis) may closely resemble *H. farciminosum* and produce a similar disease and lesions. Usually *Sporothrix schenckii* is oval in shape.

Geotrichosis

This is **a rare, opportunistic mycosis of humans and animals** caused by *Geotrichum candidum.* It is a fungus common on fruits, vegetables, and dairy products. It has been reported to cause mastitis and abortion in **cattle,** lymphadenitis in **pigs,** and systemic infection in **dogs.** In **humans,** it causes chronic bronchitis, stomatitis, enteritis, conjuctivitis, dermatitis and disseminated mycosis.

Lesions

Lesions are mainly necrotizing and suppurative with variable numbers of macrophages and multinucleated giant cells, or may occur as well-defined **granulomas**. The disseminated disease in dogs may affect lungs, kidneys, lymph nodes, myocardium, liver, spleen, bone marrow, eyes, and brain. The organisms in lesions appear as round, yeast-like cells, 3-7 μm in diameter, or as chains of yeast cells forming pseudohyphae, or as true septate hyphae branching at acute angles.

Diagnosis

Diagnosis requires demonstration of the fungi in tissue section and differentiation from *Candida albicans*. Isolation of the organism is necessary for positive identification.

Histoplasmosis

Histoplasmosis is a disease caused by the fungus *Histoplasma capsulatum*. It occurs both in **humans** and a wide variety of animals, which include **dogs, cats, cattle, horses,** and **monkeys**. It is **most common in dogs**. *H. capsulatum* is a dimorphic fungus. It grows readily in culture media and soil that bears **spores of two types**: 1. Spherical, spiny **microconidia** 3-4 μm in diameter, and 2. Spherical, or rarely clavate (club-shaped) **macroconidia**, 8-12 μm in diameter with finger-like projections over the surface. The parasitic phase in the host develops from either of these conidia into yeast-like form.

Infection occurs through inhalation of spores from infected soil. The infection is first established in the lung, where the yeast form of the **fungus proliferates within macrophages** and later may be spread throughout the mononuclear phagocyte system. Although the disease in human occurs as a fatal, disseminated infection, it is now known that **an acute non-fatal form** is much more common both in humans and animals. **The disease is not spread by direct contact between animals,** but it may appear in animals and humans sharing the same environment. Both the **benign inapparent** and the **fatal disseminated forms** of the disease occur in animals.

The **benign form** of the disease in animals is usually not recognized, unless pulmonary lesions are present, or organisms are recovered at postmortem. Benign histoplasmosis **in humans** may be seen as an acute febrile pneumonitis with weight loss. The **fatal disseminated form in animals**, seen mostly in **dogs**, runs a prolonged course with progressive weight loss, lymphadenopathy, diarrhoea, weakness, anaemia, hepatomegaly, and ascites.

Lesions

The main feature of tissue changes is the **extensive proliferation of reticulo-endothelial cells** (macrophages, endothelioid and epithelioid cells). **Many of these cells contain a large number of yeast forms of the fungus**. It is the proliferation of reticulo-endothelial cells that causes displacement of normal tissues, interference with function, **and gross enlargement of organs**. The disease has been studied extensively **in dogs. The following description of lesions applies particularly to the dog**.

Primary disease in the lung may take the form of **classical granulomas**, composed of epithelioid cells and **multinucleated giant cells**, which may contain organisms, with or without central caseous necrosis. With recovery, these lesions regress to fibro-calcareous nodules that remain in the lungs for years. **In the disseminated form**, the alveoli and interstitial stroma are full of lymphocytes, plasma cells, and epithelioid cells, **many containing organisms as yeast-like bodies**. They reproduce with tiny buds. **In sections stained with H & E**, a central, spherical basophilic body is surrounded by an unstained zone, which is encircled by a thin cell wall. But the organism has no true capsule; the clear halo is within the cell wall. With **PAS, Bauer, GMS, or Gridley fungus method**, the wall is stained selectively, leaving its contents unstained. Thus, the organism appears as an empty red or black ring.

The **lymph nodes** in the disseminated disease are **greatly enlarged** by the proliferation of reticulo-endothelial cells. Necrosis, purulent inflammation, calcification, and giant cells are rarely seen. The predominant cell is mononuclear, often packed with organisms. Lymphocytes and plasma cells are present in small numbers.

Spleen is enlarged several times to its normal size, and is firm as a result of the reticulo-endothelial proliferation. **Liver is also enlarged** and firm. Intestine, when involved, has a thickened rugose (wrinkled, corrugated) or nodular mucosal surface. Its wall is thickened by the proliferation of mononuclear phagocytes in the lamina propria and submucosa. The adrenal glands may be largely replaced by macrophages filled with organisms. This is particularly noticeable in fatal cases. Other organs are less severely affected, but may be involved by the characteristic proliferation of mononuclear phagocytes.

Diagnosis

In the living animal, diagnosis can be established by demonstration of **typical mononuclear phagocyte proliferation and organisms in tissue biopsy** (tonsils, lymph node, liver). In some cases, monocytes, neutrophils, or eosinophils containing *H. capsulatum* can be demonstrated in blood smears. Serological tests are available, but are not reliable. **Microscopic examination** of tissue sections usually permits definitive diagnosis, but in some cases identification of the organisms in cultures is advisable. The organism of epizootic lymphangitis (*Histoplasma farciminosum*) cannot be differentiated in tissue sections. **Therefore, cultures are necessary to distinguish these two infections**.

Maduramycosis

Also known as "**Madura foot**" and "**Maduramycotic mycetoma**", maduramycosis is an age-old **disease of bare-footed people**, named after Madura, in India, where the disease was first described. "**Madura foot**" in **humans** is characterized by marked swelling (**mycetoma**) of the foot (or hand) with multiple draining sinuses. Many fungal species can cause these lesions, as well as some of the Actinomycetes. **In humans**, mycetomas have been divided into: 1. **Eumycetomas, caused by Eumycetes or true fungi**, and 2. **Actinomycetomas**, caused by organisms of the genera **Actinomyces, Nocardia, Staphylococcus** sp., **Actinobacillus** sp., *Escherichia coli*, **Proteus** sp. and *Pseudomonas aeruginosa*, and others. **Here, only those lesions in animals are described which are caused by true fungi**.

In animals, maduramycosis is a skin disease of mainly horses and also dogs. It is characterized by the formation of **cutaneous granulomas (mycetomas) caused by a variety of fungi**. These, as well as the causative agents of actinomycetomas, are **introduced through trauma into tissues**. A characteristic of **mycetoma (granuloma)** is the aggregation of fungi in masses or "**grains**" similar to the "**sulphur granules**" of **Actinomyces**. That is, in tissues, the causative fungi form definite colonies or "**grains**", composed of masses of mycelial filaments, which in most cases produce pigment. Fungi which do not produce pigment cause "**white-grained maduramycosis**", and colonies which produce pigment are seen by the unaided eye as "**black grains**".

Lesions

Lesions of maduramycosis are characterized by the presence of **distinct colonies of fungi**, which appear **grossly** as tiny black, brown "**grains**", 1-3 mm wide embedded in mass of granulation tissue. These "**grains**" (colonies of fungi) can be squeezed out by pressure from the narrow zone of pus that surrounds them. The lesions in animals (**horses, dogs**) are most common on the extremities, but may involve the nasal mucosa, peritoneum, or skin at any site. **In horses**, there are one or more lesions of 1-2.5 cm in diameter anywhere on the skin, but are most common on the **coronet**. The incised lesion drains pus which contains the fungus. **In dogs**, the coiled glands of the foot pad appear to be the site of predilection. These mycotic granulomas may become quite large and are usually resistant to any treatment except surgical removal.

The microscopic appearance is characteristic. Colonies of the fungi are

seen as brown, spherical bodies embedded within a pocket of neutrophils. These purulent centres are separated by granulation tissue richly infiltrated with macrophages, plasma cells, and lymphocytes. The organisms in the colony form an outer zone consisting of **hyphae** and thick-walled **chlamydospores**. The centre of the colony contains many branching, **septate hyphae**. The hyphae are of irregular length, but 10 μm wide. The chlamydospores have thicker walls, are spherical, and may attain a diameter of 25 μm or more. The **PAS, Bauer, and Gridley fungus stains** clearly demonstrate morphology of the fungi in tissue sections.

Diagnosis

Diagnosis can be made by demonstrating typical fungal colonies in granulomas. Organisms should be cultured to establish the identity of the causative agent.

Nasal Granuloma of Cattle

In certain parts of the world, **true granulomatous lesions** in which fungi have been observed, are seen in the **nasal cavity of cattle**. However, the aetiology of such granulomas is not clearly established. It is likely that more than one causative agent may be involved. **In India**, a form of **nasal granuloma**, caused by the fluke *Schistosoma nasalis* is seen **in cattle**.

Spherical fungi have been described in sections of nasal granulomas in cattle, and cultures of **Helminthosporum** recovered. This organism has been isolated from cases of maduramycosis, suggesting that nasal granuloma may be a form of maduramycosis.

Lesions

Lesions are confined to the external nares and appear as **nodules** that project from any part of the nasal mucosa into the nasal cavity. The nodules have a glistening surface and on incision are greyish yellow to red. **Microscopically**, the lesions consist of **granulomas**, in which epithelioid and foreign-body **giant cells** predominate. Lymphocytes and eosinophils are also present in significant numbers. Spherical bodies, with thick walls, suggesting a fungus are often seen within epithelioid and giant cells.

Protothecosis

Colourless **algae** of the genus **Prototheca** are usually saprophytic. However, at times, they have been reported to cause disease in **humans** and **animals**. **Prototheca** are considered relatives of green algae. However, their exact taxonomic position is uncertain. **In humans**, infection is mostly limited to the skin, but **in animals** systemic or generalized infection, with or without involvement of the skin, is more common. **Protothecosis in animals was first described as a cause of mastitis in cattle**, and has since been reported in **dogs, cats, and**

deer. In systemic infection of dogs, organisms have a predilection for brain and eyes. Disseminated lesions occur in the kidneys, heart, liver, gastrointestinal tract, lymph nodes, muscle, bone, and skin. In **cattle**, mastitis is the most common finding. The cutaneous form of the disease has been described in **cats**.

Lesions

In tissue sections, **Prototheca** sp. appear as round or oval cells, 8-20 μm in diameter with a distinct wall and granular cytoplasm. The cell wall stains poorly in H & E stained sections, and the organisms, if few, can be easily missed. However, the wall is strongly positive to stains for carbohydrate (**PAS, Gridley, Bauer, GMS**). **Tissue reaction is variable**. In some cases, there is little inflammatory reaction, even to large numbers of organisms. However, usually, there is diffuse pyogranulomatous reaction, or typical granulomatous response, with epithelioid cells and **multinucleated giant cells**.

Diagnosis

Diagnosis is based on finding the typical organisms in tissue section, but isolation is required for species identification.

Rhinosporidiosis

Infection with the fungus *Rhinosporidium seeberi* causes **a polypoid granulomatous lesion**, particularly in the nasal mucosa. **It infects humans, horses, cattle, dogs, and in birds ducks and geese. Rhinosporidiosis is common in India**, Sri Lanka, and south-east Asia. **The source of infection is not known**, but the disease is associated with stagnant water.

Lesions

In animals, as in humans, the fungus invades the **nasal mucosa**, and sometimes spreads even further down the respiratory tract or skin. It induces a **chronic inflammation** usually leading to **polyp formation**. The **polyps** are single or multiple, irregular in size and shape. **They may become large enough to occlude the nasal passages**.

Microscopically, polyps contain a stroma filled with spherical organisms with a thick, double-contoured wall. Mature organisms (**sporangium**, pleural **sporangia**) are up to 300 μm in diameter, and are filled with **endospores** 2-10 μm in diameter. **Endospores** are larger and round in the centre of the sporangia, and flattened and mature at the periphery. Each endospore contains several eosinophilic bodies. Endospores are released by rupture of the cell wall at the pore, and develop into **trophocytes** of 100 μm in diameter. Trophocytes contain a single nucleus with a prominent nucleolus. These, in turn, mature to sporangium containing endospores. **The tissue reaction is similar to that caused by** *Coccidioides immitis*, which resembles *R. seeberi* in morphology.

The sporangia are surrounded by an inflammatory cellular infiltrate composed of epithelioid cells, **multinucleated giant cells**, lymphocytes, neutrophils, and fibrovascular connective tissue. Released endospores incite a more purulent response.

Diagnosis

Rhinosporidiosis must be differentiated from coccidioidomycosis. **Rhinosporidia** are larger than *Coccidioides immitis*. The sporangia contain endospores which are also larger than those of *C. immitis*. In **Rhinosporidia**, complete endospores stain with fungal stains, such as PAS, wheras in *C. immitis* only the walls of endospores stain. Also, endospores of *R. seeberi* contain inner granules, but those of *C. immitis* do not

Sporotrichosis

Sporotrichosis is **a granulomatous disease** caused by the dimorphic fungus *Sporothrix schenckii* (*Sporotrichum schenkii*). It occurs in **humans, dogs, cats, horses, mules, cattle**, and other animals and **also birds**. In animals, **it is most common in horses and cats**. The fungus grows on plants, soil, and wood. **Infection is acquired by entry through skin abrasions.** Like so many other mycotic diseases, sporotrichosis is not contagious. However, **infected cats have been reported to be the source of infection for humans**. In contrast to other species, the number of fungi within lesions in the affected cats are high. This may account for their ability to serve as a source of infection.

Lesions

Lesions occur in the skin and cutaneous lymphatics, particularly over the legs, thorax, and abdomen. **Spherical nodules**, 1-4 cm in diameter, are formed **in the skin along the course of lymphatics**, which are thickened and tortuous between the nodules. Sometimes the nodules ulcerate, produce small amounts of thick, creamy pus, and then heal slowly. Spread to other tissues, particularly bones and joints, occurs, but is rare. This has been mostly reported in **humans, cats** and **dogs**. Involvement of lungs, liver, spleen, kidneys, and internal lymph nodes can occur.

Microscopically, the **nodules** reveal a **purulent centre** surrounded by a band of epithelioid granulation tissue containing **giant cells** and lymphocytes. The lesion is usually surrounded by a dense connective tissue capsule. The fungi are usually not seen in H & E stained sections, except in infected cats where they are exceptionally numerous. When stained with **GMS, PAS**, and similar techniques, they appear as small, cigar-shaped or round yeasts, 4-6 μm long, with single or multiple buds. They are located within the purulent centre of the lesions and in the cytoplasm of macrophages and multinucleated giant cells.

Diagnosis

Sporotrichosis must be differentiated from epizootic lymphangitis in horses caused by *Histoplasma farciminosum*. The two yeasts may appear similar and require animal inoculation, culture or immunological staining techniques to differentiate them.

Zygomycosis (Phycomycosis) and Pythiosis

The term "zygomycosis" includes those disorders which are caused by fungi classified in the **Class Zygomycetes**, previously classified as **Phycomycetes** and the disease referred to as "**phycomycosis**" (**Table 29**). The term "**mucormycosis**" is often used to designate diseases caused by members of this group, as the Family **Mucoraceae** contains several important pathogens, especially the genera **Absidia, Cunninghamella, Mortierella, Mucor, Rhizomucor, Rhizopus, Saksenaea,** and **Syncephalastrum** (**Table 29**). Other zygomycetes which are associated with disease belong to the Family **Entomophthoraceae**, the genera being **Basidiobolus** and **Conidiobolus**. Disease produced by them is called "**entomophthoromycosis** (**Table 29**).

Table 29. Zygomycoses and Oomycoses

Organism		Disease
Kingdom	: Fungi	
Class	: Zygomycetes (Phycomycetes)	
Family	: **Mucoraceae**	**Mucormycosis (Phycomycosis)**
Genus	: **Absidia**	Seen in most animal species.
	Cunninghamella	Common manifestations include:
	Mortierella	cutaneous granulomas, rumenitis,
	Mucor	gastritis, enteritis, placentitis,
	Rhizomucor	pneumonia, disseminated
	Rhizopus	infections
	Saksenaea	
	Syncephalastrum	
Family	: Entomophthoraceae	**Entomophthoromycosis**
Genus	: **Basidiobolus**	Cutaneous and nasal
		granulomas in horsess
	Conidiobolus	
Kingdom	: Protista	
Class	: Oomycetes	
Family	: Pythiaceae	**Oomycosis (Pythiosis)**
Genus	: **Pythium sp.**	Cutaneous granulomas
		in horses ("**leeches**");
		rarely in cattle

A third group is the **Pythium** sp. **These are not true fungi**, but are members of the **Kingdom Protista, Class Oomycetes, Family Pythiaceae, Genus Pythium (Table 29)**. Since they belong to a separate kingdom, they should be considered separately. However, they have been included here because of the similarity of the lesions and also because of their identical appearance to that of zygomycetes in tissue sections. Infections with **Pythium** sp. are called **"oomycosis"** or **"pythiosis"**. These organisms produce disease mainly in **horses**, but infection also occurs in **calves** and **cats**.

Zygomycetes, in nature, grow on decaying vegetation and are usually not very pathogenic. However, under certain conditions, such as intercurrent disease, long-term administration of antibiotics, or immunosuppression, they can produce serious disease. Many species of animals and also humans may be infected. Lesions usually involve the skin or mucous membranes of the oral and nasal cavities. The disease may be disseminated or restricted to a specific organ. Lungs, placenta, mammary glands, rumen, stomach, kidneys and brain are the common sites.

There are no specific clinical signs. The signs depend on the tissues and organs affected. In **cattle**, placentitis, foetal infection, abortion, and infection of the rumen and abomasum are the most common manifestations of **mucormycosis**. **Mucor** also causes placentitis and abortion in **horses**. The digestive tract is the most common location of infection in **dogs**. In **horses** and rarely cattle, a dermal mycosis known as **"leeches"**, characterized by subcutaneous granulomatous inflammation, particularly of the legs is caused by a **Pythium** sp. Cutaneous granulomas in horses may also occur from infection with fungus of the genus **Basidiobolus**.

Lesions

Lesions produced by zygomycetes are usually **diffuse and not in the form of granulomas**. The organisms are highly invasive, moving through tissues, mainly into the blood vessel walls. **This is similar to that seen in aspergillosis**. This **angio-invasive** (invading blood vessels) characteristic leads to thrombosis, haemorrhagic infarction, and dissemination of infection. The lesions are characterized by a predominance of macrophages, accompanied by **multinucleated giant cells**, necrosis and neutrophils, resembling diffuse pyogranulomatous inflammation with necrosis and pus. All species of zygomycetes look similar in tissue section. They appear as pleomorphic, **branching hyphae**, 3-25 μm in diameter. The hyphae usually stain basophilic with H & E, and are not seen any better with special staining techniques.

Diagnosis

Diagnosis is based on demonstration of characteristic organisms in granulomatous lesions. Isolation of fungi from the lesions is necessary for further identification. However, histological demonstration of the fungus within tissues which are reacting to its presence is very important in establishing the causal relationship. Identification of the organism recovered in culture is not final because these fungi grow free in nature and can easily contaminate cultures. The zygomycetes must be differentiated from **Aspergillus** sp. **Aspergillus** are regularly septate and have uniform branching pattern. **Aspergillus** sp. also do not stain as well with H & E as do the zygomycetes.

Mycotoxicoses (Mouldy Feeds)

The fungal diseases discussed so far are the disorders **in which the fungi themselves invade tissue, no matter how superficially.** Many of these are true pathogens or obligate parasites, while many others are opportunistic infections by fungi which are usually saprophytic or pathogens of plants.

There are, however, a large number of disorders in which disease or death is due to the ingestion of fungi, or their products (toxins) produced by fungi in or on the animal's feed. Collectively, these disorders are called "**mycotoxicoses**". Diseases resulting from **mycotoxins** have been known for centuries. However, with the awareness of aflatoxicosis in the 1960s, interest in mycotoxins expanded rapidly, and many new and old diseases were recognized as being caused by toxic metabolites of fungi. The search for other mycotoxins has resulted in identification of a large number of **additional mycotoxins. There are no common clinical or pathological features with mycotoxicoses.** Many are **hepatotoxic**, but changes produced are of different types, ranging from neoplasia to neurological dysfunction. Some of the more important and better studied mycotoxicoses are listed in **Table 30.**

Aflatoxicosis (Aflatoxins, Mycotoxin, Groundnut poisoning, Toxin of Aspergillus sp.)

Aflatoxins are highly toxic and carcinogenic metabolites produced by the fungi *Aspergillus flavus* and *A. parasiticus*. **Aflatoxins are produced when environmental conditions favour their growth** on certain cereal grains, groundnuts, and seeds. **At least 17 different aflatoxins exist.** All are structurally related to coumarins. **The most important are B1, B2, G1, G2 and M1,** and these are also the most widespread. The designations B and G refer to whether they **fluoresce blue or green in ultraviolet light. Of these, aflatoxin B1 is the most prevalent and most toxic.** Aflatoxin M1, a mammalian metabolite of B1, is excreted in **milk. The most commonly contaminated foods are groundnuts, maize, and cottonseed.**

Table 30. Mycotoxicoses

Disease	Fungus	Toxin	Species	Major pathological features	Principal plant
Aflatoxicosis	*Aspergillus flavus*	Aflatoxins B1, B2, G1, G2	Poultry, dogs, pigs, cattle, humans	Toxic hepatitis, cirrhosis, hepatic adenomas and adenocarcinomas	Groundnut meal, maize, cottonseed etc.
"Atypical interstitial pneumonia" of cattle	Fusarium sp.	4-Ipomeanol	Cattle	Pulmonary oedema, alveolar cell proliferation, hyaline membranes	Sweet potatoes
Convulsive or nervous ergotism	*Claviceps paspali*	Tremorigens	Cattle, sheep, horses	Unknown	Dallis grass
Facial eczema	*Pithomyces chartarum*	Sporodesmin	Sheep, cattle	Toxic hepatitis, cirrhosis, photosensitization	Pasture plants, esp. ryegrass
Gangrenous ergotism	*Claviceps purpurea*	Ergotamine, other alkaloids	Cattle, horses, pigs, humans	Gangrene, agalactia	Grains, grasses
Hepatic necrosis	*Penicillium islandicum*	Luteoskyrin, cyclochlorotine	Humans, chickens	Toxic hepatitis, cirrhosis, hepato-carcinoma	Rice
Ill-defined (diarrhoea, tremors, convulsions)	*Penicillium cyclopium*	Cyclopiazonic acid	Sheep, horses, cattle	Toxic hepatitis	Many foods
Ill-defined	*Penicillium rubrum*	Rubratoxins	Pigs, cattle	Hepatic necrosis	Maize, other foods
Lupinosis	*Phomopsis*	Phomopsin	Sheep, horses,	Toxic hepatitis, cirrhosis	Lupines

Disease	Fungus	Toxin	Animals	Lesions	Foodstuff
Mouldy maize poisoning	*leptostromiformis* *Fusarium moniliforme?*	Unknown	cattle, pigs Horses	Encephalomalacia	Maize
Mouldy nephrosis of pigs	*Aspergillus ochraceus, Penicillium viridicatum*	Ochratoxins, citrinin	Pigs, poultry	Toxic nephrosis	Maize, wheat, barley, oats, alfalfa
Neurotoxicosis	*Penicillium patulum*	Patulin	Cattle	Convulsions, oedema, haemorrhage	Malted barley, wheat
Perrenial rye grass staggers	*Penicillium sp.*	Tremorigens	Cattle, sheep, horses	Tremors, ataxia	Perrenial rye grass
Porcine vulvo-vaginitis	*Fusarium roseum*	Zearalenone (oestrogenic)	Pigs	Hyperplasia of uterus, vagina, mammary gland	Maize, barley, wheat, oats
Stachybotryotoxicosis	*Stachybotrys sp.*	Stachybotryotoxin	Horses, humans	Haemorrhagic necrosis and ulceration of mouth, stomach, intestine	Hays
Tibial dyschondroplasia	*Fusarium roseum*	Unknown	Poultry	Tibial dyschondroplasia	Unknown
Ulcerative stomatitis, gastroenteritis	**Fusarium, Cephalosporium, Myrothecium, Trichothecium, Trichoderma**	Trichothecenes	Cattle, pigs, horses, humans	Dermatitis, gastroenteritis, haemorrhages	Maize, barley, rice, many plants

The first descriptions of aflatoxicosis appeared in 1952, when an epizootic toxic hepatitis ("**hepatitis X**") was described in **dogs**. Later, in 1955, it was demonstrated to be the result of feeding commercial dog foods that contained **contaminated groundnut meal**. It was, however, investigation in 1961 into a previously unrecognized disease of **turkeys ("turkey X disease")** in Great Britain, that killed over 1,00,000 turkeys, which first led to the identification of **Brazilian groundnut meal** as the common factor in the disorder and to the ultimate chemical isolation of aflatoxins. At about the same time, outbreaks of disease in **pigs** and **calves** were traced to **Brazilian groundnut meal**. Also, the occurrence of hepatomas in hatchery-raised trout (a type of fish) in the United States was traced to cottonseed meal contaminated with aflatoxins. In 1991, an outbreak of aflatoxicosis involving 30 **Angora rabbit** farms has been recorded **in India**.

It appears that **all animals, as well as fish, are susceptible to the hepatotoxicity of aflatoxins** and also to its **carcinogenic property** which leads to **liver cancer**. Moreover, **humans are also susceptible**, and serious outbreaks of acute poisoning have occurred in **India** and **Africa**. However, **there is evidence that aflatoxins cause cancer in humans**.

Lesions

A number of factors influence the effects of aflatoxins. **Young animals are more susceptible than adults, and males are more susceptible than females**. Poor nutritional status increases susceptibility. Considerable species variation also occurs. **Young turkeys and ducklings are much more susceptible than chickens**. Rats are more susceptible than mice, particularly to the carcinogenic effects of aflatoxins. **Natural disease has been reported in dogs, cats, pigs, and cattle, but rarely in sheep and goats. Horses** are relatively resistant. The dose of aflatoxin and the duration of exposure also influence the effects of its toxicity. **Aflatoxins bind to nucleic acids and disrupt polyribosomes. This leads to interference with both nucleic acid and protein synthesis**. They also result in **impaired T cell function**. More recently animal studies have revealed **that aflatoxin can bind covalently with cellular DNA and cause mutations in proto-oncogenes or tumour suppressor genes, particularly p53**. A particularly susceptible site for aflatoxin action is the **guanosine base** in codon 249 of the **p53** gene, leading to **G to T transversion at this site**. This specific **p53** mutation is found usually in **hepatocellular carcinomas**.

Acute Aflatoxicosis

This results from **ingestion of large quantities of aflatoxins**. This leads to **severe hepatic necrosis** within hours. **Signs of liver damage** develop rapidly and include jaundice, widespread haemorrhage, and an increase in serum hepatic enzymes. **Necrosis is mainly periportal in turkeys, ducklings, chickens, cats**, and adult rats; **midzonal** in rabbits; and **centrilobular** in **pigs, cattle,** dogs, and g uinea-pigs. Oedema and haemorrhage i n gallbladder w all are consistent findings in **pigs** and **dogs**.

Chronic Aflatoxicosis

This is the more common form of the disease, and results from expo-sure to a lower dosage of aflatoxins over a period of time. The e ffects develop over several days to months, but may be seen pathologically within one week. Signs i nclude decreased g rowth rate, lowered p roductivity, a nd eventually signs of liver disease. **The most striking and consistent lesion in all species is marked proliferation of small bile ductules at the periphery of hepatic lobules.** Changes in h epatocytes include fatty change, swelling, and necrosis. Necrosis, however, is not as extensive as in acute aflatoxicosis. As the lesion progresses, proliferation of connective tissue occurs. **This leads to periportal fibrosis or cirrhosis.** This is accompanied by nodular regeneration of hepatocytes with increase in nuclear size and **megalocytic (big) hepatocytes**.

The carcinogenicity of aflatoxin is well established. However, the pre-cise conditions under w hich neoplasia d evelops are not c ompletely u nder-stood. H epatomas, hepatic c ell carcinomas, a nd cholangio-carcinomas h ave been produced experimentally by feeding aflatoxin to ducklings, turkeys, rats, guinea-pigs, trouts (fish), **sheep**, **pigs**, and **monkeys**. Also, in rats, aflatoxins produce carcinoma of the oesophagus, glandular stomach, colon, and kidneys. Among domestic animals, **hepatic cell carcinomas** have been observed **only in pigs poisoned by aflatoxins**.

Diagnosis

Diagnosis depends on the detection of aflatoxin in the feed and blood serum, and the characteristic gross and histopathological findings in the liver. Detection of aflatoxin can be done in **two ways**: 1. By **biological testing**, and 2. By **chemical testing. Biological testing includes** the detection of char-acteristic bile duct hyperplasia produced by aflatoxins in liver of ducklings; and observation of death and abnormalities; in hatched chicks given aflatoxin through a hole in shell into the airsac. **Chemical testing includes** estimation of total aflatoxins b y fluorotoxinometer. **A flatoxin B1 in mixed feeds can be detected by enzyme-linked immunosorbent screening methods.** T hese in-clude estimation by ELISA using method of AOAC for aflatoxin B1; dot ELISA for aflatoxin B1, B2, G1 in maize, cottonseed or groundnuts; and dot immunobinding assay, c olumn and t hin layer c hromatography for detection of aflatoxin in feed.

Dallis Grass Poisoning

In United States, a fungus *Claviceps paspali* grows upon Dallis grass, a pasture plant. It produces what is known as "**Dallis grass poisoning**" in **cattle, sheep**, and **horses**. This ergot (sclerotium) is much smaller than that of *Claviceps* *purpurea* and u sually o f a b rownish colour. C linical signs of Dallis g rass poisoning are mainly nervous in character and include nervous hyperirritability, excitability, and muscular incoordination. Many animals recover with a change in feed. **Gross lesions** are few, and **microscopic studies** do not appear to have been carried o ut.

Equine Leukoencephalomalacia (Mouldy Corn Poisoning)

Many different mycotoxin-producing moulds can contaminate corn. Therefore, the t erm **"mouldy corn poisoning"** covers a n umber o f different syndromes. However, usually it is used to designate a specific disorder of **horses** and **donkeys** called **"equine leukoencephalomalacia"**. The syndrome has been associated w ith the feeding of mouldy corn **in the United States** and o ther parts of the world. A ffected **horses** are d rowsy, tend to c ircle, and d evelop **paralysis. Gross lesions** consist of softening and liquefactive necrosis, **chiefly** of the white matter of the **cerebrum.** Oedema and congestion occur, but **there** is little cellular inflammatory reaction.

Ergot

Most of the small grains and many different grasses are parasitized by the fungus *Claviceps purpurea*. Each **sclerotium** (a compact collection of mycelia) of the fungus is a hard, black, elongated body. It destroys and replaces a grain **or** seed of the maturing plant. **The sclerotia constitute the substance called ergot that has poisonous properties. Ergot contains a variety of toxic substances.** These include derivatives of lysergic acid **(ergotamine)** and isolysergic acid **(ergocristine).** In past, humans got poisoned by contaminated flour. **In animals, including birds, poisoning may occur through the feeding of contaminated grain,** but **in herbivora**, it results usually from the use of hay or straw containing a considerable proportion of **parasitized plants**.

In g eneral, action o f ergot i s to stimulate smooth muscle by st imulating adrenergic n erves. This a ction on the uterus is responsible f or its use as a n **oxytocic. Long-continued contraction of the vascular musculature is the main reason for its poisonous effects.**

Clinical signs of chronic poisoning by ergot, known as **"ergotism"**, consist of **dry gangrene** of the limbs, tail, and ears. After weeks of ingestion of small amounts, the most distal parts of the extremities may drop off. The early stages are characterized by **lameness, irregular gait, and evidence of pain in the feet**. P alpation shows t he parts t o be cold a nd insensitive. S ometimes, **gangrene** is moist instead of dry, at least in the feet. A clear line of demarcation and an inflammatory zone just proximal to it usually exist. **In birds,** c omb, tongue, and beak become gangrenous. Less common signs based upon involvement o f the g astrointestinal musculature i nclude indigestion, colic, **vomiting,** and either diarrhoea or constipation. **Pregnant animals usually abort.**

Decreased milk production (agalactia) occurs. This may be the only sign in **pigs**.

The signs described above characterize the usual "**gangrenous form**". The rare "**spasmodic form**" (convulsive form, nervous form) causes toxic contractions of the flexor muscles of the limb, trembling of the muscles, opisthotonus (an arched position of the body), tetanic spasms of the whole body, convulsions, and death. This type of reaction is believed to be due to **failing blood supply** in the central nervous system.

Lesions are seen in the gangrenous cases. Also, congestion and sometimes haemorrhages are present in the visceral organs. Another related fungus, *Claviceps paspali*, produces different effects and has therefore been described separately under "**Dallis grass poisoning**". Gangrenous ergotism is identical in appearance to fescue poisoning.

Facial Eczema

Facial eczema, caused by a mycotoxin, was first described in sheep in New Zealand. **Cattle** are also affected. It results from the **mycotoxin, sporidesmin**, produced by the fungus *Pithomyces chartarum*, which is a saprophyte on certain pastures. It is usually associated with ryegrass.

Lesions

The toxin is mainly a **hepatotoxin**. The principal lesion from which the disease gets its name is the result of **hepatotoxic photosensitization** due to circulating **phylloerythrin**. **In sheep**, face and ears are the most severely affected sites, whereas **in cattle**, the udder and teats are affected. **Microscopically**, cholangio-hepatitis, characterized by necrosis of biliary epithelium, fibrosis and ductular hyperplasia, are the main hepatic lesions. Focal hepatic necrosis and regenerative hyperplasia may be seen. Haemorrhages in the wall of gallbladder and urinary bladder are common.

Lupinosis

Also known as "**phomopsis**", lupinosis is caused by a **mycotoxin, phomopsin**, produced by the fungus *Phomopsis leptostromiformis*, which grows on sweet and bitter lupines. (**Lupine** is a tall garden plant). Lupinosis occurs in New Zealand, Australia, Europe, and South Africa.

Lupinosis is usually seen in **sheep**, caused by greater use of lupines as a forage crop. However, the disease has also been reported in **cattle, horses, and pigs**. **Clinically**, anorexia, jaundice and death occur within a few days after exposure. Serum glutamic oxaloacetic transaminase, lactic dehydrogenase, alkaline phosphatase, and bilirubin are elevated in serum. Jaundice is pronounced. **Photosensitization** may accompany lupinosis.

Lesions

Liver is enlarged, yellow, and friable. Hepatic lesions in the early stages are characterized by focal necrosis, mainly in the central and midzonal regions. The lesions then progress to scarring, resulting in distortion of the normal lobular pattern. Hyperplasia of the bile ductules occurs.

Ochratoxicosis

Also known as "**mouldy nephrosis/nephropathy of swine**" and "**citrinin toxicity**", in ochratoxicosis several nephrotoxic mycotoxins, which are isocoumarin derivatives of phenylalanine, are involved. These are produced by species of **Penicillium** and **Aspergillus**, especially *P. viridicatum* and *A. ochraceus*. In India, prevalence of *A. ochraceus* and ochratoxicosis has been widely reported. Ochratoxin A is the most important toxin in natural poisonings in pigs and poultry. Horses are suspected to suffer. Dogs are especially susceptible to ochratoxin A experimentally, but natural poisoning has not been described.

The fungi can grow on a variety of animal feeds, including **maize, oats, wheat and barley**. The same fungi also produce **another nephrotoxin, citrinin**, which produces a similar syndrome in **pigs** and **birds**. Citrinin is believed to contribute to nephropathy in pigs and birds, but does not appear to be the primary cause. The **important clinical signs** are polydipsia (excessive thirst), polyuria (excessive urination), and dehydration. **Growth rate is significantly retarded**.

Lesions

Lesions are restricted to the kidneys. Grossly, kidneys are enlarged, grey-yellow, and firmer than normal. Ochratoxin in **pigs** is particularly toxic to the proximal covoluted tubule. **Microscopically,** epithelial cells lose their brush border and become shorter than usual, with enlarged vesicular nuclei. Later, pyknosis and necrosis of the cells occur, and cells may slough into the lumen. Peritubular fibrosis occurs secondarily, which progresses until most of the kidney, including the glomeruli, are sclerotic (hard). These lesions have been reproduced in experimentally poisoned **pigs**.

Experimentally, ochratoxin is also nephrotoxic in **dogs** and **chickens**. The effect is mainly on the proximal convoluted tubule. In contrast to pigs, lesions also develop in other tissues in these species. These include fatty change and focal necrosis of the liver, ulcerative enteritis and colitis, and proctitis and necrosis of lymphoid tissues.

Ochratoxin is suspected to be a cause of **abortion in cattle** fed mouldy hay. It is also suspected to cause fatal chronic nephropathy **in humans**.

Oestrogenic Mycotoxicosis

Fungus *Fusarium roseum* and other species of **Fusarium** produce a **mycotoxin, zearalenone,** also known as **F-2 toxin,** which has oestrogenic activity. **These fungi are contaminants of maize.** A disease of **sow, vulvovaginitis,** is known to result from ingestion of this toxin. The toxicosis (condition resulting from poisoning) stimulates oestrus, and results in enlarged vulvae, mammary glands and teats, and sometimes prolapse of the vagina. **Sows** are infertile and may show nymphomania, or pseudopregnancy. Ovaries are atrophic, and uterus and cervix grossly enlarged. Ingestion in early pregnancy leads to embryonic death. In young male pigs, feminization occurs with testicular atrophy and gynecomastia (abnormally large mammary glands in the male, sometimes secreting milk.)

Lesions

Microscopic lesions include ovarian follicular atresia (degeneration of follicles), oedema and cellular proliferation of all layers of the uterus, and ductular proliferation in the mammary glands. Stillbirths, small litters, and neonatal mortality may also occur. In males, signs of feminization include testicular atrophy, swelling of the prepuce, and enlargement of the mammary gland.

Zearalenone toxicity is suspected to be responsible for similar events and reduced fertility in **cattle.**

Trichothecenes

Trichothecenes are a group of highly toxic mycotoxins produced by several species of Fusarium and certain other fungi. These fungi **affect grains** in the field. However, toxin production is increased by storage at cool temperatures. Therefore, natural poisonings are most common in areas with cooler climates. Many different trichothecenes have been identified, but only a few appear to cause disease. **No well-defined clinical or pathological syndromes are associated with specific trichothecenes.** This is because there are many toxins, and more than one toxin usually exists in the same contaminated grain. Besides, there is also difficulty of identifying the involved toxins in a clinical syndrome.

The best studied toxins include **T-2 toxin, DAS** (diacetoxyscirpenol), **vomitoxin,** (DON or deoxynivalenol), and **satratoxin. T-2 toxin and DAS are highly toxic,** and cause necrosis of skin and mucous membranes (mouth, pharynx, oesophagus, rumen, stomach) on contact. These toxins are potent inhibitors of protein synthesis, which accounts for their cytotoxicity. Ingestion of **vomitoxin** leads to anorexia and vomiting, especially in **pigs,** but most species are susceptible. It acts on central nervous system receptors without producing morphological lesions. Rapid recovery occurs following removal of the toxin from the diet.

Various syndromes are believed to be caused by trichothecene toxicity, especially in **cattle, pigs, horses**, and **poultry**. **Clinical signs** include oral ulceration, anorexia, vomiting, diarrhoea, haemorrhage, leukopaenia, jaundice, and incoordination. **Specific lesions** include necrosis of all lymphoid organs, bone marrow, and gastrointestinal epithelium. There may also be necrosis in the liver, kidney, heart, and pancreas. **In cattle**, a condition called "**mouldy corn poisoning**" is believed to result from **T-2 toxin**. This disorder is characterized by extensive haemorrhage.

Satratoxin (stachybotryotoxin), a trichothecene produced by **Stachybotrys** sp. and other fungi, on ingestion, causes a disease known as "**stachybotryotoxicosis**". It has occurred in **horses, cattle, sheep, pigs, poultry**, and **humans** in the USSR, Hungary, Czechoslovakia, Finland, France, and South Africa, following consumption of mouldy straw or hay. The disease and lesions are similar to those of **T-2 toxin**.

Avian Fungal Diseases

As discussed earlier, **fungi and yeast produce disease in two ways. First,** they invade and destroy body tissues. **Secondly**, fungi can infect growing grain or finished feeds, and produce toxic chemicals (**mycotoxins**). These mycotoxins produce disease or a decrease in growth (**mycotoxicosis**) when they are consumed.

The respiratory tract, nervous system and eyes of poultry are commonly infected by fungi. **Infections are usually due to Aspergillus species. Infections with other fungi are less common.** Fungal infections such as **histoplasmosis** and **cryptococcosis** are not common pathogens of poultry, **but are included because they are of public health importance.**

Avian Aspergillosis

When avian aspergillosis is mentioned, it usually means "**pulmonary or respiratory aspergillosis**". Thus, other synonyms of pulmonary aspergillosis are "**brooder pneumonia**" or "**mycotic pneumonia**". Although the primary target of the agent is the respiratory system, other manifestations of the disease also occur in poultry. Pulmonary aspergillosis is common in commercial poultry. **Newly hatched chickens**, turkeys, and ducks are highly susceptible to infection. **Stress of cold, high ammonia and dusty environments increase the incidence and severity of infection, as also the conjunctivitis produced by Ranikhet disease vaccination.** Older birds are constantly exposed from the environment, but due to their increased resistance, rarely develop the disease.

Aetiology

The two major species of fungus **Aspergillus** which cause aspergillosis in poultry are: *Aspergillus fumigatus* and *A. flavus*. Other species that may be involved are: *A. niger, A. glaucus*, and *A. terreus*. These organisms are common soil saprophytes, occurring in decaying vegetative matter and feed grains. They grow on organic matter in warm humid environments. Fungal hyphae are 4-12 μm in diameter and bear conidiophores producing conidia (spores) 2-6 μm in diameter that are easily spread in air.

Transmission

Infection is by inhalation of spores. Spores usually originate from infected eggs. If opened during incubation or hatching, infected eggs release large number of spores and contaminate hatchmates. **The fungus may penetrate through the eggshell during incubation, and the hatched chicks can be infected**. Egg embryos are quite susceptible to infection by *A. fumigatus* during incubation. Infection within the hatchery may also occur from contaminated equipment or air ducts. After infection in the hatchery, lateral spread is not usually an important source of new infection. Aspergillosis can also occur from inhalation of spores from contaminated feed or poultry house litter. Fungal growth in wet litter produces a large number of spores which become aerosolized as this litter is dried. In such instances, new cases continue to appear for some time.

Pathogenesis

Airborne conidia (spores) are deposited on conjunctival, nasal, tracheal, parabronchial and airsac epithelium, and **initiate granulomas** at these sites. After inhalation, spores are rapidly spread haematogenously to other tissues, producing lesions in the brain, pericardium, bone marrow, kidney, and other soft tissues. This **haematogenous spread** explains the frequent distribution of brain lesions in the meninges, causing large superficial white plaques, and leading to fungal ophthalmitis and iridocyclitis.

Clinical Signs

Within the first **3-5 days chicks** infected in the hatchery show dyspnoea, polypnoea (very rapid breathing), and begin open-mouthed breathing (gasping, 'gaspers') due to airway obstruction. When these signs are associated with other respiratory diseases such as infectious bronchitis and infectious laryngotracheitis, they are usually accompanied by gurgling and rattling noises, **whereas in aspergillosis there is usually no sound**. Those birds which survive become lethargic and stunted, develop conjunctival swelling, blindness, and exhibit torticollis and other central nervous system abnormalities. **Older birds** may remain subclinically affected initially, but gradually develop respiratory problems. They may also become asphyxiated due to the blockage of the trachea or syrinx. (Syrinx is the vocal organ of birds which is a special modification of the lower part of the trachea, or of the bronchi, or both).

Infected poultry flocks usually show a **biphasic mortality pattern** with aspergillosis. **Acute respiratory disease** may cause 5-50% mortality in the first 1-3 weeks of age. Survivors usually develop chronic disease with up to 5% mortality due to chronic pulmonary insufficiency, ascites, blindness, or neurological fungal metastasis.

Lesions

Grossly, granulomas appear as separate 1-15 mm diameter **white plaques or caseous nodules**. They are composed of necrotic centres containing branching, septate, 4-7 μm diameter hyphae. Older lesions may contain pleomorphic hyphae up to 12 μm in diameter. Older lesions in air-filled cavities may appear green to black due to development of pigmented conidiophores. Fungi tend to proliferate within the granulomas and rarely invade adjacent tissue in immunocompetent birds. Aspergillosis-induced exudate becomes lodged in the trachea or syrinx producing acute respiratory difficulty in chronically infected individuals.

The **ocular form** of aspergillosis is characterized by extensive keratoconjunctivitis. In pulmonary (respiratory) aspergillosis, besides lungs showing large and extensive **caseous nodules, caseous nodules are also present in the airsac**.

Diagnosis

Aspergillosis is usually diagnosed at postmortem examination, often based on observation of **white caseous nodules in the lungs, or airsacs**. However, these lesions are highly suggestive but not specific for aspergillosis. **Tracheal exudate plugs can be produced by severe respiratory virus vaccination reactions**, or poor air quality in the hatchery or brooding house. Pulmonary and ocular granulomas cannot be differentiated grossly from those produced by some other fungal, coliform, staphylococcal and salmonella infections.

Diagnosis depends on the demonstration of branched, septate **Aspergillus hyphae** in the lesions. They can be seen **microscopically in impression smears of lesions** after the addition of 1-2 drops of 10% potassium hydroxide (KOH) and heating to clear. Also, **hyphae** are routinely observed in H & E stained sections. However, special fungal stains, such as **Periodic Acid-Schiff (PAS), Grocott's Methenamine-Silver (GMS), or Calcofluor white**, may be required in some cases. Confirmation should also be made by cultural isolation and identification of the causative fungus. Although *A. fumigatus* is the most likely agent of avian aspergillosis, other species of fungi can cause the disease. Therefore, isolates should be identified. Granulomas or plaques may be cultured on Sabouraud dextrose agar with antibiotics. Serological tests are of limited value due to the nonspecific nature of the antigen.

Thrush (Crop Mycosis, Candidiasis)

Also known as "**moniliasis**", "**oidiomycosis**", "**sour crop**", and "**mycosis of the digestive tract**", oral, oesophageal or crop candidiasis occurs quite commonly, **but only rarely causes clinical signs**. Fungi causing candidiasis are usually associated with concurrent disease, immunosuppression, or altered microflora. They cause mostly opportunistic rather than primary infections.

Aetiology

Crop mycosis is usually caused by *Candida albicans*, a dimorphic yeast. It appears as round to oval 3-4 μm budding yeasts (**blastospores**) on epithelial surfaces, or as branching septate hyphae or pseudohyphae in deeper tissues. *Oidium pullorum* and *Candida krusei* are also sometimes isolated, but may not be involved in lesion development.

C. albicans is ubiquitous in the environment, and is usually **present in the upper gastrointestinal tract of normal birds**. Candidial overgrowth occurs in prolonged administration of antibiotics. Antibiotics suppress normal bacterial flora, thus allowing **Candida** to proliferate. **Other risk factors** include highly contaminated drinkers or feeders, eating litter, immunosuppression, environmental stress, or nutritional disease. Infections are more common in birds under 3 weeks of age. This suggests acquired or age resistance. **Mortality directly due to candidiasis is almost non-existent**. Most signs are due to other concurrent diseases, or reduced feed intake.

Clinical Signs

Infections are common, but clinical signs are seen in only severely affected birds. Birds with superficial oral, oesophageal or crop infections **fail to gain weight**. In rare cases there is systemic invasion, and signs of neurological, renal, or intestinal disease may be present.

Pathogenesis and Lesions

Candida are acquired by ingestion. They then become part of the normal flora of the mouth, oesophagus, and crop. With inhibition of competing microflora (by antibiotics) or immunosuppression, fungi proliferate on the surface, and hyphae or pseudohyphae penetrate superficial epithelial layers. This penetration stimulates epithelial hyperplasia, and **pseudomembrane or diphtheritic membrane formation**. The membrane appears grossly as multifocal to confluent layers of **white cheesy material in the crop** and sometimes in the oesophagus and pharynx. Candidial thick tangled mass and membranes are usually **adherent**. They cannot be washed away like normal accumulations of mucus. Inflammatory response to mucosal candidiasis is mild, unless ulceration is produced.

Diagnosis

Pseudomembranes and diphtheritic membranes in the crop, oesophagus and mouth **are highly suggestive of candidiasis**. However, they are also produced after ingestion of caustic substances, trichothecene mycotoxins, and in severe cases of oral trichomoniasis. Demonstration of hyphae and pseudohyphae microscopically, in either scrapings or histological sections, confirms the diagnosis. Identification of the species requires culture on Sabouraud dextrose agar or other fungal culture media. However, many normal birds may be positive.

Favus

This disease is no longer important in commercial poultry. It is sometimes seen in backyard or hobby flocks. Infections are superficial, chronic and either self-limiting or slowly progressive. Favus is usually caused by *Trichophyton megninii* (*T. gallinae*) a dermatophytic fungus. Other fungi have also been isolated. Favus usually affects only individual birds and progresses slowly. It is transmissible to other birds by contact or fomites, **but only rarely to humans**.

Pathogenesis and Lesions

Lesions appear in unfeathered skin (comb, wattle, shank) by superficial invasion of the stratum corneum by hyphae. This results in epidermal hyperplasia and hyperkeratosis. Infection is confined to the epidermis, and therefore inflammatory reaction to infection is minimal. **Grossly**, infected sites are dry, white and scaly. With time lesions may regress, remain static, or progress to adjacent superficial feathered skin. **Lesions** in feathered skin may develop depressions around follicles. These are known as "**favus cups**". There is no significant systemic invasion or signs, other than loss of feathers and scaliness of the skin.

Diagnosis

Trichophyton infections are diagnosed by histological demonstration of hyphae, or spores in skin lesions and feather follicles. This may be followed by culture on Sabouraud dextrose agar, or selective dermatophyte media.

Dactylariosis

This is **a new fungal disease of chickens** caused by the thermophilic fungus *Dactylaria gallopava*. Young chickens and turkey poults rapidly develop neurological disease. Sometimes, pulmonary lesions similar to those of aspergillosis are seen. Usually, there is also involvement of the nervous system. Infected chicks and poults develop torticollis, paresis, and incoordination. In rare cases, pulmonary granulomas develop and cause dyspnoea as in aspergillosis.

Pathogenesis and Lesions

Spores reach the brain haematogenously and produce the main lesions of meningeal and encephalitic necrosis. This lesion is most common in the cerebellum, but can appear anywhere in the brain. It differs from the mycotic encephalitis of aspergillosis by having more malacia and haemorrhage and having far greater number of giant cells. **Grossly,** ocular and pulmonary lesions appear similar to aspergillosis, but **microscopically** are less well organized and have greater number of giant cells.

Diagnosis

Clinical signs and gross lesions are not specific enough to allow diagnosis. Brain lesions should be examined microscopically. Those containing pigmented 2 μm diameter hyphae and large number of giant cells are diagnostic for dactylariosis. The fungus can be cultured from brain lesions on Sabouraud dextrose agar with added antibiotics.

Histoplasmosis

This disease is not of economic importance to the poultry industry, **but it is considered because of its public health significance.** It is caused by the fungus *Histoplasma capsulatum*, and has been reported usually in **zoo birds,** and sometimes, **in chicken** and turkey. It is an infectious and not contagious disease of **human** and lower animals. The disease occurs worldwide.

Cryptococcosis

Cryptococcosis is **a disease of humans and animals,** and has been discussed earlier. It is caused by the fungus *Cryptococcus neoformans*. In **humans,** it is characterized by a meningitis. Although the disease is not of economic importance in poultry, there are many sporadic cases from **zoo birds.**

Avian Mycotoxicoses

As discussed, **a mycotoxicosis is a disease caused by a toxic fungal metabolite known as "mycotoxin".** Mycotoxins drew attention in the early 1960s when **aflatoxin,** a mycotoxin produced by **Aspergillus** sp., was discovered to be the cause of disease in **poultry and fish.** The importance of aflatoxin further increased by the disclosure of its **carcinogenicity.** Diseases of humans and animals caused by consumption of mouldy food, however, have been recognized long before the discovery of aflatoxin. Ergotism, mouldy corn poisoning of horses, various haemorrhagic syndromes, and certain acute food poisonings are just some of the historically significant mycotoxicoses of **humans and animals.**

Fungal growth is required for mycotoxin production in grain. Fungi can infect and grow in grain prior to harvest, during storage, or after inclusion in finished feeds. Many mycotoxins are stable during milling and feed storage. **Therefore toxins can be present in grains after the fungi that produced them are dead**.

Thousands of chemically distinct mycotoxins exist. Individual fungal strains usually synthesize more than one mycotoxin, and these toxins often act synergistically. Thus, naturally occurring mycotoxicoses can occur with only one-tenth the levels required to produce intoxications in the laboratory with individual purified chemicals.

Aflatoxicosis, ochratoxicosis and trichothecene mycotoxicosis are the most commonly seen mycotoxicoses in poultry. Other mycotoxicoses are rare.

Aflatoxicosis

Aflatoxin is the most prevalent, and also economically the most important mycotoxin likely to be consumed by poultry. Aflatoxins are highly toxic and carcinogenic mycotoxins produced by *Aspergillus flavus, A. parasiticus*, and *Penicillium puberulum*. However, **most of the toxin is produced by** *A. flavus*, **and gives it its name (afla-toxin)**. Mycotoxin is found in maize, groundnuts, cottonseed, millet, sorghum, and other feed grains. Both *A. flavus* and *A. parasiticus* are ubiquitous in environment, and produce aflatoxin in warm (30⁰-35⁰ C), high humidity conditions. Aflatoxin contamination is thus more common in grains grown or handled **in tropics or subtropics**. Handling or storage of grains in these conditions anywhere would stimulate aflatoxin production.

Naturally occurring aflatoxin contains aflatoxins **B1, B2, G1** and **G2, but aflatoxin B1 is usually in the highest concentration and is also the most toxic. Aflatoxin is stable once formed and is not destroyed during normal milling and storage. Young poultry** are more sensitive to aflatoxin than are **adults**. There are also big species differences, **ducks being 10 times more sensitive than chickens,** and turkeys intermediate between the two. **Aflatoxicosis is widely prevalent in India, and is an extremely important condition in poultry**.

Pathogenesis

After ingestion, aflatoxin B1 undergoes **biotransformation** into numerous **highly reactive metabolites** having a variety of negative effects on metabolism. **Metabolites bind to DNA and RNA**, reduce protein synthesis, and decrease cell-mediated immunity, and to a lesser extent humoral immunity. These metabolic alterations lead to **liver, kidney** and **spleen enlargement,** and **bursal, thymic and testicular atrophy**.

Pathology

Aflatoxicosis in chickens causes **yellow discoloration of the liver, with multifocal haemorrhage**. In time, the livers are **enlarged**, friable, and develop **white foci** as lipid content increases. Fat accumulates in the hepatocytes. **Microscopic lesions** include clear vacuoles in the cytoplasm of hepatocytes, karyomegaly (enlargement of the nucleus), and prominent nucleoli, proliferation of bile ducts, and fibrosis. There is also **extramedullary haematopoiesis in the liver**, which is in response to a toxin-induced anaemia.

Aflatoxicosis produces marked immunosuppression and is associated with increased susceptibility to infectious diseases. In chickens, aflatoxin increases susceptibility, or increases severity of, caecal coccidiosis, Marek's disease, salmonellosis, inclusion body hepatitis, and infectious bursal disease. **Vaccination failures** are also emerging as a result of aflatoxicosis in chickens. **Immunosuppression** is, in part, due to the **atrophy of bursa of Fabricius, thymus, and spleen.** Aflatoxin is toxic for B lymphocytes in the late-stage embryo. **Cell-mediated immune responses are also decreased**.

Aflatoxin causes **anaemia** characterized by reduction in packed cell volume, erythrocyte count, haemoglobin concentration, and mean corpuscular volume. **Young birds are more susceptible to anaemia. Aflatoxin also damages coagulation in chickens by interfering with several coagulation factors,** mainly prothrombin, and thus affects the extrinsic and common pathways. Aflatoxin alters coagulation more than either ochratoxin A or T-2 toxin, but the effects of ochratoxin A last longer. **Petechial haemorrhages, or bruises after trauma, are increased due to decreased clotting factor synthesis and increased capillary fragility.**

In Leghorn chickens, **aflatoxin blocks ova maturation and reduces feed efficiency and egg production. Hatchability** is more sensitive than egg production. Egg production may be spared despite lesions of hepatotoxicity. However, some decline in production lingers on and requires several weeks to return to normal. Aflatoxin impairs egg production by reducing synthesis and transport of yolk precursors in the liver. Egg size, yolk weight, and yolk as per cent of total egg size, are decreased. **However, aflatoxin is rapidly excreted in the bile and urine and does not accumulate or persist in body tissues.** This may explain the rapid recovery of egg production and hatchability after cessation of toxin ingestion.

Aflatoxin decreases total serum protein, lipoprotein, cholesterol, triglycerides, uric acid, calcium, phosphorus, iron, copper, and zinc. Poultry reared on diets contaminated with aflatoxin **constitute a minimal aflatoxin source in the human food chain.**

Clinical Signs

Aflatoxicosis does not cause mortality directly, **although high levels (> 10.0 ppm) may be lethal**. Economically most significant effects of aflatoxicosis in growing birds are **decreased growth and poor feed conversion (> 1.0 ppm)**. There is also **a marked decrease in resistance to infections**, such as salmonellosis, coccidiosis, infectious bursal disease and candidiasis. Chickens suffering from aflatoxicosis may also have a failure of normal pigmentation and increased bruising **(> 0.5 ppm)**. Affected adult **hens** have **decreased egg production**, and the **hatchability of eggs is reduced (> 2.0 ppm). In adult breeder males testicular weights and sperm counts are reduced**. Insemination of hens with semen from affected males has shown decreased fertility.

For **diagnosis** of aflatoxicosis, or detection of aflatoxins in the feed, refer to diagnosis on mammalian aflatoxicosis, and also diagnosis of mycotoxicosis at the end of this section.

Ochratoxicosis

Ochratoxicosis is less common in poultry than aflatoxicosis, **but is more lethal. Ochratoxins are among the most toxic mycotoxins of poultry**. These **nephrotoxic metabolites** are produced mainly by *Penicillium veridicatum* and *Aspergillus ochraceus* **on different grains and feedstuffs**. The name "ochratoxin" is derived from *A. ochraceus*, **the first fungus shown to produce it**. Ochratoxins are designated as **A, B, C, and D. Ochratoxin A is the most common and most toxic**; and is also produced in greater quantities and is relatively stable. Environmental conditions favouring ochratoxin production are similar to those for aflatoxin, and concurrent contamination with both is common. Some ochratoxin-producing fungi produce other mycotoxins toxic to poultry, including **citrinin**.

Ochratoxin A occurs in maize, most small grains and in animal feeds. Ochratoxin A forms readily in poultry feed under conditions of high temperature and high moisture. **Ochratoxin A is the main toxin in naturally occurring disease**. Ochratoxin B and C occur only with high concentrations of ochratoxin A. **Young chickens are most sensitive to ochratoxin ingestion, and ducks are 7 times more sensitive to ochratoxin than chickens**. Acute ochratoxicosis induces **mortality due to acute renal failure**, with **immunosuppression** and **decreased growth** rates in the survivors. **In India,** ochratoxicosis caused by *A. ochraceus* in poultry, has been widely reported

Pathogenesis

Ochratoxin A inhibits protein synthesis, produces acute proximal tubular epithelial necrosis in the kidneys, and **inhibits normal renal uric acid excretion**.

Pathology

Gross lesions in acute lethal ochratoxin A mycotoxicosis in chickens include **pallor** (paleness) of the **liver, pancreas,** and **kidneys.** Affected **kidneys** are white to tan (yellowish-brown), swollen, hard, and have **white urate deposits** in the ureter. If damage is extensive enough to cause renal failure, there is dehydration, hyperuricaemia (increased uric acid in the blood), and **urate deposits on kidneys, heart, pericardium, liver and spleen (visceral gout).** Usually, birds survive in compensated renal failure and kidneys appear enlarged, fibrotic, and pale. **The main microscopic lesion is acute tubular necrosis characterized by proteinaceous and urate casts,** heterophil infiltration, and focal necrosis of tubular epithelium. In addition to the renal lesions, there is mild to moderate fatty change and glycogen deposition in hepatocytes, resulting in yellow enlarged livers. With time, focal necrosis of hepatocytes develops, followed by foci of **fibrosis.** There is also slight decrease in the size of bursa and thymus consistent with immunosuppression.

Subacute ochratoxin A mycotoxicosis has been studied in **turkeys, ducklings,** and **chickens.** It is characterized by increased weight of liver and kidney, and decreased weight of lymphoid organs. **Microscopic changes in kidney** include hyperplasia of tubular epithelium and interstitial inflammation, which account for the enlargement seen grossly. **Lesions in the liver** comprise vacuolar change (**fatty change**) in hepatocytes, associated with an **increase in glycogen content of liver and skeletal muscle. Chronic ochratoxicosis in** hens causes reduced renal function.

Clinical Signs

Acutely intoxicated **birds** are depressed, dehydrated and polyuric (**> 4.0 ppm**), and **die in acute renal failure.** Survivors become stunted, are poorly feathered, and have increased clotting time, anaemia, and immunosuppression (**> 0.6 ppm**). There may be loss of pigmentation and reduced weight gain (**>2.0 ppm**). Laying hens may have delayed sexual maturity. **There is also a decrease in egg production and hatchability (> 2.0 ppm).** Ochratoxicosis in broilers causes mortality and failure to gain weight. Growth rate, feed conversion efficiency, and pigmentation are affected.

Trichothecene Mycotoxicosis

This mycotoxicosis is fairly common in poultry, but does not usually cause mortality. Losses, on the other hand, are due to reduced feed intake, decreased growth and immunosuppression. Trichothecene mycotoxins are produced by many species of **Fusarium, Stachybotrys, and at least three other genera.** These mycotoxins usually occur in wheat, maize, and other grains used for poultry feed production. Environmental conditions favouring **Fusarium** and **Stachybotrys** and trichothecene production are different from those of aflatoxin or ochratoxin production. Thus concurrent contamination with these toxins is rare. Trichothecene-producing fungi produce maximum toxin in cold (< 20⁰ C), moist conditions. Trichothecenes are therefore associated with grain harvests **in the winter months,** or when infected grain has been stored in cold conditions.

There are **about 80 chemically related trichothecene mycotoxins,** but most is known about the effects of only these four: 1. **T-2,** 2. **Hydroxy T-2 (HT-2),** 3. **Diacetoxyscirpenol (DAS),** and 4. **Deoxynivalenol (DON, vomitoxin).** However, it is not known if these four compounds cause most field cases of trichothecene mycotoxicosis.

Clinical Signs

Chickens suffering from trichothecene mycotoxicosis develop **ulcers** at the commissures of the mouth, on the hard palate near the beak, and on the dorsal surface of the tongue (> 2.0 ppm T-2). Ulcers are not produced in the oesophagus unless birds eat large amounts of feed rapidly. Ulcerative stomatitis leads to decreased feed intake, reduced gain, and decreased feed efficiency. Affected birds have poor feathering, become anaemic, immunosuppressed, and have decreased growth rates. **Adult birds are more resistant,** but develop oral ulcers and **decreased egg production, shell quality and hatchability.**

Other Mycotoxicoses

Other mycotoxicoses are rare in poultry, and their economic importance is also less. These include:

1. **Citrinin toxicosis: Citrinin is a nephrotoxin** produced in a variety of cereal grains (mainly maize and rice) by *Penicillium citrinum.* In citrinin toxicosis, mortality is rare, but water consumption is increased, and there is diffuse polyuria manifested as **wet droppings.** Grossly, **kidneys are slightly swollen,** but there are no microscopic lesions except at very high dosages.

2. **Oosporein: Oosporein is a nephrotoxic mycotoxin produced by** *Chaetomium trilaterale.* Ingestion by chicks produces acute proximal tubular necrosis and acute renal failure in severe cases. Effects are particularly severe in birds less than 1 week old, and lead to **visceral and articular urate deposits** and **mortality** up to 20%.

3. **Fumonisins: Fusarium fungi** produce a wide variety of other mycotoxins. *Fusarium moniliforme* also produces **fumonisins,** a group of water-soluble mycotoxins. They cause **equine leukoencephalomalacia** (mouldy corn poisoning) and **porcine pulmonary oedema syndrome.** Fumonisin B1 is the most common of this group. **Chickens are more resistant than turkeys.**

4. **Moniliformin**: Moniliformin is another mycotoxin produced by some strains of *Fusarium moniliforme*, and **is cardiotoxic in poultry**. It has been associated with acute myocardial necrosis and death in ducks, chickens, and turkey poults.

5. **Fusarochromanone**: Also known as TDP-1, fusarochromanone is produced by **Fusarium** sp. and causes **leg deformities and tibial dyschondroplasia in chicks**. It is a rarely encountered mycotoxin.

6. **Ergotism**: Ergotism is caused by **Claviceps** sp., fungi that attack **cereal grains. Rye** is especially affected, but wheat and other cereal grains (barley, oats, rice) are also affected. *Claviceps purpurea* is the usual cause of ergotism. Ergotism causes reduction in feed intake and growth, necrosis of the beak, comb, and toes; and diarrhoea. Leghorn birds develop vesicles and crusts on the comb and wattles, face, and eyelids (**vesicular dermatitis, sod disease**). Laying hens show **reduction in feed consumption and egg production**, but no consistent lesions occur other than those on the skin.

7. **Zearalenone**: This mycotoxin is produced by the fungus *Gibberella zeae (Fusarium graminearum)* in infected grains. Also known as "**F-2**", it is a mycotoxin with **oestrogenic activity**. Chickens are more tolerant to zearalenone than are turkeys. In fact zearalenone is relatively nontoxic for chickens.

Diagnosis of Mycotoxicosis

Clinical signs, gross lesions and microscopic changes help in the differential diagnosis of most mycotoxicoses affecting poultry. However, a definitive diagnosis (i.e., confirmation) requires isolation and identification of specific toxins. This is usually difficult. This can be achieved in **two ways. Firstly, by feeding trials** with the suspected feed to reproduce the feed toxicosis. **Secondly, by chemical analysis of poultry rations**. Analytical techniques for mycotoxins include thin layer chromatography, high performance liquid chromatography, gas chromatography, or mass spectrometry and monoclonal antibody-based technology.

Feed and ingredient samples should be properly collected and promptly submitted to a feed testing laboratory for analysis. Samples of suspected feed for feeding trials and analysis should be collected directly from the trough in the poultry house. Mycotoxin formation may not be uniform in a batch of feed or grain, **and multiple samples from different sites increase the likelihood of confirming the presence of a mycotoxin**. Samples should be collected at all possible sites in the chain of ingredient, namely, storage, feed manufacture and transport, feed containers, and feeders within poultry houses.

Rickettsial Diseases

The order **Rickettsiales** has **three important families** containing pathogens for domestic animals. These are **Rickettsiaceae, Anaplasmataceae,** and
Bartonellaceae, having **eight, five,** and **two genera,** respectively **(Table 31).**

Table 31.   Classification of order Rickettsiales

Order	:	Rickettsiales
Family	:	Rickettsiaceae
Genus	:	**Rickettsia**
		Rochalimaea
		Coxiella
		Cowdria
		Ehrlichia
		Neorickettsia
		Cytoecetes
		Colesiota
Family	:	Anaplasmataceae
Genus	:	**Anaplasma**
		Paranaplasma
		Aegyptianella
		Haemobartonella
		Eperythrozoon
Family	:	Bartonellaceae
Genus	:	**Bartonella**
		Grahamella

Diseases caused by Rickettsiaceae

Micro-organisms classified in the Family **Rickettsiaceae** include several
agents which c ause disease in humans and animals. T he group i s n amed
after t he American p athologist **Howard Taylor Ricketts** who e xcellently
described features of **Rocky Mountain spotted fever** (a rickettsial disease of
humans), in 1907. **Rickettsiae** are minute, **Gram-negative, obligate
intracellular parasites. The rickettsiae and chlamydiae, in contrast to other**

bacteria, only multiply within cells. R ickettsiae are t ransmitted from o ne vertebrate species to another b y **arthropod vectors** in w hich **t ransovarian transmission** is common. **Rodents** can carry certain of the pathogens in this group and serve as reservoirs of infection. **Eight pathogenic genera are cur-rently included in the family Rickettsiaceae (Table 31).** Species comprising the genus **Rickettsia** are divided into **three groups based on their effect in humans: 1. Typhus group, 2. Spotted fever group, and 3. Scrub typhus group (Table 32).** T hese organisms a re s pread by a rthropods, a nd although m ice, rats, squirrels, and rabbits are susceptible, **the above three groups of diseases are mainly diseases of humans.** Dogs are susceptible to *Rickettsia rickettsii*, but clinical signs of R ocky Mountain sp otted fever are not usually seen. **In humans,** the d iseases are c haracterized by f ever, rash, and haemorrhage. **Rickettsia species have a predilection (affinity) for growth in endothelial cells and vascular smooth muscle cells, which accounts for most lesions.** They cause a **vasculitis** which may be **complicated by thrombi and haemor-rhages.**

Table 32. Diseases caused by Rickettsiaceae

Genus and Species	Vectors	Hosts	Disease
Genus : Rickettsia			
I. Typhus Group			
Rickettsia prowazekii	Louse	Humans	Typhus fever (epidemic typhus)
R. typhi	Rat louse	Humans, rats, mice	Murine typhus of humans
II. Spotted Fever Group			
R. rickettsii	Ticks	Humans, dogs	Rocky M ountain spotted fever
R. conorii	Dog ticks	Humans, dogs	Boutonneuse fever
R. akari	Mites	Humans, mice	Rickettsial p ox
III. Scrub Typhus Group			
R. tsutsugamushi	Mites	Humans, monkeys	Tsutsugamushi fever
Rochalimaea quintana	Louse	Humans, monkeys	Trench fever
Neorickettsia helminthoeca	Fluke	Dogs, foxes, bears	Salmon disease of dogs (neorickettsiosis)
Coxiella burnetii	Ticks, aerosol transmission	Humans, cattle, sheep, goats, birds	Q fever
Cowdria ruminantium	Ticks	Cattle, sheep, goats	"Heartwater" or cowdriosis

Ehrlichia phagocytophila Ticks		Cattle, sheep, goats	Tickborne fever
E. risticii	Unknown	Horses	Potomac horse fever
E. equi	Ticks suspected	Horses	Equine ehrlichiosis
E. bovis	Ticks	Cattle	Bovine ehrlichiosis
E. ovina	Ticks	Sheep	Ovine ehrlichiosis
E. canis	Ticks	Dogs	Canine ehrlichiosis
E. sennetsu	Unknown	Humans	Glandular fever
E. platys	Ticks suspected	Dogs	Severe thrombocytopaenia
Cytoecetes ondiri	Unknown	Cattle	Bovine petechial fever (Ondiri disease)
Colesiota conjunctivae	Unknown	Sheep, goats, cattle, pigs	Kerato-conjunctivitis

Pathologically, the main lesion is a vasculitis of capillaries, arterioles, and venules. The changes comprise endothelial hypertrophy and hyperplasia, cuffing with leukocytes, and **thrombosis**. This may lead to necrotic foci in the skin, and in typhus and spotted fever, in visceral organs as well. Necrosis of the vessel wall is common in spotted fever, because the organisms extend from endothelial cells and invade vascular smooth muscle.

Genera within **Rickettsiaceae** which are of interest as causes of disease in domestic animals are:

Neorickettsia : It contains **a single species** *N. helminthoeca*, the cause of **salmon disease of dogs**. The organism has a predilection for reticulo-endothelial cells.

Coxiella : This also contains **a single species** *C. burnetii*, the cause of **Q fever**. It is mainly of importance as an infection of **humans**. It localizes in many tissues.

Cowdria : This also contains **a single species** *C. ruminantium*, the cause of **bovine heartwater**. These organisms localize in endothelial cells.

Ehrlichia : This genus contains **several species** which affect animals, usually causing a **mild disease**. These organisms localize in various leukocytes.

Cytoecetes   :   The exact position of this genus is uncertain. It contains **a single species** *C. ondiri*, the cause of **bovine petechial fever.**

Colesiota   :   This genus is very poorly defined. Organisms termed *Colesiota* have been associated with **keratoconjunctivitis in ruminants and pigs.**

Rocky Mountain Spotted Fever

Rickettsia species cause diseases mainly in **humans**. Only *R. rickettsii*, the cause of Rocky Mountain spotted fever, is of significance as a cause of disease in domestic animals. **Dogs** are susceptible from inapparent to fatal infection. The disease is transmitted by **ticks.**

Signs

These include fever and anorexia followed by mucocutaneous lesions and ocular and nasal discharge. There is hyperaemia with petechiae and ecchymoses of the ocular, oral, and genital mucous membranes. Hyperaemia is seen in the skin, particularly on the abdomen, muzzle and ears. Lymph nodes are enlarged. Some dogs show signs of central nervous system dysfunction, such as ataxia, paresis, seizures, or coma. Bleeding time is prolonged.

Lesions

Gross lesions include hyperaemia and haemorrhages on mucous membranes, skin, gastrointestinal mucosa, serosa, and pleura. Lymph nodes are enlarged and haemorrhagic. Splenomegaly is seen. **Microscopically**, the underlying lesion is a **generalized necrotizing vasculitis of venules and veins.** This reflects the natural tendency rickettsial organisms have for vascular endothelium. Vessels are surrounded by accumulations of neutrophils and lymphocytes. Vasculitis is seen in almost all organs.

Diagnosis

Diagnosis is made on the basis of a history of tick bites and the characteristic signs and lesions. It is confirmed by detecting the causative rickettsia through intraperitoneal inoculation of guinea-pigs with blood, or by culture techniques. In recovered animals, a rise in serum antibodies can be measured by an indirect fluorescent antibody test and other serological procedures.

Salmon Disease of Dogs (Canine Neorickettsiosis)

Also known as "**salmon poisoning**", this is a febrile, often fatal, disease of **dogs** and **foxes**. It has been known to occur in association with a diet that includes **salmon, trout, and other fish.** Salmon disease is caused by

Neorickettsia helminthoeca, a rickettsial-like organism which is **carried by a fluke**. The fluke parasitizes the small intestine of dogs. Eggs, excreted in the faeces, first develop in a snail, with subsequent development of encysted metacercariae in fish (salmon, trout). Adult flukes mature in the small intestine of dogs consuming infected fish and allow *N. helminthoeca* to invade. **The disease is limited to the United States**.

Signs

The signs usually appear five days after the **ingestion of infected fish**, and begin with a fever which continues for 4-8 days. Anorexia is accompanied by depression, weakness and weight loss. Vomiting and diarrhoea, accompanied by tenesmus (spasmodic contraction of anal sphincter), are prominent symptoms.

Lesions

Lymphoid tissues are particularly affected in this disease. The visceral nodes of the abdomen may be enlarged to six times normal size. These **enlarged lymph nodes** are usually yellowish with prominent white follicles in their cortex. The **spleen** is usually enlarged. The lymphoid tissue of the intestinal tract is especially hyperplastic. Petechiae are usually seen in the intestinal mucosa, particularly over the enlarged lymphoid follicles. **Microscopic lesions** are prominent in the lymph nodes and are dominated by hyperplasia of reticulo-endothelial elements and depletion of small lymphocytes. Foci of necrosis are common, and many present haemorrhages. **Elementary bodies of Neorickettsia** (organisms) in reticulo-endothelial cells can be demonstrated by **Giemsa or Macchiavello's stain**. The **thymus**, in younger dogs, is the site of prominent changes. In the **intestine**, flukes may be demonstrated deep in the villi and occasionally in duodenal glands. The brain may show microscopic lesions in 91% of fatal cases.

Diagnosis

The small intracytoplasmic **"elementary bodies"** in reticulo-endothelial cells in lymphoid tissues and sometimes in large mononuclear cells of liver, lungs and blood are important in the diagnosis of this disease. These bodies are coccoid or coccobacillary in shape and about 0.3 μm in diameter. With Giemsa's stain, these bodies are purple; with Macchiavello's stain, red or blue; with Levaditi's method, black or dark brown; and with H & E, pale bluish-violet. They are **Gram-negative**. The presence of adult flukes in the small intestine, or their eggs in the faeces, must be confirmed.

Q Fever

This is a febrile disease of slaughterhouse workers. It was originally described in Queensland, Australia, by Derrick in 1937, who named the disease **"Q" fever** ("q" for query, i.e., of questionable or unknown cause). The disease has since been reported worldwide. The infectious agent is a rickettsial organism called *Coxiella burnetii* (*Rickettsia burnetii*), and is harboured by **cattle, sheep, goats, dogs, cats,** and other species. But, as a rule, **the infection in animals is inapparent or mild.** Although the organism can be transmitted by ticks, an intermediate vector is not required. This is in contrast to other **Rickettsia** species.

Human beings usually acquire the infection by contact with freshly slaughtered infected **cattle or sheep,** or by consuming raw **milk or butter** in which the organisms are present. Particularly high concentrations of the organism are present at parturition, and the placenta may contain millions of organisms per gram. **There have been several cases of Q fever in laboratories employing sheep as research projects.** The organisms are demonstrable in tissues stained by Giemsa or Macchiavello mthods, where they appear as minute pleomorphic organisms in the form of rods. Clusters of these orgahisms appear in the cytoplasm of tissue cells, and sometimes are seen extracellularly.

Lesions

Organisms have been recovered from **cows** that exhibited no signs of infection, and postmortem examination of such animals has revealed few, if any, specific lesions. In **humans,** the lesions in the natural infection are those of an interstitial pneumonia and disseminated epithelioid granulomas.

Diagnosis

Diagnosis of infection in cattle depends on isolation and identification of organisms, usually by inoculation of guinea-pigs. A complement-fixation test is also used.

Heartwater (Cowdriosis)

This disease is important in the **ruminant population (cattle, sheep and goats) of the African continent.** It is named after its characteristic lesion: **hydropericardium.** The causative agent, *Cowdria ruminantium* (previously *Rickettsia ruminantium*), is an intracellular parasite **transmitted by ticks.** The rickettsia, a tiny, rod-shaped, often diplococcoid organism, can be demonstrated with **Giemsa's stain** in endothelial cells of the jugular vein, vena cava, renal glomerular capillaries as well as in reticulo-endothelial cells and neutrophils.

Cattle, sheep, goats, and wild ruminants are susceptible, but there is significant variation in susceptibility between breeds. The disease may be peracute and fatal, or inapparent. Usually, there is fever characterized by signs of central nervous dysfunction, such as unsteady gait, twitching of muscles, circling, aggressive behaviour, convulsions, and coma. The characteristic **lesions** include hydropericardium, pulmonary oedema, hydrothorax, ascites, and lymphadenopathy. **Microscopically,** tissues are oedematous, and there is generalized perivascular leukocytic infiltration. As indicated, the organisms invade vascular endothelium and can be demonstrated there.

Ovine and Bovine Ehrlichiosis ("Tick-borne Fever")

This is **a febrile disease of a mild, non-fatal nature**, associated with tick infestation in **sheep** and **cattle**. The disease is caused by a rickettsial organism called *Ehrlichia phagocytophila* (*Cytoecetes phagocytophila*, *Rickettsia phagocytophila*). It is transmitted by tick *Ixodes ricinus*. Goats and other ruminants are also susceptible. **The disease has also been recorded in India.**

The **main clinical finding is fever** of several days duration. Lymphopaenia followed by neutropaenia and thrombocytopaenia are consistent findings. The lymphopaenia is mainly the result of a drop in B lymphocytes with an accompanying suppression of humoral response.

Diagnosis is made by identifying the organisms in circulating granulocytes and monocytes. They are visible in up to 50% of circulating cells, and may remain visible for periods as long as two years. **Giemsa and Wright-Leishman stains are best for identification**. The disease is not fatal, and no significant lesions are associated with the disease other than splenomegaly.

Potomac Horse Fever (Equine Monocytic Ehrlichiosis)

This disease is caused by *Ehrlichia risticii*. It was first recognized near the **Potomac River, USA**, in 1979. Potomac horse fever is seasonal, occurring in the summer months. This suggests an arthropod vector as with other **Ehrlichia** organisms, but an intermediate host has not yet been identified.

The **signs** are initially characterized by fever, followed by anorexia, colic, and diarrhoea. **The fever can be biphasic**. There is leukopaenia, with a decrease in neutrophils, lymphocytes, and eosinophils, and thrombocytopaenia. The organisms are visible in circulating monocytes, but they are small, not numerous, and easily missed. There may also be anaemia. Diarrhoea can be very severe, leading to dehydration and shock. Mortality rate is as high as 30%.

There are no diagnostic lesions. Usually, the caecum and colon are congested, haemorrhagic, and often eroded or ulcerated. The contents are watery. The stomach and small intestine are less severely affected. Organisms occur in the colonic epithelium, and macrophages in the lamina propria. Mesenteric lymph nodes are enlarged and congested and may show haemorrhage.

The **diagnosis** is confirmed by demonstrating the organism in circulating monocytes or colonic epithelium. An indirect fluorescent antibody test has been developed but may not be positive during the acute phase of the disease. Recovered horses have positive results on the test.

Equine Ehrlichiosis

The disease is caused by *Ehrlichia equi*, and **occurs in the United States.** The disease can be transmitted through blood-containing organisms, and ticks are suspected but not yet proved to transmit the disease in nature.

The infection is more serious in **horses over 3 years of age.** The **clinical signs** include fever, anorexia, oedema of the legs, and ataxia. Clinical laboratory findings include leukopaenia, thrombocytopaenia, increased plasma icterus index, decreased packed cell volume, and lymphopaenia. The organisms appear as granular bodies in neutrophils and eosinophils.

Gross lesions include petechiae, ecchymoses, and oedema in muscles, fascia, and subcutis. Jaundice and orchitis are common. The microscopic lesions consist of arteritis and phlebitis, particularly in muscles and fascia, but also in kidneys, heart, brain, and lungs.The blood vessels undergo necrosis as well as swelling of endothelium and smooth muscle cells. This is accompanied by accumulation of lymphocytes, plasma cells, and sometimes neutrophils.

Diagnosis is made on the basis of clinical findings and may be confirmed by the demonstration of organisms in neutrophils or eosinophils. They stain blue with Giemsa or Wright-Leishman's stain and are Gram-positive. The organisms are spherical, single or multiple.

Canine Ehrlichiosis (Canine Rickettsiosis)

This disease is caused by *Ehrlichia canis*. **Canine ehrlichiosis is of importance in India.** The disease is transmitted by the tick *Rhipicephalus sanguineus*. The organism multiplies in reticulo-endothelial cells, lymphocytes, and monocytes, and may be seen in stained smears of peripheral blood or tissue impressions. However, visualization if often difficult. The life cycle of the parasite is not yet completely understood. However, **three intracellular forms** are recognized: 1. **Initial bodies** are small (1-2 μm) spherical structures. These develop into larger bodies described as 2. **Mulberry bodies** or **morulae.** The morula is thought to dissociate into small granules called 3. **Elementary bodies.**

The disease is usually mild, except in **young puppies** or when complicated by another disease, such as infection with *Babesia canis*. In Asia, the disease has been called, **"canine tropical pancytopaenia". Most infections in dogs are subclinical.** Reports indicate that up to 50% of dogs in USA have antibodies to *E. canis*. **Human infection** with *E. canis* has been reported. Concurrent ehrlichiosis and babesiosis in dogs also occur; the signs of babesiosis usually overshadow those of ehrlichiosis.

Signs

Clinical signs include recurrent fever, serous nasal discharge, photophobia (intolerance to light), vomiting, splenomegaly, and signs of central nervous sysyem derangement. Leukopaenia, t hrombocytopaenia and anaemia, with increased levels of gamma globulin in the serum, are clinical features observed late in the disease. The clinical course runs from 4 weeks to several months. **Subclinical chronic infection** may last for five years, and may result in severe chronic disease.

Lesions

Gross lesions consist of haemorrhage in the mucosae of the gastrointestinal and urogenital tracts and kidneys, oedematous and haemorrhagic enlargement of m ost l ymph n odes, a nd oedema o f t he l imbs. T he **microscopic lesions** consist of w idespread perivascular a ccumulations of l ymphoreticular and plasma cells, particularly in the meninges, kidneys, liver, and lymphopoietic tissues. The b one marrow i s usually h ypoplastic. Degeneration a nd acute necrosis are common in the centre of lobules of the liver. In the central nervous system, haemorrhages and plasma cell accumulations occur in the meninges.

Ehrlichia platys has also been identified recently as a cause of disease in dogs. It c auses severe but transient thrombocytopaenia.

Diagnosis

The diagnosis may be confirmed by identifying the organisms in sections of tissues in fatal cases. Serological identification of specific antibodies can be d one b y an i ndirect immunofluorescence t est. The organisms in tissues may also be identified by electron microscopy.

Bovine Petechial Fever (Ondiri Disease)

This is an uncommon disease confined to high altitudes of Kenya. It resembles ehrlichiosis in clinical signs and g ross lesions. T he causative o r-ganism, *Cytoecetes ondiri*, is a member of the family **Rickettsiaceae**, but its exact characterization and classification are unclear. The organism is suspected to be carried by an **arthropod vector.**

Disease is usually mild, may be latent, and is only rarely fatal. There is fever, and petechiae may be visible on mucosal surfaces. Leukopaenia, charac-terized by a drop in neutrophils, lymphocytes, and eosinophils, and thrombocytopaenia are present. In severe cases, extensive haemorrhage and en-largement of lymph nodes are more extensive than in milder cases. Organisms can be demonstrated in circulating neutrophils and monocytes during infection.

Colesiota Conjunctivitis

A rickettsia-like organism called *Colesiota conjunctivae* (*Rickettsia con-junctivae*) has been found in association with conjunctivitis in sheep, goats, cattle, and pigs **in South Africa.** Organisms may be visualized in conjuctival epithelial cells.

Diseases caused by Anaplasmataceae

The Family **Anaplasmataceae** (order **Rickettsiales**) now contains **organisms grouped in five genera (Table 31)**. Of these **only three are important**, namely, **Anaplasma, Haemobartonella**, and **Eperythrozoon**. Organisms of the genus **Aegyptianella produce disease in birds**. These organisms are obligate parasites found on or within erythrocytes, or free in the plasma of domestic and wild animals. With Giemsa stain the organisms appear rod-shaped, spherical, coccoid, or ring-shaped; reddish-violet, and 0.2-0.4 μm in diameter. Each organism is enclosed in a membrane with an internal structure that resembles rickettsiae. The organisms may occur in short chains or irregular groups within erythrocytes or in plasma. They are **Gram-negative**, multiply by binary fission, and are transmitted by arthropods. Anaemia is the usual clinical sign in infected animals.

Anaplasmosis

The organisms which cause anaplasmosis are at present grouped into a single genus - **Anaplasma. Three species are of pathogenic importance**: 1. *Anaplasma marginale*, 2. *A. centrale*, and 3. *A. ovis*. With Giemsa stain, these organisms appear as dense, bluish-purple, homogeneous round structures within erythrocytes near the margin or near the centre of the cell. With the electron microscope, these structures are separated from cytoplasm of the erythrocyte by a membrane that encloses 1-8 subunits, or "**initial bodies**", **which are the parasitic bacteria**. The organisms are 0.3-0.4 μm in diameter.

Within the genus **Paranaplasma** are two organisms: *P. caudatum* (*Anaplasma caudatum*) and *P. discoides* (*A. discoides*). These are found in cattle infected with *Anaplasma marginale* and may be differentiated by their predilection for infection of cattle over sheep or deer and by their characteristic morphology. However, the pathogenic effects of these organisms are not clearly established.

A. marginale **parasitizes the red cells of cattle and buffaloes**, and causes an important disease of worldwide distribution. **Deer, antelope** and a number of other **wild ruminants** are susceptible. **Sheep** and **goats** can be infected **but do not develop disease. In cattle, the infection results in overt (visible) disease only in adult animals (similar to babesiosis).** Most **young calves** undergo an inapparent infection unless splenectomized before exposure. Parasitaemia, however, may remain in these animals (also in recovered adults), and they can serve as a source of infection for other animals. *A. centrale* also affects **cattle** but causes mild anaplasmosis. *A. ovis* affects **sheep** and **goats**. It can produce mild to severe anaplasmosis.

A marginale, which causes severe anaplasmosis, is a tiny, spherical body of 0.3 to 0.8 μm in diameter. It is found within the cytoplasm of erythrocytes

near the periphery of the cell. It is best demonstrated in blood smears with Giemsa's stain. **Four developmental stages of Anaplasma are recognized in infected erythrocytes**: **1.** Early stage, consisting of "**initial bodies**", the infective form, **2.** Mixed population with **marginal and initial bodies**, **3.** Vigorous growth and t ransfer, and **4.** Massive m ultiplication with a predominance of **marginal bodies**. The organisms reproduce by binary fission and pass through the four stages of development after penetration of the erythrocyte by initial bodies. Then, they are transferred to other mature erythrocytes by direct contact between cells. The initial body is spherical and surrounded by a double membrane. The **marginal body** contains up to si x subunits (**initial bodies**), and is su rrounded by a single membrane.

Transmission

The infection can be transmitted to a normal animal by c arrying over a minute amount of blood. This can occur by the use of improperly sterilized phlebotomy (opening of a vein, v enesection) needles, o r by d ehorning or castration without previous aseptic precautions. **However, in nature, it is usually spread by bites of ticks (*Boophilus annulatus* and others), biting flies (Tabanus species), and less often by mosquitoes (Psorophora species). Ticks are the most important vectors**, because they carry the organisms for a long period of time. The transfer in uterus between bovine mother and foetus has also been reported. The presence of carriers has posed a problem in the control of disease. The detection of such carriers is difficult by examination o f blood smears, but a complement fixation test can be used.

Pathogenesis

Anaplasma are obligate intra-erythrocytic bacteria. They **infect mature erythrocytes** by a n endocytic process called "**endocytosis**" ('**endocytosis**' i s uptake of extracellular substances by cells), and reproduce by binary fission to produce 2 -8 infective **initial bodies** which l eave by **exocytosis** (opposite o f endocytosis) to infect other erythrocytes. The number of infected erythrocytes doubles every 24-48 hours, and the infection becomes patent (visible) 2-6 weeks after infection. Depending upon the st rain and the susceptibility of the h ost from 10-90% of erythrocytes may be parasitized in the acute stage of the infection. **At least 15% have to be parasitized before there is clinical disease**. Parasitized erythrocytes are removed by phagocytosis in the reticulo-endothelial system with release of acute-phase inflammatory reactants and the consequent development of fever. **Continued e rythrocyte destruction o ccurs and anaplasmosis is primarily an anaemia**. The degree of anaemia varies with the proportion of erythrocytes which are parasitized. The first appearance of organisms in the blood coincides with a fall in the haematocrit and erythrocyte levels, and the appearance of immature erythrocytes in blood smears and the development of fever. Acutely affected animals may die soon after this phase is reached. The appearance of **antierythrocyte antibodies** late in the acute stage may worsen anaemia.If the animal recovers from the initial acute attack, periodic attacks of parasitic invasion of mature erythrocytes occur, but with diminishing intensity. **The degree of anaemia varies widely in young cattle** up to 3 years of age, but is always **severe in adults** and in splenectomized animals. **Cattle that survive the disease become carriers, and serve as reservoirs of infection**.

Signs

Clinical signs include fever, and anaemia is manifested by weakness, pallor (paleness) of mucosae, increased respiration, jaundice, decreased red cell count and decreased haemoglobin. Anaemia results from increased destruction of parasitized erythrocytes by the reticulo-endothelial system **and not by haemolysis. Therefore, haemoglobinuria is not seen. Immune mechanisms are involved in phagocytosis and destruction of erythrocytes.** Sometimes, there may be muscular trembling, anorexia, and excessive salivation. Death occurs in many cases, but recovery is not unusual. **Recovered animals remain carriers of the infection for some time.**

Lesions

Gross findings in fatal cases are those of severe anaemia, with pallor (paleness) of the tissues and sometimes with jaundice. **The spleen is usually greatly enlarged. The liver is also enlarged**, has round edges, and is yellowish in cases with jaundice. The gallbladder is usually distended. Petechiae may be seen on the pericardium, and catarrhal inflammation in the gastrointestinal tract. **Microscopic findings** indicate great demands on the haematopoietic system, with hyperplasia of the bone marrow, and extramedullary haematopoiesis in the spleen and other organs. A naplasma organisms can be demonstrated with difficulty in erythrocytes in tissue sections.

Demonstration of the organisms in the blood smears is highly variable. Before the onset of anaemia, majority of erythrocytes may harbour organisms, but with sudden removal from the circulation, their numbers decrease. Immature erythrocytes (**reticulocytes**) which enter into the circulation in response to anaemia, **are resistant to the parasites.**

Importance of *Anaplasma centrale* as a separate species is doubtful; it may be a variant of *A. marginale*. It produces a mild infection in cattle, and has been employed to immunize cattle to *A. marginale*. *A. centrale* usually localizes near the centre of the red blood cell.

Anaplasma ovis is infectious for **sheep** and **goats. Cattle are not susceptible**. The disease is mild, only rarely resulting in clinical signs of anaemia.

Diagnosis

Diagnosis is made on the basis of clinical signs, and demonstration of **Anaplasma** organisms in erythrocytes. The complement-fixation test can be used for the detection of clinically silent carriers.

Haemobartonellosis

Organisms of the genus **Haemobartonella** are at present classified in the family **Anaplasmataceae** (**Table 31**). The organisms are obligate parasites found on the surface of erythrocytes. The organisms occur as cocci or chains of coccoid, in pairs or in groups, in indentations on the surface of erythrocytes. They stain well with Giemsa stain, are **Gram-negative**, and have a limiting membrane but not a cell wall or nucleus. **Haemobartonella** organisms have not been cultivated outside the host.

The genus **Haemobartonella** has **three** recognized **species**: *H. muris*, *H. felis*, and *H. canis*. In most other species, except **cat**, the disease is mild or without clinical signs. Removal of the spleen is followed by anaemia in most infected animals.

Feline Infectious Anaemia (Feline Haemobartonellosis)

This disease of **domestic and wild cats** is caused by *Haemobartonella felis*. **It is the only Haemobartonella infection of importance in animals.** Even here, infection usually does not lead to disease in the absence of complicating factors, such as concurrent infection with feline leukaemia virus or factors that compromise (damage) the immune system. The organisms are seen as small coccoid, ring-shaped, or rod-shaped bodies on erythrocytes of affected cats. They are best seen in blood smears stained with **Giemsa or Wright** stain. The mode of transmission is not known. Blood-sucking insects, such as fleas, are suspected. Experimentally, injection of a small amount of blood containing parasitized erythrocytes can transmit the disease.

Clinical signs include fever, anorexia, depression, and macrocytic, haemolytic anaemia. The **anaemia** is revealed by pale, sometimes icteric, mucous membranes, weakness, and a characteristic blood picture in which haemoglobin and packed cell volumes are severely decreased. **The haemoglobin levels usually decrease from a normal of 11 g/dL of blood to as low as 1.5 g/dL in severe cases.** Levels of 6.0 g/dL of blood or lower are considered typical of this disease. **Macrocytosis** (having large erythrocytes) and **anisocytosis** (having erythrocytes of varying size) are usually prominent features. In the early stages, nucleated erythrocytes are present in large numbers. **Reticulocytes** (immature erythrocytes) are also increased in number, and some of them may contain *H. felis*. These organisms are not readily demonstrable in all stages of the disease. This makes the **diagnosis** difficult in many cases. **Severely affected animals may die**, others may recover, and still others undergo relapses and eventually die after a prolonged illness.

Lesions

The **lesions** are those of **haemolytic anaemia**. Jaundice is a feature in acute cases. **The spleen is enlarged many times**, and its cut surface bulges. **Microscopically**, there is congestion and extramedullary haematopoiesis. Haemoglobin may stain the urine in the bladder, and haemorrhages may be present on serous surfaces. **Microscopically**, liver reveals fatty change, and also central or paracentral necrosis. These changes are secondary to the anaemia. The bone marrow is usually solidly red in the long bones and contains a large number of haematopoietic cells. The lymph nodes are usually grossly enlarged. **Microscopically**, the enlargement is caused by reactive hyperplasia.

Eperythrozoonosis

The genus **Eperythrozoon** is at present grouped in the family **Anaplasmataceae (Table 31)**. The organisms are similar to **Haemobartonella** species and are often difficult to differentiate from them. The main features which differentiate **Haemobartonella** from **Eperythrozoon** are that eperythrozoa occur both in the erythrocytes and plasma, whereas **Haemobartonella** organisms are rarely found in the plasma and also rarely in the ring forms, which are common in eperythrozoa. **Five species of Eperythrozoon are currently recognized**. Of these, *E. suis* and *E. parvum* affect **pigs**. *E. parvum* is not associated with disease, whereas *E. suis*, when parasitaemia is high, produces clinical signs of anaemia - a disease known as "ictero-anaemia". Most infections are, however, subclinical. The mode of transmission is not established, but probably involves insect vectors. Infection with *E. wenyonii*, a parasite of cattle, can also cause mild anaemia, but is usually latent. In sheep, *E. ovis* infection is associated with haemolytic anaemia. *E. coccoides* is a parasite of mouse.

Eperythrozoon organisms in blood smears stained with **Giemsa** are seen as tiny pleomorphic structures within the erythrocytes, lying on their surface or free in the plasma. The organisms are pale purple to pinkish-purple and are mostly ring-shaped, 0.5-1.0 μm in diameter. One to a dozen organisms may be present in a single red blood cell, and large numbers are uniformly distributed throughout the plasma. Organisms are much more numerous in blood smears taken at the height of infection.

The mode of **transmission** is not clearly established, but **arthropods** are generally suspected.

Signs

Clinical disease occurs only in **sheep** and **pigs**. Infection with other eperythrozoa only causes anaemia in splenectomized animals. In sheep and pigs, infection is seen particularly in young animals exposed to harmful influences, such as helminthic parasitism, or may be brought about by splenectomy of animals already harbouring the infection. The natural disease in pigs is called "ictero-anaemia", and somewhat resembles anaplasmosis of herbivora. It is, however, difficult to differentiate from anaplasmosis when sheep are involved. The symptoms begin with fever (104°-107° F). This is accompanied by depression and weakness. The total red cell count drops suddenly to 1-2 million/mm3, haemoglobin is decreased to 2-4 g/dL, and the packed red blood cell volume falls between 4-7%. **Haemoglobinuria** has been noticed **in sheep, which indicates that anaemia is haemolytic**. The icteric index is raised between 18-25, and the sedimentation rate is greatly increased, reaching 75 mm/min in some cases. The white blood cell count is usually not changed. Death may occur in the acute stage, but animals usually recover and then are prone to repeated relapses. **In cattle**, the most common sign of eperythrozoonosis is **oedema of the hind limbs and teats**.

Lesions

The **gross lesions** are those of haemolytic anaemia resulting from the effect of **Eperythrozoon** infection on the red blood cells. **Jaundice is a persistent feature**. Blood is thin and watery. Liver is yellowish brown, and the gallbladder contains thick gelatinous bile. Hydropericardium and ascites are present in some cases. Petechiae may be seen in the mucosa of the urinary bladder. Bone marrow is mainly red rather than fatty.

Microscopic changes are seen in the bone marrow which is hyperplastic. **Liver** shows some fatty change and central and paracentral necrosis of lobules. Necrosis is due to the effect of anoxia. The organisms are difficult to demonstrate in tissue sections.

Diagnosis

Eperythrozoonosis must be differentiated from anaplasmosis, haemobartonellosis, babesiosis, and other haemolytic anaemias. The differentiation is made by accurate identification of the causative organisms in the erythrocytes.

Diseases caused by Bartonellaceae

Organisms classified in the family **Bartonellaceae** are small, very pleomorphic and found in erythrocytes of several species. They stain well with Giemsa, are **Gram-negative**, and are differentiated from protozoa by the absence of recognizable cytoplasm around their nucleus.

Two genera at present make up this family: **Bartonella** and **Grahamella**. Each of these contains parasitic species. *Bartonella bacilliformis*, the only species now recognized in this genus, causes a disease syndrome in **humans**

called "**Oroya fever**", also known as "**Carrion's disease**". This organism parasitizes erythrocytes, reticulo-endothelial system, and vascular endothelium. **Human bartonellosis** is of great importance in South America, but also occurs in Central America.

The second genus **Grahamella** consists of rod-shaped or club-shaped organisms, which occur in the erythrocytes of several hosts, mainly voles (small rodents) and deer mice, **and are of no significance in veterinary medicine**.

6

Chlamydial Diseases

The organisms previously placed under the psittacosis-lymphogranuloma-trachoma group are now classified in a separate Order Chlamydiales. It has only o ne family C hlamydiaceae, and one g enus Chlamydia. In this genus t here are f our species: 1) *C. trachomatis* which mainly affects humans and also other mammals, 2) *C. psittaci* which affects humans and other mammals and birds, including poultry, 3) *C. pneumoniae* which affects only humans, and 4) *C. pecorum* which affects ruminants (cattle and s heep) and perhaps other a nimals (pigs). H owever, currently only two species are accepted as valid : *C. trachomatis* and *C. psittaci*.

Chlamydiae are minute bacteria (0.2-1.5 μm). However, i n contrast to other bacteria, they multiply only within host cells of vertebrates, including humans, other mammals, and birds. The organisms are non-motile, spherical, Gram-negative, and have a cell wall. Morphologically, there are two distinct forms of Chlamydia: 1. elementary body (EB) and, 2. reticulate (or reticular) body (RB). EB is the basic unit which is a small dense, spherical body about 0.2-0.4 μm in diameter. The EB never divides but is the infectious form of the organism, w hich attaches t o host c ells through s pecific receptors and gains entry. The reticulate body is the intracellular, metabolically active non-infectious form and divides by binary fission. It is larger than the EB (about 0.6-1.5 μm). Elementary bodies have a cell wall that is made rigid by disulphide bonds rather than by cross-linked peptidoglycans found in bacteria. Therefore, chlamydiae are not susceptible to penicillin. Chlamydiae have adhesins on their surface which b ind to microvilli o n host columnar epithelial cells.

Developmental cycle

Chlamydiae have an unusual d evelopmental cycle consisting of an obligatory intracellular m ode of r eplication (growth) within cytoplasmic vacuoles of the host cells. The cycle consists of basically five major phases: 1) attachment and penetration by the elementary body, 2) transition of the metabolically inert EB into the metabolically active reticulate body, 3) multiplication of the RB by binary fission, producing many progeny (chlamydiae), 4) maturation of the non-infectious RBs into infectious EBs, and 5) release of EBs from the host cell (Fig. 11).

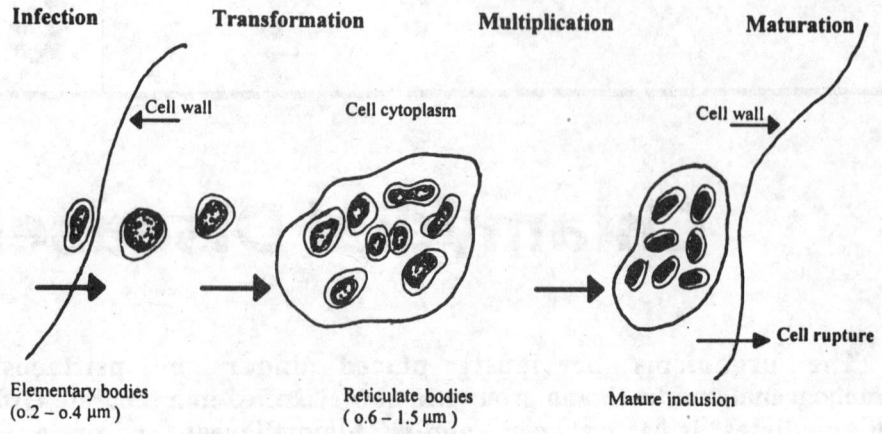

Fig. 11. Developmental cycle of Chlamydiae.

The **first event** in the infectious process begins with the **attachment of C. psittaci elementary bodies to host cells through specific receptors**. The elementary body then enters the cell in a phagosome (Fig. 11). Thus, uptake is similar to an endocytosis-like process. **The phagosomes do not fuse with lysosomes. Thus, chlamydiae remain surrounded and protected by the phagosome membrane throughout their intracellular development**. Once inside the cell, the **elementary body undergoes morphological changes**. It becomes larger (0.6-1.5 µm) and gains more ribosomes, and the nucleus becomes reticular (resembling a net, or reticulum) and is termed a **reticulate body** (Fig. 11). That is, **these changes result in conversion of the EB to the RB form**. The daughter reticulate bodies divide by binary fission. The resulting chlamydial microcolony is termed an "**inclusion**", and may contain anywhere from 100-500 progeny, depending on the species of chlamydia. In some cases multiple inclusions appear in *C. psittaci*-infected cells. In contrast, *C. trachomatis*-containing phogosomes fuse with one another early in the developmental cycle. This results in the appearance of usually only one inclusion. Reticulate bodies ultimately re-organize into elementary bodies, which are then released from the cell (Fig. 11). It is believed that when nutrients (glycogen) are depleted, the RB progeny mature and condense into EBs and are released. The released EBs infect neighbouring cells. Release mechanisms are not understood, but the cell can simply burst, liberating its entire contents. **The developmental cycle (i.e., time from infection to release) within the host takes about 30 hours**. The released elementary bodies survive extracellularly to infect new hosts.

Staining Characteristics

Chlamydiae are large enough to **be seen with a light microscope using special stains**. The intracellular organisms can be stained with **Giemsa**,

Macchiavello, Castaneda, or Gimenez methods after appropriate fixation. They appear **dark purple** with Giemsa, **blue** with Castaneda, and **red** with Macchiavello and Gimenez stains. They can also be demonstrated in unstained preparations (**wet mounts**) of infected cells with a phase-contrast microscope. They are readily seen by dark-field illumination.

As stated earlier, **only two species of chlamydiae are currently recognized:** *C. trachomatis* and *C. psittaci*. There are, however, multiple strains of each species. These are host-specific, and associated with characteristic diseases. These are listed in **Table 33**.

Table 33. Diseases caused by Chlamydiae

Chlamydia	Disease	Species affected
C. trachomatis	Trachoma	Humans
	Inclusion body conjunctivitis	"
	Urogenital inflammatory disease	"
	Lymphogranuloma venereum	"
	Pneumonia	"
	Murine pneumonitis	Mice
C. psittaci	Psittacosis (ornithosis)	Humans, **birds**
	Sporadic bovine encephalomyelitis	Cattle
	Polyarthritis	Cattle, sheep, horses
	Enzootic bovine abortion	Cattle
	Enzootic ovine abortion	Sheep
	Abortion	Horses, pigs
	Feline pneumonitis and rhinitis	Cats
	Pneumonia	Cattle, sheep, goats, horses, dogs
	Conjunctivitis	Sheep, cats
	Enteritis	Cattle, pigs

Chlamydial Infections in Humans

Chlamydia trachomatis strains cause several diseases **in humans**, including **trachoma** and **lymphogranuloma venereum (Table 33). These strains are highly specific for humans.**

Avian Chlamydiosis (Psittacosis, Ornithosis, Parrot fever)

Avian chlamydiosis is caused by *Chlamydia psittaci*. It is a **Gram-negative**, coccoid organism. It multiplies intracellularly within **phagosomes**. Multiplication is characterized by change from a small (250-300 nm diameter) rigid-walled **infectious form** (**elementary body**) to a larger (400-600 nm diameter) flexible-walled **non-infectious form** (**reticulate body**) that divides by binary fission. The daughter reticulate bodies then re-organize into elementary bodies. These are shed extracellularly to infect new cells (see Fig. 11).

C. psittaci causes disease **both in birds and humans. In human,** it occurs as a febrile pulmonary disease. Since the disease was contracted from sick **parrots,** it was called **"parrot fever".** It is now known that the causative agent is harboured not only by parrots, but also by a wide variety of other birds. Chlamydiosis is referred to as "**psittacosis**" when it affects humans, mammals, and psittacine birds (e.g., parrots, parakeets etc). **'Psittacus'** in Latin means **a parrot.** The disease is called "**ornithosis**" when it affects **birds other than psittacines. The disease is worldwide in prevalence.**

There is **considerable variation in virulence** among strains and also among species of host. **Among domestic poultry, turkeys** are most susceptible and then **ducks** and **pigeons, while chickens are rarely affected.** The **serotypes** of *C. psittaci* **which infect birds are different from those associated with chlamydiosis in mammals.** Currently, six **serotypes of** *C. psittaci* are known to **infect birds.** However, avian strains of *C. psittaci* can infect humans, and precautions should be taken when handling infected birds, or contaminated materials. The disease in humans contracted from turkeys is usually more severe than that from psittacine birds. **Avian chlamydiosis in birds is usually systemic and sometimes fatal.**

Spread

Spread of infection occurs **by direct means** when birds are in close contact, **and indirectly** through fomites and perhaps biting insects, and mice and lice. The sources of infection include birds in the incubative stage of infection, sick birds and carriers, and infected inanimate material. **Elementary bodies** are found in faeces and also in respiratory excretions. **Spread occurs mainly through the inhalation of infected, contaminated dust. The elementary form** of the organism is **highly resistant** outside the host and **can survive in dried faeces for many months.** Egg transmission is not known to occur. Factors which may contribute to precipitation of disease, or increase its severity, include stress due to movements of birds, crowding, change of diet or environment, and concurrent infection with other organisms such as **Salmonella** or *Pasteurella multocida*.

Pathogenesis

After entry into the body, **mainly through inhalation,** the organisms multiply in the lungs, airsacs and pericardium. By **haematogenous spread** they reach the liver, spleen and kidneys where further replication occurs, along with the production of reticulate and elementary bodies.

Signs

The disease **in humans** is manifested by sudden onset of a febrile illness with upper respiratory involvement, pneumonia, and severe debility. Although the disease is not usually fatal, significant deaths occur in some outbreaks. Antibiotic therapy has reduced the death rate markedly. **In birds**, clinical signs vary greatly in severity and depend on the species and age of the bird and on the strain of chlamydia. **Thus, clinical signs may be absent, mild, or severe**. In the turkey, duck and pigeon signs include depression with ruffled feathers, anorexia, purulent nasal discharge and conjunctivitis, sometimes tracheitis with rales, and grey-green diarrhoea which may contain blood. In a flock the disease may be sporadic or a number of birds may be affected at the same time. **The mortality is likely to be higher in parrots than in parakeets**. Recovered birds may excrete the organism for long periods of time. **Chickens, although susceptible, are rarely affected**.

Lesions

Gross lesions vary and are dependent on the severity and acute nature of the disease. Serofibrinous exudate covers serosal surfaces. There is pericarditis, congestion of the lungs, clouding of airsac walls, and enlargement of liver and spleen. Both liver and spleen are softer than normal and may show small necrotic foci and petechiae. **Mortality varies from 0 to 30%.**

Microscopically, various tissue cells in acute psittacosis reveal presence of the organism. The **spleen** is infiltrated by mononuclear cells containing organisms. Hyperplasia of the reticulo-endothelial cells is usually observed. **Liver** often contains **focal lesions of necrosis**. The portal areas are rich in lymphocytes and plasma cells. The epithelium of the **kidney** may be packed with large numbers of "**LCL bodies**". These are minute, spherical basophilic bodies. They were discovered by Levinthal, Coles, and Lillie, **hence the acronym "LCL"**. (An **acronym** is a word formed from the first letters). **In the lungs**, a few alveoli may contain serous exudate, but frank pneumonic consolidation is rare. The mucosa of the **intestine** is usually eroded, and the underlying lamina propria and submucosa are infiltrated with lymphocytes and plasma cells. Within macrophages and epithelial cells, cytoplasmic bodies, which represent the organism, may be seen. They are best observed with **Giemsa, Macchiavello, Castaneda, or immunofluorescent techniques**.

Diagnosis

The clinical signs and gross lesions are usually insufficient for definitive diagnosis. **Confirmation depends on demonstration of the causal organism, or its isolation and identification, or serological examination**. It is emphasized that **due to the zoonotic nature of the organism, great care should be taken in handling birds or carcasses suspected of being infected with *C***.

psittaci. This also includes the wrapping of carcasses for dispatch to a laboratory. Microscopic examination of smears, or sections of peritoneal, pericardial, liver and spleen lesions, appropriately stained, show intracellular organisms in most acute cases. **Other techniques** for detection of the causal organism include demonstration of chlamydial antigens, and chlamydial DNA. Antigen can be demonstrated by fluorescent antibody or immunoperoxidase staining, whereas DNA probes and reagents for the **polymerase chain reaction (PCR)** can be used to demonstrate chlamydial DNA.

Isolation and identification of chlamydia is one of the more common and reliable methods of diagnosis. It involves isolation of organisms in cell culture or embryonated hen's eggs. Experimental mice inoculation with susceptible material can also be used. **Serological tests** can be used to detect current or past chlamydial infections. Serological methods of detecting and measuring antibodies include complement fixation test (CFT), ELISA, immunofluorescence and gel diffusion tests. The standard CFT was the most widely used serological test for the chlamydial group antigen. However, because the sera of many avian species interfere with this test, a modified CFT or an indirect CFT (complement fixation inhibition test) is used. **The ELISA is more sensitive and faster than CFT, and is now widely used for the recognition of antibody and antigen.** More recently, **monoclonal antibodies (MAbs)** have been developed and are available to detect chlamydiae in clinical specimens.

Zoonotic Importance

The avian strains of *C. psittaci* can infect humans, and precautions should be taken when handling infected birds, or contaminated materials. Human infections are common following handling or processing of infected turkeys or ducks. **Most infections are through inhalation of infectious aerosols.** Therefore, processing plant employees are especially at risk. Also at risk are farm workers and poultry inspectors at processing plants. Personnel who are employed to process turkey meat have also become infected. **Pigeons** also may pose public health threats, mainly to their producers. **Chickens are of lesser importance as potential health hazards.**

Strains of *C. psittaci* which cause psittacosis and are spread directly from human to human **without an avian host** have been identified. These organisms, termed **TWAR strains** (*C. pneumoniae* strain), **are** considered **primary human pathogens.**

The diseases of domestic animals listed in **Table 33**, as being caused by *C. psittaci*, are not to be confused with psittacosis.

Chlamydial Infections of Domestic Animals

Organisms identified as *Chlamydia psittaci* have been recovered from

several different disease syndromes of cattle. These include enteritis of calves, latent intestinal infection, pneumonia, polyarthritis, placental infection, and abortion. As strains of the organisms are being studied more extensively, it is becoming clear that only one causative organism may be involved, even though many organs and systems are affected. If this proves to be true, the disease should be described as **"psittacosis"** or **"chlamydiosis"**, which may have different clinical and pathological manifestations. **In India,** chlamydiae have been reported to cause **abortion in sheep and goats** and have been also associated with **pneumonia, arthritis, and encephalitis.**

Sporadic Bovine Encephalomyelitis

This is a disease of **young calves** and, less often, **older cattle.** It is caused by an infectious agent currently designated as *Chlamydia psittaci* (*C. pecoris*).

Signs

The onset is sudden, with fever (105°- 107° F), anorexia, depression, excessive salivation, and nasal discharge. Dyspnoea with cough is observed in some cases, but diarrhoea, either mild or severe, is more common. Within a few days, calves have difficulty in walking and exhibit stiffness in the fetlock joints. They move aimlessly in circles, stagger, and fall with the head extended. In the final stages, the limbs appear paralyzed. **Death usually occurs within 5-7 days.**

Lesions

The most constant lesion in fatal cases is **sero-fibrinous peritonitis.** Excessive amount of clear yellow peritoneal fluid is present in the early stages. In more prolonged cases, adhesive strands of fibrin form an exudate over the omentum, liver, and spleen. A similar fibrinous exudate lies over the pleura and peritoneum. The brain and spinal cord usually appear oedematous and their blood vessels are congested. The **microscopic lesions** consist of fibrinous peritonitis, pericarditis, and severe, diffuse meningo-encephalomyelitis. The entire brain and spinal cord are involved in an intense inflammatory reaction. The meninges at the base of the brain are particularly affected. Severe damage to neurons, both in brain and cord, has been described. Minute elementary bodies are demonstrable in mononuclear cells in the serosal exudates, and in the brain and spinal cord.

Diagnosis

The gross and microscopic lesions are characteristic, although not diagnostic. Demonstration of the typical elementary bodies is helpful.

Polyarthritis of Calves

A variety of organisms can cause polyarthritis in calves. *Mycoplasma mycoides* infection can cause polyarthritis, as also several other species of

Feline Pneumonitis

Feline pneumonitis, a chlamydial infection (**C. psittaci**) of **cats** starts as **an acute upper respiratory infection**, with sneezing and catarrh. Later symptoms are nasal and conjunctival mucous discharges, and transitory fever. **The disease runs a short course and may terminate fatally.** Chlamydial infection has also been associated with peritonitis. Organisms have been identified in and recovered from mucus-producing cells of the gastric mucosa of **healthy cats**.

Lesions

Apart from catarrhal inflammatory changes in the upper respiratory passages, the main lesions are usually found in the **lungs**. Sharply demarcated patches of consolidation may be seen in various lobes. **Microscopically**, these affected areas are distributed around terminal bronchioles, and consist mainly of alveolar collapse rather than consolidation. **Of diagnostic significance** is the presence of **elementary bodies** in the cytoplasm of epithelial and mononuclear cells. They usually appear in loose aggregates as tiny structures, about 0.5 μm in diameter. In smears they stain selectively with Macchiavello stain, and appear brightly eosinophilic usually as coccoid. Sometimes, the elementary bodies coalesce into a plaque and form a solid eosinophilic body, which distends the cytoplasm of epithelial cells.

Zoonotic Importance

A case of acute kerato-conjunctivitis has been described in **humans** caused by the feline pneumonitis agent.

Other Chlamydial Infections

Chlamydial Polyarthritis in Foals

In one case, chlamydiae were cultured from joint exudate from **a young foal** with spontaneous polyarthritis. However, this disease is much less common in foals than in **lambs** and **calves**.

Chlamydial Infection in Dogs

Although chlamydial antibody titres have been demonstrated in as many as 50% of dogs in some surveys, clinical disease is reported much less often in this species. However, dogs are susceptible to experimental infection.

Follicular Conjunctivitis of Sheep

A specific ocular disease of sheep in Australia is known as contagious conjunctivo-keratitis, **pink eye**, or **snow blindness**. **This has been compared to trachoma of humans.** Chlamydiae have been isolated from affected sheep. Chlamydiae have also been isolated from the conjunctival sac of sheep suffering from a similar disease, follicular conjunctivitis, in the United States.

7

Mycoplasmal Diseases

Mycoplasmosis

The infectious agent involved in **bovine pleuropneumonia** was recognized more than a hundred years ago, in 1898. This organism is now called *Mycoplasma mycoides*, (or *M. mycoides* subsp. *mycoides*), and is the type species of the genus **Mycoplasma**.

Mycoplasmas are the smallest free-living microbes 300-800 nm in diameter. They c an be p assed through b acteria-retaining filters. **I n contrast to bacteria, they have no cell wall but are bounded by a plasma membrane.** They a re found i n humans, many animal s pecies, birds, p lants and i nsects. Mycoplasmas tend to be quite host specific. In general, mycoplasmas colonize mucosal surfaces, and most s pecies a re non-invasive. **T hey grow on agar media without living cells**, and form small, microscopically visible, disc shaped colonies with a dark, thick centre and lighter periphery. Mycoplasma belong to the Order **Mycoplasmatales**, Family **Mycoplasmataceae**, and genus **Mycoplasma** (Table 34). **Two genera** in the Family **Mycoplasmataceae** are of veterinary interest: **Mycoplasma** and **Ureaplasma**. **Acholeplasma** species belong to genus **Acholeplasma**, Family **Acholeplasmataceae**, Order **Acholeplasmatales**.

Table 34. Classification

Order	Mycoplasmatales
Family	Mycoplasmataceae
Genus	Mycoplasma
	Ureaplasma
Order	Acholeplasmatales
Family	Acholeplasmataceae
Genus	Acholeplasma

For many years the cumbersome name "**pleuropneumonia-like organism**" or "**PPLO**" was applied to all **Mycoplasma** organisms, other than the causative agent of bovine pleuropneumonia. Specific names are now available for most organisms in this genus. However, PPLO still remains in the older literature and may confuse the newcomer.

A large number of different Mycoplasma species have been isolated from animals. Many of these are nonpathogenic commensals living on mucosal surfaces, especially of the respiratory and genital tracts. Some are of low pathogenicity, producing only mild disease; or they may become pathogenic only in association with another injury, particularly viral and bacterial infections. There is no easy distinguishing feature that can differentiate pathogenic from non-pathogenic mycoplasmas. Certain respiratory pathogens (*M. mycoides* subsp. *capri, M. hyorhinis, M. dispar*) inhibit the activity of epithelial cilia, which helps in production of disease. **There are, however, mycoplasmas which are true pathogens producing both acute and chronic disease.**

Spread may be by **aerosol (droplet infection), venereal (sexually transmitted),** or *in utero*. Organisms remain and are shed from animals after clinical disease has subsided. This provides a reservoir for the spread of infection. Many mycoplasmas may remain alive in the environment for several days. **In general, mycoplasmas are species-specific.** Most pathogenic mycoplasmas are associated with farm animals, particularly **cattle, sheep, goats, pigs, and poultry.** They are of much less importance as a cause of disease in horses, dogs, and cats. **Table 35** presents important mycoplasmas of animals.

Table 35. Diseases caused by Mycoplasmas

Mycoplasma	Disease
BOVINE MYCOPLASMAS	
M. mycoides subsp. *mycoides* [SC type]	Contagious bovine pleuropneumonia
M. alkalescens	Arthritis in calves; isolated from mastitis
M. bovigenitalium	Mastitis, arthritis in calves, chronic seminal vesiculitis, endometritis, vulvo-vaginitis; suggested as a cause of infertility
M. bovirhinis	Mild mastitis; often isolated from pneumonia
M. bovis	Severe mastitis, arthritis; associated with pneumonia
M. bovoculi	Conjunctivitis; kerato-conjunctivitis usually in association with *Moraxella bovis*

M. californicum	Acute mastitis
M. canadense	Mastitis; recovered from cases of calf arthritis
M. verecundum	Possible cause of conjunctivitis in calves

OVINE AND CAPRINE MYCOPLASMAS

M. mycoides subsp. *capri* and strain F38	Contagious caprine pleuropneumonia
M. mycoides subsp. *mycoides* [LC type]	Pneumonia, arthritis, mastitis, septicaemia
M. agalactiae	Contagious agalactia (mastitis), arthritis, pneumonia, kerato-conjunctivitis, vulvo-vaginitis
M. capricolum	Polyarthritis with septicaemia in goats, conjunctivitis, mastitis, vulvo-vaginitis, balano-posthitis
M. conjunctivae	Conjunctivitis and kerato-conjunctivitis
M. ovipneumoniae	Chronic interstitial pneumonia, mastitis
M. putrefaciens	Mastitis in goats

MYCOPLASMAS OF PIGS

M. flocculare	Mild focal mononuclear pneumonia
M. hyopneumoniae	Enzootic pneumonia
M. hyorhinis	Arthritis and polyarthritis
M. hyosynoviae	Polyarthritis

OTHER MYCOPLASMAS

M. cynos	Pneumonia in dogs
M. canis	Possibly not pathogenic
M. felis	Conjunctivitis in cats

Ureaplasma species differ from Mycoplasma species in that they hydrolyze urea with the production of ammonia. Two species, *Ureaplasma diversum* and *U. urealyticum*, have been recovered from humans and animals, including **cattle, sheep, goats, horses, pigs, dogs, cats, monkeys, and birds**. They are associated with bovine mastitis, enzootic pneumonia, bovine abortion, and infertility in cattle and sheep.

Members of the genus **A choleplasma** differ from **M ycoplasma** species and **Ureaplasma** species in that **they do not need serum or cholesterol for growth**. They can occur as saprophytes in soil and sewage, but some species are mucosal commensals of animals (pigs, cattle, and horses). They have been detected in association with **kerato-conjunctivitis, pneumonia, and abortion**.

Table 36 presents important ureaplasmas and acholeplasmas of animals.

Table 36. Diseases caused by Ureaplasmas and Acholeplasmas

Organism	Disease
UREAPLASMAS	
U. diversum	Host specific strains recovered from many animal species, including cattle, horses, pigs, cats. Associated with pneumonia, conjunctivitis, mastitis, vulvo-vaginitis, and infertility
U. urealyticum	Commensal of humans; associated with urethritis, endometritis, infertility
ACHOLEPLASMAS	
A. equifoetale	Recovered from normal respiratory mucosae and aborted equine foetuses
A. hippikon	Recovered from aborted equine foetuses
A. oculi	Kerato-conjunctivitis and pneumonia in goats; recovered from cases of infectious bovine kerato-conjunctivitis, and from nasal cavity of normal calves, horses, and pigs

Contagious Bovine Pleuropneumonia (CBPP)

Contagious bovine pleuropneumonia is a highly infectious septicaemia characterized by localization of organisms in lungs and pleura. It is one of the important diseases of **cattle**, c ausing heavy l osses i n many parts o f the w orld, **including India**. *Mycoplasma mycoides* subsp. *mycoides* (small colony type) is the cause of the disease in cattle. It is not communicable to other species. This i s the only mycoplasma w hich is d ivided into a nother subspecies: *M. mycoides* s ubsp. *capri*, cause of **contagious c aprine p leuropneumonia (CCPP)**.

The two groups, or strains of *M. mycoides* subsp. *mycoides*, **are differentiated in culture: a small colony (SC) strain and a large colony (LC) strain**. The SC strain causes contagious bovine pleuropneumonia. The LC strain resembles *M. mycoides* subsp. *capri*, and is associated with **contagious caprine pleuropneumonia (CCPP)**, arthritis, mastitis, and septicaemia in **goats**.

Spread

The focus of infection is usually provided by **recovered "carrier" animals** in which a **pulmonary sequestrum** (a segregated area) preserves a potential source of organisms **for periods as long as 3 years**. Conditions of stress due to starvation, exhaustion, or intercurrent disease can cause the sequestrum to break down and convert the animal into an active case. The **principal method of spread** of this disease is by the **inhalation** of infective droplets from active, or carrier cases of the disease.

Pathogenesis

Contagious bovine pleuropneumonia is **an acute lobar pneumonia and pleurisy**, which develop from **localization of organisms in lungs and pleura** from an initial **septicaemia**. An essential part of the pathogenesis of the disease is **thrombosis in the pulmonary vessels**, prior to the development of pneumonic lesions. The mechanism of development of thrombosis is not known. **Death results from anoxia and toxaemia.**

Signs

Although **the disease can be acute, leading to death within a week**, the common course is two to several weeks after a prolonged incubation period of 3-6 weeks. There is a sudden onset of high fever (105° F) and the affected animal shows signs of pneumonia. **In the acute stage**, dry and painful cough, which later becomes moist, is followed by laboured respiration. When the lungs are extensively involved, respiratory distress is shown by dyspnoea (laboured or difficult breathing) so severe that the animal stands with its elbows out. In the later stages, mucopurulent discharge from the nose may be seen. Weakness and emaciation usually become noticeable, and swelling of the joints **(polyarthritis)** is sometimes seen in **young calves**. The organism may invade the placenta and foetus, resulting in **abortion**. Morbidity is high, although clinical signs may develop in only 50% of affected herds. Mortality varies from 10-90%.

Lesions

In the typical case, lesions are **characteristic**. They are **usually limited to one lung**, but sometimes are bilateral. However, they never symmetrically involve contralateral lungs (i.e., similar parts on the opposite lung). The pleural cavity over the affected lung contains an excess of pleural fluid, which may be blood-stained and contains strands of fibrin. The parenchyma does not collapse when the thorax is opened, but remains raised. **The cut surface of the lung has a marbled appearance** with red and greyish areas of parenchyma separated by **thick yellowish interlobular septa**. The presence of unequally distended lymph spaces usually give a **"beaded" appearance** to these septa. In cases of long standing, zones of necrosis within groups of lobules become sequestrated from the adjacent lung and are surrounded by a dense layer of connective tissue. Within these sequestra, which are usually large, the original shape of lung parenchyma is retained for a time. Eventually, **abscesses** form in the encapsulated tissue, and their rupture may cause an acute aggravation of the symptoms, or the entire sequestrum may be converted to **scar tissue**.

Microscopically, the characteristic lesion is separation of the lobules into distinct compartments by the heavily thickened interlobular septa. The septa have not only oedema but organization as well. The lobules contain areas of consolidation. An intense infiltration of mainly lymphocytes and plasma cells is seen around blood vessels and bronchi. Similar focal collections of leukocytes are found within the interlobular septa.

Lesions in other organs are not specific. Liver may be infiltrated by round cells in the hepatic triads, with necrosis of individual liver cells near central veins. The necrotic cells are acidophilic and have dark pyknotic nuclei. In the **spleen**, the germinal centres are enlarged, mature lymphocytes decreased in number, and plasma cells increased.

Diagnosis

Diagnosis may be established by the history, clinical symptoms, gross and microscopic lesions, and recovery of the organism. Immunofluorescent staining techniques are particularly useful. Results are often positive, even in the absence of positive culture. Serological tests (mainly **complement fixation test**) and a skin test (**single intradermal allergic test**) can be used to identify chronically affected and recovered animals. An ELISA test developed has been found accurate.

Other Bovine Mycoplasmal Infections

Several other mycoplasmas of bovine origin can serve as primary pathogens, or participate along with other infectious agents in several diseases. These include **mastitis, urogenital infections, kerato-conjunctivitis, enzootic pneumonia, and arthritis**.

Bovine Mastitis

Mycoplasma bovis (*Mycoplasma agalactiae* var. *bovis*) is the most important agent in primary mycoplasma mastitis in cows. The second is *M. californicum*. Bovine mastitis is also caused by several other species of

Mycoplasma and **Acholeplasma**. *M. bovis* has also been recovered from calves with arthritis.

Disease caused by *M. bovis* occurs worldwide, in an acute, highly contagious form. The disease is characterized by a sudden onset of **agalactia** (absence of milk secretion) **with a swollen firm udder**. All four quarters are affected. Morbidity rates within a herd are high. Systemic signs are usually absent, although the organism can c ause arthritis a nd pneumonia along with mastitis. The milk c ontains a l arge number o f neutrophils. On keeping, i t rapidly separates into a flaky deposit and a clear supernatant. Recovery usually occurs in 2-3 weeks with a marked decrease in size of the udder, **but mycoplasmas are excreted for months**.

Lesions

Lesions i nvolve acini, i nterlobular ducts, a nd interstitial s troma. In t he beginning, all acini in the lobule get filled with purulent exudate. The interlobular ducts may also become filled with neutrophils, and the epithelium becomes hyperplastic. As the disease progresses, the ductal epithelium undergoes squamous metaplasia. The interstitial stroma is initially oedematous and infiltrated b y l ymphocytes and p lasma cells, b ut eventually undergoes fibrosis. Eosinophils are a common component of the e xudate.

Bovine Genital Infections

Several **Mycoplasma** species a re normal c ommensals o f the u rogenital tract of **cows** and **bulls** and may cause disease. *M. bovigenitalium*, which is also associated with **mastitis and arthritis**, is the Mycoplasma species usually recovered from animals with inflammatory disease of the urogenital tract. It may also cause sterility or low fertility in cattle.

Lesions

No gross lesions are seen. M icroscopically, l esions are l imited to t he uterus, oviducts, and related peritoneum. T he e ndometrium is o edematous, and infiltrated with lymphocytes and plasma cells.

M. bovigenitalium and **Ureaplasma** species are also associated with **bovine granular venereal disease (granular vulvo-vaginitis)** and **infertility**. The **gross lesions** consist of mucopurulent discharge and the appearance of tiny granular elevations of the vulvar and vaginal epithelium. **Microscopically**, these elevated nodules consist of aggregations of lymphocytes. The epithelium is necrotic and the stroma is oedematous and infiltrated by eosinophils. **Seminal vesiculitis and epididymitis in bulls** may be the result of infection by *M. bovigenitalium*.

Infectious Bovine Kerato-Conjunctivitis

This disease is caused by *Moraxella bovis*. However, *Mycoplasma bovoculi* is also usually recovered from cases of infectious bovine kerato-conjunctivitis. The organism appears to increase severity of the disease. By itself, *M. bovoculi* causes a mild conjunctivitis. Ureaplasmas have also been recovered from animals with conjunctivitis.

Enzootic Pneumonia of Calves

Enzootic pneumonia is a term used for pneumonias occurring not only in **calves**, but also in **lambs** and **young pigs. Usually, it is not a severe or fatal disease**. However, it is important as a cause of subnormal growth. It is not a specific disease with a single cause. It is the result of a combination of infectious agents, which include respiratory viruses, bacteria, acholeplasmas, mycoplasmas, and ureaplasmas. *Mycoplasma dispar*, *M. mycoides* subsp. *mycoides* and *M. bovis* are recognized as **primary respiratory pathogens**.

Gross lesions are usually limited to a few lobules in apical or cardiac lobes. They are characterized by consolidation of small groups of lobules, sharply demarcated from adjacent ones. **Microscopically,** lesions are present around bronchioles, with purulent exudate and debris in the lumen. Nodules of lymphocytes distort the bronchial wall. This is consistent with the fact **that mycoplasmas grow on epithelial surfaces of the respiratory tract**.

Bovine Mycoplasmal Arthritis

Polyarthritis in calves and cows can be caused by several species of bovine mycoplasmas (e.g., *M. bovis*, *M. canadense*, or *M. alkalescens*). **Mycoplasmas, when they gain entry into the bloodstream of any species, usually tend to localize in synovial membranes** and mesothelial surfaces. Affected joints become swollen and painful, leading to lameness. Pathologically, there is increased synovial fluid, which is cloudy and may contain fibrin. The synovial membrane is thickened as a result of villous hyperplasia and infiltration of mononuclear cells, mainly lymphocytes.

Mycoplasmal Diseases of Goats and Sheep

Contagious Caprine Pleuropneumonia (CCPP)

This respiratory disease of goats is very similar to contagious bovine pleuropneumonia (CBPP). The disease is caused by *Mycoplasma mycoides* subsp. *capri*. However, a basically similar disease is caused by *M. mycoides* subsp. *mycoides* (**LC type**) and a mycoplasma known as **strain F38**. The disease occurs in many parts of the world, **including India**.

The disease is readily spread by inhalation, but the organism does not survive for long outside the animal body. The infection is brought into the flock by a carrier or infected animal. The **clinical signs** include fever (104.5°-106°F), nasal discharge, cough, and dyspnoea; and in the terminal stages, mouth-breathing, tongue protrusion and frothy salivation with death in 2 or more days. **The mortality rate is high, usually reaching 100% in an outbreak**.

The **pulmonary lesions** resemble those of contagious bovine pleuropneumonia, except that sequestration of lung tissue is less common or absent. In the **peracute form**, lungs are uniformly consolidated with fibrino-purulent exudate on the pleura. In the **less severe form**, pulmonary lobules have a variegated appearance, i.e., having markings of different colours. Oedema is extensive in the interlobular septa and under the pleura. There is fibrinous pleuritis and pericarditis. In addition to pneumonia, the infection may also cause arthritis or mastitis. Serological tests to identify carrier animals include **complement fixation, ELISA**, and a **latex agglutination test**.

Contagious Agalactia of Goats and Sheep

This is caused by *Mycoplasma agalactiae*. However, other species, namely, *M. putrefaciens*, *M. ovipneumoniae* and *M. mycoides* subsp. *mycoides* (LC type) may also be involved. Infection with *M. agalactiae* results in bacteraemia, followed by excretion of organisms in milk within 6 days. Mammary infection persists for months, and the organisms may be isolated from blood, milk, or joint fluid.

The **signs** appear in females first at lambing time as mastitis. **The infection may be very acute, leading to septicaemia and death in ewes** and kids before clinical mastitis is seen. The milk may become greenish-yellow, and the solids tend to sediment. Polyarthritis (particularly in males), pneumonia, and kerato-conjunctivitis usually appear.

In India, *M. agalactiae* has been associated with **granular vulvo-vaginitis of goats**. The lesions consist of multiple tiny nodules of lymphocytes and plasma cells in the lamina propria and muscularis of vagina and vulva. These aggregations of lymphocytes are seen grossly as **tiny granules** which raise the mucosa. This appearance gave the descriptive term granular vulvo-vaginitis.

Ureaplasmas have also been associated with vulvo-vaginitis in **sheep** as well as mastitis in **ewes**.

Other Mycoplasmoses in Goats and Sheep

Apart from *M. mycoides* var. *capri* and *M. agalactiae* several other mycoplasmas have been isolated from sheep and goats. *M. capricolum* causes different lesions in goats ranging from **acute septicaemia** to fibrino-purulent **arthritis, conjunctivitis, mastitis, vulvo-vaginitis**, and **balano-posthitis** (inflammation of the glans penis and prepuce). Interstitial pneumonia of sheep and goats can result from *M. ovipneumoniae* infection. Kerato-conjunctivitis (**pink eye**) in sheep and goats may be caused by *M. conjunctivae*.

Ureaplasmas have been associated with granular vulvitis and infertility in sheep.

Mycoplasmal Diseases of Pigs

Mycoplasmal Arthritis and Polyserositis in Pigs

Two mycoplasmas are important causes of **polyarthritis in young pigs**: *Mycoplasma hyosynoviae* and *M. hyorhinis*. Both organisms are common commensals of the nasopharynx. Young pigs are infected by their mothers at an early age. Infection with *M. hyorhinis* also results in polyserositis. Clinical disease usually follows infection with either organism. Mostly the infection is subclinical. Stress of some kind appears to allow the mycoplasma to enter the bloodstream and localize in joints, and in the case of *M. hyorhinis*, serous surfaces.

Lesions

Pericarditis, pleuritis, and peritonitis (collectively referred to as "**polyserositis**") are **characteristic**. Fibrino-purulent exudate may be seen grossly on serous surfaces. Underlying the serosal lining cells are lymphocytes, macrophages, and plasma cells. With time, the exudate may organize, particularly over the pleural and peritoneal surfaces. This results in adhesions, which may persist for a long time.

The lesions of **arthritis** usually follow those of polyserositis. **Both *M. hyorhinis* and *M. hyosynoviae* produce similar lesions in the joints**. One or more joints may become involved, with swelling, congestion, and pain resulting in **lameness**. The synovial fluid becomes yellow or turbid, and contains numerous neutrophils, and sometimes, strands of fibrin. Fibrous thickening of the joint capsule may result in partial or complete **ankylosis** (immobility) of the affected joint.

Diagnosis is made on the basis of gross and microscopic lesions, and demonstration of the organism by cultural methods, immunofluorescence, or electron microscopy.

Enzootic Mycoplasmal Pneumonia of Pigs

This pulmonary disease is mainly caused by *M. hyopneumoniae*, although in some cases *M. hyorhinis* or *M. flocculare* are recovered. The **clinical signs** include a prolonged course with subnormal weight gain, chronic cough, and high morbidity and low mortality rates.

Gross lesions are seen mainly in the apical and cardiac lobes of the lung, with lobular consolidations and atelectasis, and enlarged peribronchial lymph nodes. **Microscopic lesions** include peribronchial and peribronchiolar accumulations of lymphocytes and plasma cells in large numbers. **Diagnosis** can be established by finding characteristic microscopic lesions, and by demon- strating mycoplasma on the bronchial or bronchiolar surface epithelium with immunofluorescence.

Mycoplasma in Other Species

Dogs

Mycoplasmas have been recovered from conjunctiva, respiratory systems, and genital tracts of dogs; and include various species. Some organisms have been recovered from lesions, such as those of **pneumonic lungs, balano- posthitis, vaginitis, and urinary tract infections**. The organisms may have a causative relationship to these diseases. However, the pathogenic significance of mycoplasma in dogs still remains to be established.

Cats

Several **Mycoplasma** species and one **Acholeplasma** species are often recovered from sick and normal cats. Although an association with severe conjunctivitis appears to have been established with *Mycoplasma felis*, in many other instances a causative relationship has not been clearly established.

Horses

No specific disease caused by a mycoplasma has been identified in horses.

Avian Mycoplasmosis

Of the 22 species of mycoplasma recovered from birds, **only four of them are established pathogens** for domestic poultry. These are: 1. *M. gallisepticum*, and 2. *M. synoviae* for chicken and turkey, and 3. *M. meleagridis* and *M. iowae* for turkey.

Mycoplasma gallisepticum Infection

M. gallisepticum infection is commonly known as **"chronic respiratory disease (CRD)"** of chickens, and **"infectious sinusitis"** of turkeys. It is characterized by respiratory rales, coughing, and nasal discharge in chickens, and by sinusitis in turkeys. Clinical signs usually develop slowly and the disease has a long course. It occurs worldwide. Among domestic poultry, **chicken and turkey are natural hosts. The turkey is more susceptible** than the chicken, and **very young birds** are **more susceptible**.

Spread

Spread occurs from direct contact of susceptible birds with infected carrier chickens or turkeys. Spread may also occur from contaminated airborne dust, droplets, or feathers. The organism is fragile outside the body of the host and its survival is limited to a few days. However, if protected by exudates and/or cold environment, the organism may survive longer. **Spread** can also occur **through the infected eggs** of chickens and turkeys.

Signs

The appearance of disease depends upon the presence of other pathogens or debilitating factors. Other pathogens include the viruses of Ranikhet disease and infectious bronchitis (including the live vaccine strains), infectious bursal disease, turkey rhinotracheitis **and the pathogenic strains of *E. coli*** and *Haemophilus paragallinarum*. Debilitating factors include nutritional deficiency, excessive environmental **ammonia and dust,** and the stress associated with intensive management. **Uncomplicated infections usually cause no clinical signs or mortality, except in very young.**

The most common clinical signs occur with disease of the respiratory tract, and include coryza, sneezing, moist rales and breathing through the partly open beak. Coryza is more severe in turkeys than in chickens. In turkey, sinusitis with swelling of one or both infraorbital sinuses, may occur. Swelling of the infraorbital sinuses is rarely seen in chickens. **If airsacs alone are affected there may be no respiratory signs. Lowered egg production** may occur in larger chickens. Other clinical signs are rare and include swelling of the hock and lameness in chickens.

Lesions

Gross lesions of the respiratory tract may be so **mild that they may not be visible,** or consist only of excess mucus or catarrhal exudate in the nares, trachea and lungs and oedema of the airsac walls. **Caseous exudate may appear later in the airsacs,** or be attached to their walls. Dilatation of the infraorbital sinuses, particularly in turkeys, is caused by excess mucus which may be replaced by caseous material. **When the disease is aggravated by other pathogens,** lesions are more severe and prolonged, giving rise to **a chronic condition. With *E. coli* infection in young chickens, colisepticaemia may result with pericarditis, perihepatitis, and disease of the respiratory tract, including airsacculitis. Microscopic lesions** in chickens and turkeys include marked thickening of the mucus membrane of the affected tissues from infiltration with mononuclear cells and hyperplasia of the mucous glands. Focal areas of lymphoid hyperplasia are commonly found in the submucosa.

Diagnosis

There are no clinical signs or gross or microscopic lesions which are pathognomonic in either the chicken or turkey. Isolation and identification of the causal organism is the most certain method of confirming infection. Samples can be taken from live birds or fresh carcasses. From live and dead birds swabs may be taken from the oropharynx, oesophagus, trachea and cloaca, and exudates may be aspirated from the infraorbital sinuses and joints. If mycoplasmas are isolated, identification may be made by using specific sera for immunofluorescence. Methods for **detection of *M. gallisepticum* DNA** have been developed and c ommercial kits utilizing the p olymerase chain reaction (PCR) are a vailable. There are also a number o f serological t ests which are used for the demonstration of specific antibody. These include the rapid serum agglutination test, the haemagglutination inhibition test, and the ELISA.

Mycoplasma synoviae Infection

This disease occurs both in chickens and turkeys. The infection usually does not result in either clinical signs or gross lesions, but may cause mild upper respiratory disease. However, it may produce a more severe respiratory condition in association with predisposing factors. It may also cause a reduction in egg p roduction.

Spread

Spread occurs readily by direct contact. That is, spread of infection is similar to *Mycoplasma gallisepticum*. Haematogenous spread of *M. synoviae* occurs and, in a ddition to d isease of the articular a nd/or respiratory t issues, there may be anaemia and vasculitis. **Vertical transmission also occurs.** However, many flocks hatched from infected hens remain free of infection.

Signs

Both in chicken and turkey usually there are no clinical signs. When clinical signs occur they may take a respiratory or arthritic form. In the **acute arthritic form**, there is pallor (paleness) of the face and comb, rapid loss of condition, and swelling of the joints. The feet and hock joints are particularly affected with accompanying lameness. In the **respiratory form**, w hich may occur independently o f joint lesions, there may be mild r ales a nd c oryza. More severe respiratory conditions may be seen when *M. synoviae* infection is associated with viruses, bacteria and other predisposing factors as described for *M. gallisepticum*.

Lesions

Gross lesions involving the j oints include o edema and t hickening of periarticular tissues, especially in the synovial membranes. The **foot and hock joints** are usually affected, but others may also be involved. Erosion of articular cartilage has also been observed. The lesions in the respiratory form are similar to those of *M. gallisepticum*.

Diagnosis

Neither the respiratory signs are specific nor the joint lesions are pathognomonic. Diagnosis depends on the isolation and identification of the organism, or demonstration of antibodies by serology. Trachea, lungs and airsacs and joint lesions are the best sites for the isolation of the organism. For serology, rapid serum agglutination test, or ELISA are commonly used. A monoclonal antibody-blocking ELISA is being developed, and a commercial PCR test has been shown to be sensitive and specific for *M. synoviae*. This may prove to be a useful tool in diagnosis.

Mycoplasma meleagridis Infection

M. meleagridis infects turkeys only. In young turkey poults it causes poor growth, airsacculitis, osteodystrophy, and abnormalities of wing feathers. It usually occurs as a silent infection in adult birds. However, infection in breeding birds may result in reduced hatchability.

Mycoplasma iowae Infection

M. iowae infects turkeys and sometimes chickens. In the turkey, it can cause reduced hatchability and poor quality poults.

8

Protozoal Diseases

The Subkingdom **Protozoa** (Kingdom **Protista**) is composed of various single-celled "**eukaryotes**". ('**Eukaryotes**' are cellular organisms, such as protozoa, that have a distinct, visible nucleus, whereas "**prokaryotes**" are cellular organisms, such as bacteria, that do not have a distinct nucleus.) The vast majority of these eukaryotes are free-living and not pathogenic to either animals or humans. However, a number of important diseases are caused by the **pathogenic protozoa**. A classification of only the important species is presented in **Table 37**.

Table 37. Classification of important pathogenic protozoa

Kingdom	:	Protista
Subkingdom	:	Protozoa
Phylum	:	Sarcomastigophora
Subphylum	:	Mastigophora
Family	:	Trypanosomatidae
Genus	:	**Leishmania**
		Trypanosoma
Family	:	Hexamitidae
Genus	:	**Giardia**
Family	:	Trichomonadidae
Genus	:	**Tritrichomonas**
		Trichomonas
Family	:	Monocercomonadidae
Genus	:	**Histomonas**
Subphylum	:	Sarcodina
Family	:	Entamoebidae
Genus	:	**Entamoeba**
Phylum	:	Apicomplexa (previously **Sporozoa**)

Family	:	Klossiellidae
Genus	:	**Klossiella**
Family	:	Haemogregarinidae
Genus	:	**Hepatozoon**
Family	:	Eimeriidae
Genus	:	**Eimeria**
		Caryospora
		Isospora
Family	:	Cryptosporidiidae
Genus	:	**Cryptosporidium**
Family	:	Sarcocystidae
Genus	:	**Besnoitia**
		Neospora
		Toxoplasma
		Sarcocystis
Family	:	Plasmodiidae
Genus	:	**Plasmodium**
Family	:	Babesiidae
Genus	:	**Babesia**
Family	:	Theileriidae
Genus	:	**Theileria**
		Cytauxzoon
Phylum	:	Microspora
Family	:	Pleistophoridae
Genus	:	**Encephalitozoon**
Phylum	:	Ciliophora
Family	:	Balantidiidae
Genus	:	**Balantidium**
Unknown Classification		
Genus	:	Pneumocystis

The Subphylum **Mastigophora** includes those protozoa whose **trophozoites** have one or more **flagella**. These may occur as **extracellular parasites**, for example, **Giardia** in the digestive tract, **Trichomonas** in the digestive tract or reproductive tract, and **Trypanosoma** s p. in the vascular system; or as **intracellular parasites,** such as **Leishmania** and **Histomonas** (a parasite of turkey). Their life cycles allow their spread from host to host. **The life cycles**

may include : 1. direct transmission with no extra-host stage, 2. direct transmission with a resistant cyst stage outside their mammalian hosts (**Giardia**), 3. indirect transmission with a parasitic stage in some insect, which serves as an intermediate host (**Leishmania, Trypanosoma**), or 4. in the case of **Histomonas**, the **trophozoites** enter and live in eggs of the roundworm *Heterakis gallinae*.

The Subphylum **Sarcodina** includes those protozoa which **utilize pseudopodia for locomotion**. These protozoa are **extracellular parasites** of the intestinal lumen. They are capable of invading the intestinal wall and spreading to other organs, e.g. **Entamoeba**. Their life cycles are direct with a cyst stage outside their hosts.

The Phylum **Apicomplexa** (previously **Sporozoa**) includes several families which contain some of the most important pathogenic protozoa. They **lack means of locomotion** (e.g., cilia, flagella, or pseudopodia). Their **life cycles** may be: 1. **direct** with an encysted extra-host form, as in the case of **Eimeria, Isospora, Klossiella**, and **Cryptosporidium**, or 2. **indirect** with an intermediate host, as in the case of **Sarcocystis, Toxoplasma, Babesia, Plasmodium, Besnoitia**, and **Neospora**. **Babesia, Plasmodium**, and **Theileria** are **all intracellular parasites**.

The Phylum **Microspora** contains only a single parasite of importance, *Encephalitozoon cuniculi*. It is transmitted directly through spores in the urine, and may also be transmitted *in utero*.

The Phylum **Ciliophora** contains dikaryotic protozoa (i.e., having two nuclei) with **cilia** or other ciliary structures for locomotion. The macronucleus is concerned with cell metabolism, and the micronucleus with genetics. Most are free-living or commensals. *Balantidium coli* is the only pathogen of importance. It is transmitted directly through cysts.

In this chapter, besides describing the effects of protozoa upon hosts and the life cycles of some, **emphasis is given on those features that influence pathogenesis**. In some cases, the effects upon the host have been clearly demonstrated and the tissue changes are well understood. But, in others, practically nothing is known.

The diseases are discussed genus-wise in the order presented in Table 37.

Genus: Leishmania
Leishmaniasis

Protozoan organisms of the genus **Leishmania** cause infections in humans and animals. Several pathogenic species of **Leishmania** are recognized. However, they cannot be differentiated from one another in tissue section.

They have different geographic distributions, or the diseases they produce are relatively different. The diseases, however, may overlap in clinical signs or lesions.

Leishmania occur **in vertebrate hosts** within parasitophorous vacuoles in **macrophages** and **reticulo-endothelial cells** as **amastigotes (leishmanial forms)**. These are small oval protozoans about 1-2 μm wide and 2-4 μm long, without a flagellum. In Romanovsky-stained (**Leishman, Giemsa, or Wright**) preparations, they have pale blue cytoplasm containing, near the posterior end, a reddish nucleus. Anterior to the nucleus is a deep violet, rod-shaped body, the **kinetoplast**. In the invertebrate hosts (sand flies), or in cultures, the organisms take shapes which vary from the **leishmanial to the leptomonad form**. The leptomonad forms are slender and spindle-shaped, 14-20 μm in length and 1.5-4 μm in width. This form is motile by means of a flagellum.

Life Cycle

Leishmania reproduce in the vertebrate host by **binary fission**. However, the complete life cycle and maintenance of virulence depend upon an intermediate host or vector. Many species of sand flies (**Phlebotomus**) are involved in the transmission of **Leishmania**, and are necessary for their perpetuation. However, certain flies, such as *Stomoxys calcitrans*, may transmit the infection mechanically.

Clinical Forms

Leishmaniasis is divided into **three major clinical forms** : 1. **visceral**, 2. **cutaneous**, and 3. **mucocutaneous. Each form is associated with specific species of Leishmania**. The most important difference between the forms is the generalized spread of organisms in the visceral leishmaniasis and their confinement locally in the other forms.

Visceral Leishmaniasis

Also known as "**Kala-azar**" and "**Dum-dum fever**", this form is caused by *L. donovani*. It occurs naturally in **humans, dogs, cats, cattle, horses, and sheep**. It has a wide geographical distribution and is **quite prevalent in India.** Visceral leishmaniasis **in animals** occurs usually **as a chronic debilitating disease** with periods of fever, gradual weight loss, anaemia, and leukopaenia. Lymph nodes are enlarged, and there is splenomegaly and hepatomegaly. Usually the infection slowly progresses to death.

The lesions are characterized by massive infiltration of various organs with huge macrophages whose cytoplasm is filled with leishmaniae. The architecture of the lymph nodes and spleen, which are particularly affected, may be completely obscured by the phagocytic cells. Large numbers of plasma cells are also usually present. Liver, bone marrow, kidneys, lungs, gastrointestinal tract, and less often, other organs and skin, may be affected.

Gross lesions at postmortem consist of enlarged lymph nodes, spleen and liver, pallor (paleness) of mucosal and serosal surfaces, soft red bone marrow, and ulcers of the intestine.

Cutaneous Leishmaniasis

This is caused by *L. tropica* or *L. major*, and occurs mainly in countries bordering the Mediterranean. It is also known as **'Old World cutaneous leishmaniasis'**, **'Oriental sore'**, **'Delhi sore'**, or **'Baghdad boil'**. The reservoirs for human infection are various **wild rodents**. The infection is characterized by **single or multiple** very slowly developing **nodules or ulcers of the skin** which usually heal spontaneously, but only over a period of months. The **lesions** are characterized by infiltration of the skin with macrophages accompanied by lymphocytes, plasma cells and rarely eosinophils. Numerous parasites are present within the macrophages. Lesions of long-standing are surrounded by fibroblastic connective tissue. This gives them the appearance of a typical granuloma.

Mucocutaneous Leishmaniasis

Also known as **'New World cutaneous leishmaniasis'** or **'American leishmaniasis'**, mucocutaneous leishmaniasis is caused by *L. braziliensis* or *L. mexicana*. It occurs in Mexico and Central and South America. Animals are usually not found infected, although **dogs**, **cats**, and **monkeys** are susceptible. The infection resembles cutaneous leishmaniasis, but in addition to the skin, chronic ulcers often occur at mucocutaneous junctions and may occur in oral and nasal cavities. The lesions are similar to those of cutaneous leishmaniasis.

Diagnosis

Diseases which also cause proliferation of reticulo-endothelium, such as toxoplasmosis, histoplasmosis, blastomycosis, and epizootic lymphangitis, present problems in differential diagnosis. Final diagnosis must be based upon demonstration and identification of the causative organisms in tissue sections, smears or cultures. Identification of the kinetoplast and the nucleus, which are not present in the organisms of the diseases mentioned above, allows differentiation. Tissues taken by biopsy are most useful in demonstrating the organisms in a living animal or human patient.

Genus: Trypanosoma

Trypanosomiasis

Trypanosomiasis is **a very serious disease of humans and animals** in certain regions of the world, **which includes India**. The disease trypanosomiasis is divided into **two major forms**: 1. *American trypanosomiasis* caused by *Trypanosoma cruzi*, and 2. *African trypanosomiasis* caused by the other pathogenic trypanosomes. Most species of trypanosomes do not produce serious effect upon their host, but a few are important pathogens (**Table 38**).

Trypanosomes are **flagellated** motile protozoan parasites that live in blood and body fluids of their host and localize in tissues, sometimes in a non-**flagellated form**. Trypanosomes have certain common features, such as an ovoid or rounded body in the non-flagellate stage and a slender elongate body when it becomes flagellated; a flagellum which arises from the **blepharoplast**; an **undulating membrane** which extends along the border of the trypanosome, with the **flagellum** forming its margin; and the **parabasal body** (Fig. 12). A relatively large **nucleus** is usually located near the middle of the body. Trypanosomes can usually be identified by their morphological features, such as size, shape, position, arrangement, and development of the organelles.

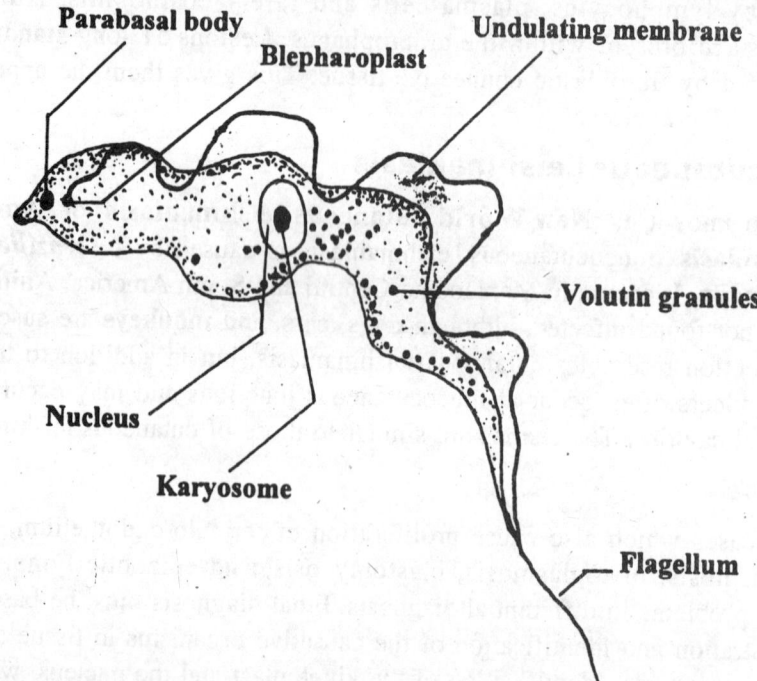

Fig. 12. Diagram showing the morphology of a trypanosome.

Table 38. Important Trypanosomes of Man and Animals

Species	Definitive host	Intermediate hosts (vectors)	Geographic distribution	Disease
T. brucei	Man, domestic and wild mammals, except goats	Tsetse fly	Tropical Africa	Nagana
T. caprae	Horse, sheep, cattle	Tsetse fly	Tanzania, Malawi	Trypanosomiasis

T. congolense	Cattle, horse, goat, sheep, pig, ass, dog, camel	Tsetse fly	Tropical Africa	Trypanosomiasis
T. cruzi	Man, dog, cat, armadillo, opossum	"Kissing bug" (**Triatoma** sp.)	South America	American trypanosomiasis
T. equiperdum	Horse, ass	Transmitted by coitus	Worldwide	Dourine
T. evansi	Horse, mule, ass, cattle, buffalo	Horse flies (**Tabanidae** and **Stomoxys**)	Africa, Asia, South America Far East	Surra
T. gambiense	Man, antelope	Tsetse fly	Tropical Africa	Chronic "sleeping sickness"
T. rhodesiense	Man, antelope	Tsetse fly	East Africa	Acute "sleeping sickness"
T. simiae	Monkey, pig, horse, sheep	Tsetse fly	East Africa	Trypanosomiasis
T. vivax	Cattle, sheep, horse, goat, camel	Tsetse fly	Central and South America, Mauritius and Africa	Souma

Life cycle

Almost all trypanosomes are **transmitted by arthropods**, which act as biological vectors. The only exception is *Trypanosoma equiperdum*, cause of **dourine**, which is **transmitted by coitus**. Mechanical transmission of trypanosomes may be done by certain biting flies (**Tabanus, Stomoxys**), but this is not an important means of spread, except for *T. evansi*, the cause of **surra** in horses, cattle and buffaloes. **Definite cyclic development occurs in the body of true invertebrate hosts. In these hosts,** trypanosomes multiply in various forms in the digestive tract, finally migrate as infective forms to the salivary glands and are injected into the **mammalian host** with the vector's saliva at the time of the bite. *T. cruzi*, the cause of American trypanosomiasis, is an exception. In this case, the infectious stage is located in the hind gut and is excreted in the faeces of the arthropod (**Triatoma** sp.), when the arthropod defecates at the time of its bite. When transmitted through vector saliva, trypanosomes are referred to as **salivarian**, and when through arthropod faeces as **stercorarian**.

Pathogenesis

The pathogenesis of trypanosomiasis in humans and animals is **not fully understood**. The mechanisms that induce disease or cause death are basically unknown, with the exception of **Chagas disease** (American trypanosomiasis) caused by *T. cruzi*. **This trypanosome invades cells, whereas trypanosomes of the African trypanosomiasis do not.** Following entry into the mammalian host, t rypanosomes of A frican trypanosomiasis (salivarian) rapidly m ultiply by binary fission (as **trypanomastigotes**) within the bloodstream, leading to **parasitaemia**. The parasitaemia remains mostly unaffected and **is not diminished by the host's immune response. This is because of the parasite's unique ability to undergo almost endless antigenic variations through changes in surface glycoproteins** (see evasion of the immune response by trypanosomes, discussed next). Because of their variability, these **surface antigens** are called **variant** or **variable surface glycoproteins (VSGs)**. Trypanosomes may also enter the interstitial space and multiply there.

Continued stimulation of the immune system by **VSGs** explains the reticuloendothelial, lymphocytic, and plasmacytic (of plasma cells) hyperplasia seen in the spleen and lymph nodes of many affected animals. **Glomerulonephritis** and **vasculitis**, which may occur in chronic trypanosomiasis, can also **result from the continuous immune response and the formation of antigen-antibody complexes. Anaemia** is a common finding. Although its pathogenesis is not settled, it may also be immunologically mediated. It is in part **haemolytic** and in part due to **erythrophagocytosis**. Just as a drug can adsorb (adhere to the surface) o n r ed cells and m ake them i mmunologically f oreign, s o also the trypanosomes. These altered cells, being regarded as foreign, are either lysed by antibody and haemolytic complement, or are phagocytosed by mononuclear phagocytes. **Clinically**, severe anaemia is, therefore, characteristic of trypanosomiasis. **Hypersensitivity** to trypanosomal antigens may explain some acute deaths. The **pathogenesis** of inflammatory reactions in various tissues is also considered to be immune mediated. These reactions are mainly characterized by **proliferation and activation of macrophages**. Toxic products of trypanosomes may also play a role in the pathogenesis of tissue damage, w hich can i nclude necrosis. U sually leukocytosis, t hrombocytopaenia, and hypergammaglobulinaemia o ccur.

Evasion of the Immune Response by Trypanosomes

Most protozoan parasites h ave evolved mechanisms for escaping the effects of t heir host's immune responses. Trypanosomes may promote the development o f suppressive r egulatory cells, or stimulate the B c ell system t o exhaustion. **Trypanosome-induced immunosuppression can lead to the death of the host as a result of secondary infection.** In trypanosome infection of cattle death is usually due to **bacterial pneumonia** or **sepsis** occurring as a result of immunosuppression.

In addition to immunosuppression, trypanosomes have evolved **two other effective evasive techniques**. One involves becoming **non-antigenic**, and the other involves **ability to alter surface antigens rapidly and repeatedly (i.e., antigenic variation)**. Examples of non-antigenic trypanosomes are *T. theileri* in cattle and *T. lewisi* in rats. They can become **functionally non-antigenic** by masking themselves with host antigens. These both are non-pathogenic trypanosomes that survive in the bloodstream of infected animals, because they become covered with a layer of host serum proteins and thus are not regarded as foreign. *T. brucei*, a pathogenic trypanosome of cattle, may also adsorb host serum proteins or red cell antigens and thus become **functionally non-antigenic. Complete absence of antigenicity is the last step in the evasive process**.

Trypanosomes also successfully employ extensive **antigenic variation**. For example, if **calves** are infected with the pathogenic trypanosomes *T. vivax*, *T. congolense*, or *T. brucei* and their parasitaemia is checked at regular intervals, the numbers of circulating trypanosomes are found to fluctuate. Periods of high parasitaemia alternate regularly with periods of low parasitaemia. Each period of high parasitaemia corresponds with the development of a new surface glycoprotein antigen. The removal of this population by an **antibody response** leads to a rapid fall in blood parasite levels (i.e., periods of low parasitaemia). However, within the surviving population, some trypanosomes **express new surface glycoproteins** to escape the host's immune response and to grow without hindrance. As a result, **a fresh population arises to produce yet another period of high parasitaemia**. This **cyclic fluctuation** in parasite levels, with each peak reflecting the appearance of a population of parasites with new surface glycoproteins, **can continue for many months**.

Variant surface glycoproteins (VSGs) are the major surface antigens of trypanosomes. VSGs produced early in the infection develop in a particular sequence. However, as the infection progresses, production of VSGs becomes more random. Trypanosomes grown in tissue culture also show antigenic variation. This demonstrates that the change in surface VSG is not necessarily induced by antibody. On electron microscopy, it can be seen that the **VSG forms a thick coat over the surface of the trypanosome**. When antigenic change occurs, VSG in the old coat is shed and **replaced by antigenically different VSG. Recent studies** indicate that the trypanosomes possess **a large number of genes for** VSGs. Only one VSG gene is active at a time. This active gene is associated with a series of related genes that regulate its expression. Trypanosome also possesses a pool of about 1000 silent VSG genes. **Antigenic variation** occurs as a result of replacement of an active VSG gene with one from the silent VSG gene pool.

Specific Infections

Surra

Surra is **an acute, subacute, or chronic disease of mainly horses, mules, asses and camels,** but also occurs in **cattle, buffaloes, dogs, deer, Bengal tiger** and **elephants. In India,** besides cattle, surra is widely prevalent in **buffaloes. It is caused** by ***Trypanosoma evansi*** (syn. ***T. equinum***). Wild ruminants can act as reservoirs. ***T. evansi*** is transmitted mechanically by the bite of horse flies (**Tabanus, Stomoxys**). The disease is characterized by fever, progressive emaciation, anaemia, subcutaneous oedema, nervous signs and death. It is regarded as the **most important health problem in camels.**

T. evansi **is the first pathogenic trypanosome to be identified in 1880, in India.** As it belongs to the ***brucei*** group, it is not easy to distinguish ***T. evansi*** morphologically from ***T. brucei*** and ***T. equiperdum*** in blood smears. **In India,** the incidence of surra increases significantly during the rainy season when there are large biting fly populations, the so-called "**surra season**". **Mortality in horses and camels is nearly 100%** if untreated, but is much lower in **cattle** and **buffaloes. The survivors become carriers.**

The trypanosomes are inoculated into the host from the contaminated mouth parts of the biting insects. The parasites multiply in the blood and body fluids, including the cerebrospinal fluid, and cause inflammatory changes and anaemia. **Immune mechanisms are related to antigenic variation of the parasite and the production of antibodies by the host.**

Clinical Signs

Surra usually occurs in a severe form. The main clinical signs include intermittent fever associated with trypanosomes in the blood, oedema of dependent parts of the body (limbs, lower abdomen and thorax), gradual emaciation in spite of good appetite, nasal and ocular discharge, progressive anaemia, delirium and convulsion. **Surra is always fatal in camels and horses,** death occurring within a few days or a few months. **However, camels may exhibit chronic signs for years.** These signs include a reduction in milk yield and capacity for work, and a high abortion rate in pregnant females. **Cattle** and **buffaloes** in enzootic areas usually have mild infections, which may be aggravated by stress, such as from bad climatic conditions, work, or intercurrent disease. Surra may affect the quality of semen in **bulls,** and cause irregular oestrus, abortion and stillbirths in **cows.**

Lesions

Grossly, the carcass is emaciated and pale and may be jaundiced. There may be patchy alopecia and petechiae and ecchymoses of visible mucosae. However, as in ***T. brucei*** infection, there are **no pathognomonic gross or**

microscopic lesions, although a lymphoplasmacytic (lymphocytes and plasma cells) infiltrate of various organs, including the brain and spinal cord, is characteristic. **Trypanosomes can be detected in body fluids.**

Diagnosis

Laboratory help is required to confirm a diagnosis, and even then surra cannot be easily differentiated from *T. brucei* infection where both coexist. Trypanosomes are readily seen in blood smears from animals in the acute phase of the disease. In the **chronic phase, repeated sampling** for some days may be required, or the trypanosomes in the blood could be concentrated into the buffy coat layer by centrifugation before examination. Also, suspected blood samples could be inoculated into rodents or dogs which are highly susceptible.

Nagana

Also known as **"tsetse fly"** disease, 'Nagana' is commonly used as a collective term for **'African trypanosomiasis'** of domestic animals, particularly for infections caused by *Trypanosoma brucei*, *T. congolense*, and *T. vivax*. *T. vivax* and *T. congolense* are highly pathogenic for **cattle**. *T. brucei* is pathogenic for many domestic animals, particularly **horses, dogs** and **camels**. Cattle, sheep and goats are less susceptible and the disease in these species tends to be chronic. The local term **"Souma"** is sometimes applied to infection with *T. vivax*. A large number and variety of wild animals may serve as reservoirs of infection, but they themselves do not suffer the disease.

Nagana is transmitted mainly by the tsetse fly (**Glossina** sp.). Animals recovering from infection with one strain or species of trypanosome are not immune to infection with another strain or species. This is due to the ability of trypanosomes to readily change their surface coat antigens through a process called **antigenic variation**. The glycoprotein surface coat is continuously shed and replaced by mechanisms not fully understood (see evasion of the immune response by trypanosomes).

Pathogenesis

Nagana in all species is a progressive but not always fatal disease. **Metacyclic trypanosomes** are injected into the host by the fly during feeding. They multiply at the subcutaneous site, provoking a local skin reaction called a **chancre**. Within the chancre, metacyclic trypanosomes change to **trypomastigote form**, and enter the bloodstream directly or through the lymphatics. Their behaviour therefore depends on the species of trypanosome. *T. vivax* usually multiplies in blood and is even disseminated throughout the cardiovascular system, whereas *T. congolense* tends to be aggregated in small blood vessels and capillaries of the heart, brain and skeletal muscles from where a small proportion of trypanosomes enter the blood circulation. **On the** other hand, *T. brucei* and rarely *T. vivax*, have the ability to pass out of the capillaries into the interstitial tissues and serous fluids of body cavities where they continue to multiply.

T. vivax and *T. congolense* exert their effect mainly by causing severe **anaemia** and mild to moderate organ damage. With *T. brucei*, there is more severe organ damage in horses, small ruminants and sometimes pigs, as well as anaemia. **In very acute infections**, there is disseminated intravascular coagulations with haemorrhages resembling a septicaemia. Trypanosomes can also pass through the placenta and into the foetus in pregnant animals. **As a result, some cows abort and some calves are born prematurely**. Trypanosomes in the brain and cerebrospinal fluid are protected against the commonly used chemotherapeutic agents by the blood-brain barrier, and are believed to be the source of some relapsed infections.

Clinical Signs

Clinical signs are not diagnostic. There are no pathognomonic signs and a clinical examination is of little help in diagnosis. Nagana results in acute or chronic manifestations with irregular fever, anaemia, emaciation, subcutaneous oedema, conjunctivitis, photophobia, lachrymation, and neurological signs of tremor, hyperexcitability, incoordination, paresis, and coma. Death may occur following an acute illness or after a prolonged course, during which gradual wasting is a main feature.

Lesions

The postmortem lesions, like the clinical signs, are not pathognomonic. The carcass shows severe emaciation, with oedematous change in all fatty tissues. The lymph nodes are swollen, oedematous, sometimes with haemorrhage in the medulla. **Liver** is enlarged and congested. **Spleen** is either enlarged, normal, or atrophic. Haemorrhages are common, particularly in the subendocardial and epicardial locations. Pericardial fluid may be excessive. Congestion and haemorrhage may be prominent in the gastrointestinal tract.

Trypanosomes are found in blood and other body fluids as well as free in tissues. Here they cause an inflammatory reaction, mainly mononuclear. Inflammation characterized by mononuclear infiltration occurs virtually in every body tissue, including skeletal muscle, myocardium, brain, spinal cord, meninges, eye, liver, adrenal gland, uterus, and skin. Lymph nodes and spleen are hyperplastic. Erythrophagocytosis may be prominent throughout the reticulo-endothelial system.

Diagnosis

Nagana is difficult to diagnose without laboratory help because it resembles any other chronic disease and has no characteristic clinical signs or postmortem lesions. Because of the unpredictable and fluctuating levels of parasitaemia, repeated examination of blood may be necessary.

Dourine

Dourine is a venereal infection of horses and donkeys caused by *Trypanosoma equiperdum*. It has a worldwide distribution. Dourine is characterized clinically by inflammation of the external genitalia, cutaneous lesions and paralysis. In contrast to other trypanosomes, *T. equiperdum* **is transmitted by coitus**, rarely by biting flies.

The disease is manifested by oedematous lesions in the genital tract and ventral body wall, persistent ulcerous plaques in the genitalia and skin, and sometimes by anaemia, incoordination and paralysis. *T. equiperdum* is demonstrable in the lesions, particularly those of the genitalia. **The lesions are those of a mononuclear or granulomatous inflammation**.

Diagnosis

The clinical signs are diagnostic. No other disease has the clinical and epizootiological characteristics of dourine. However, when the full clinical picture is not developed, other diseases like coital exanthema, equine infectious anaemia and purulent endometritis should be considered.

Chagas disease

Also known as "**American trypanosomiasis**", Chagas disease is caused by *T. cruzi*. This trypanosome was shown to be the cause of **human trypanosomiasis** in 1909, by **Chagas**, in South America. Chagas disease is transmitted by blood-sucking bugs. **Dogs, cats, pigs, monkeys** and small wild animals harbour and also suffer from the disease like humans.

T. cruzi, in contrast to other trypanosomes, **multiplies within the cytoplasm of cells in the mammalian hosts**. After release of the infectious stage in the faeces of the **Triatoma** bug, trypanosomes enter the bloodstream, but do not multiply within the bloodstream. Instead, they invade host cells, particularly cardiac and skeletal muscle. Here they transform to **amastigotes**, a form closely resembling **Leishmania** and usually referred to as the leishmanial form of *T. cruzi*. The amastigotes multiply within the cytoplasm of the infected cells, forming collections of organisms called "**pseudocysts**". The amastigotes differentiate into **trypanomastigotes** (i.e. typical trypanosomes), which are released upon rupture of the infected cells into the circulation. In the circulation they are available to infect the intermediate host, or invade another cell to repeat the cycle.

Lesions

Lesions result from the growth and activity of *T. cruzi* in the blood, but are influenced by its intracellular activities, particularly in the myocardium. The initial lesion, in **humans**, following the bite of a bug is a hard, red, painful oedematous mass at the site of the bite. This soon subsides and the organisms spread. The lymph nodes become enlarged, oedematous, and sometimes may contain microabscesses. The heart is particularly affected. Myocardial fibres are penetrated by *T. cruzi*. The trypanosome proliferates fills and destroys muscle fibres, and causes severe myocarditis. The heart becomes enlarged, and the pericardial sac distended with fluid. Large cystic collections of **leishmanial forms** can be seen microscopically in cardiac muscle cells. Skeletal and smooth muscles may also be invaded. In brain, *T. cruzi* may produce oedema and congestion, particularly in the meninges. Testicle may be severely invaded by *T. cruzi*.

Diagnosis

Diagnosis depends upon demonstration of *T. cruzi* in blood or tissues of infected animals.

Mal De Caderas

This is a trypanosomiasis of tropical and subtropical South America. It affects **horses** in particular and is caused by *Trypanosoma equinum*. The disease is an acute infection similar to surra.

Genus: Giardia

Giardiasis (Lambliasis)

Protozoa of the genus **Giardia** are pyriform in shape (i.e., shaped like a pear). The anterior end is rounded and the posterior end is elongated, nearly pointed. Each organism has four pairs of flagella. **These organisms are common inhabitants of the small intestine and colon of humans and animals without producing signs of disease.**

Giardia can, however, be an important cause of **diarrhoea**, mainly in **humans**. In domestic animals, giardiasis is seen usually in **dogs** and **cats**, and sometimes in **cattle**. A separate species of **Giardia** is associated with each animal, such as *G. canis* for **dogs**, *G. cati* for **cats**, and *G. bovis* for **cattle**. However, they are not host-specific. The organisms localize in the **small intestine** on the surface of epithelial cells.

Clinically, the **diarrhoea** tends to be **chronic**. It usually lasts for several weeks, and is sometimes recurrent. The stools tend to be bulky, malodorous (foul-smelling), and light coloured. The prolonged course can lead to **malabsorption syndrome** with weight loss. Lesions in the intestinal tract may be minimal. Stunting of villi and an inflammatory infiltrate in the lamina propria can occur. Organisms may be difficult to detect in tissue section. They are better identified in faecal specimens where typical trophozoites or cysts can be found.

Genus: Tritrichomonas and Trichomonas

Trichomoniasis

Protozoa of the genus **Tritrichomonas** and genus **Trichomonas include flagellated organisms**. These are divided on the number of anterior flagellae. Genus **Tritrichomonas** has **three anterior flagellae**, and genus **Trichomonas** has **four anterior flagellae. Most are not pathogenic.**

Bovine Trichomoniasis

Tritrichomonas foetus is the cause of bovine trichomoniasis. It is an important genital infection of **cattle. The organism is transmitted by coitus.** The infection in **bulls** usually goes unnoticed. **Microscopically,** there may be a mild mononuclear and neutrophilic inflammation in the penis and prepuce, but it is of little importance.

In **cows,** on the other hand, infection leads to vaginitis, endometritis, placentitis, foetal infection, and pyometra. **Following coitus with an infected bull,** cows conceive normally, but the pregnancy terminates early in gestation. **Most abortions occur in the first half of pregnancy (between 2-4 months) or earlier,** and usually go unnoticed. However, trichomoniasis may cause abortion in the last trimester (i.e., last three months). The **main sign** of trichomoniasis in a herd is **infertilitiy** (and return to heat at 4-5 months), which can affect a high percentage of animals and result in significant economic loss. Cows ultimately usually clear the infection.

Lesions

Lesions in the female reproductive tract are usually not extensive. They consist of non-specific inflammation, unless pyometra develops, which is not the usual outcome. In the **foetus,** lesions may be absent. However, in foetuses aborted late in gestation there may be pyogranulomatous bronchopneumonia with multinucleated giant cells.

Diagnosis

Diagnosis is achieved by demonstrating *Tritrichomans foetus* in vaginal, uterine, or prepucial exudates, in association with a herd history of decreased fertility, abortions, vaginitis, metritis, and balanitis (inflammation of glans penis). Direct microscopic examination may not be sufficient if numbers of trichomonads are small, as is usually the case in bulls. Culture of the organisms is more accurate.

Trichomoniasis in other domestic animals

Trichomonas suis is found in the digestive and upper respiratory tract of pigs, but its pathogenicity is not fully established. *T. gallinae* is an important pathogen of the mouth, crop and oesophagus in pigeons. *T. vaginalis* is found in the vagina, urethra, and prostate of **women and men**. It may be carried without producing signs, especially in men, but can also result in vaginitis or urethritis. It is transmitted by coitus. *T. faecalis* (*T. equi*) is a common organism in the intestinal tract of normal **horses**. It is thought to cause gastroenteritis, but there is no good evidence to support this. **Tritrichomonas** and **Trichomonas** sp. are common inhabitants of the intestinal tract, and have been associated with enteritis and diarrhoea in a number of domestic animals. However, **there are only a few reports which present convincing evidence in support of their role as pathogens.**

Genus: Entamoeba

Amoebiasis

Parasitic protozoa of the genus **Entamoeba** (those with pseudopodia) are best known as pathogens of **humans**, but also of **monkeys** and less commonly other animals. These organisms usually inhabit the intestinal tract and may be present in the absence of noticeable effects. However, under some circumstances, severe dysentery may result from their presence. The amoeba may invade and ulcerate the intestinal wall, and can migrate to the liver or brain, resulting in "amoebic" abscesses. The most important pathogen in this group is *Entamoeba histolytica*, **the cause of amoebic dysentery in humans.**

Monkeys are susceptible to *E. histolytica* and may develop amoebic dysentery. *E. histolytica* can also infect many species of domestic animals, namely, **dogs, cats, pigs**, and **cattle**. However, the presence of the organism only rarely results in disease. **Even in humans many asymptomatic carriers exist. The life cycle is direct.** Following their proliferation in the intestinal tract, **trophozoites** become **cysts** which are excreted. The organism may be transmitted between hosts by contamination of food or water by handlers who are carriers, also by means of cysts carried by flies or cockroaches, or by consumption of contaminated water, in which amoebic cysts may survive for long periods.

Lesions

Once infection is established, reproduction is by binary fission. Under appropriate conditions, trophozoites invade mucosa and **produce ulcers of various sizes.** The trophozoites may be found deep in the wall of the colon, usually associated with a **flask-shaped ulcer** of the mucosa. The parasite is believed to secrete a **lytic enzyme** under some as yet unknown circumstances. The trophozoites may spread to other organs, particularly **liver** and **brain**.

Here, they produce, large l ytic lesions, known as **'amoebic abscesses'**, characterized by liquefactive n ecrosis of t he parenchyma, and less c ommonly, frank suppuration. A characteristic feature of t he necrotizing l esions in the colon and other sites is the **almost total absence of a cellular inflammatory response**. This may be due to the secretion of products that inhibit leukocyte chemotaxis.

The **trophozoites** are detected in the tissue sections as irregularly spherical organisms without cilia but usually having pseudopodia. They have a nucleus, and their a bundant cytoplasm i s often v acuolated and m ay contain phagocytized **erythrocytes** or t issue debris. The size is v ariable and ranges from 10-60 μm in diameter. They may be seen in intestinal crypts, in necrotic foci in the submucosa, or at the margins of ulcers.

Diagnosis

A t entative diagnosis m ay be m ade by i dentifying trophozoites o f *E. histolytica* in the faeces in the presence of dysentery. Diagnosis may be confirmed by demonstrating the organisms in ulcers or abscesses.

Genus: Klossiella

Klossiella Infection

Among these protozoa, the only species of some importance is *Klossiella equi* which occurs in **horses, asses,** and **zebras**. These **coccidia** localize in the convoluted tubules of the kidney. Schizogony occurs in endothelial cells and epithelium of B owman's capsule, r eleasing merozoites w hich infect tubular epithelial cells, where gametogenesis o ccurs. Oocytes are shed i n the urine. Although these organisms destroy some renal epithelium, their total effect is slight. **Usually there are no clinical signs. The parasites are generally found incidentally at necropsy**.

Genus: Hepatozoon

Hepatozoon Infections

Protozoa of t he genus **H epatozoon** contain s everal pathogenic s pecies, the most important being *Hepatozoon canis*. *H. canis* occurs in **dogs, c ats, jackals**, and a number of wild felidae.

Life cycle

The developmental cycle of *H. canis* involves the brown dog tick, *Rhipicephalus sanguineus*, which when infected, carries sporocysts in its body cavity. I ngestion of the infected v ector tick by the host results i n release of **sporozoites**. Sporozoites p enetrate the intestinal wall to r each t he s pleen, liver, lungs, lymph nodes, myocardium, and bone marrow through the bloodstream. The parasites enter tissue cells to become **schizonts**, and reproduce several generations in these cells. Finally, **merozoites** are produced, which parasitize erythrocytes or leukocytes and become **gametocytes, or gamonts**. These gametocytes become differentiated into macro- and micro-gametocytes in the body of the vector tick. Sexual union results in a motile zygote, the **ookinete**. This **ookinete** migrates to the haemocoel of the tick, where it grows into a large oocyst, in which large numbers of sporozoites are formed within **sporocysts**. The sporozoites are released from the oocyst after the tick is ingested by the vertebrate host.

Clinical signs

Usually, the parasites are encountered as an incidental finding in the absence of clinical signs, or tissue reaction. Clinical signs include fever, anaemia, splenomegaly, progressive emaciation, and sometimes paralysis. Death may occur 4-8 weeks following onset of clinical signs.

Lesions

Lesions are those of anaemia and focal necrotizing granulomas in affected tissues.

Diagnosis

Diagnosis is based on demonstration of the organisms, gametocytes in the leukocytes in blood smears, or schizonts in biopsy or necropsy specimens of liver, spleen, bone marrow, or other tissue.

Genus: Eimeria and Isospora

Coccidiosis

Coccidiosis is the name given to the disease produced by protozoa of genera of the order **Eucoccidiorida**. Clinically, "coccidiosis" is applied to the diseases produced by protozoa of the genera **Eimeria** and **Isospora**, in the family **Eimeriidae**, order **Eucoccidiorida**. The order **Eucoccidiorida,** however, includes many additional parasitic protozoa that are referred to as **coccidia,** but the diseases produced by them are usually named after that particular genus, such as, toxoplasmosis, sarcosporidiosis, and besnoitiosis. Most of these additional parasitic protozoa of **Eucoccidiorida** were once thought to have only a tissue phase in their life cycle. **However, it is now known that these also have an enteric cycles. Thus, the enteric phases of Toxoplasma, Sarcocystis, Besnoitia, and other protozoa are also included under the disease classification of coccidiosis.**

Many coccidia affect animals and birds. The species and the tissues attacked depend upon the obligate preferences of each parasite (i.e., preferences biologically essential for their survival). Coccidiosis is particularly common in **cattle, sheep, and poultry** (see avian coccidiosis), **and is a disease of great economic importance**. Some of the important coccidial parasites of animals are shown in **Table 39**.

Table 39. Important Eimeria and Isospora of Animals

Cattle	*Eimeria bovis* *E. zuernii* *E. ellipsoidalis*	Small intestine, caecum, colon
Sheep	*E. ovina* *E. ovinoidalis* *E. parva*	Intestine
Goats	*E. arloingi* *E. caprovina* *E. faurei*	Intestine
Pigs	*E. porci* *E. scabra* *Isospora suis*	Intestine
Dogs	*Isospora canis* *I. burrowsi* *I. neorivolta*	Intestine
Cats	*Isospora rivolta* *I. felis*	Intestine
Horses & donkeys	*E. leuckarti*	Intestine
Rabbits	*E. stiedae* *E. perforans*	Bile ducts Intestine
Monkeys	*Isospora sp.*	Intestine
Man	*Isospora belli (hominis)* *I. natalensis*	Intestine

Life cycle

The life cycles of coccidia are similar. It is, however, important to understand the life cycles in order to get a clear idea of their effects upon the host. The **oocysts** are the thick-walled forms of the organism. These resist drying and provide the means of spread of infection from one host to another. The **oocysts** of each species are different morphologically, but basically have similar features. In the genus **Eimeria, each** fully-matured **oocyst** contains **four** sporocysts. Each sporocyst has **two sporozoites**. Thus, **each oocyst has a total of eight sporozoites**. Oocysts of **Isospora** contain **two sporocysts**, each with **four sporozoites**. **Thus, the total number of sporozoites in Isospora is also eight.** **Isospora** oocysts are similar in appearance to those produced by the sexual, intestinal phase of **Toxoplasma, Sarcocystis**, and **Besnoitia**. Each oocyst has at one pole a tiny pore, the **micropyle**. The micropyle is sealed by a substance that, like the rest of the wall, is resistant to drying and to many chemical substances. **When oocysts are ingested and reach the small intestine, the trypsin-kinase of the pancreatic juice digests the seal of the micropyle, and through this opening the tiny sporozoites, now actively motile, escape from the oocyst.**

Infection occurs by direct invasion of the intestinal epithelium. **Each sporozoite enters a single epithelial cell**, where it undergoes **asexual development** known as **schizogony** (Fig.13). The **sporozoite** gradually increases in size, becomes first a **trophozoite** and finally **a schizont**. The schizont completely fills the cytoplasm of the epithelial cell, displacing the nucleus to one side. Each mature schizont contains many elongated structures (spores), which are similar morphologically to sporozoites, but are known as **merozoites**. The schizont then ruptures its own wall and also that of the epithelial cell's, **liberating the merozoites**. The merozoites infect other epithelial cells and continue **this asexual life cycle**.

Then, at certain stage, some of the merozoites enter into the **sexual phase** of the cycle, known as **gametogenesis** or **gametogony**. Each of these merozoites develops within an individual epithelial cell into a **female form**, a **macrogamete**, or into a **male counterpart**, a **microgametocyte**. The microgametocyte finally ruptures to release a large number of tiny motile **microgametes**. One of the microgametes unites with a single macrogamete. Once thus fertilized, the macrogamete soon becomes an **oocyst**. When oocysts are passed in faeces they contain an undifferentiated spherical body. **These oocysts become infective only after undergoing sporulation**. Further development within the oocyst, known as **sporogony**, requires oxygen and certain other conditions. These are met outside the body of the host. **When the oocysts are taken with food or water by a new host, the cycle is repeated.**

This cycle, which occurs usually in the intestine (i.e., **enteric**) is shown in **Fig. 13.** Life cycle is the same for all species of **Eimeria** and for most species of **Isospora**. However, the cycle in certain species of **Eimeria** occurs **in tissues other than the intestine**. For example, in rabbits, *Eimeria stiedae* multiplies in the intrahepatic bile ducts. The sporozoites reach these ducts through portal veins or lymphatics, and not through the common bile duct. **Hepatic coccidiosis is a very common disease of rabbits**. Intrahepatic biliary coccidiosis has been reported in a **dog** (probably **Isospora**) and a **calf**. **Eimeria** sp. have also been found in the gallbladder and mesenteric lymph nodes of **goats** and **sheep**.

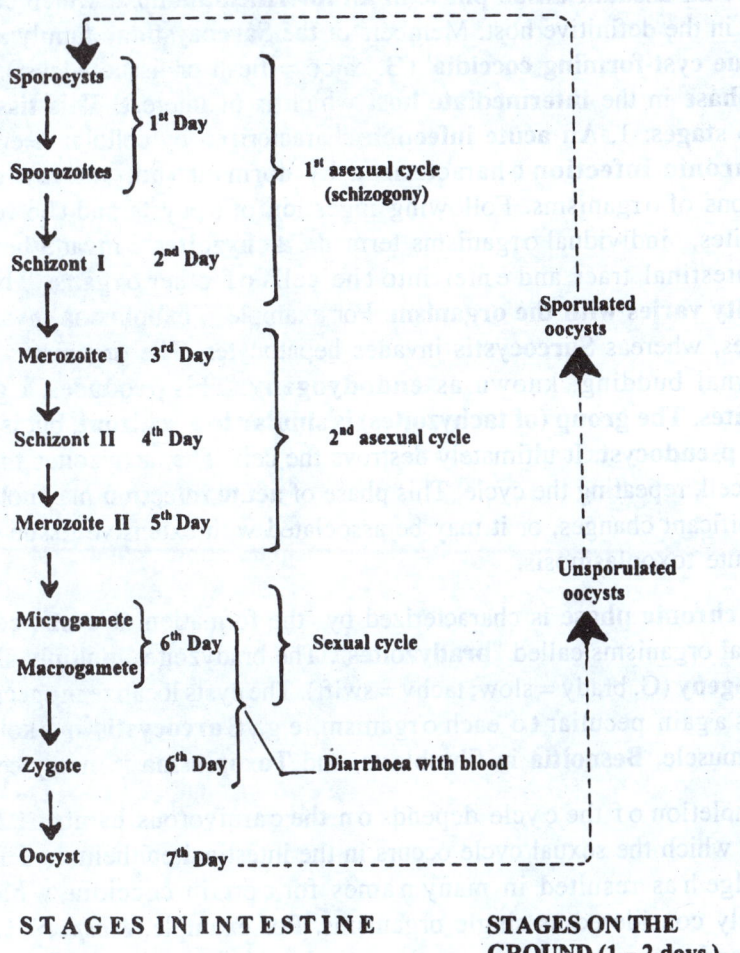

STAGES IN INTESTINE   **STAGES ON THE GROUND (1 – 2 days)**

Fig. 13 Diagrammatic life cycle of **Eimeria**.

The life cycle is also the same for the genus **Caryospora** of the family **Eimeriidae**, and genera of the Family **Sarcocystidae**, namely, **Besnoitia, Neospora, Toxoplasma,** and **Sarcocystis** (see **Table 37**). However, coccidia of all these genera utilize an intermediate host. The intermediate host ingests the oocyst. The released sporozoites enter internal organs where they remain as a small cyst containing a single sporozoite, known as cystozoite. Upon ingestion by the definitive (final) host, the released sporozoite enters intestinal epithelium to repeat the cycle described earlier.

Members of the genera **Besnoitia, Neospora, Toxoplasma** and **Sarcocystis** of the Family **Sarcocystidae** also have an **enteric asexual and sexual cycle** in their definitive hosts which is almost the same as that of coccidia (Eimeria), and their oocysts are similar to those of **Isospora**. However, in addition, these also have **an asexual tissue phase in an intermediate host,** which can be the same as in the definitive host. Members of the **Sarcocystidae** family are called the 'tissue cyst-forming coccidia' (G. sarco = flesh or tissue + cyst). It is the **tissue phase** in the **intermediate host** which is of interest. **This tissue cycle has two stages:** 1. **An acute infection** characterized by cellular necrosis, and 2. **A chronic infection** characterized by dormant (not active), or latent collections of organisms. Following ingestion of oocysts and the release of sporozoites, individual organisms termed "**tachyzoites**", invade beyond the gastrointestinal tract and enter into the cells of other organs. **The tissue specificity varies with the organism.** For example, **Toxoplasma** invades most cell types, whereas **Sarcocystis** invades hepatocytes. The organisms multiply by internal budding, known as **endodyogeny.** This produces a group of **tachyzoites. The group (of tachyzoites) is similar to a schizont,** but is wrongly called a **pseudocyst.** It ultimately destroys the cell. The tachyzoites then infect another cell, repeating the cycle. This phase of **acute infection** may not produce any significant changes, or it may be associated with extensive tissue necrosis, as in acute toxoplasmosis.

The **chronic phase** is characterized by the formation of **cysts,** containing individual organisms called "**bradyzoites**". The bradyzoites multiply **slowly by endodyogeny** (G. brady = slow; tachy = swift). The cysts localize in specific sites, which is again peculiar to each organism, e.g., **Sarcocystis** in skeletal and cardiac muscle, **Besnoitia** in fibroblasts, and **Toxoplasma** in many cell types.

Completion of the cycle depends on the carnivorous habits of the final hosts, in which the sexual cycle occurs in the intestinal epithelium. This newer knowledge has resulted in many names for certain coccidia, which were previously considered as single organisms. For example, *Isospora bigemina* of **dogs** and **cats** is now known as the sexual stage for species of **Toxoplasma, Sarcosporidia (Sarcocystis),** and **Besnoitia.**

Methods of transmission

As mentioned, the source of infection is the **faeces** of clinically affected or carrier animals. The **infection is acquired by ingestion** of contaminated feed and water, or by licking the hair coat contaminated with infected faeces. Also as mentioned, **oocysts** passed in the faeces require suitable environmental conditions if they are to become sporulated. Moist, temperate or cool conditions favour sporulation, whereas high temperatures and dryness hinder it. **Ingestion of the sporulated oocysts results in infection,** but very large numbers must be taken before clinical disease occurs.

Pathogenesis

Coccidia of domestic animals pass all the stages of their cycle in the alimentary mucosa and do not invade other organs, although schizonts have been found in the mesenteric lymph nodes of **sheep and goats**. The different species of coccidia show a tendency to localize in different parts of the intestine. *E. bovis* and *E. zuernii* occur mainly in the caecum, colon and last part of the ileum, whereas *E. ellipsoidalis* parasitizes the small intestine.

The coccidial life cycle is self-limiting. As described under life cycle, **sporozoites** are released from the ingested **oocysts. Sporozoites** invade the intestinal epithelium, and develop into **asexual schizonts**. After the schizont matures, **merozoites** are released by rupture of the epithelial cell. New epithelial cells are again invaded and **second generation schizogony** occurs in the large intestine. This is followed by the release of second generation of merozoites which invade epithelial cells and produce the sexual stages, the **macrogametocyte** and **microgametocyte**. The second generation schizogony and fertilization of the macrogametocyte by the microgametocyte **(gametogony) are the stages of the life cycle which cause functional and structural lesions of the large intestine.** As the second generation schizonts **(gamonts)** mature, the cells containing them slough from the basement membrane, **and cause haemorrhage and destruction of the caecum and colon.** The oocysts are the result of fertilization of the gametocytes and are discharged at the time of rupture of the cells. **This usually coincides with the onset of clinical signs of dysentery.** The prepatent period varies with the species of coccidia. With *E. bovis* it is 15-20 days and with *E. zuernii*, 15-17 days. **(Prepatent period** is the period between the time of introduction of parasitic organisms into the body and their appearance in the blood, tissues, or faeces).

The **two species of coccidia** which are considered **most pathogenic to cattle are** *E. bovis* **and** *E. zuernii*. Their life cycles are similar. **The gametocytes are the pathogenic stages and cause rupture of the cells they invade.** This results in exfoliation of the epithelial lining of the intestine. The oocyst count is usually low when the disease is at its peak. This is because the oocysts have not yet formed. **Exfoliation of the mucosa causes diarrhoea.** In severe cases, haemorrhage into the intestinal lumen and the resulting haemorrhagic anaemia, **may be fatal**. If the animal survives this stage, the life cycle of the coccidia terminates without further damage. **The intestinal mucosa regenerates and returns to normal.**

Immune Mechanisms

Immunity against intestinal coccidia appears to have **both cellular and humoral** components. **Cellular immunity** is probably **more important** in resistance against infection than humoral immunity. **Coccidiosis in cattle is immunosuppressive** which increases their susceptibility to other common infections. Neutrophil function may be inhibited. Specific immunity to each coccidial species develops after infection so that young animals exposed for the first time are usually more susceptible to a severe infection and clinical disease than other animals.

Clinical Signs

Coccidiosis affects the host in many ways. This depends on the tissue affinity of the particular coccidia, and the **number of oocysts** present in the initial infection. Most coccidia attack the mucosa of the intestinal tract. Therefore, symptoms are mainly enteric. **Clinical signs include** sudden onset of **bloody diarrhoea**, with fever, followed by dehydration, emaciation, and sometimes death. However, usually little or no evidence of infection is observed in the living animal. **In rabbits**, hepatic coccidiosis is rarely accompanied by diarrhoea and young rabbits may die suddenly without showing any signs. However, jaundice and emaciation may be seen in older animals.

Lesions

Coccidia are obligate intracellular parasites. (An **obligate parasite** is one that can exist only at the expense of another organism. Biologically this is essential for its survival). Development of coccidia within the cytoplasm of epithelial cells results in the death of each cell which is parasitized. The **total effect on the animal depends on: 1. The initial infecting dose of oocysts.** This determines the number of cells invaded at the outset by sporozoites, and **2. Spread of infection during schizogony.** This is affected to a great extent by immunity acquired by the host. As increasing numbers of organisms enter the sexual phase (gametogenesis), infection of new cells by merozoites decreases **and the disease gradually becomes less intense.**

When many cells of the intestinal epithelium are attacked at one time, **the denuded mucosa bleeds freely.** An intense inflammation involves the lamina propria and sometimes the submucosa. As large numbers of epithelial cells are destroyed, the remaining epithelium regenerates to replace that which was lost. This leads to hyperplasia of the intestinal epithelium, which is cast into long papillary folds (fronds). This is because replacement of epithelial cells exceeds their loss. In lesions showing hyperplasia, coccidia in various stages of gametogenesis are present in large numbers. This is in contrast to the erosive, haemorrhagic stages, in which coccidia in various stages of schizogony are most common.

Certain coccidia attack cells other than those of the intestinal tract. The most important of these is **hepatic coccidiosis in rabbits due to E. stiedae**, which affects the **intrahepatic biliary epithelium**. In the early lesions, there is destruction of the biliary epithelium, but when course of the disease, is somewhat longer, proliferation of this epithelium is the main feature. The bile ducts become greatly enlarged by proliferation of epithelium, which is thrown up into papillary folds resembling **adenomatous hyperplasia**. These greatly enlarged portions of the bile ducts displace the adjoining liver parenchyma and appear grossly as irregular greyish areas, seen as depressions in the surface of the capsule. A similar hepatic coccidiosis has been reported in a **dog, a calf**, and in the gallbladder of a **goat**.

Gross lesions include intensely congested, eroded, and bleeding areas of certain portions of the small intestine. Sometimes these alternate with, or are replaced by, areas in which the mucosa is thickened.

Diagnosis

The clinical diagnosis is usually based on the presence of **oocysts in faecal samples**, associated with sudden onset of typical bloody diarrhoea. The microscopic lesions are characteristic. These are confirmed by demonstration of the organisms in tissue sections.

Genus: Caryospora

Caryospora

Caryospora are **coccidia** and belong to the Family **Eimeriidae. Little is known about their importance in domestic animals.** However, infection has been recorded in **dogs**. These coccidia have a complicated life cycle. Asexual and sexual cycles occur in both primary (definitive) and secondary (intermediate) hosts. The primary hosts are reptiles and raptors (birds of prey), in which a coccidian life cycle occurs in the intestinal tract. This leads to production of oocysts. **Sporulated oocysts** contain **a single sporocyst** with **eight sporozoites**. Ingestion of sporulated oocysts by the **primary host** results in repetition of the intestinal cycle.

When sporulated oocysts are ingested by the **secondary (intermediate) hosts**, which are rodents and **dogs** (see **Table 40**), the sporozoites enter tissues and begin schizogony and gametogony. This leads to production of oocysts which sporulate. Sporozoites released in tissues, in turn, develop into a stage known as a **"Caryocyst"**. It contains a single sporozoite. The most common site is the dermis or tongue. Upon ingestion of caryocyst-containing tissue by another **secondary host**, this tissue cycle is repeated. When ingested by the **primary hosts**, the intestinal cycle is repeated. Thus, the tissue phase in secondary hosts can be continued without the need of the primary host. This situation is similar to that which can occur in **Toxoplasma**. **Caryospora infection in dogs** is characterized by pyogranulomatous dermatitis and lymphadenitis. The lesions contain schizonts, macrogamonts, microgamonts, unsporulated and sporulated oocysts, and caryocysts. The presence of oocysts and the unique unicellular caryocysts allows differentiation from other tissue coccidia.

Genus: Cryptosporidium

Cryptosporidiosis

Cryptosporidiosis is a disease of most domestic and wild animals, birds, and humans. It is caused by members of the genus **Cryptosporidium**. **Cryptosporidia** are members of the Order **Eucoccidiorida** and closely resemble the non-tissue cyst coccidia **Eimeria** and **Isospora**. In contrast to coccidia, however, cryptosporidia are extremely small. Like coccidia, the organisms are located **intracellularly**. They have a typical coccidian life cycle of trophozoites, schizonts containing merozoites, macrogametocytes and microgametocytes, and oocysts. **Transmission** is direct through sporulated **oocysts which contain four sporozoites**. In contrast to most coccidia, cryptosporidia are not host specific. However, some twenty different species have been described, which are named after the host from which they are recovered. For example, *C. bovis* from cattle, *C. felis* from cats, and *C. muris* from mice. However, species identification cannot be made from tissue section or simple examination of oocysts. Therefore, most cases of disease due to **Cryptosporidium** are called only as **cryptosporidiosis**.

The majority of cryptosporidia of animals parasitize intestinal epithelial cells, usually of the distal small intestine, but also of the caecum and colon and sometimes bile ducts, trachea, and bronchi. Cryptosporidiosis of abomasum has also been described in **cattle**. Various species of birds are susceptible to intestinal and gastric cryptosporidiosis, and also to infection of the respiratory mucosa and conjunctiva (see avian cryptosporidiosis). **In humans**, intestinal tract is also the most frequent site, but cryptosporidia have been found in the respiratory tract as well.

Cryptosporidiosis is usually subclinical. **Clinical** disease is characterized by diarrhoea and is most common in young animals, or occurs in association with immunosuppressive disorders. The disease is of greatest importance in **calves** and **lambs**.

Lesions

In sections of small intestine or colon, small basophilic organisms are found fixed deeply in microvilli of the intestinal cells. Lesions may be few. Infected cells are slightly more eosinophilic than normal, but extensive necrosis is not a feature. There may be villous atrophy and fusion, dilatation of crypts and infiltration of the lamina propria with lymphocytes and plasma cells and some neutrophils and eosinophils.

Diagnosis

Diagnosis in tissue section depends on demonstration of the organism. Use of **Giemsa stain** and thin sections are helpful. Oocysts are acid-fast. This characteristic is useful in identification in both tissue section and faecal flotation preparations. **Phase-contrast microscopy** is also helpful in the identification of oocysts, which are brightly refractile in faecal flotations.

Zoonotic Implications

Since the parasite can cross host species barriers, infected domestic animals and pets may act as reservoir of infection for susceptible humans. **In humans, Cryptosporidium** is a non-viral cause of self-limiting diarrhoea, particularly in **children.** In immunologically compromised persons, clinical disease may be severe. This is particularly serious in human patients with acquired immunodeficiency syndrome (AIDS). Animal handlers on a calf farm can be at high risk of diarrhoea due to transmission of cryptosporidiosis from infected calves. Immunocompromised people should be restricted from contact with young animals and possibly from entry to farms.

Genus: Besnoitia

Besnoitiosis

Besnoitiosis is **a chronic debilitating and sometimes fatal disease of cattle,** associated with cutaneous and systemic manifestations. It has been described from South Africa, and is called 'besnoitiosis' after the cyst-forming protozoa, *Besnoitia besnoiti*. Genus **Besnoitia** comes under the family **Sarcocystidae,** i.e., family of **'tissue cyst-forming coccidia'.** Earlier, the organism was wrongly named as *Globidium besnoiti*, and the disease as 'globidiosis'. *B. bennetti* is the name given to the species which occurs in horses and burros (small donkeys).

Life cycle

Besnoitia has a **two-host life cycle** like **Toxoplasma** and **Sarcocystis** which also belong to the same **Sarcocystidae** family. Sexual reproduction occurs in the intestinal tract of the final host, leading to production of oocysts. Cats serve as the definitive (final) host for *B. besnoiti*. Upon ingestion of oocysts by intermediate hosts (**cattle, horses;** see **Table 40**), organisms attack many types of cells and produce small groups of tachyzoites, very similar to those of **Toxoplasma. This acute infection can be severe and can cause death.** Tachyzoites later attack fibroblasts and produce large cysts filled with **bradyzoites.** This is the infective stage for the final host. The cysts are large (up to 2 mm in diameter) and therefore visible to the unaided eye.

The organisms in **cattle, horses,** and burros usually occur in the cyst **form.** The cysts are surrounded by a dense, uniformly eosinophilic wall which appears to come from host tissue. Inside this wall are one or more giant nuclei, which become compressed against the periphery by the spores within. These tiny crescentic spores are similar to those of **Toxoplasma** in size and

host cat, but has a wide range of **intermediate hosts (Table 40)**. Toxoplasmosis is caused by **Toxoplasma gondii**, a small crescentic (sickle-shaped) protozoan parasite. **T. gondii** was first recorded in 1908 in material from a small rodent, the **gondi** (hence the name **gondii**) and belongs to the family **Sarcocystidae**, the family of '**tissue cyst-forming coccidia**'.

The recent discovery of **Neospora** has complicated the diagnosis of toxoplasmosis in all species. **Neospora** is similar in appearance to **Toxoplasma** and produces similar lesions, especially in the central nervous system. **Clinically**, toxoplasmosis is manifested mainly by abortion and stillbirths in ewes, and in all other species by encephalitis, pneumonia, and neonatal mortality. **Its major importance is as a zoonosis.** Toxoplasmosis occurs in most parts of the world, **including India.**

Life Cycle and Transmission

The **sexual cycle** of Toxoplasma occurs in the **cat** which is the **definitive (final) host** and the most important source of infection for other animals. After eating infected meat or sporulated oocysts, the organism undergoes **schizogony in the cat's intestine with a typical coccidian cycle.**

Table 40. Characteristics of important tissue cyst-forming coccidia

Organism	Definitive* (final) host	Intermediate host	Initial proliferative form	Cyst
Caryospora	Birds of prey	Rodents, dogs	Gamogony in definitive and intermediate host	Sporulated oocysts and caryocysts in tongue, skin, and other tissues
Besnoitia	Cats, others unknown	Cattle, horses	Tachyzoites	Restricted to connective tissue
Neospora	Unknown	Dogs, cats, cattle sheep, horses	Tachyzoites	Restricted to CNS
Sarcocystis	Cats, dogs, humans, etc.	Mainly herbivores, but seen in most species	Merozoites	In myofibres
Toxoplasma	Cats	All species	Tachyzoites	In multiple tissues

*Coccidial cycle in gastrointestinal tract

This leads to the production of oocysts. After 1-2 weeks cats shed millions of oocysts which are resistant to environmental influences. They are infective after sporulation (sporogony). The **sporulated oocysts** contain eight sporozoites and are capable of infecting a wide variety of **intermediate hosts**. This leads to either subclinical, acute or chronic infection characterized by formation of groups of **tachyzoites** in acute infection and **cysts of bradyzoites**

in chronic cases in a variety of tissues.

Most mammals and birds, as well as cats, serve as intermediate hosts (Table 40). Infection of intermediate hosts and cats occurs following exposure to **cat faeces**, or materials contaminated by cat faeces (e.g., soil), or by the consumption of, or exposure to, infected tissues of intermediate hosts containing tachyzoites or bradyzoites. **Congenital transmission** may also occur in intermediate hosts during the acute phase by invasion of tachyzoites across the placenta. **Toxoplasma** have also been identified in **milk** and **semen**, which are also potential source of infection. Released sporozoites, ingested tachyzoites, or bradyzoites first multiply locally intracellularly in the intestine and lymph nodes. **By endodyogeny** they produce **two tachyzoites** per cell. These spread to other organs and tissues where they continue to reproduce. This leads either to tissue damage and clinical disease, or encyst (form cyst) as a **collection of bradyzoites**. The sexual stages in the intestinal tract have been observed so far **only in cats**, but the **disease caused by the asexual parasites is known to occur in humans and almost all wild and domesticated mammals and birds.**

Characteristics of Toxoplasma

T. gondii **is the single species of Toxoplasma which infects all varieties of animals, as well as humans.** The organism is maintained in the laboratory by cultivation in the peritoneal cavity of the mouse, or in tissue cultures. In these situations, the organism is crescentic (sickle-shaped), with one end rounded and the other pointed. It is 2-4 μm wide and 4-7 μm long. It has a **nucleus** which is best demonstrated with **Giemsa stain**. It is located near one pole of the cell. The cytoplasm contains mitochondria, microtubules, endoplasmic reticulum, and a number of organelles. Among the organelles are structures called "**rhoptries**". These are dense, vase-shaped, gland-like structures. Their function is unknown, **but are useful in differentiating various members of the Sarcocystidae family. Toxoplasma** have 4-6 rhoptries. **Toxoplasma** lack a kinetoplast. The organisms are usually found **in parallel pairs** due to reproduction by longitudinal division (**endodyogeny**). These organisms, so far considered as the only form of **Toxoplasma, now appear to be tachyzoites,** which have the ability to multiply in animal tissues and form collections of organisms. Under certain conditions, especially in brain, these collections of organisms become encysted collections of **bradyzoites**.

In tissue sections, tachyzoites besides being crescentic, may also occur in rounded or oval form. Because of shrinkage of fixation, the organisms usually appear smaller in sections than in smears, about 2 μm wide and 4 μm long. They are usually found in the cytoplasm of cells, but may also be free. A large number of organisms may be present in a single cell. **Within the cell, the tachyzoites are contained within a vacuole called a "parasitophorous vacuole".** It does not fuse with lysosomes and is seen only with electron microscopy. This characteristic is helpful in differentiating **Toxoplasma** from **Neospora** which is free in the cytoplasm. **Chronic infection** is characterized by larger cysts filled with **bradyzoites**, which represent the **resting stage of the parasite**. This is because they are usually seen in the absence of reaction in the neighbouring tissues.

Transmission

As mentioned, the only source of infection for **cattle, sheep** and **horses** is the **oocyst** passed in the **faeces of the cat.** Oocysts are also the major source of infection for **pigs.** The pigs can also get infected by the ingestion of tachyzoites or bradyzoites present in meat. Cats become infected, and shed oocyst in the faeces, as a result of ingesting tissues of intermediate hosts infected with the parasite. **Oocysts are extremely resistant to external influences and can survive in the environment for at least one year.**

Pathogenesis

T. gondii is an **intracellular parasite**. It attacks most organs with predilection for the reticulo-endothelial and central nervous systems. **Sporozoites** from oocysts, or **bradyzoites** from tissue cysts, penetrate and multiply in the intestinal epithelium. After invasion of a cell, the parasite multiplies, **and eventually fills and destroys the cells. Released toxoplasma reach other organs through the bloodstream.** The stage of parasitaemia begins about 5 days after initial infection, and lasts until the development of immunity 2-3 weeks after infection. At this stage the organism localizes in tissue cysts. **The clinical picture of the disease varies with the organs affected.** This itself depends on whether the disease is congenital or acquired. **In general the development of the disease in animals is the same as it is in humans.** The main manifestations are **encephalitis** when infection is **congenital,** and **febrile exanthema** (skin eruptions) **with pneumonia and enterocolitis in acquired infections. However, the vast majority of infections occur without any clinical signs; and tissue cysts can be found in many animals and appear to cause no harm.** When immunity of the animal falls because of stress, disease, or immunosuppressive therapy, tissue cysts rupture, and large numbers of inflammatory cells invade surrounding tissue. The characteristic granulomatous lesions are thought to be the result of a hypersensitivity reaction.

Immune Responses in Toxoplasma

Normally both antibody-mediated and cell-mediated immune responses occur on exposure to **Toxoplasma.** The antibodies together with complement, destroy organisms found **free in body fluids (Fig. 14)** .Thus, they reduce the spread of the organisms between cells **but have no effect on the intracellular forms of the parasite.** *T. gondii* is an obligate intracellular parasite whose tachyzoite stages grow within cells. **Tachyzoites which invade normal macrophages are not destroyed.** *T. gondii* **can survive and multiply inside normal macrophages (Fig. 14). As a result, antibodies are ineffective against the organisms.** When the number of tachyzoites within the cell becomes excessive from growth, the cell ruptures. **The released tachyzoites invade other cells.** They penetrate these cells by a mechanism similar to phagocytosis. In the normal phagocytosis, once a particle has been enclosed in a phagosome, lysosomes move through the cytoplasm towards the phagosome, fuse with it, and empty their enzymes around the particle. **This does not happen in macrophages which phagocytose Toxoplasma.** The lysosomes may move towards the phagosome, but they fail to fuse with it. **As a result, Toxoplasma tachyzoites can grow inside cells in an environment free of antibodies or lysosomal enzymes.**

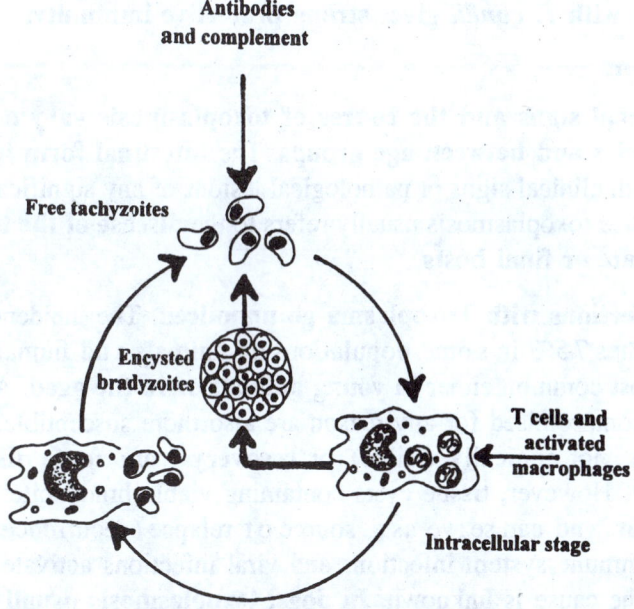

Fig. 14. The points in the life cycle of *T. gondii* at which the immune system can use its controlling influence.

The intracellular organisms are destroyed by a cell-mediated immune response. Sensitized helper 1 (Th1) T-cells secrete cytokines gamma-interferon (IFN-gamma) and interleukin-2 (IL-2) in response to **Toxoplasma** ribonucleoproteins. **IFN-gamma activates macrophages, enabling them to kill otherwise resistant intracellular toxoplasma by permitting lysosome-phagosome fusion (Fig. 14). Activated macrophages** have an increased ability to kill intracellular organisms by **generating the free radical nitric oxide (NO). Nitric oxide can destroy intracellular parasites.**

Some T-cells may also release cytokines which interfere directly with toxoplasma replications. In addition, cytotoxic CD8+T-cells can destroy **Toxoplasma** tachyzoites and toxoplasma-infected cells. **In these ways, antibody-mediated and cell-mediated immune responses act together and eliminate the tachyzoite stage of this organism.** However, *T. gondii* tachyzoites can transform themselves into **a cyst form** containing **bradyzoites (Fig. 14)**. The cysts appear to be non-immunogenic and do not stimulate an inflammatory response. Also, this cyst stage does not appear to be as foreign.

T. gondii has also evolved mechanisms for escaping the effects of host's immune responses. For example, it can **avoid neutrophil attachment and phogocytosis**. Also, *T. gondii* can become **non-antigenic**. The **cyst stage** of *T. gondii* is an example of its **non-antigenic form**, which, as mentioned, does not appear to stimulate a host response.

Infection with *T. gondii* gives strong protective immunity.

Clinical signs

The clinical signs and the course of toxoplasmosis vary a great deal between species and between age groups. The **intestinal form in cat** is not associated with clinical signs or pathological lesions of any significance. Therefore, the disease toxoplasmosis usually refers to the **disease of the tissue phase in intermediate or final hosts**.

Most infections with Toxoplasma go unnoticed. The incidence of infection approaches 75% in some populations of animals and humans. Clinical disease is most common either **in young animals or in the aged**. Animals that are immunocompromised for any reason are also more susceptible. Inapparent infection (i.e., not clinically visible), or **recovery from acute disease, leads to immunity**. However, tissue cysts containing viable bradyzoites remain for over one year, and can serve as a source of relapse (recurrence) for active infections. Immune system infections and viral infections activate such cysts, but usually the cause is unknown. **In dogs, toxoplasmosis usually accompanies canine distemper.**

As toxoplasma can infect a variety of cells, a great diversity of clinical signs can occur in toxoplasmosis. The organisms most commonly affect the brain, myocardium, lymph nodes, lungs, intestinal muscularis, pancreas, liver, uterus, placenta, and foetus. As a result, symptoms may relate to involvement of any one or more of these organs.

In dogs, toxoplasmosis is most common in **puppies**, and is usually characterized by neurological signs, diarrhoea, or pneumonia. It usually occurs in association with canine distemper virus infection. **In cats**, the most common manifestations are pneumonia, encephalitis, and pancreatitis. **In sheep and goats**, toxoplasmosis is an important cause of **abortion**, associated with necrosis and inflammation in the cotyledons of the placenta. It is also associated with infection of the foetus, especially the central nervous system. Congenitally infected lambs and kids may be born with encephalitis. **Toxoplasmosis is not common in cattle or horses.** Many cases of protozoal abortion in cattle are the result of infection with **Neospora,** or a similar as yet unidentified, protozoan. **Monkeys** are very susceptible to infection and develop disseminated disease. **In humans,** toxoplasmosis occurs usually as a congenitally acquired infection of the newborn, manifested by encephalitis, chorioretinitis, macroencephaly (enlarged brain), microencephaly (small brain), cerebral calcifications, convulsive disorders, and mental retardation. **In adults,** chorioretinitis, lymphadenopathy, myocarditis, pneumonia, and meningo-encephalomyelitis have been associated with Toxoplasma.

Lesions

After initial multiplication, usually in the intestine and associated lymph nodes, **parasitaemia** spreads the protozoa to **various tissues.** Here, **Toxoplasma** actively penetrate a variety of cell types. Most types of cell are susceptible. In all affected tissues, besides the main parenchymal·cell, **Toxoplasma** can be found in macrophages, fibroblasts, and smooth muscle cells. **Their continued intracellular multiplication leads to cell death.** Thus, the lesion is characterized by the presence of intracellular **tachyzoites,** foci of necrosis, and an associated inflammatory reaction composed mainly of mononuclear cells. As indicated, **most infections are subclinical.** In these cases, the organisms form **tissue cysts,** especially in the brain, but also in the liver, kidney, and skeletal muscle. **The cysts remain viable for years in the absence of any host reaction.**

In brain, **Toxoplasma** mainly attack **neurons** and **astrocytes.** This leads to diffuse necrotizing and non-suppurative infiltration of brain parenchyma. Lymphocytic cells accumulate within the Robin-Virchow spaces, and are scattered singly or in pairs in the parenchyma. Vacuoles may occur in the white matter. **Toxoplasma tachyzoites** may be found scattered, singly or in pairs, in the parenchyma. Or, they may be present in aggregations containing up to 50 organisms. The **liver** contains large, sharply well-defined areas of coagulative necrosis. The necrotic areas are surrounded by normal liver cells with little or no cellular reaction. **Tachyzoites** may be found within liver or Kupffer's cells, in cysts containing a large number of organisms, or scattered thinly in both the necrotic and normal tissues. Organisms may be few in number even when severe necrosis is present.

In the **lung, Toxoplasma attack type I and II pneumocytes** and bronchial epithelial cells, as well as macrophages, fibroblasts, endothelial cells, and smooth muscle cells. This leads to foci of necrosis and prominent proliferative reaction, particularly in **cats.** The changes are particularly noticeable in the alveolar walls. Lining of the alveoli becomes cuboidal or columnar and rich in cells, suggesting the appearance of foetal lung ("**foetalization**" **of lung**). This feature also r esembles pulmonary a denomatosis. T he alveoli are filled w ith l arge mononuclear cells and leukocytes, and cells lining the alveoli with aggregations of **Toxoplasma**. These lesions have a nodular distribution throughout the lung. **Grossly**, they appear as small, grey, tumour-like masses.

Lymph nodes of t he affected organs are usually involved. They are e n-larged to several times their normal size, are firm in consistency, and severely congested. **Extensive coagulative necrosis is seen microscopically**. Tachyzoites may be found near these necrotic areas, particularly in endothelial cells of v eins. They m ay also b e found w ithin the c ytoplasm of m onocytic cells, o r free i n the tissues. T he **i ntestine** shows u lcers. These r esult from necrosis of submucosal lymph nodes. At times, toxoplasma invade muscularis where a chronic necrotizing lesion, followed by granulation tissue formation, results in large, grossly visible **granulomatous nodules**. These may r eplace the wall o f t he i ntestine and e ncroach upon t he lumen. The organisms are clearly demonstrable in the muscularis and the granulation tissue. In **pancreas** acute necrotizing lesions incite intense lymphocytic infiltration, oedema, and swelling.

The **eye** may be infected in **human adults**. Ocular infection has also been reported in **animals**. The lesion is a granulomatous chorioretinitis in w hich toxoplasma are demonstrable. **Myocardium** is usually invaded by toxoplasma, which may be present in large or small groups within the cytoplasm of cardiac muscle cells. Invasion of the **placenta** causes focal necrosis in the cotyledons, usually accompanied by calcification. Tachyzoites are found free and within trophoblasts. **Abortion** usually follows acute infection of the pregnant animal. **In the infected foetus**, lesions are most common in brain. Placental transmission may also cause stillbirth and neonatal death.

Diagnosis

Diagnosis of toxoplasmosis in the living animal is more of a problem than at postmortem. A large number of tests are used to detect antibodies. These include c omplement fixation, h aemagglutination, latex a gglutination, indirect fluorescent antibody, ELISA, and several others. Although these are valuable to detect antibodies, but d ue to t he high p ercentage of s erological positivity, **demonstration of antibody cannot differentiate between present and past infection**. The combined testing for both IgM and IgG class antibody can eliminate this problem. **This is because IgM develops earlier and decreases more rapidly than do IgG antibodies**. D etection of circulating antigen, o r isolation of organisms by mouse inoculation can detect active infection.

At postmortem, demonstration of toxoplasma in tissue sections in char-acteristic lesions should be supported by isolation of the organisms, or by use of immunological staining techniques. In tissue sections, microscopic appearance of other members of the family **Sarcocystidae** is similar. *Neospora caninum* is the most similar in appearance. In fact, until its discovery in 1988, it has usually been misdiagnosed as **Toxoplasma**.

Zoonotic implications

Humans are intermediate hosts for *T. gondii*, and about one-half the population of the United States is infected. Most infections arise from the ingestion of **oocysts** from **cat faeces** that contaminate food, or which are accidentally ingested because of poor hygienic practices. However, human infection can also occur from **ingestion of tachyzoites and bradyzoites in meat** or tissues which are eaten or handled. **The risk is with raw or undercooked meat.** Beef is a minor source of infection, whereas **risk with pig, sheep and horse meat is greater**. Usually there is no clinical disease in humans infected with *T. gondii*, or the disease is mild and self-limiting. However, significant disease can occur **in humans suffering from acquired immunodeficiency syndrome (AIDS) or cancer**, and also in the very young and the very old. There is also the risk in pregnant women for **abortion**, or congenital infection of the foetus, which result in hydrocephalus and intracranial calcification. **Toxoplasmosis poses an occupational risk for veterinarians, farmers, and slaughterhouse workers who handle infected material.**

Genus: Sarcocystis

Sarcocystosis (Sarcosporidiosis)

For over a century it has been known that **tiny tubular cysts filled with crescentic (sickle-shaped) bodies** are extremely common in the skeletal and cardiac muscle fibres of most mammals, particularly **herbivora**. Sarcocystis sp. were once considered of little pathological significance. However, they are now recognized as **important pathogens** which cause **encephalitis, generalized disease**, and **abortion**. They were first described by Miescher in 1843 in the musculature of **mouse**, and were later called "**Miescher's bodies, sacs, or tubules**". However, their classification, life cycle, source of infection, and significance remained a complete mystery until 1976, when it was demonstrated that parasitic cysts in muscle represent intermediate stages of intestinal coccidia, and that their life cycle is similar to that of **Toxoplasma**. They are currently classified in the Family **Sarcocystidae**, to which genera **Toxoplasma, Neospora**, and **Besnoitia** also belong (see **Table 37**). Only a few sarcosporidia have been studied in any detail.

Over the years, numerous species names have been given to members of the genus Sarcocystis. However, usually the proliferating or encysted organisms look exactly similar, and techniques which can differentiate them in tissue sections are not available. This makes species identification ordinarily not possible. A type, called **Sarcocystis gigantea** found in the tongue, oesophagus, and sometimes other muscles of **sheep**, forms large, grossly visible, multinucleated saccules. The saccules have a fibrillar network within which innumerable crescentic spores are found. Some important **Sarcocystic** species affecting domestic animals are given in **Table 41**.

Quiescent (inactive, dormant) **sarcocysts** are seen in myofibres in many other species, besides **sheep**, usually as incidental findings. Quiescent sarcocysts also occur in **dogs** and **cats**, which are usually definitive hosts for various species of **Sarcocystis**. Generalized infection with extensive proliferation of merozoites causing necrosis and inflammation in many different organs is the important form of disease in animals. **In wildlife**, sarcocystosis has been reported in deer, mule deer and wild boars.

Table 41. Some important Sarcocystis species affecting domestic animals

Intermediate host	Species	Definitive host	Comments
Cattle	S. cruzi	Dog, wolf, fox,	Highly pathogenic
	S. hirsuta	Cat	Low pathogenicity
	S. hominis	Man, monkey	Low pathogenicity
Sheep	S. gigantea	Cat	Very large
	S. ovicanis	Dog, fox	Pathogenic
	S. tenella	Cat	Low pathogenicity
Goat	S. capracanis	Dog, fox	Can cause disseminated disease in goats
	S. orientalis	Unknown	-
Pig	S. miescheriana	Dog, wolf	-
	S. suihominis	Man	-
	S. porcifelis	Cat	Pathogenic
Horse	S. bertrami	Dog	Thin-walled cyst
	S. fayeri	Dog	Thin-walled cyst
	S. neurona	Unknown	Associated with meningo-encephalitis in horses
Dog	S. canis	Unknown	Disseminated disease in dogs

Life Cycle

Sarcocystis has an obligatory **two-host life cycle**. After ingestion of **sporulated oocysts** by an **intermediate host, sporozoites** are released.

Sporozoites invade beyond the intestinal tract, and first multiply by **endopolygony** in endothelial cells of arteries into groups of **merozoites** (first-generation **meronts**). Released merozoites undergo a second cycle in capillary endothelium in many tissues. This results in the production of second generation **meronts**, whose released merozoites parasitize circulating mononuclear cells. Merozoites then undergo **endodyogeny** (division in two), and are released to enter myofibres of skeletal muscle or heart. Here, the **metrocytes** divide into large numbers of **bradyzoites** forming typical **sarcocyst**. The cycle is completed when the **definitive (final) host** ingests muscle. The released bradyzoites develop directly into microgamonts and macrogamonts. These, in turn, form **oocysts** to be released in the faeces as infective sporulated oocysts. **The sporulated oocysts of Sarcocystis are exactly similar to those of Isospora with two sporocysts each containing four sporozoites.**

The final hosts for many species of Sarcocystis have not been determined. Both **dogs** and **cats** have been identified as final hosts for cattle, sheep, pig, and horse sarcosporidia. The intestinal stage in dogs and cats was previously called *Isospora bigemina*. **Humans** are hosts for the sexual stage of sarcosporidia of cattle and pigs. The intestinal stage in humans was previously called *Isospora hominis*. Based on the two hosts involved in the life cycle of sarcosporidia, new nomenclature (names) have been given to them as listed in **Table 41**.

The sarcocysts within muscle fibres vary in size, but are usually slightly wider than a muscle fibre and several times longer than their width. The wall of the cyst appears clear or hyaline. Usually septae extend from the wall, which divide the cyst into tiny subcompartments, which contain bradyzoites. The **bradyzoites** are strongly basophilic, and elliptical (oval-shaped) or banana-shaped, each measuring about 4 by 8 µm. Usually degeneration occurs in the centres of larger sarcocysts.

Pathogenesis

Individual species vary in their pathogenicity and in their ability to produce clinical disease in the intermediate host. For example, in **cattle**, *S. cruzi* is much more pathogenic than *S. hominis*. **There is a strong correlation between the number of sporocysts ingested and the severity of disease.** Sarcocys'' *p.* are organisms with a two-host cycle. The species from the dog undergo schizogony in the endothelial cells of the arterioles and capillaries of the ntermediate host. This causes **widespread haemorrhage** and **anaemia**. Fever is associated with parasitaemia, and coincides with the time of maturation of the first and second generation schizonts. The vascular lesions appear to be an essential part of the pathogenesis.

Clinical Signs

Natural infections of **sheep, goats, buffalo calves,** and **cattle calves** are characterized by anorexia, fever, emaciation, nervousness, hypersalivation, lameness, anaemia, and abortion. There is a loss of tail switch, creating a **'rat-tail' appearance.** Infection and disease can occur at all ages. The clinical illness begins 23-26 days after infection and a rise in temperature is noticed first. This is followed by anorexia, weight loss, fall in milk production, muscle twitching, and in heavy infections, death. **The course of the disease depends on the dose of sporocysts,** and less serious forms of the disease may occur. For example, in **sheep** a reduction in growth rate may be the only manifestation.

Chronic sarcocystosis in cattle is manifested by poor weight gains and loss of hair of the neck, rump, and the switch of the tail. A non-suppurative encephalomyelitis of **lambs** has been suspected to be caused by sarcosporidia. Affected lambs showed ataxia and then flaccid paralysis. The main clinical sign of sarcocystosis in the **horse** is associated with infestation of nervous tissue.

Lesions

Sarcocysts distort myofibres of the heart or skeletal muscle without any inflammatory reaction. Purkinje fibres (lying beneath endocardium) may also be affected, but whether this has any effect on the conduction system is not known. **Smooth muscle is not affected.** The **mature sarcocysts,** filled with their bradyzoites, **represent the final stage in the life cycle,** awaiting ingestion by the definitive (final) host. These mature sarcocysts are more of an incidental finding than of pathological significance. Sometimes, rupture of a sarcocyst stimulates an inflammatory reaction, which may be granulomatous in nature. Usually, no clinical sign or lesion precedes maturation of the sarcocyst.

Sarcocystosis can, however, cause more serious disease and clinical signs during its early cycle in the intermediate host. If infection is heavy, multiplication of merozoites in endothelial cells and their invasion and proliferation in parenchymal cells, including neurons and myocardial fibres, is associated with fever, anaemia, thrombosis, haemorrhage, and even death. This results from extensive proliferation of merozoites, which cause arteritis and capillary damage, tissue necrosis and inflammatory reaction. The organisms have an affinity for the vascular tree of the central nervous system, where they cause encephalitis. But they may also produce pneumonia, hepatitis, dermatitis, polymyositis, and necrotizing and inflammatory lesions in other organs and tissues.

Sarcocystosis is also an important cause of **abortion in cattle, sheep, goats, and pigs.** Extensive multiplication of merozoites in endothelial cells throughout tissues of the foetus and within the placenta causes death of the foetus and its expulsion. The organisms cause vasculitis and necrosis of affected tissues in many organs, but especially in the brain. The aborted cows may be otherwise normal.

Diagnosis

Diagnosis in clinical cases is very difficult because of the non-specific signs. Sarcocystosis should be considered in problems of fever and anaemia of undetermined origin in cattle, and in cases of unthriftiness in cattle and sheep. At necropsy, microscopic examination of muscles can diagnose the cysts, and this helps in grading severity of the infestation.

Genus: Plasmodium

Malaria

Malaria is an important disease of **humans**. Its name comes from the **Italian words "mala"** (bad) and **"aria"** (air) (malaria). This had a reference to the **"miasmic vapours"**, which were believed to come from swamps and cause malaria ("Miasma" is a Greek word and means a foul, unhealthy smell or atmosphere). One of the parasites was discovered by a French army physician, Laveran, who in 1880 found what we now know as microgametocytes, probably of *Plasmodium falciparum*. However, it was not until after the turn of the century in 1910 that Sir Ronald Ross, an English physician **working in the Indian army,** demonstrated **mosquitoes to be "miasmas"** arising from swamps to spread the disease. The causative protozoa are all members of the genus **Plasmodium,** which includes many pathogenic species.

Although malaria is most important as a disease of humans, many species of animals are susceptible to their own specific species of **Plasmodium,** including **monkeys** and **birds. In general, however, malaria is not of veterinary importance.** Natural infections in animals are not associated with significant clinical disease, or pathological findings. Malaria in **monkeys** is sometimes an exception, but even here malaria in monkeys is usually an incidental finding.

Life Cycle

The life cycles of different species of **Plasmodium** are quite similar. **Two hosts are required:** 1. **Vertebrate hosts** (humans, other mammals, birds). In these **schizogony** takes place in erythrocytes and other cells; and 2. **Invertebrate hosts.** These are blood-sucking insects (**mosquitoes**). The life cycle begins when a **female mosquito** penetrates the skin of the vertebrate host, introducing the **sporozoites** into circulation. After a few days of exo-erythrocytic (i.e., outside the erythrocytes) development in the endothelial cells, or hepatocytes as schizonts, **merozoites** are released. Merozoites then enter red blood cells. Here, at first, they appear as ring forms which enlarge to a stage called **trophozoites**. The trophozoites, in turn, divide into **schizonts** containing up to 24 or more merozoites. On rupture of the infected erythrocytes, released merozoites reinfect other red blood cells. This repeated schizogony results in the recurrent paroxysms (attacks) of fever and anaemia. Some of the merozoites ultimately develop into **gametocytes**. They remain in the blood as macrogametocytes and microgametocytes until ingested by a mosquito, or eliminated by phagocytosis as their life cycle is completed. The organisms catabolize haemoglobin only incompletely. This leaves a brownish pigment, **haemozoin**, easily visible in stained smears.

The **macrogametocytes** and **microgametocytes** ingested by female mosquitoes (**the males do not ingest blood**), undergo further development in the **stomach of the mosquito**. The macrogametocyte becomes one **macrogamete** and the microgametocyte becomes 4-8 **microgametes**. Fusion of gametes results in a **motile zygote**, called **ookinete**. The ookinete enters the gastric mucosa of the mosquito and becomes an **oocyst**, which then lies in the stroma close to the gastric epithelium. Repeated nuclear divisions result in the formation of many **sporozoites**. These are set free by rupture into the haemolymph, permitting migration to the salivary glands of the mosquito. From salivary glands, sporozoites are available to a new vertebrate host when the female mosquito bites the skin to suck blood.

Clinical Signs

Signs in malaria are related to the number of parasites in the blood. Signs appear 5-15 days after infection. The incubation period depends to some extent upon the exo-erythrocytic period of the parasites. Attacks of chills and fever appear at intervals which roughly correspond to the periods of reproduction of the malaria parasite. The terms **tertian** (third) and **quartan** (fourth) apply to the interval between paroxysms. In **tertian malaria** in *Plasmodium vivax* and *P. falciparum* infection, the **signs appear on the third day** after a 48-hour cycle. In the case of **quartan malaria**, cycle of *P. malariae* is about 76 hours, and the **signs reappear each fourth day**. Relapses usually occur in human malaria, sometimes after long intervals. This provides them a **carrier state. This state also appears to occur in animals**.

Lesions

Destruction of parasitized erythrocytes results in haemolysis and anaemia, which are responsible for most of the clinical and pathological findings. Marked **splenomegaly** and **hepatomegaly** result from congestion, haemorrhage, hyperplasia of reticulo-endothelial cells, and an influx of macrophages. Both reticulo-endothelial cells and macrophages contain phagocytized free parasites.

Diagnosis

The diagnosis of malaria is usually established by demonstrating the organisms in erythrocytes in thin or thick smears stained with Giemsa or Wright-Giemsa stain.

Genus: Babesia

Babesiosis

Also known as 'piroplasmosis', 'tick fever', and 'red water fever', babesiosis includes diseases caused by **Babesia** (Family **Babesiidae**) species. Organisms of the genus **Babesia** parasitize the erythrocytes of a wide range of vertebrate hosts, namely, **cattle, buffaloes, sheep and goats, pigs, horses, and dogs and cats**. They multiply in the erythrocytes by **binary fission**, giving rise to two or four daughter individuals. **Blood-sucking ticks act as intermediate host-vectors in which the parasites reproduce**. Sometimes, they penetrate the eggs and infect the young tick. Babesiosis is characterized by fever and intravascular haemolysis causing a syndrome of anaemia, haemoglobinaemia, and haemoglobinuria. **Babesia**, were first described in 1888 by **Babes** in Roumania. However, they were not recognized as important pathogens until 1893 when Smith and Kilborne reported them to be the cause of "**Texas cattle fever**". Their work demonstrated for the first time that an infection of any kind could be transmitted by an arthropod vector. **This was a major scientific achievement and a milestone in the control of disease.**

Aetiology

A large number of **Babesia** sp. have been identified (**Table 42**), **all of which are pathogenic**. However, there is considerable variation in the severity of disease caused by the different species and strains of organisms. In **cattle**, severity of infection also depends on the breed. *Bos indicus* (i.e., Zebu-type cattle) breeds are relatively resistant because of their resistance to heavy infestations with ticks. Infection in young animals is mild due to the effects of **colostrum**. The disease may have a **seasonal incidence** if the tick population varies with climate. **Recovery from infection in adults confers relatively good immunity.** The infection is more severe following splenectomy. Of the 71 species in the genus **Babesia**, only a few affect domestic animals. **Babesia** sp. are relatively **host-specific**. Recently, however, cross-species infections have been recognized. Cattle, buffaloes, horses, sheep, goats, pigs, monkeys, and even humans are susceptible to one or more species of **Babesia**. However, **the general features of the disease are similar in all hosts.**

Of the several species that affect **cattle**, *B. bigemina* and *B. bovis* are the most prevalent and important. In **equine babesiosis**, *B. caballi* is reportedly less pathogenic than *B. equi*. In **canine babesiosis**, *B. gibsoni* principally occurs **in India**. In **humans**, babesiosis was first reported in 1957 in a patient in

Yugoslavia affected with *B. bovis*. Additional reports have followed from various parts of the world.

Table 42. Babesia Infections

Babesia	Animals affected	Remarks
B. argentina	Cattle	-
B. bigemina	Cattle, zebu, buffalo, deer	-
B. bovis	Cattle, buffalo, deer, stag	Recorded in India
B. caballi	Horse, donkey, mule	Recorded in India
B. canis	Dog, wolf, jackal	Recorded in India
B. divergens	Cattle	-
B. equi	Horse, mule, donkey, zebra	Recorded in India
B. felis	Domestic cat, wild cat, **lion,** **leopard**	-
B. gibsoni	Dog, wolf, fox, jackal	Recorded in India
B. major	Cattle	-
B. motasi	Sheep, goats	Recorded in India
B. ovis	Sheep, goats	Recorded in India
B. trautmanni	Pig, warthog, bush pig	

Domestic animal-wise classification of Babesia sp. is as follows:

Cattle	*B. argentina, B. bigemina, B. bovis, B. divergens, B. major*
Buffaloes	*B. bigemina, B. bovis*
Sheep and goats	*B. motasi, B. ovis*
Horses	*B. caballi, B. equi*
Pigs	*B. trautmanni*
Dogs	*B. canis, B. gibsoni*
Cats	*B. felis*

Babesia occur in circulating erythrocytes as pyriform (pear-shaped) or ovoid (egg-shaped) bodies, usually in pairs, or multiples thereof. They can be **divided into two groups based on their size: 1. The larger group (*B. bigemina*, *B. major*, *B. caballi*, *B. motasi*, *B. canis*, *B. trautmanni*),** measuring 4-5 µm long by 2-3 µm wide; and 2. **The smaller group (*B. bovis*, *B. argentina*, *B. ovis*, *B. gibsoni*, *B. felis*, *B. divergens*, *B. equi*),** which are 1-2 µm long and about 0.5 µm wide. **Babesia** are easily differentiated from **Plasmodium** sp. by the absence of haemoglobin-derived pigment. **Babesia** completely catabolize haemoglobin, whereas **Plasmodia** retain the brownish pigment (**haemozoin**).

Babesia are well demonstrated by Romanovsky-type stains.

Transmission

Ticks are the natural vectors of babesiosis. Babesia persist and pass part of their life cycle in the ticks. When adult animals become infected they act as carriers for a variable period. If they are constantly reinfected, as they are in an endemic environment, **they act as carriers for life.** Contaminated needles and surgical instruments can transmit the infection physically. This depends largely on the degree of parasitaemia which occurs with each species.

Pathogenesis

The main pathogenic effect of **Babesia** is **intravascular haemolysis.** The effect of the haemolysis is to produce **a haemolytic anaemia which could be acutely fatal due to anoxia.** In longer surviving animals, there are ischaemic changes in skeletal and heart muscle. When an animal becomes infected, protozoa **multiply in the peripheral vessels (*B. bigemina*, *B. ovis*), or in the visceral vessels (*B. bovis*).** The multiplication reaches a peak with the development of clinically detectable haemolysis. The **haemolysis** results in prolonged **anaemia, jaundice,** and **haemoglobinuria. Death is due to anaemic anoxia.** If the animal survives, it becomes a **carrier.** A harmless, subclinical infection is then maintained by a delicate immunological balance between protozoa and antibodies. In the carrier state, the animal is resistant to infection and it persists for about a year. **When cows become infected during pregnancy** there is no apparent infection of the calf *in utero*, but there is a transfer of passive immunity through colostrum to the newborn calf.

Immune Responses in Babesia

In babesiosis, the infective stages of the organisms (**sporozoites**) attack red blood cells. This invasion involves **activation of the alternate complement pathway.** Infected erythrocytes incorporate **Babesia** antigens into their membranes. These, in turn, induce **antibodies** which **opsonize the red cells and lead to their removal** by the mononuclear-phagocyte system (MPS). In addition to the humoral response, infected red cells may also be destroyed by **antibody-dependent cell-mediated cytotoxicity (ADCC).** The **Babesia antigen-opsonizing antibody complex** on the surface of infected erythrocytes can be recognized by **macrophages and cytotoxic lymphocytes.** The cytotoxic lymphocytes are important early in infection when the number of infected erythrocytes is small.

Many factors contribute to the resistance of animals against babesiosis, including **genetic factors** and **age.** For example, Zebu cattle are more resistant to disease than European cattle, and cattle show a significant resistance to babesiosis in the first six months of life. Animals that recover from acute babesiosis are resistant to further clinical disease. **This immunity has been** considered to be a form of preimmunity.

For many years it was thought that a common feature of many protozoan infection was **premunition**. **Premunition** is a term used to describe resistance that is established after the primary infection has become chronic. It is effective only if the parasite persists in the host. In other words, **premunition is a form of immunity that is dependent on the continued presence of parasite in the host.** With **B abesia**, it was believed t hat only c attle actually i nfected w ere resistant to clinical disease. If all organisms were removed from an animal, resistance decreased immediately. **However, recent studies have shown that this is not entirely true.** For example, cattle c ured of **Babesia** infection by chemotherapy have been shown to be resistant to challenge w ith the similar strain of that organism for several years afterward. Nevertheless, the presence of i nfection does appear to b e essential for protection a gainst other s trains. Also, splenectomy of infected animals will cause the development of clinical disease. The spleen not only serves as a source of antibodies in this disease, but it also removes infected erythrocytes. **Removal of these functions through splenectomy is sufficient to allow the clinical disease to develop.**

It has been observed that **parasite-induced immunosuppression** may promote parasite survival. *Babesia bovis* **is immunosuppressive for cattle**. As a result, its host vector, the tick **Boophilus**, is able to survive better on an infected animal. Thus, infected cattle h ave more ticks that non-infected animals and the efficacy of transmission of *B. bovis* is increased. **The parasite-induced immunosuppression can lead to the death of the host as a result of secondary infection.** Therefore, it is not necessarily always beneficial to the parasite.

Babesia sp. **may show antigenic variation to evade the immune response of the host.** Thus, it has been observed that in babesiosis strains which cause relapse o f the d isease appear t o be a ntigenically different from t he original strains.

Clinical Signs

Clinical signs vary, but include f ever, listlessness, anorexia, a naemia, **jaundice, haemoglobinuria**, and ascites. Coma may appear prior to death. In cattle, the disease is characterized by an acute onset of high fever (106^0 F), anorexia, depression, w eakness, cessation o f rumination, a nd a f all in m ilk yield. The brick-red conjunctivae and mucous membranes soon become extremely pale d ue to **severe anaemia**. I n the terminal stages, there is **severe jaundice** and the urine is dark red to brown in colour. **Many severely affected animals die suddenly** at this stage, after an illness of only 14 hours. In those that survive, the febrile stage lasts for about a week and the total course about 3 w eeks. **Pregnant animals usually abort**. Animals t hat survive recover gradually from the severe emaciation and anaemia. In **horses**, there is sudden onset of immobility and reluctance to move. There is complete anorexia and a fever of 104⁰ F, which usually subsides after one day. Oedema of the fetlock occurs and m ay also b e present o n the head and v entral abdomen. U sually **there is no haemoglobinuria**. T he mucosae a re pale p ink a nd tinged w ith jaundice. In young horses and newborn foals the signs are more severe; jaundice, m ucosal p allor (paleness) and weakness are m arked. Affected h orses may die w ithin 24-48 hours after t he first si gns appear. C hronic cases m ay survive for months, and 'carriers' may persist for up to 4 years. In all **other species**, the signs observed are clinically similar to those described for cattle.

Lesions

Postmortem examination of animals died from babesiosis shows the **blood** to be **thin and watery**, and t he plasma i s red-tinged. T he subcutaneous, subserous, and intramuscular connective tissue is oedematous and yellow. Fat is similarly affected. **Icteric discoloration is clearly seen in all organs**. The **spleen** is usually **enlarged 4-5 times the normal size**, and its parenchyma is soft and d ark red. T he splenic c orpuscles are prominent. **Lymph nodes** are usually enlarged. The **liver** is enlarged, and the **gallbladder** distended w ith dark green bile. The **lungs** are slightly oedematous, and the urinary b ladder contains red-coloured u rine.

The **microscopic lesions** are characteristic **of severe haemolytic anaemia**. Haemoglobinuric nephrosis, centrilobular and paracentral necrosis of the liver, oedema, excessive fluid in the peritoneal, pericardial and pleural cavities, and serosal haemorrhages are usual findings. **Babesia** can be demonstrated in large numbers in capillaries in brain. They are both free in the lumen and present in packed erythrocytes. The organisms may be associated with small thrombi, foci of haemorrhage and necrosis.

Diagnosis

Clinically, j aundice with h aemoglobinuria a nd f ever are suggestive o f babesiosis. The diagnosis is confirmed by identification of **Babesia** in blood smears. The organisms can be identified by their morphology, and their stimulation of specific antibodies in the serum of infected animals. The antibodies can be detected by haemagglutination, agglutination, complement fixation, fluorescent antibody, and microplate **enzyme immunoassay** (EIA) tests. **Of all these tests, EIA is probably the most sensitive**. The latest thing in cattle is an ELISA using a recombinant **B. bovis** antigen. **DNA probes** are also being used, and can detect specific parasitaemias at very low levels of infection.

Genus: Theileria

Theileriasis

Theileriasis is a tick-borne protozoan disease caused by **Theileria** sp. in **cattle, buffaloes, sheep and goats**, as well as in wild and captive animals. The disease i s characterized b y fever a nd lymphoproliferative disorders w hich may be associated with leukopaenia a nd/or anaemia. E uropean breeds of cattle are more susceptible than Zebu breeds. Like Babesia, protozoan para-sites of the genus **Theileria** (Family **Theileriidae**) are found in the **erythro-cytes**, but reproduce by s chizogony (not b inary fission) in lymphocytes or histiocytes. Members of a related genus (of the **Theileriidae** family) **Cytauxzoon** multiply by schizogony in histiocytes and by binary fission in erythrocytes. **Table 43** presents important pathogenic **Theileria**.

Table 43. Important Pathogenic Theileria

Theileria	Animals affected	Remarks
T. annulata (*T. dispar*)	Cattle, Zebu cattle, buffaloes	Recorded in India
T. hirci	Sheep, goats	-
T. lawrencei	Cattle, buffaloes	-
T. mutans	Cattle, deer	-
T. ovis	Sheep, goats	Recorded in India
T. parva	Cattle, Indian buffaloes, African buffaloes	Recorded in India

Transmission and Life Cycle

Theileria parva, the c ause of E ast Coast fever, a disease of cattle of great importance in Africa (**and now also in India**) is transmitted by several species of ticks, the most important of which is **Rhipicephalus**. The life cycle in the m ammalian hosts c attle and **buffaloes** is s till not f ully understood. However, following introduction into the host by saliva of the tick, **Theileria invade lymphocytes and histiocytes**, first in the regional l ymph nodes, b ut later in all the l ymph nodes, spleen, liver, a nd other o rgans, as w ell as t he circulating c ells. Here, t hey develop i n the cytoplasm of a ffected cells i nto **macroschizonts**, w hich are up to 16 μm in diameter a nd contain 8 or more nuclei of 1 μm in diameter. These large bodies, known as "**Koch's bodies**"after their discoverer, **are considered characteristic and diagnostic of the disease.** After about 10 days, forms known as "**microschizonts**" appear in **lymphocytes and histiocytes**. These are characterized by more nuclei (up to 100 or more). It is not clear whether microschizonts f orm following release of m erozoites fro m macroschizonts, or through another mechanism. Released **'micromerozoites'** (they destroy t he cell i n the process), parasitize e rythro-cytes as tiny rod, comma, or ring-shaped bodies. They are smaller than **Babesia** and do not undergo further division. Their pleomorphism distinguishes them from **Babesia**.

Pathogenesis

In general, **the pathogenesis of various forms of theileriasis is dependent on the production of schizonts in lymphocytes and piroplasms in erythrocytes**. Thus, *T. parva*, *T. annulata* and *T. hirci* produce numerous schizonts and piroplasms **and are very pathogenic**. *T. mutans*, *T. orientalis*, and *T. ovis* rarely produce s chizonts but m ay cause v arying degrees o f anaemia w hen piroplasms are many in red blood cells. With *T. velifera* and *T. separata*, no schizonts have been described, the parasitaemia i s usually s canty, and t he infection is mild or subclinical.

Sporozoites (e.g., of *T. parva*) a re **introduced into bovine host by the vector tick in its saliva when it is feeding**. Ticks m ust feed f or 2-4 d ays before the sporozoites in their salivary glands mature and become infective to cattle. **One tick can transmit sufficient sporozoites to cause a fatal infection in a susceptible animal**. T he sporozoites then e nter lymphocytes and develop into **schizonts** in the lymph node draining the area of attachment of the t ick, usually the parotid node. Infected **lymphocytes** are transformed to lymphoblasts, which divide a long with the schizonts **so that each daughter cell is also infected**. Finally, infected lymphocytes are disseminated throughout the lymphoid system. Later, some schizonts, differentiate into **merozoites**, are released from the lymphoblasts, and they **invade erythrocytes**. In the red blood cells, the parasites transform to become **piroplasms** which are infective to t he tick w hen it f eeds. The i ngested parasite u ndergoes several developmental stages a nd eventually f orms sporozoites i n the t ick salivary g lands, thus completing the cycle.

The main pathological lesion is the damage caused to the lymphoid system by rapidly multiplying schizonts, a nd the a ssociated proliferation o f lymphocytes in parenchymatous organs. As a result, the disease is less virulent in indigenous breeds of cattle because of their inherent ability to limit the rapid multiplication of schizonts during the acute phase.

Immune mechanisms

Animals that survive an infection have a solid immunity. In *Theileria parva* infection o f cattle, sporozoites preferentially attack lymphocytes. **The parasite can invade both T cells and B cells**. The parasite then triggers certain pathways which result in the **production of interleukin-2 (IL-2) and its receptors**. IL-2, i n turn, st imulates the growth of these lymphocytes. Their growth stops if IL-2 production is stopped. As the schizont stage of **Theileria** develops within lymphocytes, the infected l ymphocytes enlarge to form **lymphoblasts**, and begin to proliferate. Since the parasite divides along with the host cell, this leads to very rapid clonal expansion of parasitized cells. **In most cattle, this results in overwhelming infection and death**. Some cattle, however, r ecover and b ecome solidly i mmune. In t hese animals, **c ytotoxic**

CD8+ T cells kill the infected lymphoblasts.

T. parva **is immunosuppressive. It attacks and destorys T cells**. Cattle can be made resistant to *T. parva* infection by infecting them with virulent sporozoites, and treating them simultaneously with tetracycline.

Clinical Signs

The clinical signs begin with **fever**, which appears about 15 days **following the bite of infected ticks**. After several days, **Theileria** become demonstrable in the blood. The appetite is then gradually lost, rumination ceases, and milk secretion decreases. **The superficial lymph nodes become visibly enlarged**, the muzzle dry, the hair coat rough, and salivation and lachrymation become excessive. **Respiratory distress may follow pulmonary oedema, and death may result from asphyxia**. As the disease progresses, severe leukopaenia of all white blood cell types develops, and enlarged lymph nodes may regress to less than normal size. Anaemia, believed to be of immunological origin, may be present. In some cases, death follows gradual emaciation, delirium, and coma. **Mortality is high, and may approach 100%**.

Lesions

The most constant and most important gross lesion is **generalized enlargement of lymph nodes**, although in some animals enlarged lymph nodes may have regressed to smaller than normal. **Lymph nodes** are oedematous and may show haemorrhage. **Spleen** may be normal, large, or small. Usually, pulmonary oedema and emphysema, subcutaneous and intramuscular oedema, and excessive pericardial and pleural fluids are present. The **liver** is usually enlarged, yellowish, and mottled. White foci of various sizes may be seen in the renal cortex. The meninges may be congested and focal haemorrhages are present in the brain.

The main **microscopic lesion** is **proliferation of lymphocytic cells** in lymph nodes, spleen, Peyer's patches, liver, kidneys, and elsewhere. Blood vessels, including cerebral vessels, are filled with parasitized lymphocytes. These obstruct the blood flow and cause focal infarction. **Koch's bodies may be found in tissue sections of many organs**.

T. annulata, the cause of tropical theileriasis in cattle, is similar to East Coast Fever caused by *T. parva*, but less severe. *T. lawrencei* affects cattle and buffaloes and causes what is known as "**Buffalo disease**" in Africa. If severe, it resembles East Coast Fever. *T. mutans* also affects cattle, but is of little pathogenic importance. Sheep are affected by *T. hirci*, which can cause a disease resembling East Coast Fever. *T. ovis* rarely causes clinical disease. Other species of **Theileria** are of no pathological significance.

Diagnosis

The d iagnosis of t heileriasis depends u pon demonstration o f the o rganisms in erythrocytes and in lymphocytes (**Koch's bodies**). Koch's bodies (i.e., **schizonts**) are seen only sometimes in circulating lymphocytes, but mostly in biopsy smears of enlarged lymph nodes stained with **Giemsa**. Piroplasms are seen easily in erythrocytes from day 16 after tick attachment, and they increase in number until death. **Babesiosis is the most important disease from which it must be differentiated**. Various tests for antibodies have been used with success. These i nclude complement fixation, i ndirect haemagglutination, immunofluorescence, and ELISA. **The ELISA test** is being used increasingly for seroepidemiological studies.

Genus: Cytauxzoon

Cytauxzoonosis

This disease, caused by the species of genus **Cytauxzoon** within the Family **Theileriidae (Table 37)**, is **an infection limited to various wild animals in Africa**. However, a disease pathologically similar has now been recognized to occur in domestic **cats** in the United States. The life cycle is not known, but the organism is believed to be transmitted by ticks, similar to that known for **Theileria** sp. Schizogony occurs in macrophages with a piroplasm form in erythrocytes. **The disease in domestic cats is always fatal**.

Clinically, the disease in cats is characterized by fever, dyspnoea, anorexia, enlargement o f lymph nodes, anaemia, and jaundice, leading to d eath in 3-6 d ays. **Gross lesions** include pale mucous m embranes, with petechiae and ecchymoses in and on the l ung, heart, lymph nodes, and mucous membranes. Lymph nodes and spleen are enlarged. The characteristic **microscopic lesion** is the presence of **numerous large schizonts within the cytoplasm of macrophages**. Each s chizont contains n umerous small m erozoites. The affected macrophages are very big (up to 75 μm in diameter) and may occlude the lumen of the vessels. Such cells are found in almost any tissue, including lung, heart, lymph nodes, spleen, liver, kidneys, brain, and bone marrow.

Genus: Encephalitozoon

Encephalitozoonosis

Protozoon *Encephalitozoon cuniculi* is best known as a cause of encephalitis and nephritis in **rabbits**, but also affects **dogs, cats, monkeys**, wild carnivores, and **humans**. **Infection is usually subclinical**, even in rabbits. The infection i s acquired b y ingestion o f spores e xcreted in u rine. **Ingestion of infected tissues containing spores is another source of infection. T rans-**

placental infection of the foetus is also an important means of transmission. Encephalitozoon attacks a variety of cell types. **Clinical signs are usually not detected.** In d ogs, g ranulomatous meningo-encephalomyeiitis a nd nephritis are the chief findings. **Diagnosis** depends upon demonstration of the organisms in tissue section, isolation in tissue culture, or mouse inoculation.

Genus: Balantidium

Balantidiasis

The only member of the ciliated **Protozoa** which is of pathologic significance (and this is questionable) is *Balantidium coli* (*B. suis*). This large (50-200 µm) single-celled organism is a natural inhabitant of the digestive tract of **pigs, monkeys,** and **humans.** It lives in the lumen, or between the villi and causes no visible effect on the host. Under some imperfectly understood circumstances, *B. coli* invades the i ntestinal mucosa. It penetrates i nto the submucosa and localizes particularly in lymphoid nodules. Sometimes, it may reach the genital tract. This tissue penetration r esults in varying degrees of acute inflammation in the vicinity, and may result in some clinical manifestations of enteric disease.

Genus: Pneumocystis

Pneumocystosis

A protozoan organism of **uncertain classification,** *Pneumocystis carinii,* **inhabits the pulmonary alveoli of human and animals,** a nd under c ertain conditions causes severe disruption of the respiratory function. **Pneumocystis pneumonia** has b een recognized i n **humans, dogs, h orses, p igs, goats,** and **monkeys.** The disease is seen in animals and humans suffering from immunodeficiency. **Pneumocystis pneumonia is the most common opportunistic infection in patients with AIDS.** Although the organisms in various tissues a re morphologically i ndistinguishable, it a ppears that e ach may b e specific for the respective species.

The organisms are located in alveoli in close contact with type I, and sometimes, type II pneumocytes. **Microscopically,** there is little inflammatory reaction, but t ype II a lveolar lining cells may b e enlarged. T he ai veoli a re filled with pink material w hich represents vast collections of organisms. *P. carinii* proliferates as t rophozoites, which in t urn become c ysts. Each cyst contains up to eight intracystic bodies or **sporozoites.** Neither form stains well in H and E stained sections. The trophozoites are best seen with **Giemsa stain,** the n ucleus staining red and the cytoplasm blue. The wall of the cyst stains well with **Gomori silver stain or PAS.** Immunoperoxidase and immunofluorescent staining techniques are the most scientific methods for positive identification. **If the infection cures, it does not confer any immunity**.

Avian Protozoal Diseases

Coccidiosis

Coccidiosis is one of the most important diseases of poultry worldwide, and is characterized by enteritis. It is caused by protozoa of the Phylum **Apicomplexa (Table 37)**. These protozoa undergo a direct life cycle and spread between hosts through resistant oocyst. In the host, the parasite grows and multiplies intracellularly in epithelial cells usually in the **intestine**. Most coccidia of poultry belong to the **genus Eimeria, Family Eimeriidae (Table 37)**.

The Eimeria are highly host specific. Within each host, there may be several species of varying pathogenicity which are specific to it. Coccidiosis is **largely a disease of young birds** because immunity quickly develops after exposure and gives protection against later disease outbreaks. **However, there is no cross-immunity between species of Eimeria in birds**, and later outbreaks may be the result of different species. The disease occurs under conditions of **high stocking density**. This favours the build-up of potentially pathogenic populations of the parasite. **Thus, coccidiosis is especially important in intensive poultry operations**. The disease may be **mild**, resulting from ingestion of a few oocysts, and may escape notice, or may be **severe** as a result of ingestion of millions of oocysts. Apart from causing disease, **subclinical infections cause impaired feed conversion**, and since feed costs comprise some 70% of the cost of producing broiler chickens, **the economic impact of coccidiosis can be considerable**.

Aetiology

Nine species of Eimeria have been described from chickens, Of these **seven are important** as shown in **Table 44**, but the other two species are of doubtful validity, namely, *E. hagani* and *E. mivati*. All seven species appear to be distributed throughout the world. *E. tenella* **is the commonest of the highly pathogenic species**, whereas *E. acervulina* and *E. maxima* are the most prevalent. **Characteristics useful in the identification of species are: 1**. Location of the lesions in the intestine, **2**. Appearance of the gross lesions, **3**. Oocyst size, shape, and colour, **4**. Size of schizonts and merozoites, **5**. Location of parasites in tissues, **6**. Minimum prepatent period in experimental infections, **7**. Minimum time for sporulation, and **8**. Immunogenicity against pure strains.

Table 44. Characteristics for Seven Species of Chicken Coccidia

Characteristics	High pathogenicity; dysentery, high mortality, high morbidity			Medium pathogenicity; lesions present but low mortality, high morbidity		Low pathogenicity; no lesions	
	E. brunetti	E. necatrix	E. tenella	E. acervulina	E. maxima	E. mitis	E. praecox
Portion parasitized	Lower small intestine	Middle small intestine; same as in E. maxima	Caeca and adjacent intestinal tissues	Duodenum	Middle small intestine; same as in E. necatrix	Duodenum	Duodenum
Macroscopic lesions	Coagulative necrosis; mucoid, bloody enteritis	Ballooning; white spots (schizonts); petechiae; mucoid, blood-filled exudate.	At onset: haemorrhage into lumen. Later: thickening, whitish mucosa; clotted blood	Light infection: whitish round lesions, sometimes in ladder-like streaks. Heavy infection: plaques coalescing; thickened intestinal wall	Thickened intestinal walls; mucoid, blood-tinged exudate; petechiae	No lesions; mucoid exudate	No lesions; mucoid exudate
Oocyst Length x width (Average in microns)	24.6 x 18.8	20.4 x 17.2	22.0 x 19.0	18.3 x 14.6	30.5 x 20.7	16.2 x 16.0	21.3 x 17.1
Schizont (size in microns)	30.0	65.9	54.0	10.3	9.4	11.3	20.0
Minimum prepatent period (hrs)	120	138	115	97	121	99	83
Sporulation minimum (hrs)	18	18	18	17	30	18	12

Life Cycle

The life cycle of *Eimeria tenella*, which is typical of all **Eimeria**, is shown in **Fig. 15**. However, some species vary in the number of asexual genera-tions and the time required for each developmental stage. After ingestion of the **sporulated oocyst (infective stage)**, the oocyst wall is crushed in the gizzard, and the **sporozoites** are released from **sporocysts** by the action of chymotrypsin and bile salts in the small intestine. Sporozoites enter into the epithelial cells of the intestinal mucosa, and begin the cell cycle leading to reproduction. **At least two generations of asexual development**, called **"schizogony"**, lead to a **sexual phase**, where small, motile **microgametes** find out **macrogametes** and unite with them **(fertilization)** The resulting **zygote** matures into a n **oocyst**, which i s released from t he intestinal mucosa a nd **shed in the faeces**. An important feature of the cycle is that it is quite rapid, with a prepatent period of about 4-6 days, depending on the species, and involves tremendous multiplication. The d egree varies w ith the species, **but may result in hun-dreds of thousands or even millions of oocysts produced from one ingested oocyst**.

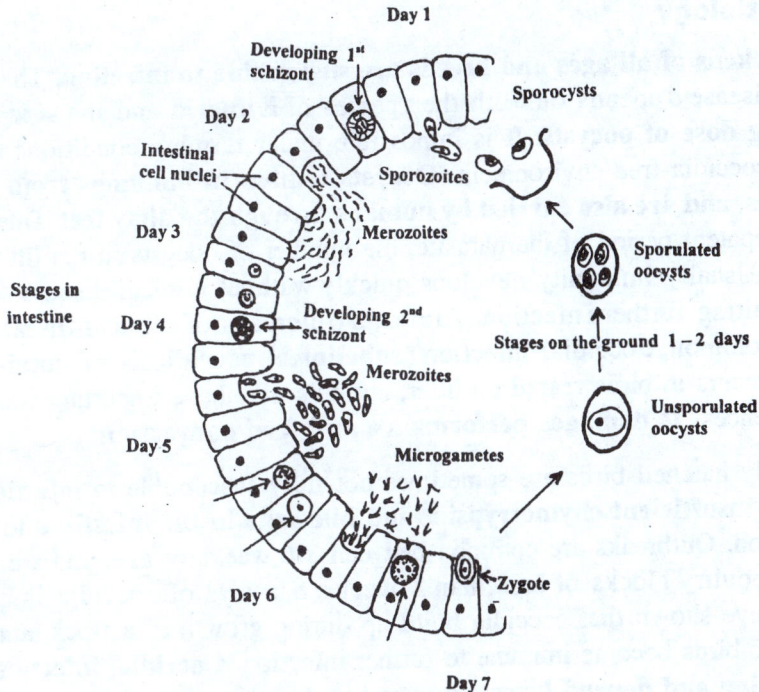

Fig. 15. Life cycle of *E. tenella*, typical of the genus **Eimeria**. The **7-day life cycle** includes t wo or more **asexual and one sexual cycle** during the 6 days after an oocyst has been swallowed by the host. The new generation of oocysts must sporulate (day 7) after being passed by the host before becoming infective.

In some species (*E. tenella*, *E. necatrix*), the maximum tissue damage occurs when second-generation schizonts rupture to release merozoites. Other species may have small schizonts, which cause little damage. However, gametocytes may produce a strong reaction with cellular infiltration and thickened, inflammed tissues.

The **oocysts** become infective only after undergoing sporulation. This requires subdivision into **four sporocysts** (Fig. 15), each of which contains **two sporozoites. Sporulation requires three conditions: warmth, moisture, and oxygen.** Under optimal conditions, around 25-30° C, this takes 1-2 days. **Sporulated oocysts**, protected by the thick oocyst wall, **are fairly resistant** to a wide range of environmental conditions. **Some even survive for months or years**, which is a key factor in the epidemiology of coccidial infections. Temperatures above 56° C and below freezing are lethal, as is drying, but **oocysts are able to tolerate most disinfectants.** Only small molecular weight compounds, like ammonia and methyl bromide, effectively kill oocysts. However, as these are highly toxic gases they are of little practical value for cleaning poultry premises.

Epizootiology

Chickens of all ages and breeds are susceptible to infection. The severity of disease depends on both the species of Eimeria and the size of the infecting dose of oocysts. It is impossible under farming conditions to produce a coccidia-free environment. **Oocysts remain in buildings from previous birds, and are also carried by humans through the dirty feet.** Due to the short prepatent period of the parasite, the number of oocysts in the litter rises rapidly. Usually immunity develops quickly without clinical disease occurring, limiting further infection. Although outbreaks of clinical disease may not be common, coccidial infection (**subclinical coccidiosis or coccidiasis**) always occurs in birds reared on litter, and this may have important economic consequences. **It damages performance and feed conversion.**

Newly hatched birds are sometimes not fully susceptible to infection **because of insufficient chymotrypsin and bile salts in the intestines** to cause excystation. Outbreaks are common between 3-6 weeks of age, and are rarely seen in poultry flocks of less than 3 weeks. Surveys of coccidia in broiler houses have shown that coccidia build up during growth of a flock, and then decline as birds become immune to further infection. **Coccidial infections are self-limiting and depend largely on the number of oocysts ingested and on the immune status of the bird.** This "self-limiting" nature of coccidial infections is widely known in chickens and other poultry. **There is no production of cross-immunity between species of coccidia. Therefore, several outbreaks of coccidiosis can occur in the same flock, with different species involved in each.** Breeder pullets and layer pullets are at greatest risk because they are k ept on litter for 20 w eeks o r m ore. Usually, infections with *E. acervulina*, *E. tenella*, and *E. maxima* are seen between 8-18 weeks of age. **Coccidiosis rarely occurs in layers and breeders because of prior exposure to coccidia and resulting immunity.**

To summarize, the key factors in the epizootiology of coccidiosis are: 1. Persistence of the oocysts in the environment, 2. **Absence of maternally derived protective immunity** in chicks, 3. **Short prepatent period** of the parasite, 4. **Dependence of the disease on oocyst dose and species**, and 5. **Acquirement of immunity by infection** and its m aintenance by continued reinfection.

Transmission

Ingestion of viable sporulated oocysts is the only natural method of transmission. Infected chickens may **shed oocysts in the faeces** for several days or weeks. The oocysts in faeces become infective through the process of **sporulation within 2 days**. Susceptible birds in the same flock may ingest the oocysts. The oocysts can be spread mechanically by different animals, insects, contaminated equipment, wild birds, and dust. As already mentioned, **oocysts are resistant to environmental extremes and to disinfectants**. Oocysts may survive for many weeks in soil, but their survival in poultry litter is limited to a few days because of the **ammonia** released by composting and the action of moulds and bacteria. Spread from one farm to another is facilitated by **movement of people and equipment between farms** and by the migration of wild birds, which may mechanically spread the oocysts. **Threat of coccidiosis is less during hot dry weather and greater in cooler wet weather.**

Relationship with Other Poultry Diseases

The tissue damage and changes in intestinal tract function may allow colonization by various harmful bacteria, such as *Clostridium perfringens*, causing **necrotic enteritis**, or *Salmonella typhimurium*. Immunosuppressive diseases m ay act i n association w ith coccidiosis t o p roduce a more s evere disease. Marek's d isease may i nterfere with d evelopment of i mmunity to coccidiosis, and infectious bursal disease (Gumboro d isease) may aggravate coccidiosis.

Pathogenicity and Clinical Findings

E. brunetti is found in the l ower small intestine (**Table 44**). I n severe cases, the lesions may extend from the gizzard to the cloaca and extend into the caeca. Although less serious than *E. tenella* or *E. necatrix*, *E. brunetti* is capable of producing **moderate mortality, loss of weight gain, poor feed conversion**, and other complications. Infection with 100,000 - 200,000 oocysts causes 10-30% mortality and reduced gain in survivors. **Light infections** can cause reduced weight gain and poor feed conversion even though gross lesions are not clearly visible.

E. necatrix is found in the **middle small intestine**, in approximately the same location as *E. maxima* (**Table 44**). Probably because of its low reproductive capability, *E. necatrix* is not able to compete with other coccidia and **is diagnosed mostly in older birds**, such as brooder **pullets or layer pullets 9-10 weeks old**. The **intestine is usually distended to twice its normal size (ballooning)** and the **lumen may be filled with blood**. Infection with 75,000 - 100,000 oocysts is sufficient to cause **severe weight loss, morbidity and mortality**. Survivors may be emaciated and suffer secondary infections. Droppings of infected birds usually contain blood, fluid, and mucus. **This species and *E. tenella* are the most pathogenic.** Naturally occurring infections have caused **more than 25% mortality in commercial flocks.**

E. tenella inhabits the **caeca and adjacent intestinal tissues**. It causes a **severe disease** characterized by **bleeding, high morbidity and mortality, reduced weight gain, and emaciation**. Infection with 100,000 sporulated oocysts can cause morbidity, mortality and greatly reduced weight gain, **making this one of the most pathogenic species in chickens**. Infection with 1 000-3000 oocysts is sufficient to cause blood droppings and other signs of infection. **The most pathogenic is the second-generation schizont**, which matures at 4th day. Like *E. necatrix*, it produces colonies of large schizonts, which contain hundreds of merozoites. The schizonts develop deep in the lamina propria so that the mucosa is badly disrupted when the schizonts mature and merozoites are released. **Onset of mortality in a flock is rapid.** Most of the mortality occurs between 5 and 6 days following infection. In acute cases it may follow the first signs of infection by only a few hours. **Blood loss may reduce the erythrocyte count and haematocrit value by 50%.** The maximum effect on weight gain is seen at 7 days. The exact cause of death is not known, but toxic factors are suspected. Blood loss does not alone account for mortality

E. acervulina is found in the **duodenum**. Ingestion of 1 000, 30,000, 100,000 or 1,000,000 oocysts results in mild to severe coccidiosis. **Reduction in the rate of weight gain is also proportional to the infective dose.** In heavy infections sometimes mortality may result. Light to moderate infections may produce little effect on weight gain and feed conversion. The intestinal mucosa may be thickened, resulting in poor feed conversion. **Egg production may be reduced in laying birds.**

E. maxima usually parasitizes **middle small intestine (same as in *E. necatrix*)**. *E. maxima* is an easy species to recognize because of the **characteristic large oocysts**, which have distinctive yellowish/brownish walls. This species can be differentiated from *E. necatrix* **by the absence of large schizonts in the lesions**, and from *E. brunetti* by the larger oocysts and the appearance of the lesions. *E. maxima* is **moderately pathogenic**. Infection with 200,000 oocysts is usually sufficient to cause **poor weight gain, morbidity, diarrhoea, and sometimes mortality.** There is usually **extreme emaciation**, roughening of the feathers, and anorexia.

E. mitis is found in the **duodenum.** The lesions are usually very slight. Infection with 1,000,000 to 1500,000 oocysts reduces weight gain and causes morbidity. The lack of distinct gross lesions causes this species to be over-looked.

E. praecox is also found in the **duodenum.** This species is named from the **short prepatent period** (about 83 hrs); hence a 'precocious (i.e., develop-ing or maturing early) **parasite.** Although *E. praecox* is usually overlooked because there are no prominent lesions, there may be **reduced weight gain,** extreme loss of fluids, and **poor feed conversion.**

Lesions

E. brunetti: In the early stages mucosa of the **lower small intestine** is covered with **tiny petechiae. In heavy infections,** the mucosa is badly dam-aged. **Coagulative necrosis** appears between 5-7 days of infection, and there is a caseous eroded surface over the entire mucosa. The coagulated blood and mucosa are seen in the droppings. Oedematous swelling and thickening of the mucosa occur in severe infections. **Histopathology** on the 4th day of infection reveals **schizonts** and cellular infiltration. By the 5th day, tips of many villi are broken off. **Merozoites** invade the epithelium, and develop into sexual stages in the lower small intestine and caeca. In severe cases, the villi may be completely denuded, and only the basement membranes remain.

E. necatrix: Some gross lesions occur in the **first-generation schizogony** between 2-3 days of infection. **By the 4th day, the mid-small intestine may be ballooned,** the mucosa thickened, and the lumen filled with fluid, blood, and tissue debris. From the serosal surface, foci of infection appear as **small white plaques,** or **red petechiae.** Smears examined microscopically between 4-5 days **may contain clusters of large schizonts (66 µm), containing hun-dreds of merozoites.** Schizonts, present deep in the mucosa, usually pen-etrate submucosa and smooth muscle layers and destroy blood vessels. **No significant pathologic effects are seen with the invasion of the caecal mucosa by the third-generation** schizonts and gametocytes. The **third-generation schizonts** produce only 6-16 merozoites, compared to the hundreds of merozoites produced by the **second-generation schizonts.**

Lesions may extend throughout the small intestine in severe infections, causing dilation (**ballooning**) and thickening of the mucosa. **The lumen may be filled with blood and pieces of mucosal tissue.** From the serosal surface, the infection is seen as white or red foci. In dead birds foci are white and black, giving the appearance of "**salt and pepper**". **Microscopic examination**

of smears from the mucosal surface reveals numerous clusters of large schizonts. These are characteristic for this species and distinguish *E. necatrix* from others. Also, oocysts are never associated with lesions in this species. The oocysts are found only in the caeca. The sexual stages do not develop in the intestine where the lesions are found, but in the caeca.

E. tenella: Even during maturation of the **first-generation schizonts**, small foci of denuded epithelium may be seen. By the 4th day of infection, **second-generation schizonts** mature and haemorrhages are noticeable. The **caecal pouch may become greatly enlarged, and distended with clotted blood** and pieces of caecal mucosa in the lumen. By 6th and 7th day, the caecal core becomes hardened and dry. **Finally, it is passed in the faeces.** Regeneration of the epithelium is rapid and may be complete by the 10th day. The infection is usually seen from the serosal surface of the caeca as dark petechiae and foci. The caecal wall is usually thickened because of oedema and infiltration, and later scar tissue.

Microscopically, the **first-generation schizonts** are widely scattered. Heterophil infiltration of the submucosa occurs rapidly as the large **second-generation schizonts** develop in the lamina propria. These are found in clusters and are usually progeny of a single first-generation schizont. Maturation of the second-generation parasites is accompanied by **excessive tissue damage, bleeding, disruption of the caecal glands,** and often complete destruction of the mucosa and muscularis layer. **Oocysts are seen on microscopic examination on the 6th and 7th day.** Regeneration of the epithelium and glands may be complete by the 10th day in light infections, but the epithelium may never completely recover in severe infections. Lost muscularis mucosa is not replaced, and the submucosa becomes fibrosed.

E. acervulina: Lesions can usually be seen from the serosal surface of the **duodenum and small intestine.** The mucosa may at first be covered with **white plaques,** which tend to arrange in transverse fashion and cause **a ladder-like appearance** because of the striations. The intestine may be pale and contain watery fluid. **The gross lesions in light infections are limited to the duodenum,** with only a few plaques, but in heavy infections lesions may extend some distance through the **small intestine,** and plaques may overlap or coalesce. The **lesions** contain schizonts, gametocytes, and oocysts. **Microscopic examination** of smears from intestinal lesions usually reveals **numerous oocysts. H**istopathology **of the small intestine** reveals ovoid gametocytes lining the mucosal cells on the villi. In moderate to heavy infections, the tips of villi are broken off, leading to fusion of villi and thickening of the mucosa.

E. maxima: With the first two asexual cycles, tissue damage is minimal, since these cycles occur superficially in the epithelial cells of the mucosa. When the **sexual stages** develop in deeper tissues between 5th to 8th days of infection, lesions develop due to congestion and oedema, cellular infiltration, and thickening of the mucosa. *E. maxima* causes **distinct focal haemorrhagic lesions. The mid-small intestine may be flaccid and filled with fluid, containg mucus and blood.** The condition has been described as "ballooning". **Microscopic changes** are characterized by oedema and cellular infiltration, developing schizonts (day 4), and sexual stages (macrogametes and microgametes) between days 5-8, and distinctive oocysts. **The oocysts are the most characteristic. They are the largest of all chicken Eimeria** sp. **and have a golden brown-tinted oocyst wall.**

E. mitis: **The gross lesions are very slight and can be easily overlooked.** The **duodenum and lower small intestine** appear pale and flaccid. **Microscopic examination** of smears from the mucosal surface may reveal **numerous tiny oocysts.** The infection can be differentiated from *E. brunetti* by the smaller, round oocysts. In light infections, gross lesions may be similar to those of *E. brunetti.* **The lesions in this species are not prominent** because the developing parasites do not localize in colonies as do other species. Moreover, the schizonts and gametocytes are superficial in the mucosa.

E. praecox: The gross lesions consist of watery intestinal contents, and sometimes mucus and mucoid casts. **Most of the infection is confined to duodenum. Small pinpoint haemorrhages** are seen on the mucosal surface by the 4th and 5th day of infection. **Dehydration** may result from the extreme fluid loss caused by severe infections. **Little tissue reaction has been described.**

Immunity

Day-old chicks usually do not get passively transferred protective immunity from the hen, and birds of any age are susceptible to coccidiosis. Most birds acquire infection in the first few weeks of life, and this infection produces a **good immunity.** This immunity mostly persists for life due to frequent low-grade re-exposure to infection. However, **in the absence of infection, immunity may decrease.** A main feature of **immunity** is that it **is species specific. For example, immunity to** *E. maxima* **does not give resistance against** *E. tenella* **and so on.** However, within species, there is little strain variation, and strains of the same species provide substantial cross-protection, important exceptions being *E. maxima* and *E. acervulina.*

Immunity is best produced by repeated exposure to low numbers of oocysts. This is the usual situation in the field. The mechanisms of immunity are not yet fully known, but **cell-mediated responses appear to be the most important.** Secretory IgA may also contribute to protective immunity, but **circulating antibodies,** although produced, **play only a minor role.**

Diagnosis

The presence of dysentery, diarrhoea, or soft mucoid faeces suggests coccidiosis. With less pathogenic species, however, the only signs will be poor growth and impaired feed conversion. The earliest signs with the pathogenic species may be a sudden increase in daily mortality.

Postmortem examination is essential to confirm diagnosis. A few sick birds should be sacrificed for this purpose so that fresh material is available. Lesions can be seen from the serosal surface, but the mucosal surface should be examined carefully. In fact, the entire intestinal tract should be examined. It is important to demonstrate the parasite in association with lesions by examination of mucosal scrapings. Examination of wet smears diluted with isotonic saline under a coverslip with appropriate lighting is normally sufficient to detect schizonts, gamonts, and oocysts. At high power, merozoites can be distinguished. If required, thin smears can be stained to identify all stages. The finding of a few oocysts by microscopic examination of smears from the intestine indicates the presence of infection, but not a diagnosis of clinical coccidiosis. Coccidia are usually present in the intestines of birds 3-6 weeks old in most flocks. Coccidiosis should be diagnosed if the gross lesions are serious.

Cryptosporidiosis

Cryptosporidiosis is caused by protozoa of the Phylum **Apicomplexa**, genus **Cryptosporidium** (Table 37), which have similarities with **Eimeria**, but also a number of important differences. In **mammals**, infections of the **intestine** and diarrhoea are characteristic, but in **birds** the disease is usually associated with infection of the **respiratory tract**.

Cause

Two species have been described in birds, *C. baileyi* and *C. meleagridis*. *C. baileyi* causes both respiratory and intestinal disease, whereas *C. meleagridis* is associated with enteric disease only. Cryptosporidia infect chickens, turkeys, ducks, geese, and several others. Isolates do not have rigid host specificity.

Transmission

Respiratory infections result from inhalation or aspiration of oocysts that are present in the environment. Oocysts of *C. baileyi* are infective at the time they are passed, and no vectors have been identified. Since *C. baileyi* can infect a variety of birds, it is possibe that wild birds may serve as carriers. Although less common, respiratory cryptosporidiosis can be a major cause of morbidity and mortality. *C. baileyi* also produces intestinal cryptosporidiosis (cloaca and bursa of Fabricius). Oocysts are picked up from heavy faecal contamination of the litter or cages.

Life Cycle

In the parasitic phase, cryptosporidia parasitize the margin of epithelial cells. They are enclosed within the host epithelial cell membrane. In this site, asexual multiplication (schizogony) followed by gametogony (gametogeny) occur with the release of merozoites and microgametes, respectively. Following zygote formation, oocysts are shed which are already sporulated. The prepatent period is very short (3 days). Oocysts have a tough wall and are environmentally resistant.

Pathogenicity, Symptoms, and Lesions

Infections can occur in very young chicks. Disease has been reported in chickens, turkeys, ducks, quail, pheasant and others. Disease associated with enteric infection is rare. Also, intestinal disease is usually mild. No clinical signs of gastrointestinal disease occur in chickens. By contrast, respiratory infection produces a variety of clinical signs depending on the particular site involved. There may be airsacculitis, pneumonia, sinusitis or conjunctivitis, with coughing, nasal discharges, and high morbidity and mortality. In addition to increased mortality, the performance of birds with respiratory infections is also affected by lower weight gains and higher feed/gain ratios.

Histopathology of the affected chicks shows a large number of parasites throughout the epithelium lining the trachea and bronchi. Microscopic lesions include epithelial cell hyperplasia, thickening of the mucosa by mononuclear cell infiltrations with some heterophils, loss of cilia, and discharge of mucocellular exudate into the airways. Intestinal cryptosporidiosis (i.e., of cloaca and bursa of Fabricius), caused by *C. baileyi*, may produce microscopic lesions, but these do not result in gross lesions or in clinical signs of the disease.

Diagnosis

Both, respiratory and intestinal infections, can be diagnosed by identifying oocysts from fluid obtained from the respiratory tract, or from the faeces. Diagnosis can also be made from demonstration of the organisms in sections of the affected mucosal epithelium, and of cysts in stained smears from the respiratory mucosa. With a modified Ziehl-Neelsen stain, oocysts stain red, are 4-6 μm in diameter, subspherical; and should be searched using a high-power objective.

Histomoniasis

Also known as "blackhead", "infectious enterohepatitis", histoplasmosis is a disease of caeca and liver caused by the protozoan parasite *Histomonas meleagridis*. Although the disease is called "blackhead", the signs are neither pathognomonic nor characteristic of the disease, since many other diseases may produce a similar appearance. Although histomoniasis occurs in several species of birds, **it is primarily a disease of turkeys.** The turkey is considered **the most susceptible host** because **most affected turkeys die.** Sometimes, the disease **also occurs in chickens but in a milder form.** The disease is characterized by **necrotic foci in the liver** and **ulceration of the caeca.**

Life Cycle

The existence of *H. meleagridis* is closely associated with caecal nematode *Heterakis gallinarum* and several species of earthworms common in the soil of poultry premises. **Histomonads cannot survive outside the host for more than a few minutes unless protected by the heterakid egg or earthworm.** Earthworms serve as transport hosts in which heterakid eggs hatch, and the young worms survive in tissues in an infective stage. The earthworms thus serve as a means for collection and concentration of heterakid eggs from the poultry premises environment.

The parasite invades the caecal mucosa and then spreads through the blood to the liver. In **caeca** and **liver**, the parasite grows and **multiplies intracellularly,** leading to the formation of **necrotic foci** surrounded by colonies of organisms. In the caecal lumen, the parasite is flagellated and pleomorphic, but in tissues it rounds up and loses its flagellum. Histomonas does not form cysts, and there is no direct faeco-oral transmission.

Transmission

The most important natural route of transmission is within the egg of *Heterakis gallinarum.* Parasites are ingested by worms in the caecal lumen. In females, they enter into the nematode eggs which are ultimately shed in the host faeces and are available to infect further hosts. **The role of heterakids as vectors for histomonads is very important,** because they are also parasites of birds and protect the histomonad within their egg during transmission from bird to bird. The **earthworms** may also act as a transport host in which *Heterakis* larvae may hatch but remain viable and infected with histomonads in the earthworm tissues. Besides the earthworms, **insects** such as flies, grasshoppers, and crickets may serve as mechanical vectors.

Clinical Signs

In turkeys signs include anorexia, drowsiness, dropping of the wings, closed eyes, and **sulphur-yellow droppings. Blackhead** is an inaccurate term, since the head may or may not be **cyanotic,** nor it is unique to histomoniasis. It was a sign observed by those who gave the disease the name blackhead. **Mortality may be high,** reaching a peak about a week after the onset of signs. Infection in chickens may be mild and go unnoticed, or may be severe and cause high mortality. **Sulphur-coloured droppings seen in turkeys are**

seldom found in chickens, but blood caecal discharges have been observed. Sometimes, **gross pathology** in chickens may resemble caecal coccidiosis.

Lesions

Lesions first occur in the **caeca** and then in the **liver.** After tissue invasion by histomonads, caecal walls become thickened and hyperaemic (i.e., **typhlitis,** inflammation of caeca). Serous and haemorrhagic exudate from the mucosa fills the lumen of caeca and distends the walls with a caseous or cheesy core. **Ulceration of the caecal wall may lead to perforation of the organ and cause generalized peritonitis. Liver lesions** in turkeys appear as **circular depressed areas of necrosis** up to 1 cm in diameter, and are surrounded by a raised ring. **These lesions are pathognomonic.** The liver may be enlarged and discoloured green. **Microscopically,** early changes in the caecal wall include hyperaemia and heterophil infiltration. Later, large numbers of lymphocytes and macrophages infiltrate the tissues. There is a core in the caecal lumen composed of sloughed epithelium, fibrin, erythrocytes, and leukocytes along with trapped caecal ingesta. The earliest microscopic changes are seen in the **liver** by about 6-7 days of infection, and consist of small clusters of heterophils, lymphocytes, and monocytes near portal vessels. Later, hepatocytes in centres of the lesions necrose and disintegrate. Necrosis becomes increasingly severe, resulting in large areas consisting of only reticulum and cellular debris.

Diagnosis

Diagnosis can usually be made **from the characteristic gross lesions** which remain clearly visible long after death. If confirmation is required, stained sections from the periphery of liver lesions will reveal rounded up organisms. Identification of living organisms in wet preparations from caecal lesions is a little difficult. It requires fresh material and a heated microscope stage.

Avian Malaria

Avian malarial infections are caused by parasites of the genus **Plasmodium.** A number of species infect domestic poultry. Of these *P. gallinaceum* and *P. juxtanucleare* are pathogenic for **domestic fowl.** The commonest **vectors are the mosquitoes** of the genera **Culex** and **Aedes,** and to a lesser extent **Anopheles. Sporogony occurs in the vector host.**

The **clinical signs** of disease are depression, weakness, anorexia, and sometimes ataxia and incoordination. The severity of the disease varies from inapparent infection to mortality as high as 90% of the flock. The **lesions** include anaemia, splenomegaly, nephritis, oedema of the lungs, and hydropericardium. **Diagnosis** is confirmed by the recognition of the parasite in stained blood films. **Trophozoites, schizonts, and gametocytes all occur in erythrocytes.**

9

Helminthic Diseases

Parasitic helminths, or worms, are important causes of disease in all species of animals. Although in many cases they cause no serious damage to the host, these parasites are never beneficial. In some cases, they can produce severe and even fatal disease. **Their life cycles are complex;** most alternate between sexual reproduction in the **definitive (final) host** and asexual multiplication in an **intermediate host or vector.** Adult worms, once residing inside the hosts, do not multiply in number but produce eggs or larvae for the next phase of the cycle. An exception is **Strongyloides**, the larvae of which can become infective inside the intestine. **There are two important consequences of this lack of multiplication by the adult worms: 1. Disease** is usually **caused by** inflammatory r esponses against the eggs or larvae rather than the adults (e.g., **schistosomiasis**), and 2. **Disease is in proportion to the number of parasites** that affect the individual (e.g., 10 hookworms can cause little damage, whereas 1000 hookworms cause severe anaemia by consuming 100 ml of blood per day). **The effect of various helminths upon animal hosts is given main consideration in this chapter.** Life cycles, host range, immunity, and infectivity are also briefly discussed.

The parasitic helminths are classified in three phyla, as follows:

1. Phylum - **Platyhelminthes:** This includes **trematodes** or **flukes**, and the **cestodes** or **tapeworms,**

2. Phylum - **Nemathelminthes:** This i ncludes **nematodes** or **round-worms,** a nd

3. Phylum - **Acanthocephala:** This includes the **thorny-headed worms.** A few of these are important parasites of animals.

Effects of Helminthic Parasites on the Host

Helminths produce harmful effects on the hosts in a variety of ways. They may:

1. **Mechanically interfere with function**

a. Obstruct blood vessels or lymphatics

1. Right ventricle and pulmonary artery - *Dirofilaria immitis* (dogs)

2. Carotid arteries - *Elaeophora schneideri* (sheep)

3. Lymphatics - *Dracunculus insignis* (dogs)

4. Mesenteric arteries - *Strongylus vulgaris* (horses)

5. Aorta - *Spirocerca lupi* (dogs); *Strongylus vulgaris* (horses)

6. Vena cava - *Schistosoma bovis*; *S. haematobium*

b. Obstruct ducts or tracts

1. Bile duct - Liver flukes, ascarids, fringed tapeworms

2. Oesophagus - *Spirocerca lupi* (dogs)

3. Intestinal lumen - Ascarids, tapeworms

4. Respiratory tract - *Filaroides osleri, Metastrongylus apri*

5. Urinary tract - *Dioctophyma renale*

c. Attach to, or use functional tissue

1. Stomach mucosa - *Trichostrongylus axei* (sheep, cattle), *Draschia megastoma* (horses)

2. Small intestine - Hookworms

3. Caecum and large intestine - Strongyles (horses), caecal worms (dogs)

d. Act as foreign bodies, with resultant tissue reactions displacing normal structures

1. Schistosome ova (flukes)

2. Dead larvae of many nematodes - *Toxocara canis, Dirofilaria immitis*

2. Invade and displace cells and tissues, producing necrosis, loss of function and hypersensitivity reactions

a. Skin - Hookworm larvae, **Habronema** larvae, **Onchocerca** larvae, **Stephanofilaria stilesi, Elaeophora schneideri** larvae, **Rhabditis** sp.

b. Liver - Giant liver flukes, kidney worm larvae, cysticercus, echinococcus and coenurus cysts, ascarid larvae

c. Intestinal wall - Nodular worms (**Oesophagostomum** sp.), larvae of strongyles (horses)

    d. Brain and spinal cord - Coenurus, echinococcus, filaria, other helminth larvae

    e. Lung - Lungworms, ascarid larvae, hookworms

    f. Musculature - Trichinae, cysticerci

3. Suck blood and thereby cause anaemia

    a. Hookworms (dogs, cattle)

    b. Stomach worms (cattle and sheep)

4. Use food needed by the host

    a. Tapeworms

    b. Ascarids

5. Induce, or predispose to neoplasia

    a. Oesophagus - *Spirocerca lupi* (dogs)

    b. Urinary bladder - *Schistosoma haematobium* (humans)

    c. Liver - *Cysticercus fasciolaris* (rats)

6. Introduce bacterial or other infection into tissues of the host

    a. Lungs - Lungworms, ascarid larvae

    b. Intestinal wall -Hookworms, nodule worms, salmon flukes (dogs)

    c. Perirenal tissues - *Stephanurus dentatus* (pigs)

    d. Caecum - Caecal worms (histomonads of turkeys)

7. Eat up tissues of the host

    a. Ascarids

    b. Stomach worms

8. Secrete toxic products (haemolysins, histolysins, anticoagulants)

    a. Hookworms, nodule worms

    b. Stomach worms

    c. Strongyles

Identification of Helminths in Tissues

    The importance of the presence of one or more fragments of a helminth in tissue sections is difficult to interpret. To properly evaluate the significance of such a finding, it is essential to know about potentialities of the parasite. That is, about its origin, where it was going when trapped by the fixative, and what its total effect upon the host could be. Whenever possible, it is important to obtain complete, well-preserved specimens for reference to a parasitologist, if required. However, presumptive identification of the parasite can usually be made from fragments of the organism in tissues. Although not fully dependable, **information on the appearance of helminths in tissue sections is now considered sufficient to permit the identification of many species.**

In identifying a parasite in tissue, **several factors may be used** to narrow the field of consideration. These include, the host and its usual parasites; the anatomical location of a parasite; the nature of the tissue reaction; **and most important, the morphological features of the parasite.** Helminths must also be differentiated from arthropods and pentastomids (see "**arthropod diseases**", Chapter 10).

Nematodes have an **external cuticle** supported by a thin membrane, the **hypodermis.** Within the hypodermis is a muscular wall surrounding the **body cavity.** Nematodes have an alimentary canal **and the sexes are separate. All these features can be seen in cross sections of the adults,** and in some cases, of the larvae. The mid-somatic muscular wall of the nematodes has some distinguishing features. The muscle cells are arranged longitudinally in a single layer just within the hypodermis. In cross section of most species, **muscle cells** are visibly divided into four groups by **chords** (cords of cells) **of the hypodermis.** These chords project towards the centre. Thus, **one dorsal, one ventral, and two lateral chords** are formed by the hypodermis. These cells differ characteristically in size and number in different species. When numerous long slender muscle cells, running lengthwise along the body wall, protrude into the body cavity and are divided into four longitudinal units (by dorsal, ventral, and lateral chords), **nematodes** are said to have a **polymyarian somatic musculature** (**Ascaris, Filaria,** and **Dracunculus**). Those **nematodes** with closely packed, somewhat flattened muscle cells in units of three or four cells are classified **meromyarian,** and include such genera as **Ancylostoma, Enterobius,** and **Necator.** In a **third group of nematodes,** the muscle cells, although closely packed, are not divided by chords, and the body cavity is completely surrounded by longitudinally running muscle cells. This group is classified as **holomyarian,** and includes the genus **Trichuris.**

The eggs or larvae can be helpful in the identification of some adult parasites in tissues. Sections are usually made through the **ovary or uterus of adult worms,** in which numerous **ova or larvae** are present. The size, shape, and shell of many ova are characteristic for the species; for example, the ovoid egg with double-contoured shell of **Strongylus,** the single polar eminence of ova of **Oxyuris,** and the double polar eminence of ova of **Capillaria.** Nematodes in which the ova embryonate and hatch in the uterus and the larvae escape as free forms, are called **viviparous (Dirofilaria).** Others are **ovoviviparous.** That is, they produce ova which are embryonated, but the larvae are still within the eggshell when they are expelled from the parasite

(Spirocerca).

Trematodes and cestodes can be usually differentiated from nematodes in tissue sections. They are flat dorso-ventrally and they do not have a body cavity. However, some of the forms may be suspended in a bladder (see cysticerci). **Most of them are hermaphroditic.** Therefore, **male and female sex organs** can usually be seen in tissue sections of a single parasite. The anatomical site in which cestodes and trematodes are found, the nature of the tissue reaction they produce, and their structural forms are often useful in the tentative identification of these parasites in tissues. **Thus, knowledge of their life cycle, host range, and morphology are an asset to the pathologist.**

The **cestodes** possess a specialized structure, the **scolex.** This can usually be detected in larval forms and also in adults in sections. The scolex may have two or more elongated suctorial (i.e., adapted for sucking) grooves, or they may have cup-shaped sucking discs and a proboscis. **In some species, the proboscis is armed with characteristic hooklets.** An external cuticle, from which **scolices** or **brood capsules** containing scolices may arise, also serves to identify cestodes in tissue sections. The **body of cestodes** is almost always **segmented.** The outer longitudinal muscles are separated from the inner circular muscles by parenchyma. Within parenchyma are suspended calcareous corpuscles. **Cestodes lack a digestive tract.**

In contrast to cestodes, trematodes are leaf-shaped and non-segmented. They contain a digestive tract, lack calcareous corpuscles, and the longitudinal and circular muscle layers are close to one another. Their **cuticle** is usually thinner than that of cestodes. **The eggs of trematodes are also characteristic.** They are usually **pigmented, operculated,** and anisotropic (birefringent). The presence of some trematodes in the body should be determined by the identification of the **ova of the parasite,** even though the adult is not found. This is particularly important in schistosomiasis, in which many ova are carried by the bloodstream to various organs, where they become embedded in small granulomas. Some of the filarid worms are rarely seen in adult form in the tissues, **but their larval forms are sufficient for diagnosis.**

Evasion of the Immune Response by Helminths

Although there are a number of mechanisms by which animals resist helminth infection, **these responses are not very effective. Successfully adapted helminths can survive and function in the presence of a fully functional host immune system.** Several mechanisms play a role in this adaptation. These include **loss of antigenicity by molecular mimicry or absorption of host antigens, interference with antigen presentation, antigenic variation, shedding of the glycocalyx, and immunosuppression.**

Helminths become gradually less antigenic as they adapt themselves in

the presence of a functioning immune system. Natural selection favours parasites which show reduced antigenicity. *Haemonchus contortus* has become less antigenic for sheep, its natural host, than for rabbits, which it does not normally infect. Also, to bring about the loss of antigenicity, helminths may synthesize and express host antigens on their surface ("**molecular mimicry**"). (Molecular mimicry is development by parasites of molecules whose structure closely resembles molecules found in their host. **In this way the parasites may be able to escape destruction by the host's immune system**). For example, they may synthesize blood group antigens in order to match those of their host. Many trematodes and cestodes can synthesize blood group antigens. Tissue helminths reduce their antigenicity by adsorbing host antigens onto their surface and thus mask (hide or disguise) parasitic antigens. This is seen in adult *Taenia solium* infestations in pigs, where the parasites are coated with IgG.

Other helminths interfere with antigen presentation. Thus, macrophages from schistosome-infected animals are incompetent as antigen-presenting cells. Filarial worms secrete inhibitors that can block macrophage proteases. *Taenia taeniaeformis* secretes **taeniastatin**, a protein inhibitor which inhibits neutrophil chemotaxis, T cell proliferation, and interleukin-2 production. Some parasites, such as *Fasciola hepatica*, can secrete proteases that destroy host immunoglobulins.

Another mechanism of evasion of the immune response involves **antigenic variation**. Although helminths have not developed a system similar to that seen with trypanosomes, **gradual antigenic variation does occur**. For example, the circulating antigens of *Trichinella spiralis* larvae are extensively altered following each moult. Some parasites, such as *Fasciola hepatica*, shed their glycocalyx and thus their surface antigens, when exposed to specific antibodies.

Yet another mechanism that contributes to the survival of parasitic helminths is **immunosuppression**. Sheep infected with *Haemonchus contortus* may become specifically suppressed so that they are unreactive to *H. contortus* even though they remain responsive to unrelated antigens. The mechanisms involved in this immunosuppression are unknown. *Ostertagia ostertagi* and *Trichostrongylus axei* infestations result in depressed lymphocyte blastogenic responses in calves. *Oesophagostomum radiatum* secretes soluble factors that inhibit the responses of lymphocytes to antigens and mitogens.

Host Response to Parasites

It is obvious from the above that **parasites are very clever at avoiding the host's immune system**. This allows their development and persistence. **Most infections with helminths are chronic**. Those parasites which live in the lumen of the intestinal tract or in airways, such as **adult ascarids or**

Paragonimus, do not come in direct contact with humoral and cellular immune mechanisms. **Therefore, they escape the immune attack.** However, even intravascular parasites, which should be the most prone to attack, may escape immune destruction. Adult *Dirofilaria immitis* may remain viable within pulmonary arteries for long periods of time. Those parasites which live in tissue, or spend part of their life cycles migrating through tissue, also usually remain free from immune attack.

As discussed, **there are several mechanisms which allow parasites to escape immune destruction.** Like certain protozoa (e.g., trypanosomes), helminths change their appearance, that is, disguise themselves, **through antigenic variation.** They thus deceive the humoral and cellular immune responese by presenting their false appearance or camouflage. **This allows them to complete their maturation.** The migrating larvae proceed without interference **on first encounter,** producing tissue damage mainly from mechanical injury. However, on **repeated exposure** this mechanism begins to fail, and fewer larvae reach their final destination as adults. **Parasites may also acquire surface antigens that are very similar to those of their hosts, which help them escape immune destruction.** Exposure to helminths *in utero* also imparts a degree of unresponsiveness on the part of the host's immune system. Certain parasites also **secrete substances that suppress immune function and the inflammatory response. Thus, helminths may migrate through tissues or live as adults with a minimal tissue reaction.**

This does not mean that an immune response does not exist, nor that it is not important. Helminths contain a wide range of antigens that do produce both humoral and cellular immunity. It is this response which provides some degree of immunity to challenge in previously exposed individuals. These antigens also promote expulsion of adult worms from the intestinal tract, and the formation of the inflammatory lesions which surround helminth eggs, larvae, and adults in tissue. Severity of the response depends on the parasite, its site, and whether or not there has been previous exposure. The type of inflammatory response is highly variable, and **includes all forms of inflammatory reaction, from purulent to granulomatous.** A unique feature of many parasitisms is the occurrence of eosinophils both in the inflammatory and immune responses, and in the circulation. **Eosinophils seem to be particularly important to the host's defence against helminthic parasites,** releasing their cytotoxic granules on the parasite's surface.

Destruction of Parasitic Helminths by Eosinophils

One of the functions of eosinophils is the destruction of parasitic helminths. Eosinophils contain two major types of granule: small, **primary granules,** and crystalloid granules. The main protein in the crystalloid granule is **major basic protein (MBP),** which is **directly toxic to a number of**

helminthic and protozoal parasites. The eosinophil is able to recognize parasites after they a re coated w ith complement (**C3b), IgG, or even IgE** (i.e., **antibody-coated**) through **specific membrane receptors** for these molecules. **Eosinophils possess Fc receptors** which specifically bind to antibody. Binding occurs between the parasite and eosinophil through these **receptor-ligand interactions.** In other words, because eosinophils possess Fc receptors, they bind to antibody-coated parasites. O nce bound, eosinophils degranulate a nd release their granule contents onto the worm cuticle, which include **superoxide, hydrogen peroxide and other free radicals and lytic enzymes,** s uch as **lysophospholipase** and **phospholipase D.** The p arasite is then k illed by eosinophil d egranulation. T he c rystalloid granule contents, s uch a s **MBP, eosinophil cationic protein, and eosinophil-derived neurotoxin are directly toxic to parasites and d estroy them.** MBP can damage the cuticles of schistosomula, **Fasciola,** and **Trichinella** at vey low concentrations. **Eosinophil cationic protein** is a ribonuclease which is lethal for helminths. **Eosinophil-derived neurotoxin** is also a ribonuclease which is slightly toxic for parasitic helminths.

Trematodes (Flukes)

Trematodiasis (Distomiasis)

Trematodes are flat worms in the Phylum **Platyhelminthes.** Most a re **leaf-like in shape and have one or two suckers.** T he term "distoma", t he former name of a specific genus, is now synonymous with trematode. There are three sub-classes of the trematodes, but all that are parasitic in domestic animals, lie within the subclass **Digenea. Each has an indirect life cycle.**

Life Cycle

In the typical life cycle, the hermaphroditic parasites (i.e., having reproductive o rgans of b oth sexes) deposit **ova** which pass through t he faeces. Fluke **eggs** are **usually operculated** and yellow-brown. These features help in their i dentification in tissue sections. **Each ovum,** under warm moist conditions, produces a free-living ciliated larva **(miracidium).** The miracidium either bores into the body (i.e., enters by making a hole), or is ingested by one of the several varieties of **snails.** In the snails, they encyst (i.e., form a cyst) to become **a sporocyst.** The sporocyst reproduces asexually to produce **daughter sporocysts,** or several generations of **rediae.** These begin to look like an adult fluke. The final stages in the snail are m otile **cercariae.** These l eave the intermediate host and usually encyst on plants to become the infective stage **(metacercariae).** M any flukes r equire **a second intermediate host** (e.g., *Dicrocoelium dendriticum*) in which the metacercariae are formed. **Infection in the final host occurs by ingestion of the metacercariae. T hose flukes which live in the liver are the most important for animals.** Flukes may **also live in the intestinel tract, pancreatic ducts, lungs, and veins** (schistosomes or blood flukes). **Tables 45** and **46** present important trematodes of animals.

Table 45. Important species of trematodes (flukes) in domestic animals

Trematode	Host	Site of Adult	Intermediate Host(s)
Family: Fasciolidae			
Fasciola hepatica	Cattle, sheep, goat, dog, cat, horse, humans	Bile ducts	Snail
Fasciola gigantica	Cattle, sheep	Bile ducts	Snail
Fascioloides magna	Cattle, sheep, horse, pig	Liver	Snail
Family: Dicrocoeliidae			
Dicrocoelium dendriticum	Sheep, goats, pig, dog, deer	Bile ducts	Snail, ant
Eurytrema pancreaticum	Sheep, goat, cattle	Pancreatic and bile, ducts duodenum	Snail, grasshopper, crickets
Family: Paragonimidae			
Paragonimus westermani	Dog, cat, pig	Lungs	Snail, crayfish
P. kellicotti	Dog, cat, pig	Lungs	Snail, crayfish
Family: Paramphistomatidae			
Paramphistomum cervi and other species	Cattle, sheep, goat	Rumen	Snail
Calicophoron calicophorum	Cattle, sheep, goat	Rumen	Snail
Cotylophoron cotylophorum	Cattle, sheep, goat	Rumen	Snail
Ceylonocotyle streptocoelium	Cattle, sheep, goat	Rumen	Snail
Family: Schistosomatidae	-	see Table 46	

Hepatic Distomiasis

Hepatic distomiasis includes **"fascioliasis"** or **"liver fluke disease"**, **"fascioloidiasis"**, and **"dicrocoeliasis"**. Liver flukes are important pathogens of domestic animals, particularly sheep and cattle, and are widely prevalent in India.The most important species are *Fasciola hepatica* (common liver f luke), *Fasciola g igantica* (large A frican l iver f luke), and *Dicrocoelium dendriticum* (lancet fluke). Many other species also infect the liver of various animals. Some of these are briefly discussed under "hepatic distomiasis in dogs and cats".

Fascioliasis

Fascioliasis is a very important disease of cattle in India. *Fasciola hepatica* in its adult form is found in the liver, bile ducts, and gallbladder in cattle and sheep. However, it may also occur in the horse (rarely), goat, dog, cat, pig, deer, and even humans. The adult fluke is 20-30 mm long and about 13 mm wide. It is flattened and leaf-like, and usually reddish-brown. It is a hermaphrodite and reproduces by d epositing o va in t he b iliary passages, through which they reach the intestine and are then passed in the faeces. The life cycle, which is typically the same described earlier, uses several species of snails of the genus Lymnaea. Following ingestion, infective metacercariae encyst in the duodenum, penetrate the wall, and migrate through the abdominal cavity to the liver. The immature flukes in the liver migrate for about six months and begin to reach the bile ducts, where they become adults during the seventh w eek.

Fasciola gigantica resembles *Fasciola hepatica*, but is larger. The adults measure up to 75 mm in length and about 12 mm wide. These flukes are common parasites of cattle and sheep. The intermediate hosts are also species of Lymnaea.

Fascioloides magna, the large liver fluke, occurs in the liver of cattle, sheep, horse, deer, and rarely pig. It has been reported in the lungs of some of these hosts. The fluke is similar in appearance to *Fasciola hepatica*, except that it is larger (30 by 80 mm in greatest dimension), and has more rounded ends. It is a hermaphrodite, and its life cycle is similar to that of *Fasciola hepatica*. Snails are required as intermediate hosts. The infective forms penetrate the intestinal wall, and wander around in the peritoneal cavity before invading the liver.

Clinical Signs

Fascioliasis occurs in three forms: 1. Chronic, which is rarely fatal in cattle, but is usually fatal in sheep, 2. Subacute, and 3. Acute. Subacute and acute forms mainly occur in sheep and are usually fatal. Fascioliasis in cattle and sheep ranges in severity from a fatal disease in sheep to an asymptomatic infection in cattle. The course is usually determined by the numbers of metacercariae ingested o ver a s hort p eriod. In s heep, a cute fascioliasis i s manifested by a d istended, p ainful abdomen, a naemia, a nd s udden death. Deaths can occur within 6 weeks of infection. In subacute disease, survival is longer (7-10 weeks), even in cases with great damage to livers, but deaths occur due to haemorrhage and anaemia. **In chronic fascioliasis of cattle** signs include anaemia, unthriftiness, **submandibular oedema**, and reduced milk secretion. **But even heavily infected cattle may show no clinical signs.** Heavy chronic infection is fatal in **sheep**.

Lesions

Lesions produced **by** *F. hepatica* are most constant and **important in liver**, although occasional parasites may wander into the **lungs** or other tissues. **The lesions in the liver can be divided into**: 1. Those **caused by the migrating larvae**, and 2. Those **caused by the adults. However, the effects of both may occur together**. After penetration of the liver parenchyma by the flukes, hepatic cells are destroyed as the larvae migrate, **and produce tracts of blood, fibrin, and cellular debris**. These tracts soon become filled with neutrophils, eosinophils, and lymphocytes. Macrophages, epithelioid cells, and multinucleated giant cells become numerous in older lesions, particularly around the dead larvae. **The lesions finally heal by the growth of granulation tissue, causing random scarring (scar formation).** If the animal is exposed to a large number of **metacercariae**, this early migration results in **extensive liver damage**, causing an **acute disease** characterized by anaemia, eosinophilia, peritonitis (due to initial migration), and **sudden death. This acute syndrome is more common in sheep than in cattle.**

Flukes that reach the bile ducts, start producing eggs by the tenth week following oral infection. Their presence in the biliary passages stimulates considerable tissue reaction, leading to **cholangio-hepatitis** (inflammation of the bile ducts and liver). The biliary epithelium is stimulated to papillary and glandular hyperplasia. The walls of the ducts become infiltrated with eosinophils, lymphocytes, and macrophages, and ultimately become thickened from fibrous proliferation. Partial or complete occlusion of the bile ducts is a common effect. **Extensive fibrosis and calcification of the bile ducts**, most common **in cattle**, gives rise to the term "pipe-stem liver". Small granulomas may form around **eggs** that become lodged in small bile ducts.

Extensive infection interferes with liver function. This causes **weight loss, or failure to gain normally**. Raised hepatic serum enzymes, eosinophilia, hypoproteinaemia, and anaemia are common findings. **Anaemia** results from haemorrhage both into the migrating larval tracts, as well as from blood-sucking by the adults and haemorrhage into the bile ducts. The anaemia may be normocytic, normochromic, macrocytic, or have the characteristics of iron deficiency anaemia. The effects of *Fasciola gigantica* are similar to those caused by *Fasciola hepatica*.

The migration of *Fascioloides magna* within the liver parenchyma produces severe damage in some animals, and less in others. In the **"true" host** (deer), the parasite is well-tolerated. Although it soon becomes encysted, the cyst wall is thin and its lumen communicates with bile ducts. Thus, ova of the fluke escape with its excreta into the intestinal lumen of the host. This favours the completion of the life cycle of the parasite.

In cattle, the flukes wander briefly through the liver parenchyma. They destroy tissue and stimulate a reaction which encapsulates the parasites. A cyst soon forms, but its lumen rarely communicates with the bile ducts. **As a result, excreta and ova accumulate around the fluke.** Black granular pigment collects in the cyst, and is phagocytized by the macrophages of the host. This characteristic pigment is part of the excrement of the fluke. **The black pigment** is usually grossly visible in affected liver. **In sheep**, migration of this large liver fluke (**F. magna**) through the liver is virtually unchecked. Therefore, **severe tissue destruction and marked clinical disease result.** A severe neutrophilic and eosinophilic tissue reaction, with little encapsulation, is the rule in the liver of infected sheep. **Even a few flukes**, by their migrations through the liver, **produce severe symptoms and death in sheep.** They also migrate in and out of the vascular system. This causes phlebitis, arteritis, and thrombosis, which further aggravate hepatic damage. The death of the animal brings to a halt the life cycle of the parasite. **Therefore, sheep is not considered a true host for *F. magna*.**

Diagnosis

Fascioliasis can be diagnosed in the living animal **by the identification of characteristic ova in the faeces.** The **oval, operculated, golden brown eggs** must be differentiated from those of **paramphistomes (rumen flukes),** which are larger and clear. Eggs of *F. hepatica* cannot be demonstrated in faeces during acute fascioliasis. In subacute or chronic disease, the number varies from day to day and **repeated faecal examination may be required. At postmortem, the lesions in the liver are diagnostic.** Adult flukes are easily found in the liver parenchyma or affected bile ducts. The immature stages may be squeezed from the cut surface.

Dicrocoeliasis

Dicrocoelium dendriticum (lancet fluke) is capable of infecting **cattle, sheep, goats, horses, pigs, dogs, camels, deer,** and **humans. This parasite is smaller than the other flukes.** It is 5-12 mm long and about 1 mm wide. It is slender, flat, and lancet-shaped, with pointed ends.

In the **life cycle**, the parasite requires not only a **snail** as intermediate host, but also an **ant** (*Formica fusca*) as a **second intermediate host.** The final **hosts are infected by the ingestion of ants containing encysted metacercariae.** When released in the small intestine, the **metacercariae** migrate to the liver through the common bile duct. **The adult flukes are found in the bile ducts of** the definitive (final) host. The infection is **less severe than** that of *Fasciola hepatica*. Also, because they are smaller, they are found in smaller bile ducts. Hyperplasia of bile duct epithelium occurs. **The walls of the bile ducts become thickened**, and general periportal fibrosis may be produced by the parasite. Liver parenchyma is rarely destroyed. **Clinical signs are not present**, but may be seen in massive infections. Dicrocoeliasis can be **diagnosed** by the identification of **characteristic ova in the faeces**. At postmortem, the parasite can be found in the affected bile ducts.

Hepatic Distomiasis in Dogs and Cats

Hepatic distomiasis in dogs and cats is **caused by several different flukes**. *Metorchis conjunctis* is the **most common**, and **lives in bile ducts**. It causes **cholangio-hepatitis** characterized by biliary necrosis, hyperplasia, eosinophilic and mononuclear infiltration and fibrosis. It requires two intermediate hosts: a snail and a suckerfish. Other species which affect the bile ducts include: *Platynosomum fastosum* in cats; *Metorchis albidis* of dogs; *Clonorchis sinensis* of dogs, cats, pigs, and humans; *Opisthorchis tenuicollis* of dogs, cats, foxes, and pigs; *Pseudamphistomum truncatum* of dogs, cats, foxes, and humans, **reported also in India**; and *Concinnum procyonis* of cats and foxes.

Infestation with any of these flukes may lead to **cholangio-hepatitis**. Some have a strong association with **cholangiosarcoma**, particularly *Clonorchis sinensis* infection in **humans**.

Paramphistomiasis

Also known as "**stomach fluke disease**", the intestinal phase of amphistomiasis is a common parasitic disease of **cattle**, and to a lesser extent, **sheep**. It is caused by **paramphistome flukes**, and characterized by **severe enteritis**. As a serious disease, **intestinal amphistomiasis has been recorded in cattle, sheep, and also goats in India. Cattle are most commonly affected**, and the mortality rate in heavily infected animals may be as high as 96%. The mortality rate in **sheep** has been as high as 90%. **Cattle, sheep**, and **goats** of all ages may be affected, **but young cattle are the usual subjects**. It appears that some degree of immunity develops. Perhaps that is why the disease is uncommon in adults. *Paramphistomum cervi* and other species, *Calicophoron calicophorum*, *Cotylophoron cotylophorum*, and *Ceylonocotyle streptocoelium* are the commonly recorded species in **cattle, sheep**, and **goat** (**Table 45**).

Life Cycle

All these flukes have aquatic planorbid (fresh water) **snails** as hosts. The **immature flukes** excyst (come out of the cyst) in the **duodenum**, and as they mature, migrate through the abomasum to the **rumen** and **reticulum**. The period required for maturation varies from 6 weeks to 4 months.

Pathogenicity

Adult (or mature) flukes in the rumen and reticulum appear to cause little harm and do not produce clinical disease, even though present in large numbers. Clinical illness is produced only when there are numerous numbers of the immature flukes in the duodenum and abomasum. The migrating flukes set up an acute enteritis. The immature worms attach to the duodenal, and at times, ileal mucosa by means of a large posterior sucker and cause severe enteritis, possibly necrosis, and haemorrhage.

Clinical Signs

Immature flukes cause a persistent fetid diarrhoea which is characteristic. It is accompanied by weakness, depression, dehydration, and anaemia. There may also be submaxillary oedema and visible paleness of the mucosa. Death usually occurs 15-20 days after the first signs appear.

A syndrome has also been described in heavy infestations with adult flukes. The disease is chronic, and signs include loss of weight, anaemia, rough dry coat, and a drop in production.

Lesions

There is subcutaneous oedema, and accumulation of fluid in the body cavities. The fat depots are gelatinous. Mucosa in the upper part of the duodenum is thickened, covered with blood-stained mucus, and there are patches of haemorrhage under the serosa. A large number of small, flesh-coloured flukes are present in this area, but decrease towards the ileum. There may be none in the abomasum and forestomachs, but a few in the peritoneal cavity. On microscopic examination, the young (immnature) flukes are present not only on the mucosal surface, but are also embedded in the mucosa and deeper layers.

Diagnosis

The large, clear, operculated eggs are easily recognized, but in acute paramphistomiasis there may be no eggs in the faeces. Thus, intestinal amphistomiasis can be easily missed because immature flukes, which usually cause disease, do not lay eggs. Diagnosis is therefore usually possible at postmortem. Even at postmortem, the small parasites can be missed.

Paragonimiasis

Small reddish-brown, egg-shaped flukes of the genus Paragonimus are important parasites of humans and animals (Table 45). These flukes are 8-12 mm long and 4-6 mm in diameter. They are hermaphroditic and have a spiny cuticle. Two species are important: *Paragonimus westermani* which occurs in a variety of animal species, including humans; and *P. kellicotti* which occurs in cats, dogs, and pigs. The adults of *P. kellicotti* are found in pairs in lung

cysts, and m ay or m ay not c ommunicate with b ronchi. The c ysts are l ined with b ronchial epithelium, a nd surrounded b y granulomatous i nflammation. Released eggs lodge in the **pulmonary p arenchyma** and stimulate an **eosinophilic granulomatous response**. Eggs c an also e nter the c irculation and lodge in a variety of organs producing **granulomas**. Rarely, adult flukes lodge in other tissues, such as brain.

The **life cycle** involves **two intermediate hosts: snail** and **crayfish. Eggs** that reach the bronchi are coughed up, swallowed, and expelled with the faeces. The eggs are thick-walled and operculated. **Miracidia** develop slowly in these ova, hatch into water, and then burrow into freshwater **snails. Cercariae** that escape the snail then penetrate **crayfish. Metacercariae** released from ingested crayfish encyst in the duodenum. Immature flukes bore through the duodenal wall and reach the lungs through migration in the peritoneal and pleural cavities. This migration can lead to peritonitis and pleuritis.

Eurytrema pancreaticum

Eurytrema pancreaticum is **a small red fluke** which **lives in the pancreatic duct of sheep, goats, cattle,** and b uffaloes. I t may also parasitize **humans.** The flukes are slightly over 1 cm long. When present in large numbers, they may cause fibrosis of the duct and the acinar tissue. Erosion of the mucosa may allow **eggs** to enter tissue, where they stimulate **granulomas**.

Schistosomiasis

The schistosomes, or blood flukes, affect both humans and animals, causing serious disease worldwide. The adults of most schistosomes live i n **portal** and **mesenteric veins**, others reside in **pelvic veins.** *Schistosoma nasalis* resides in **veins of the nasal cavity. Table 46** presents certain characteristics of important blood flukes of humans and animals.

Table 46. Important Schistosomes of Humans and Animals

Species	Host	Location	Remarks
Schistosoma bovis	Cattle, sheep, goat, horse, mule, antelope	Portal and mesenteric veins	Africa, India
S. haematobium	Humans, monkey	Pelvic veins	Africa, Western Asia, Europe, Australia
S. hippopotami	Hippopotamus	Cardiovascular system	South Africa
S. incognitum	Dog, pig	Mesenteric and portal veins	India

S. indicum	Cattle, sheep, goat, horse, camel	Mesenteric, portal and pelvic veins	India
S. intercalatum	Humans, horse, cattle, sheep	Mesenteric and portal veins	Africa
S. japonicum	Humans, dog, cat, cattle, sheep, buffalo, goat, horse, pig	Mesenteric and portal veins, haemorrhoidal plexus	China, Japan, Taiwan, Philippines
S. mansoni	Humans, monkey	Mesenteric and portal veins, haemorrhoidal plexus	Africa, South Africa
S. mattheei	Cattle, sheep, goat, horse, and rarely humans	Mesenteric and portal veins	Africa
S. nasalis	Cattle, goat, horse	Nasal veins	India
S. spindale	Cattle, sheep, goat, buffalo, dog, antelope	Mesenteric and portal veins	India, Africa, Indonesia
Ornithobilharzia bomfordi	Zebu cattle	Mesenteric veins	India
O. turkestanicum	Cattle, sheep, goat, horse, camel, cat	Mesenteric veins	Eurasia (i.e., Europe and Asia)

These worms **are small trematodes** which **live in the blood vessels** of their hosts. Their **ova**, which **circulate as emboli** and lodge in tissue as foreign bodies **produce the main pathological changes** in the host. The females are slender round worms, 1.4-2.0 cm in length. **The characteristic feature of the slightly shorter male is a long gynecophoric canal**, a canoe-shaped structure in which the female is held during coitus. Schistosomes are grouped in the Family **Schistosomatidae (Table 45)**.

Life Cycle

All blood flukes have similar life cycles. The adult female first copulates with the male within the lumen of a vein. **After copulation**, she moves against the venous bloodstream into small venules, where she **deposits the ova**. Schistosomes which live in the **mesenteric veins** (*S. bovis, S. japonicum*, and *S. mansoni*) deposit their ova in the venules of the intestine. Those which live in the **pelvic veins** (*S. haematobium*, and sometimes *S. mansoni*) use venules of the urinary bladder (vesical veins). The deposited ova secrete cytolytic fluid through p ores of t he eggshell. T his fluid a nd movement o f the h ost's tissues enable ova to rupture the capillary walls. The **ova** then move through the tissues towards t he l umen of t he intestine or the urinary b ladder. The successful ova leave the body o f the h ost with the faeces (*S. japonicum*, *S. bovis*, and *S. mansoni*). Unsuccessful ova may remain in those tissues through which they are unable to pass. Or, they may b e transported through the bloodstream to other organs, **where they produce lesions. Fertile ova do not hatch in the tissues of the host.** However, upon reaching a favourable external environment, a **miracidium** (an ovoid ciliated organism) quickly escapes from the ovum. The miracidium swims in the water until it finds a suitable **intermediate host, a snail,** whose body it penetrates by a boring action with the aid of **proteolytic enzymes** secreted by its cephalic glands.

Within the body of the snail, the miracidium soon becomes a thin-walled **sporocyst** which reproduces several **daughter sporocysts.** Each of these secondary sporocysts releases thousands of tiny fork-tailed organisms, **cercariae.** The c ercariae wander t hrough the t issues of t he snail, s ometimes killing i t, and finally emerge i nto the surrounding water. T hese cercariae m ust find a suitable definitive host in order to carry their life cycle further. On meeting such a host, cercariae penetrate the skin, where they undergo structural changes to become immature flukes, called "**schistosomula**". These are **carried by the venous circulation to the lungs,** and then through the arterial system to the **liver.** Within the intrahepatic portal system the flukes grow in size, **and then depending upon the species, migrate to the portal, mesenteric, or pelvic veins.** Here, they attain their adult form and continue the reproductive cycle.

Clinical Signs

The main clinical signs associated with the **intestinal and hepatic forms of schistosomiasis in ruminants** develop after the ova begin to pass out in the faeces, and consist of h aemorrhagic enteritis, anaemia, and emaciation. **Severely affected animals** deteriorate rapidly, and **usually die within a few months of infection.** Those less heavily infected develop chronic disease and may r ecover eventually. Many o lder cattle i n e ndemic areas may h ave a n effective level o f immunity a gainst reinfection. N asal schistosomiasis is a **chronic disease of cattle, horses, and sometimes buffaloes.** In severe cases, there i s a c opious mucopurulent discharge, s noring, a nd d yspnoea. M ilder cases are usually asymptomatic.

Lesions

It is obvious from the life cycle that **damage to the host can result from three factors:** 1. from the **presence of adults in the veins,** 2. from the **presence of ova in veins or tissues,** and 3. from **penetration of cercariae in the skin.**

The adult blood flukes, which live within the veins, may produce phlebitis, with intimal proliferation and sometimes venous thrombosis. **Vascular lesions are severe when the adult worms die**, or are trapped in unusual sites. The adult schistosomes also consume erythrocytes and discharge **blood pigment**. The pigment is engulfed by macrophages, and may be found in reticuloendothelial cells in the **liver** and **spleen**. This **pigment** appears in the cytoplasm of macrophages **as black granules**, somewhat similar to that seen in association with certain liver flukes.

The ova are the most important factors in the production of lesions. The ova deposited in the venules reach venous capillaries. **They adhere to the endothelium and become embedded within it**. Then they rupture the basement membrane by means of enzymes secreted through the pores of the eggshell by the **miracidium** within, and escape into the tissues to make their way to the lumen of the intestine or urinary bladder. **This migration causes small haemorrhagic ulcers**, which in extensive infestations may lead to frank **haemorrhage, anaemia**, and **hypoproteinaemia**.

However, most eggs do not escape to the outside. Instead, they become embedded in tissues and **stimulate an extreme immunological response to carbohydrate antigens released by the eggs**. The carbohydrate antigens from eggs induce macrophage accumulation and granuloma formation. **Thus, the hypersensitivity reaction** leads to the formation of **granulomas** composed of neutrophils, lymphocytes, macrophages, and multinucleated giant cells. The **granuloma formation is mediated by tumour necrosis factor (TNF) and Th1 and Th2 helper cells. These granulomas or "pseudotubercles" are a characteristic feature of schistosomiasis**. They may be widespread, and lead to **extensive tissue damage**. They are especially prominent in the wall of the **intestine** and throughout the **liver**, as ova move up the portal veins into the hepatic parenchyma. **Cirrhosis** follows extensive hepatic involvement. Other ova may enter into the general circulation to be distributed widely throughout the body. These ova also stimulate **granuloma** which may be found in the **spleen, lungs, brain**, or **any other organ of the body**.

With time, the eggs die and the host response diminishes. This leads to **healing**, which may leave **a small scar**. Within each granuloma lies an ovoid, **schistosome egg**, with a thick, hyaline, unstained, or yellow wall. Sometimes a single **spine** may be seen protruding from this wall. This spine is located along the lateral surface in ova of *S. mansoni* and at one terminal pole in *S. haematobium, S. bovis, S. indicum, S. intercalatum, S. nasalis*, and *S. spindale*. Spine is lateral, small, and not prominent on the ova of *S. japonicum*. The nature and location of the spine can be used to identify the type of infection. Microscopic sections of ova may contain parts of the **miracidium**, but in older lesions only the eggshell may be left. The eggshell is usually ruptured, and only a fragment may be present. However, the tissue reaction and microscopic appearance of the eggshell are characteristic. The Ziehl-Neelsen stain is useful in differentiating some schistosome eggs. Eggs of **S. *mansoni*, S. *nasalis*** and **S. *intercalatum*** are **acid-fast**, whereas **S. *spindale*, S. *indicum*, S. *haematobium*, S. *mattheei*, S. *japonicum***, and **S. *bovis*** are **negative**.

Cutaneous lesions develop in humans and animals from penetration of the skin by the cercariae. The intensity of the tissue reaction depends on the sensitivity and resistance of the host to the parasite. As the cercariae reach dermis, a leukocytic reaction of varying intensity results, having neutrophils, lymphocytes, and eosinophils. This is accompanied by **urticaria, itching,** and the formation of tiny **nodules** which raise the epidermis. In sensitized animals or humans, a severe tissue reaction occurs, and death of the parasite in the dermis may produce a prolonged local tissue reaction. **Cercariae** even have the ability to **penetrate the epidermis** of hosts in which complete development of the fluke does not occur. **In such a case, cercariae die in the dermis.** This is the basis of "**cercarial dermatitis**", also known as "**swimmer's itch**" "**collector's itch**" and "swamp itch". It is a problem to individuals exposed to infected waters, such as, agricultural workers, swimmers.

In humans, carcinoma of the urinary bladder is a common complication of vesicular schistosomiasis. The carcinomas are usually squamous cell type arising in metaplastic epithelium. The exact causal relationship has not been established. **S. *japonicum*** infection of humans has also been associated with **hepatocellular carcinoma**.

Diagnosis

Clinical diagnosis can be confirmed by **demonstration of schistosome ova in the faeces, or by histopathological examination** of biopsy specimens of rectal mucosa, liver, or other affected organs. The adult parasite may be found in veins at postmortem. Typical ova in granulomas can be demonstrated by microscopic examintion of specimens collected at postmortem, or biopsy.

Cestodes (Tapeworms)

Cestodiasis

Cestodiasis, also known as "**tapeworm disease**" and "**taeniasis**", is caused by cestodes. **Cestodes**, or **tapeworms** (Phylum **Platyhelminthes**, Class: **Cestoda**) are common **parasites of all vertebrate animals, and also humans.** The adult forms in the intestinal tract of the definitive (final) host are **flat worms** made up of a chain of independent, hermaphroditic segments (**proglottieds**). The proglottides are joined together, and usually they attach to the intestinal mucosa by a specialized segment (scolex) at the anterior end. **Each proglottid contains male and female genitalia and is complete in other respects.** As a result, the tapeworm is in reality a group of individuals attached to one another in a tape-like chain. As proglottides of most tapeworms mature, those of the caudal end are shed and expelled from the body with the faeces, **to release their countless ova**.

All tapeworms have one or more larval stages. Through these they pass in various **intermediate hosts**, including insects and mammals. Some tapeworms require more than one intermediate host. **Only one tapeworm,** *Hymenolepis nana*, a parasite of rodents, **has a direct life cycle.** Here, the definitive host serves also for the stages of development that are usually completed within the intermediate host. These larval forms invade host's tissues and produce serious effects upon the host.

Certain tapeworm larvae were known for a long time before their connection with the adult form was understood. For this reason, the larval form came to have a separate well-established name. For example, *Cysticercus cellulosae*, the bladderworm of 'measly pork', is the larval form of *Taenia solium*, a tapeworm of humans.

The Class **Cestoda** is divided into **eleven orders**, nine of which contain parasites of fishes, reptiles, or amphibia. **Only two, Pseudophyllidea and Cyclophyllidea, contain all tapeworms parasitic for humans and other mammals.** The **Pseudophyllidea** are mostly parasites of fish. However, the adult of one species, *Diphyllobothrium latum*, is parasitic in mammals. Species of this order have a scolex which has no hooks, and instead of suckers, contain narrow, deep grooves and **bothria**. The **eggs are usually operculated**, resembling those of trematodes. All the rest of the **species of tapeworms parasitic for mammals belong to the order Cyclophyllidea**.

Life Cycles

The adult tapeworms produce little serious effect upon the host except in heavy infections, in which case they interfere with digestion, or cause partial obstruction. **All adults live in the intestine**, with the exception of a few species, such as, *Thysanosoma actinoides* and *Stilesia hepatica* (limited to Africa), which live in the bile ducts in ruminants.

The parasites in their intermediate stages produce more serious effects upon the host. As these intermediate stages of tapeworms are encountered in host's tissues, their identifying features are of diagnostic significance. **The larvae usually develop in two ways:** either to become **solid larvae**, or to become **bladder larvae. In the first (solid) type**, the egg-shaped operculate ovum is passed out of the uterus to hatch into a ciliated motile embryo, the **coracidium**. The coracidium escapes through the operculum and becomes free-living. The coracidium is ingested by a freshwater crustacean (an aquatic arthropod), in whose tissues it develops into an elongated form, the **procercoid larva**. Development of this larva continues after the arthropod is swallowed by a second intermediate host (usually a fish), until it becomes an elongated solid larva (**plerocercoid**) with a head resembling that of the mature tapeworm. The fish tapeworm *Diphyllobothrium latum* is an example of larval development of this type. The bladder type of larvae are usually termed "**tetrathridia**"

In the development of the **second (bladder) type**, the **larvae originate from eggs** which are usually round. The proglottid releases the larvae from the uterus when it breaks, or by discharge through one or more uterine pores by those species which have them. The eggs are fully developed when they escape from the uterus. That is, they contain a larva, the **hexacanth embryo**, or **onchosphere**, surrounded by a dense membrane. In the intestine of the intermediate host, the hexacanth larva is released. It then migrates through the intestinal mucosa, enters into the lymph or blood vessels, and circulates to other tissues. **In tissues**, it gets transformed into **a bladder-shaped structure** with one or more inverted scolices in an invaginated portion of the wall.

When the **larvae** has a solid caudal portion and a bladder-like proximal portion, it is called a "**Cysticercus**". Modifications of the cysticercus include: **1. Strobilocercus.** This has an invaginated scolex attached to a bladder by a segmented portion, **2. Coenurus** or **multiceps.** It has a germinal layer capable of producing multiple scolices beneath the bladder wall, and **3. Echinococcus** or **hydatid cyst.** This has a germinal layer which produces brood capsules within which scolices develop. "**Cysticercoid**" is a form that is usually found in invertebrates. It consists of a small vesicle with a tiny cavity and one scolex. The scolices in all these larval stages possess **suckers**, and in armed species **hooklets** similar to those of the adult stage. When ingested by the definitive host, the scolex evaginates and attaches itself to the intestinal mucosa. **Growth of the tapeworm then takes place by proliferation of segments at the posterior extremity.**

Some of the features of important tapeworms of domestic animals are presented in Table 47.

Table 47.   Features of some important tapeworms

Tapeworm	Final Host	Intermediate Stage		
		Site	Type of Larva	Intermediate Hosts
Taenia hydatigena	Dog	Peritoneal cavity	*Cysticercus (tenuicollis)*	Cattle, wild ruminants, sheep, goat, pig
T. multiceps (Multiceps multiceps)	Dog	Brain, spinal cord	*Coenurus (cerebralis)*	Sheep, goat
T. ovis	Dog, fox, wolf	Muscles	*Cysticercus (ovis)*	Sheep, goat

T. pisiformis	Dog, cat, fox, wolf	Liver capsule, peritoneum	*Cysticercus (pisiformis)*	Rabbit, squirrel, other rodents
T. saginata	Humans	Heart, skeletal muscles	*Cysticercus (bovis)*	Cattle
T. serialis	Dog, other carnivores	Subcutis	*Coenurus (serialis)*	Rabbit
T. solium	Humans	Muscle, heart, viscera	*Cysticercus (cellulosae)*	Pigs
T. taeniaeformis	Dog, cat, fox	Liver	*Cysticercus (fasciolaris)*	Rats, mice, rabbits
Echinococcus granulosus	Humans, dog, fox, wolf	Liver, lungs, other viscera	*Echinococcus (granulosus)*	Humans, cattle, pig, sheep, horse, deer
E. multilocularis	Humans, dog, fox wolf, jackal	Liver, lungs, other viscera	*Echinococcus (multilocularis)*	Humans, cattle, pig, sheep, horse, deer
Diphyllobothrium latum	Humans, bear, dog, cat, pig, fox	Muscles	Procercoid and plerocercoid	Microcrustacea, freshwater fish
Dipylidium caninum	Dog, cat	-	Cysticercoid	Dog flea, biting lice
Moniezia expansa	Sheep, goat, cattle	-	Cysticercoid	Mites
M. benedeni	Sheep, goat, cattle	-	Cysticercoid	Mites

Cysticercosis

The **presence of larvae** of certain tapeworms **in the tissues of animals and humans** results in a disease known as "cysticercosis", also known as **beef or pork "measles"**, and **"bladderworm disease"**. **The effect on the host depends upon the organs involved and the degree of parasitism.** In some sites, such as peritoneum and subcutis, the cysticerci are tolerated and there is no tissue reaction, **but those species which invade the critical organs (liver, heart, brain) can produce serious signs and even death.**

Cysticercus bovis

Cysticercus bovis (larva of *Taenia saginata*, **beef bladderworm**) is found in the muscle, liver, heart, lungs, diaphgram, lymph nodes and in other parts of the body of **cattle**. *C. bovis* is important because this bovine parasite is the intermediate stage of the **human tapeworm, *Taenia saginata*. Few symptoms are produced in cattle**, but in cases of massive infection **death** may occur following a febrile course. The **cysticerci** are usually found on postmortem examination as **small cysts**, up to 9 mm in diameter. They occur in **musculature**, or in the **heart**, partly embedded and partly projecting from the surface. The cysts are white or grey. The main tissue change is displacement of normal cells, with little inflammatory reaction surrounding the viable bladderworm. In long-standing cases, however, death of the parasite is followed by dense encapsulation, which ultimately forms a scar. **Microscopic sections** through the lesion may reveal thin bladder wall and the invaginated scolex of the cysticercus bearing hooklets.

Cysticercus cellulosae

Cysticercus cellulosae (the **pork bladderworm**, or worm of "**pork measles**") is the intermediate stage of *Taenia solium*. The tapeworm *Taenia solium* **occurs in the small intestine of humans**. Apart from **pigs**, *C. cellulosae* in some cases, has been found in **cattle, sheep, deer** and **humans**. The **cysticerci** resemble *C. bovis* and are most common in striated muscles, particularly of the neck, cheek, shoulder, and tongue. However, heart, abdominal wall, liver, lungs, brain and eye may be involved. This bladderworm closely resembles *Cysticercus bovis*, except that the scolex bears a double row of hooklets.

Taenia solium is a serious tapeworm in **humans** because of the possibility of autoinfection, with cysticerci developing in tissues. **Diagnosis in humans** is usually possible by radiography because of the frequent calcification of mature cysts.

Cysticercus ovis

Cysticercus ovis is the intermediate stage of *Taenia ovis*, a tapeworm of **dogs, foxes, wolves** and other carnivores. *C. ovis* is the **cause of sheep "measles", or ovine cysticercosis**. The bladderworms are found in the connective tissue of the heart, skeletal muscles, diaphragm, oesophagus, and rarely, the **lungs of sheep and goats**. The effect of this parasite on its intermediate host is similar to that of the other cysticerci which invade the same tissues. Heavy infections are the cause of condemnation of animals slaughtered for food.

Coenurus cerebralis

Coenurus cerebralis is the larval stage of a **dog tapeworm, *Taenia multiceps* (*Multiceps multiceps*)**. It causes an uncommon disease in the central nervous system of **sheep** known as "gid" or "sturdy". It may also infect other herbivorous animals, a nd rarely c arnivores, monkeys, a nd humans. Symptoms indicating c entral nervous s ystem involvement d epend upon l ocalization of the bladderworms in the brain or spinal cord. **Symptoms** vary from incoordination to paralysis. The larvae wander in the body before localizing in nervous tissue in the form of **cysts**. Each cyst is filled with clear fluid and contains as many as 500 scolices. These are visible through the thin walls of the cyst as small white foci. The "**coenurus**" is a modified cysticercus with a germinal layer and the ability to produce many scolices.

Cysticercus tenuicollis

Cysticercus tenuicollis is the i ntermediate stage of a t apeworm of dogs and o ther carnivores, *T aenia h ydatigena*. It i s found mainly in t he liver, mesentery, a nd omentum o f **cattle**, wild r uminants, **sheep,** a nd **pigs**. The cysticerci a re large, usually of 80 mm in diameter, b ut they c ontain only a single scolex armed with a double row of hooklets. The effect upon the intermediate host i s not s ignificant. The c ysticerci may b e noticed o nly d uring postmortem examination. The migration of larvae through the liver results in necrotic tracts similar to those caused by *Fasciola hepatica.*

Other Cysticerci

The other cysticerci include *Cysticercus pisiformis*, which occurs on the peritoneum a nd liver capsule of **rabbits**, sq uirrels, and other small r odents. The adult stage of this parasite (*Taenia pisiformis*) is attached in the **small intestine of dog**, **cat**, wolf, and other carnivores.

A similar parasite, *Cysticercus fasciolaris*, i s found in t he l iver of **rats, mice,** and **other rodents**. T he adult form (*Taenia taeniaeformis*) i s a tapeworm of the **cat**, less often of the **dog**, fox, and other carnivore s. A **bladderworm** found in the subcutis of **rabbits** is known as *Coenurus serialis*. It is the intermediate stage of *Taenia serialis*, a tapeworm of **dog** and closely related carnivores.

Echinococcosis

The **larval or intermediate stages of tapeworms** in the genus **Echinococcus** are known as "hydatid cysts", and the disease they produce is called "**echinococcosis**" or "**hydatid disease**". **The adult tapeworms are of no importance, but the larval forms which localize in the liver, lungs and other vital organs, cause serious disease.**

Four species of Echinococcus exist, of these **only two are important:** *E. granulosus* and *E. multilocularis*. **Dogs** and wild carnivores serve as the main final hosts for *E. granulosus*, whose larvae mostly occur in **sheep**, but can also infect cattle, horses, pigs, monkeys, deer, rodents, and humans and other species. It is distributed worldwide. Several strains exist with affinity for a particular intermediate host. **Foxes** serve as the main final host for the adults of *E. multilocularis*, but **dogs** and **cats** can also serve this function. Larval forms occur in various rodents, **although humans can be infected**.

Eggs ingested by the appropriate intermediate host hatch in the small intestine. The released **hexacanth embryos (onchospheres)** invade a venule or lymphatic, pass to the liver or lungs where they may lodge. Or, they enter into the general circulation and are spread elsewhere to develop into a hydatid that grows slowly. **The hydatid of *E. granulosus* is unilocular**, consisting of a thick concentrically laminated outer membrane enclosing a germinal membrane, from which numerous **brood capsules** arise. These may be attached by a short stalk, or be free in the cyst where they are called "**hydatid sand**". Each brood capsule contains germinal epithelium from which as many as 40 scolices arise. Each scolex is egg-shaped and bears a crown of 32-40 hooklets. Daughter cysts may form within the parent cyst. The hydatids of *E. multilocularis* produce **multilocular hydatids** with external daughter cysts.

The effect on the host depends upon the organ parasitized and the size attained by the hydatid cyst, which may measure up to **several inches**. The hydatids are usually surrounded by mononuclear cells, eosinophils, multinucleated giant cells, and fibrous connective tissue. The inflammatory reaction becomes severe when the cyst ruptures. In **humans**, rupture of the cyst can lead to anaphylactic shock, or other allergic reactions. Adjacent tissues undergo pressure atrophy. Hydatids may degenerate spontaneously, in which case they undergo calcification.

Diagnosis

The presence of the adult worm in the intestinal tract can be diagnosed by the demonstration of segments and ova in the faeces. **However, the intermediate stage presents difficulties**. The hydatid cysts can be identified by histopathological examination of tissue removed at postmortem examination. Complement fixation test, delayed hypersensitivity tests, haemagglutination tests, fluorescent antibody test, and other immunological procedures have been used with varying results.

Nematodes (Roundworms)

Ascariasis

Also known as "**common roundworm infection**" and "**ascarid worm infection**", ascariasis is caused by ascarids. **Ascarids (Phylum: Nemathelminthes; Family: Ascaridae) are extremely common roundworms.** Their adult forms are **found in the gastrointestinal tracts of mammals and birds**. Ascarids occur not only in great numbers, but in many varieties. **Most of them are host-specific.** However, larval migration may occur in other than the true host, which are referred to as **"paratenic hosts"**. In other words, **a "paratenic host" is an abnormal host.** The important ascarids are presented in Table 48.

Table 48. **Important species of Ascaridae**

Species of Ascarid	Final (definitive) Hosts
Ascaris lumbricoides (suum)	Humans, pigs (var. *suis*)
Toxocara canis	Dog
Toxocara cati	Cat, wildcat, lion, leopard
Toxocara vitulorum	Cattle
Toxascaris leonina	Dog, cat, lion, tiger, fox
Parascaris equorum	Horse
Ascaridia galli	Chickens, turkeys

The adults are usually large worms found in the small intestine. The eggs are thick-shelled and unsegmented when laid. A period of incubation and two mounts within the shell are required before the embryo becomes infective. The eggs are resistant to drying, low temperatures, and many chemical agents. **Young animals are particularly susceptible to infection with ascarids.**

Ascarids are among the most common intestinal parasites of animals. They are particularly important in **dogs, cats, pigs,** and **horses. Cattle** are less frequently infected. Infection in **sheep** and **goats** is rare to non-existent.

Life Cycles

The life cycles of all ascarids are direct. However, several variations in the migratory patterns of larvae can occur. **In the typical life cycle, using** *Ascaris suum* **as the standard,** embryonated eggs containing **second-stage larvae** are ingested and hatch in the stomach wall. They then enter the portal veins and invade the hepatic parenchyma. Here, they may moult to third-stage larvae and wander for some time before entering the general circulation to be carried to the **lungs.** In the lungs, the **third stage larvae** penetrate into the alveoli, and move up the bronchi and trachea to be swallowed. In the intestine, two more moults occur before maturation to adult worms. This **tracheal migration** occurs in *Toxocara canis, T. cati, T. vitulorum, Parascaris equorum,* and *Ascaris suum.* The main difference with *T. canis, T. cati,* and *P. equorum* is that **the moult to third-stage larvae occurs in the pulmonary alveoli.**

Only *Toxascaris leonina* varies from this general migratory pattern. The second-stage larvae of *T. leonina* penetrate the intestinal wall and do not migrate further. They undergo their moults here and re-enter the lumen as **fourth-stage larvae,** which mature to adults.

Larvae of *T. canis, T. cati* and *T. vitulorum*, besides entering pulmonary alveoli, remain in the circulation and are **widely distributed in the body**. This pattern is called the **somatic migration of the larvae**. The second-stage larvae lodged in various tissues do not undergo further development, but remain live for months or years. Others die at these sites, producing **small granulomas**. Localization of such migrating larvae in the brain or retina may lead to serious complications. An important feature of **somatic migration in dogs** is that these **larvae** can migrate from their tissue location to the uterus, cross placenta, and **infect pups *in utero* during the later third of pregnancy**. Prenatal infection does not occur with *T. cati* or *T. vitulorum*. However, larvae of these species and *T. canis* **can enter the mammary glands and milk to infect pups, kittens, and calves**. Somatic migration is much more likely to occur **in older dogs**, than tracheal migration. **In cats**, tracheal migration is the more common route, regardless of the age.

There is yet another difference in the life cycles of *T. canis* and *T. cati*. It involves **infection of paratenic hosts**. A number of different species, including rodents and even humans, support initial development of these parasites. **Tracheal migration** leads to the larvae's death, because further development in the gastrontestinal tract does not occur. However, **systemic migration** in the paratenic host may lead to second-stage larvae embedded in tissues, where they stimulate an inflammatory reaction. This is known as **"visceral larval migrans"**, and is particularly important in **young children** where the larvae may locate in brain. *Toxocara canis* **is the most important cause of visceral larval migrans in humans**. However, other parasites (e.g., *Ascaris suum*, *Capillaria hepatica* and *Dirofilaria immitis*) may also cause this condition. When the tissues of a paratenic host are ingested by a dog or cat, **the second-stage larvae** develop to mature worms in the alimentary tract. **Third and fourth-stage larvae** develop in the wall of the stomach and re-enter the lumen without the need of tracheal migration.

Thus, the dogs can become infected with adult *T. canis* through: **1.** Ingestion of eggs, **2.** *In utero*, **3.** Through milk, or **4.** Through ingestion of paratenic hosts. *T. cati* also use each of these routes except *in utero* infection.

It can be seen that ascarid larvae can penetrate various tissues of the host, where they may remain for some time and produce tissue damage. While the **intestinal wall, liver, and lungs are the common routes for larval migration**, any tissue of the body can be attacked. The interval between ingestion of infective forms and the appearance of eggs in the faeces of the final host is called the **"prepatent period"**. This is a period during which the animal can suffer serious damage from the migration and development of larvae in the tissues. It can be relatively long. For example, 60 or more days for *A. lumbricoides*.

Pathogenesis

Adult ascarids usually live in the small intestine. They feed on the intestinal contents, and sometimes damage the mucosa. By a swimming movement, they maintain their position in the intestinal lumen inspite of peristaltic movement. Several factors increase their motility, such as increased temperature (fever) and starvation. On the other hand, they are unable to maintain their position against increased peristalsis which occurs in diarrhoea and after purging (evacuation of bowels by a drug). **Thus, they are swept out of the intestine.** When their motility increases, ascarids may move into the stomach, or into the hepatic or pancreatic ducts. **They may produce obstruction in the bile ducts,** resulting in **jaundice. Adult ascarids** which remain in their usual location (intestine) may become so numerous that they cause **obstruction of the intestinal lumen. This may be fatal, particularly in young animals.** Sometimes, penetration of the intestinal wall may produce **peritonitis. Inanition** (lack of adequate nutrition) and **retardation of growth** of the **young animals** are the most common effects, because ascarids deprive the host of food and interfere with the digestive processes.

Clinical Signs

In all species only the young are seriously affected. The first indication of infection in young animals is **lack of growth and loss of condition.** Infected animals have a dull coat and are "**pot-bellied**". Worms may be vomited and are usually passed in the faeces. In the early stages, **pulmonary damage** due to migration of larvae can occur. It may be complicated by bacterial pneumonia, so that respiratory distress of variable severity may occur. **Diarrhoea** with mucus may be present.

In pigs up to 4-5 months old, important clinical signs are poor growth and lowered resistance to other disease. Ascariasis during the growing phase causes permanent damage to growth potential. **Swine influenza and enzootic pneumonia of pigs are much more serious diseases when accompanied by ascariasis.** There may be cough but this is not marked. However, in severe cases, which are rare, pigs show severe dyspnoea, or die from acute hepatic insufficiency. Adult worms may be vomited up, and rarely, cases of **obstructive jaundice,** and **intestinal obstruction or rupture,** may occur. The effect in **calves** from infestation with *T. vitulorum,* and in foals with *P. equorum,* are similar to those observed **in young pigs,** and include poor coat, diarrhoea, and sometimes colic. In addition, **in foals,** convulsions, intestinal obstruction and perforation may occur. **In calves,** reduced weight gains, anaemia, and steatorrhoea (fatty stools) are additional signs. **In older animals no clinical signs are observed.** In severe infections of **puppies,** verminous pneumonia, ascites, fatty change of the liver, and mucoid enteritis are common.

Lesions

Lesions produced by the larvae during their migration and development in the tissues can be **minimal to severe.** As the larvae migrate, tissues along the route are damaged. Reparative processes then become part of the pathological changes. Larvae which penetrate the intestinal mucosa may carry bacteria into the tissues. **In the liver,** heavy infection with larvae usually produces intense inflammation, with oedema, neutrophils, eosinophils, and lymphocytes as components of the inflammatory reaction. **Larvae** can be identified in the central mass of characteristic caseous necrosis surrounded by epithelioid cells, eosinophils, lymphocytes, and neutrophils. **The portal areas are most severely involved.** However, later fibrosis may obliterate entire lobules. **In pigs,** a diffuse, subcapsular fibrosis marks the sites of previous larval invasion of the liver. Larval migration through the **lungs** sets up an inflammatory reaction that may result in mild to severe respiratory involvement. It usually heals with few residual lesions. **Haemorrhages** occur as the larvae break out of the pulmonary capillaries to enter the alveoli. In heavy infection loss of bronchiolar epithelium and infiltration of leukocytes may occur.

Ascarids may wander throughout the body and produce **granulomatous nodules** in many sites. They are usually seen in the kidney, but may occur in any tissue, including liver, lung, myocardium, brain, eye, and lymph nodes.

Diagnosis

Diagnosis of ascariasis is based upon **demonstration of ova and adults in the faeces,** and the correlation of these findings with the clinical signs. It is important to differentiate the spherical eggs of **T**oxocara sp. from the oval eggs of *Toxascaris leonina,* because of the public health importance of the former. During the prepatent period, ova are not found in the faeces, although immature forms may be present in the tissues or intestine. Ascarid larvae can be identified in tissue sections, and their relationship to lesions demonstrated. **Serological tests are useful in diagnosing visceral larval migrans.** Eosinophilia usually accompanies larval migrans. Occlusion of hepatic ducts by adult ascarids is usually detected at postmortem examination.

Ancylostomiasis

Ancylostomiasis is also known as **"hookworm disease".** Hookworms (Family: **Ancylostomidae**) are important parasites of animals and humans. These parasites are worldwide in distribution. One or more species of hookworm occur in every domestic animal, **except horse.** A few important hookworms are presented in **Table 49.**

Table 49. Important Hookworms

Hookworm	Host	Remarks
Ancylostoma caninum	Dog, fox, wolf	Recorded in India
A. duodenale	Humans	Rare infections in pig
A. braziliense	Dog, cat, fox	Infection not characterized by anaemia
A. ceylanicum	Dog, cat	Recorded in India. Rare infections in humans
A. tubaeforme	Cat	Widely distributed
Agriostomum vryburgi	Cattle	Recorded in India
Bunostomum phlebotomum	Cattle	Recorded in India. An important pathogen
B. trigonocephalum	Sheep, goat, deer	
Gaigeria pachyscelis	Sheep, goat	Recorded in India
Globocephalus urusubulatus	Pig	U.S.A., Europe, Asia
G. longemucronatus	Pig	Europe, Africa, Asia
Necator americanus	Humans, monkeys	Rare infections in dogs
Uncinaria stenocephala	Dog, cat, fox	Usually no anaemia

Life Cycle

The life cycle of each hookworm is not fully understood, but several different migratory patterns are known. For example, adults of *Ancylostoma caninum* live in the small intestine, where they attach to the mucosa with hooklet-like structures present in the well-developed buccal cavities. Eggs are passed in the faeces, and under favourable conditions of a moist warm environment, hatch and develop into **rhabditiform larvae**. Hatching may occur within the gut. Following two moults, the larvae become **filariform larvae** and may infect another host by penetration of the skin, or through **ingestion**. After ingestion, the larvae migrate briefly in the mucosa, and then develop directly to adults in the small intestine. After penetration of the skin, larvae migrate systemically to reach the lungs where they penetrate into the alveoli, are coughed up, and are swallowed to develop into adults in the small intestine.

Some species, for example *Ancylostoma caninum*, may enter the systemic circulation and are deposited in muscle **as arrested third-stage larvae**. These can become re-activated **and enter the milk of bitches, infecting newborn pups**. Rarely, they may penetrate the pregnant uterus and infect the foetus. Hookworms are host-specific. However, the larvae can penetrate the epidermis of **aberrant (paratenic or abnormal) hosts**, producing a specific dermatitis called "**creeping eruption**". These larvae do not develop into an adult stage.

Clinical signs

In young puppies, an acute normocytic, normochromic anaemia followed by hypochromic, microcytic 'iron deficiency' anaemia is the characteristic and often a fatal clinical manifestation of *A. caninum* infection. Surviving puppies develop some immunity and show lesser clinical signs. Nevertheless, debilitated and malnourished animals continue to be unthrifty and suffer from chronic anaemia. **Mature well-nourished dogs may harbour a few worms without showing signs**. These are important as they act as direct or indirect source of infection for pups. **Diarrhoea** with dark, tarry (resembling tar) faeces occurs in severe infections. **Hydraemia** (excess of watery fluid in blood), **emaciation**, and weakness develop **in chronic disease**.

Lesions

The most important effect of hookworms results from the parasite's ingestion of blood, leading to anaemia and hypoproteinaemia. Ancylostoma, which **consumes 0.2 ml of blood per day per worm**, causes severe anaemia because individuals may be infected with more than 100 worms. This illustrates the principle referred to earlier in this chapter that **the severity of infestations caused by helminths**, which do not divide within the host, **is proportional to the number of infecting worms**. Hookworms secrete **an anticoagulant protein** called "AcAP" that inactivates clotting factor Xa. The **anaemia** in severe acute infection, as occurs in **newborn pups** infected through milk, is **normocytic and normochromic**. However, in more chronic disease it is **microcytic and hypochromic**, and usually presents itself as an **iron deficiency anaemia**. Even a small number of *A. caninum* can lead to severe anaemia, although a small to moderate burden of other species of hookworms may not lead to anaemia. Certain parasites, such as *A. braziliense* and *Uncinaria stenocephala* in dogs, are not associated with anaemia. However, hypoproteinaemia may occur. Extensive oedema, hydrothorax, and ascites may accompany the anaemia and hypoproteinaemia.

Changes in the intestinal mucosa are minimal, although diarrhoea is a common clinical sign. Hookworms attach to the mucosa and usually change positions. **They leave small denuded areas in the epithelium which continue** to bleed. These areas appear as punctate (pipoint) haemorrhages at postmortem examination. There may be blunting and fusion of intestinal villi, and inflammation and fibrosis of the lamina propria. This intensifies the disease by causing malabsorption.

Larval migration occurs usually without clinical signs or lesions. However, severe infestation may lead to **pulmonary haemorrhage**, and even **pneumonia**. Entry through the skin leads to dermatitis in the natural host ("**ground itch**", or "**water itch**" **in humans**), and in aberrant (abnormal) hosts to "**creeping eruption**". The dermatitis is most severe in previously sensitized animals, and is characterized by irregular reddish patches. **Microscopically**, the tissue reaction is limited to the vicinity of the migrating path of the larvae, and is characterized by infiltration of eosinophils, lymphocytes, and macrophages.

Diagnosis

The characteristic thin-shelled, oval eggs are easily seen on flotation of fresh faeces from infected dogs.

Bunostomiasis

Bunostomiasis, also known as "**hookworm disease**" occurs in **cattle, sheep,** and **pigs**. These hookworms (**Bunostomum** sp.) are small (1-2.5 cm), reddish roundworms which live in the small intestine of their hosts. *Bunostomum phlebotomum* is the important hookworm of cattle, but *Agriostomum vryburgi* may also occur (**Table 49**). In sheep, *Bunostomum trigonocephalum* is the most important hookworm, but *Gaigeria pachyscelis* also occurs and **is prevalent in India**. Infestations with some species of hookworms occur in **pigs**, but are rarely important. Infestations with hookworms cause poor growth and blood loss manifested by anaemia and anasarca. Calves 4-12 months of age are most commonly affected, and the degree of infestation is always greater in the **winter months**.

Life Cycle

The life cycle of all the hookworms is direct. The **eggs** hatch and a larva is produced in about a week. There are two non-parasitic larval stages, and an **infective larva** which is capable of entering the body of the host through the skin. **Bunostomum sp. larvae enter through the skin**, and also through the mouth, but larvae of *G. pachyscelis* enter only through the skin. The larvae, after skin penetration, enter the bloodstream. They are then carried to the heart and lungs, enter the alveoli where the **fourth-stage larvae** develop. The larvae move up in the air passages to the pharynx, are swallowed and reach the small intestine. Larvae then penetrate the intestinal wall and return to its lumen without further migration. The prepatent period for *B. phlebotomum* is about 8 months.

Pathogenesis

Hookworms are blood suckers and cause severe anaemia in all species. Total worm numbers as low as 100 may cause clinical illness, and 2000 may also cause **death in young cattle**. There is loss of blood, and hypoproteinaemic oedema may result. Irritation of the intestinal mucosa may cause **mild or intermittent diarrhoea**.

Clinical Signs

Constipation and mild abdominal pain are seen in the early stages. This is followed by diarrhoea. The **cattle** are unthrifty and anaemic. In severe infestations, there i s paleness of mucosae, a nasarca under t he jaw and along the belly, prostation and **death in 2-3 days**. Signs in **sheep** are similar to those in cattle. Clinical signs both in cattle and sheep are usually seen in the prepatent period before eggs appear in the faeces.

Postmortem Findings

Most of the worms are found in the first few feet of the **small intestine**. The intestinal contents are usually deeply blood-stained. The number of worms present m ay be quite small. In calves, t otal counts o f 100 o r more w orms suggest a s ignificant level o f i nfestation, and c ounts o ver 2 000 i ndicate a degree of infestation likely to be fatal.

Diagnosis

The disease can be diagnosed from demonstration o f eggs in the faeces. The blunt ends a nd d eeply p igmented e mbryonic cells of h ookworm e ggs enable them to be differentiated from the eggs of other strongylid worms.

Capillaria

Genus **Capillaria** contains a large number of species which parasitize mammals and birds, but only a few are important as pathogens of animals.

C. hepatica is m ainly a p arasite of **r ats** and **m ice**, b ut may a lso i nfect **dogs, cats, horses, monkeys, and humans**. The adult worm is a thin nematode related to whipworms (**Trichuris sp.**). The adults live in the **liver parenchyma**. Here, ova and excreta accumulate, which cause tissue destruction leading to fibrosis. The **life cycle** continues only when t he infected liver is eaten by a new (intermediate) host, in which the ova are released but do not hatch. **Ova** with **bipolar plugs** (typical of the genus) are passed in the faeces of this second host, and embryonate on the ground to reach the infective stage. **Ova** ingested by a third host **contain larvae** that penetrate the intestinal wall, and **eventually reach liver**.

C. feliscati and *C. plica* are also slender, about 30-60 mm long, and are found in the urinary bladder and sometimes ureters and renal pelvis. *C. feliscati*

lymphocytes, neutrophils, o r sometimes eosinophils i s u sually observed in the pia mater. Perivascular lymphocytic cuffing may be prominent near primary malacic foci. The parasitic helminths are seen in tissue sections only by chance, unless a careful search of serial sections through the characteristic lesion i s made.

Diagnosis

Diagnosis can be made only after careful microscopic examination of the central nervous system. Typical lesions must be found, and some should contain the causative n ematodes.

Dirofilariasis

Dirofilariasis is also known as "**canine filariasis**" and "**heart worm disease**". **Animals** and **humans** can suffer from a number of **filarid parasites** (genus: **Filaria**; superfamily: **Filarioidea**). A selected list is presented in **Table 50**. The heart worm *Dirofilaria immitis* is an important filarid parasite. It infects **dogs**, **cats**, foxes, wolves, and rarely other species such as **horses and humans**.

Table 50 . Important filarial parasites of animals

Filarial parasite	Final host	Location	Intermediate host
Dirofilaria immitis	Dogs, cats, foxes, wolves	Right ventricle	Mosquitoes
Dracunculus insignis	Dogs, wild carnivores	Subcutis	Cyclops sp.
D. medinensis	Humans, dogs, horses	Subcutis	Cyclops sp.
Elaeophora schneideri	Sheep, deer	Arteries	Horseflies
Onchocerca armillata	Cattle, sheep, goats	Aorta	Unknown
O. cervicalis	Horses	Ligamentum nuchae	Culicoides sp. (biting insects)
O. gibsoni	Cattle	Subcutis	Culicoides sp. (biting insects)
O. gutturosa	Cattle	Ligamentum nuchae	Black flies
O. lienalis	Cattle	Gastrosplenic ligament	Black flies
O. reticulata	Horses	Tendons of legs	Culicoides sp.

Setaria digitata	Cattle	Peritoneal cavity	Mosquitoes
S. equina	Horses	Peritoneal cavity	Mosquitoes
Stephanofilaria assamensis	Cattle	Subcutis	Flies
S. stilesi	Cattle	Subcutis	Flies
S. zaheeri	Buffaloes	Ears	Flies

Life Cycle

The adult worms are thin, almost thread-like, **filarial parasites**. Males are 12-30 cm long and females 25-31 cm long. **They are found in the right ventricle of the heart**, and less often in the right auricle, pulmonary artery, and vena cava. The males and females copulate in these sites. The viviparous (producing living young instead of eggs) female releases highly motile **microfilariae**, which circulate in the blood. These microfilariae are taken up from the cutaneous circulation by certain biting insects (**mosquitoes**), in whose bodies they undergo stages of development. The **infective microfilariae** then enter into the tissues of final hosts through the **bite of the intermediate host**. The filarial larvae undergo further development in muscles, subcutaneous and adipose tissues of the new host. When they reach a length of about 5 cm, they enter veins and are carried to the right heart. The cycle is complete when **adult filariae** start reproduction in the right ventricle. **Trans-placental infection of the foetal pups with microfilariae may occur**. However, these do not develop into adults and disappear after two months.

Clinical Signs

In the earliest stages, there are no significant clinical signs. However, severely affected animals show shortness of breath, weakness, cardiac enlargement, hepatomegaly, ascites, sometimes hypertrophic pulmonary osteoarthropathy, **and may die from failure of the right side of the heart**. In a few cases, **death** may be the result of **pulmonary embolism** by adult **Dirofilaria**, which die and are carried away forcefully into the smaller branches of the pulmonary artery.

Lesions

The main effects of *Dirofilaria immitis* are produced by the adult worms, **which interfere with circulation through the right heart**. Mechanical interference over long period produces **compensatory hypertrophy and enlargement of the right ventricle**. Insufficiency of the right heart results in passive congestion of the lungs, liver, and spleen, as well as **ascites**. Some worms die and are transported through the pulmonary artery to the lungs where they produce **pulmonary embolisms**. Sometimes this leads to **infarction**.

Changes in the pulmonary arterial system develop over a period of months. Lesions first develop in the smaller branches of the pulmonary arteries, but ultimately involve the extrapulmonary segments. The initial damage is to the endothelial cells, which become swollen. Platelets and leukocytes adhere to the damaged endothelium and an **endarteritis** occurs with infiltration of eosinophils in intima. Hypertrophy and hyperplasia of medial smooth muscle cells extend into intima and project into the lumen. The release of **platelet-derived growth factor (PDGF)** stimulates the marked proliferation of smooth muscle. This leads to the formation of **villous projections** into the lumen. **Grossly, intima of the arteries is uneven and rough, and this is considered pathognomonic of dirofilariasis**. The proliferative lesion may occlude the lumen of the smaller pulmonary arteries. This causes pulmonary hypertension. The presence of adult worms and the damaged endothelium may lead to **thrombosis and thrombo-embolism to the lungs**, which can cause **infarction**. Fragments of dead worms may also lodge in the lungs, stimulating a granulomatous inflammatory reaction.

In heavy infestations, *D. immitis* may occupy the **vena cava**, resulting in **phlebosclerosis** (fibrous hardening of the wall) **of vena cava and hepatic veins**. Rarely, adult worms are found in the left side of the heart, aorta, or peripheral arteries, and sometimes outside the arteries in such locations as the peritoneal cavity, eye, or ventricles of the brain.

The **microfilariae**, though circulate freely in the blood, **appear to produce little tissue damage**. This is because they are found in tissue sections, usually without inflammatory or other tissue reaction. However, some microfilariae die and **a small granuloma** forms around them. Such tiny granulomas have been seen in the kidney of infected dogs. **Immune complex glomerulonephritis** is another complication of dirofilariasis.

Diagnosis

Presumptive diagnosis can be based on the symptoms. **Diagnosis is confirmed by demonstration of the microfilariae in peripheral blood**. However, absence of circulating microfilariae does not rule out infection. This is because up to 20% of the cases may be occult (hidden), without detectable circulating microfilariae. Several different tests are available for the detection of microfilariae. ELISA and indirect immunofluorescent assays, for adult or microfilarial antigens, are both sensitive.

Dracunculosis

Two species of Dracunculus or "guinea-worms" can infect animals (see **Table 50**). The classical guinea-worm *Dracunculus medinensis* is **mainly a**

parasite of humans in tropical and subtropical countries. **It may also infect dogs**, and rarely **cats, horses**, and **cattle**. *D. insignis* parasitizes **dogs** and wild carnivores.

The adult parasites live in the subcutis, particularly in the limbs. The females may reach up to 400 cm in length. Sometimes, adults may be found in other connective tissue, in a body cavity, heart, or eye. **In subcutis**, the parasites produce **painful inflammatory swellings** which tend to ulcerate, and are subject to secondary bacterial infection. **The head of the worm protrudes from the ulcer**. When the worm is in contact with water, the uterus prolapses and releases larvae. Larval development to the infective stage requires the **intermediate host, Cyclops**. The **final host** becomes infected after drinking water in which crustaceans (**Cyclops**) live. The **Cyclops** in the intestine release **infective larvae**. These migrate through tissues for several months to reach subcutis. Here, the lesions become visible 10-12 months after initial infection.

Diagnosis depends on identification of the adult parasites in the lesions. When in unusual sites, they must be differentiated from other filarial parasites.

Elaeophoriasis

Elaeophoriasis is also known as "**filarial dermatosis of sheep**", "**clear-eyed blindness**", and "**sorehead**". The disease is caused by *Elaeophora schneideri* and is **prevalent in the United States**. This "**arterial worm**" is a filarial parasite (see **Table 50**) of **sheep** and deer. Deer (white-tailed and mule) suffer no harmful effects from the parasite, and are considered the normal or reservoir hosts. **In sheep**, the parasitism results in "**filarial dermatitis**". Its life cycle is indirect, using **horseflies (Tabanus)** as **intermediate host**.

Lesions

In sheep, the adult worms are found usually in the carotid arteries, but mesenteric, iliac, and other arteries may also be involved. The adults are thin, thread-like and white. **Microfilariae** localize in the dermis and lead to **circumscribed dermatitis** over head, poll, and face. The lesion is accompanied by considerable pruritus (itching). Formation of vesicles, small pustules, and crust formation may occur. **Microscopic changes** include severe localized acanthosis with clubbing of the rete pegs. Areas of ulceration are associated with haemorrhagic and serous exudation. Superficial vesicles in the epithelium are common, and are filled with serum, red blood cells, and eosinophils. **The dermis is severely involved in an inflammatory process of granulomatous nature**. In some foci of inflammation, histiocytes and giant cells predominate, with lymphocytes and plasma cells in the surrounding tissue. In others, eosinophils are predominant. These changes are influenced by the age of the lesion, death of larvae, and sensitization of the host. **The adult worms may**

cause thrombosis of the arteries in which they are found.

Diagnosis

Diagnosis c an be made by finding characteristic microfilariae in microscopic sections of affected skin, or in smears of skin scrapings. The adult worms are found only at postmortem examination.

Equine Strongylosis

The Family Strongylidae contains more than 50 species of worms which parasitize the caecum and colon of horses. Of these, the larger strongyles of the genus Strongylus are the most important as pathogens. These large strongyles are slender worms about 1-2 inches in length. Three species, *Strongylus vulgaris*, *S. equinus*, and *S. edentatus* cause "strongylosis" or "redworm infestation" in horses. They cause disease through blood sucking by the adult worms and extensive tissue damage from larval migration. The presence of blood in their alimentary tracts is responsible for the common name "redworms". *S. vulgaris* is the most important and most pathogenic of the three strongyles. Strongylosis is a common disease of horses throughout the world.

The small strongyles include about 40 species within six or more genera. These parasites are much less injurious to the host, since they neither attach themselves to the intestinal mucosa nor ingest blood. Also, they do not undergo extensive tissue migration as larvae, as do the important larger varieties.

Clinical Signs

Clinical signs are of different types, and depend on the severity of the infection caused by the adult worms and the anatomical localization of the larval forms. General debility, emaciation, diarrhoea, and anaemia can result from the presence of numerous worms in the caecum and colon. The larvae of *S. vulgaris* are the most pathogenic, and usually give rise to lesions in the mesenteric arteries. This results in intestinal infarction which manifests as severe abdominal pain (colic). The larvae may also produce thrombi in the aorta, or iliac arteries. Thrombi may partially occlude these vessels, causing serious weakness in one or both hind limbs. This symptom is aggravated by exercise. Migration of *S. equinus* and *S. edentatus* through the liver and peritoneal cavity can cause peritonitis, colic, and in severe infections in foals, even death.

Specific Strongyles

Strongylus vulgaris

This strongyle is the most common and is double-toothed. It is found in the caecum of horses, usually attached to the mucosa. The males are about 16 mm long, the females about 24 mm, and as a rule, **the worms are red from ingested blood ("redworms").**

The life cycle is direct. Eggs pass i n the faeces and **f irst-stage larvae** hatch out. These e ventually d evelop to s **econd-stage** and f inally to t **hird- stage infective larvae.** Following i ngestion, third-stage larvae penetrate the wall of the intestine, moult in the submucosa, and penetrate terminal branches of intestinal arteries. This migration results in **small haemorrhages** through- out t he wall o f the **sm all intestine** and in a n i nfiltration o f lymphocytes, neutrophils, a nd eosinophils. The submucosal arteries also show similar i n- flammation and t **hrombosis,** a nd contain f **ourth-stage larvae.** T he f ourth- stage l arvae move up in the mesenteric a rteries, in the intima, t o reach t he **anterior mesenteric artery** at one of i ts major b ranches w ithin 2-3 w eeks after infection. Here, they produce striking arterial lesions, particularly in the anterior mesenteric artery, and less frequently in the aorta, i liac, renal, a nd other arteries. The **fourth-stage larvae** then retum through arteries to the wall of the c aecum and c olon, where t hey again c ause local h aemorrhage and inflammation. **They then enter the lumen and mature to adults.**

Lesions

Larvae after burrowing the arteries, stimulate proliferation of intima and endothelium, sometimes associated with haemorrhage and necrosis. Fi- brin and c ellular debris a ccumulate on t he roughened i ntimal areas, e xtend into the lumen and sometimes cause obstruction. In long-standing cases, the wall of the artery gets markedly thickened from the proliferation of both intimal and adventitial fibrous tissue. Collections of lymphocytes usually occur in the thickened wall of the artery. **This is the most common lesion and is called "verminous arteritis"** In a l ess common l esion, the a rterial wall b ecomes both thickened and sacculated, forming a dilated segment with a smooth lining. This is called a "verminous a neurysm". Rupture of such aneurysms is uncommon.

Thc worms are found in the artery, firmly attached to the intima, and associated with inflammation. In some cases, only a few parasites are seen in an arterial lesion, whereas in others, as many as 50 may be found. Sometimes, the worms may also be found in the **emboli** or **thrombi** that originate from the arterial lesions. **Fifth-stage larvae** have been found in the spinal cord lesions of a pony. When mature young parasites return to the intestine through lumens of arteries, they again produce local haemorrhage and inflammation.

Strongylus equinus

This is t he **triple-toothed strongyle,** o r bloodworm, f ound i n its **a dult form in the caecum, and rarely in the colon of horses.** It is usually attached to the mucosa and engorged with blood (**"bloodworm"**). The male is about 35 mm long; the females up to 55 mm. Ingested third-stage larvae penetrate the wall of the caecum or colon, and cause **small haemorrhages and inflammatory nodules** before migrating into the peritoneal cavity and entering the liver, where they wander for 6-7 weeks. Their migration leads to paths of hepatic necrosis a nd eosinophilic i nflammation. Larvae l eave the l iver through t he hepatic ligament, enter the pancreas and then peritoneal cavity, where t hey moult to the **fifth stage** and migrate directly to the intestinal lumen.

Strongylus edentatus

This is the toothless strongyle. It occurs in adult form **in the caecum and colon of horses,** usually attached to the mucosa. The males are about 28 mm long; the females are as much as 44 mm. **The life cycle is direct. Infective third-stage larvae** penetrate the wall of the intestine and reach the liver through the portal veins. The larvae d evelop to f ourth-stage larvae. These m igrate within the liver, producing necrosis and inflammation. Larvae leave the liver within hepatic ligaments, and reach the retroperitoneal tissue of the right flank. Here, they remain as **fourth-stage** and **early fifth-stage** larvae for abou. three months, and c ause small h aemorrhages and inflammatory nodules. T hey then migrate through t he mesentery to the wall of t he c aecum a nd colon, again causing nodules before re-entering the lumen t o become adults.

S. edentatus infection causes **prominent nodules in the small and large intestines.** The lesions are subserous. When fresh, these lesions are bright red from recent haemorrhage. Later, they change to shades of yellow and brown as the blood cells disintegrate to release blood pigment, which is haematoidin or haemosiderin. **Microscopically,** these **subserosal lesions** are m ade up o f connective tissue, red blood cells, leukocytes, macrophages, blood pigment, and a central area of caseous necrotic debris. It is difficult to find larvae in the subserosal l esions

Larvae of any of the three strongyles may sometimes be found in unusual locations, such as the lung or brain.

Diagnosis

Counting of the strongyle ova in the faeces is used to estimate the parasitic burden in the living animal. This is necessary because these parasites are so common that a few ova in a faecal sample have no diagnostic significance. The diagnosis of equine strongylosis must be based on proper evaluation of symptoms and ova counts. Verminous arteritis and lesions due to the migration of the parasite are usually seen at postmortem examination.

Gnathostoma

Gnathostoma spinigerum is a parasite of the **stomach of cats, dogs,** and wild carnivores. Two intermediate hosts are required, a **Cyclops** and a **fresh**

water fish or frog in which third-stage larvae encyst. The encysted larvae are released after ingestion of the intermediate host. They then migrate through the liver and other v iscera, where e xtensive damage may occur. U ltimately, the adult worms reach t he wall o f the st omach where t hey live in the large cavities within the submucosa.

Gongylonemiasis

Gongylonema pulchrum occurs in sheep, cattle, goats, pigs, buffalo, and sometimes, horse, camel, donkey, and wild boar. It has been reported in humans. *G. verrucosum* lives in the rumen of s heep, g oats, cattle, deer, a nd zebu. It is known to occur in India. The adults of both these tiny worms lie within the s tratified squamous e pithelium of t he oesophagus, r umen, and stomach. They are usually encountered in tissue sections of the organs, coiled in the e pithelium, without producing any host reaction. T he life c ycle i s indirect, using various beetles as intermediate hosts.

Habronemiasis

The stomach worms of horses are of three species: *Habronema muscae, H. majus* (*H. microstoma*), and *Draschia megastoma* (*Habronema megastoma*). The adults of *H. muscae* and *H. majus* live on the surface of the gastric mucosa, whereas *D. megastoma* penetrates t hrough the mucosa, p roducing g rossly visible l arge nodules. *H. muscae* and *H. majus* may c ause mild catarrhal gastritis and small erosions and ulcers. O nly rarely they produce significant lesions or clinical disease. Although *D. megastoma* produces **nodules or tumours**, which can cause mechanical interference, but these nodules too rarely lead to clinical disease. These nodules have a small opening on the gastric lumen, and are characterized by a granulomatous inflammatory reaction c ontaining numerous e osinophils. The centre contains the parasites and necrotic debris.

All these parasites have an indirect life cycle. Eggs passed in the faeces are ingested by larvae (maggots) of the housefly (*Musca domestica*) in the case of *H. muscae* and *H. majus*, and by larvae of the stable fly (*Stomoxys calcitrans*) in case of *D. megastoma*. The larvae undergo further development in the pupae of the fly, then migrate, as infective larvae, into the proboscis of the adult flies. The infective larvae are deposited on the lips of horses, and eventully swallowed to develop into adults in the stomach.

Cutaneous habronemiasis

Also known as "**summer sores**", cutaneous habronemiasis is a persistent disease of the skin in horses. It results from the activity of larvae of stomach worms, especially *Draschia megastoma*. The larvae are deposited on the skin by flies. The flies are attracted by a pre-existing ulcer or wound in the skin. Lesions are particularly common in the skin of the pectoral region, between the forelegs. The larvae penetrate deeply into the dermis and stimulate granulomatous tissue formation in which eosinophils are prominent. The skin loses its hair and becomes encrusted by serous exudate, which oozes from the surface. This lesion is seen in horses during the summer months ("**summer sores**"), and is **prevalent in India**. However, the true nature of the lesion can be known only when the larvae are squeezed out from the lesion and identified by microscopic examination.

Habronema larvae may be deposited in the eye and cause **granulomatous conjuctivitis**. They have also been observed in granulomas in the lung. Recently cutaneous habronemiasis has also been reported in a **dog**.

Macracanthorhynchus Infection

Macracanthorhynchus hirudinaceus is a **thorny-headed nematode** (Phylum: **Acanthocephala**) of pigs. It has an **indirect life cycle** and uses various beetles as intermediate hosts. These parasites attach to the wall of the **small intestine**. They usually move from site to site, where they penetrate the mucosa and muscularis and induce **small ulcers** surrounded by neutrophils and granulation tissue. Only rarely parasites penetrate the wall and produce peritonitis.

Oesophagostomiasis

Oesophagostomiasis is also known as "**nodule worm disease**" and "**pimply gut**". It is an important parasitic disease of **cattle, sheep, and goats** in many parts of the world, **including India**. The important species which are members of the genus **Oesophagostomum** (Family **Strongylidae**) are: *O. radiatum* in cattle, *O. columbianum* in sheep and goats, and *O. dentatum* in pigs. Several other species may infect these animals, but they are less pathogenic. **Oesophagostomum** sp. may also infect **monkeys**.

Life Cycle

The parasite is a small, thin nematode that has a **direct life cycle**. Adults in the lumen of the large intestine produce **ova** that pass out in the faeces. After a period outside the host, they develop into **infective larvae**. These larvae, when ingested by another host, penetrate the intestinal mucosa, become encysted, moult in the submucosa, and finally return to the intestinal lumen, where they reach maturity. **Infection occurs only by ingestion**.

Clinical Signs

Clinical signs are usually observed in young animals. Profuse diarrhoea is the most constant sign. It is more intense when larvae return from the submucosa to the intestinal lumen. Heavy long-standing infections usually result in **chronic diarrhoea, anaemia, emaciation, cachexia (wasting), prostration, and death**. Even though signs are mild, lesions may be found at postmortem examination.

Lesions

Mucus a nd inflammatory c ells which e xude from t he intestinal m ucosa are the **result of irritation caused by substances secreted by the adult parasite, from its cephalic or oesophageal glands.** This inflammatory exudate is the chief source of food for the worms. This is because **these worms are not blood suckers, neither do they attach themselves to the mucosa nor cause obstruction of the lumen.** A lthough the m echanism i s n ot understood, the adult parasites do cause intestinal haemorrhage, which may lead to anaemia.

The larvae, on the other hand, produce severe lesions. They penetrate the mucosa anywhere from the pylorus to the anus to reach the deeper parts of the submucosa. Here they encyst and undergo a moult. Some may encyst in the lamina propria, but most are found in the submucosa on the deeper side of the muscularis mucosae. Larvae a re capable of migrating i nto the peritoneal cavity and encysting in granulomas on the surface of various abdominal organs.

In initial (i.e., first-time) **infections,** larvae shed a restricted skin and return to the intestinal lumen as **fourth-stage larvae** in 5-6 days. They produce only mild inflammation in the mucosa and submucosa. However, their ecdysis (shedding of the skin) causes small ulcers and intestinal bleeding. Some **fourth-stage larvae** of *O. columbianum* may undergo **a second intestinal penetration,** where further penetration is usually arrested. **In contrast, in animals repeatedly exposed to these parasites, local tissue sensitivity develops, and subsequent entry of larvae into the mucosa produces an intense tissue reaction.** Large numbers of eosinophils, lymphocytes, m acrophages, and foreign body g iant cells surround the larvae and infiltrate the submucosa and mucosa. The centre of these lesions b ecomes caseated, often calcified, a nd is s urrounded by a dense capsule which p reserves the n odular character o f the l esion. A f ew larvae survive and escape by wandering through the muscularis, but most of them die without finding their way back to the lumen.

The **nodules** may become infected and enlarged, and displace the muscularis mucosae to serve as a focus for local or generlized peritonitis. However, **usually they remain as calcified, encapsulated nodules.** These lesions give the intestine a nodular appearance as they thicken the wall and project from the serosal surface. Hence the name **"nodule worm disease"** or **"pimply gut"**, that is, a gut full of pimples (pimple = a small nodule). When present in large numbers, these nodules may interfere with peristalsis and intestinal absorption.

Diagnosis

Clinical diagnosis can be made by finding eggs or fourth-stage larvae in faecal samples. At postmortem, lesions are recognized by their characteristic gross a nd microscopic features.

Chabertiasis

Another member of the Family **Strongylidae** which closely resembles equine strongyles, as well as **Oesophagostomum** sp. is *Chabertia ovina*. It is **an inhabitant of the colon of sheep, goats, cattle,** and wild ruminants. The parasites have a large buccal capsule on the anterior end, which is used to attach to the mucosa. The parasites draw in a piece of the mucosal epithelium, digest it with their oesophageal secretions, and may ingest blood. Haemorrhage and loss of blood may lead to **anaemia** and **death of the host.** The life cycle is similar to **Oesophagostomum** sp., with a tissue phase in the small intestine, but **Chabertia does not produce nodules.** Marked diarrhoea with blood and mucus may be present in severely affected animals.

Onchocerciasis

Also known as **"worm nodule disease"**, onchocerciasis is caused by filarial worms of the genus **Onchocerca** (Superfamily: **Filarioidea**) (see **Table 50**). Onchocerciasis occurs in **cattle, horses, sheep,** and **goats. Onchocerca are large parasites** whose adults usually live in connective tissue, especially of the subcutis, tendons, and fascia. **Most stimulate chronic inflammatory response leading to the formation of dense fibrous nodules.** Each worm produces **microfilariae,** many of which locate in the skin. Here they are available to **various insects,** which act as **intermediate hosts.** There are several species of importance in domestic animals.

O. gibsoni, transmitted by midges (**Culicoides** sp.), **infects cattle.** It is usually found in the subcutaneous tissue of the brisket and the hind limbs. *O. gutturosa* also infects **cattle,** usually occurring in the connective tissue close to the ligamentum nuchae, or in fascia close to major bones of the limbs. Its microfilariae concentrate in the skin. It is transmitted by black flies and occurs throughout the world. **Neither the microfilariae nor the adults produce any significant pathological change.** Another species which affects cattle is *O. lienalis,* which localizes in the gastrosplenic ligament. *O. armillata* occurs in **cattle, sheep,** and **goats,** and has been **recorded in India. The adults of this parasite form tunnels, nodules, and cysts in the aortic wall, with microfilariae concentrating in the skin.**

In the horse, the adults of *O. cervicalis* are found in the **ligamentum nuchae,** and sometimes in nodular cutaneous lesions. The microfilariae accumulate in the skin of the abdomen near the umbilicus, the flank, or in the eyelids and other ocular tissues. *O. cervicalis* **is common in horses.** The worms have some aetiological relationship to **"poll-evil", "fistulous withers",** and periodic ophthalmia. However, there is no firm evidence to attribute these conditions to onchocerciasis. *O. reticulata* lives in the suspensory ligaments of the forelimbs of horses. The incidence of infection is high. It ranges from 10% in young horses to 90% in horses over 16 years of age. The **lesions are** also more noticeable in **older horses**, and comprise **mineralization and granuloma formation** around adult worms in the nuchal ligaments. Both of these equine parasites are transmitted by black flies.

Physaloptera Infection

Several species of genus **Physaloptera** (Order: **Spirurida**, Family: **Physalopteridae**), also known as "**stomach worms**" parasitize the stomach and duodenum of **cats, dogs**, and **monkeys**. The species include: *P. felidis, P. praeputialis*, and *P. pseudopraeputialis* for cats; *P. rara* for dogs; and *P. canis* for both dogs and cats.

Infection follows ingestion of an intermediate host, which includes cockroaches, beetles, and crickets. The adults attach to the mucosa and suck blood, leaving small erosions and ulcers when they change positions. Hyperplasia of the gastric mucosa may cause nodular projections resembling tumours, especially in monkeys infected with *P. tumefasciens*. As a rule, **Physaloptera infections do not cause clinical disease.**

Pinworms

Several members of the Family **Oxyuridae** are parasitic in animals and humans. They include *Oxyuris equi* (horses), *Skrjabinema ovis* (sheep and goats), *Enterobius anthropopitheci* (monkeys and apes), and *E. vermicularis* (humans).

Life Cycle

The life cycle is direct. Fertilized adult females lay **operculated eggs** in clusters in the perianal region. The eggs reach the infectious stage within a few hours. They are either licked off by a new host, or fall off, and are later ingested. The larvae are released in the intestine and mature to adults, which live in the caecum or colon. Fertilized females migrate to the lower rectum and anus to deposit their eggs.

Lesions

Pinworms are relatively harmless parasites and are rarely associated with serious disease. Activities of the female worms result in pruritus (severe itching), and heavy infestations cause **ulcerative colitis**. The adult worms do not attach themselves to the mucosa, but in ulcerative colitis they may migrate into the mucosa along with larvae.

Diagnosis

Diagnosis is usually made by either detecting adult worms at the anus, or eggs (have single operculum) recovered from the perianal area. Cellophane, or similar clear sticky tape is useful to recover the eggs.

Pulmonary Nematodiasis (Lungworm Disease)

Pulmonary nematodiasis is also known by several other names: "**verminous pneumonia**", "**verminous bronchitis**", "**dictyocauliasis**", "**dictyocaulosis**", and "**metastrongylidosis**". This is because adults of a number of different genera of nematodes, each having several species, live in the lung, and produce "**pulmonary nematodiasis**" or "**lungworm disease**". **It is an important disease of cattle, sheep, and goats in India.** Table 51 presents the common lungworms. The lungworms usually produce disease that leads to death. However, they may live in the lungs with little noticeable effect on the host. **Serious disease is usually encountered in young animals.**

Larval migration of other nematodes may also cause lung damage, but these are not considered here. Other parasites of the lung include: flukes (**Fasciola, Schistosoma, Paragonimus** sp.); intermediate stages of cestodes (hydatid cysts); and arthropods (*Linguatula serrata*, Pneumonyssus sp.). Those which live in the upper respiratory passages include: *Linguatula serrata* (nasal passages of dogs); and the fluke *Schistosoma nasalis*.

Dictyocaulus

Species of the genus Dictyocaulus are among the most important nematodes that parasitize the lung. These include *D. viviparus* of cattle, buffalo camel, and deer; *D. filaria* of sheep and goats; and *D. arnfieldi* of horses and donkeys (Table 51).

Table 51. Common Lungworms

Parasite	Hosts	Site of adult parasite
Aelurostrongylus abstrusus	Cats	Bronchioles, alveolar ducts
Angiostrongylus vasorum	Dogs, foxes	Pulmonary arteries
Capillaria aerophila	Dogs, cats, foxes	Trachea, bronchi
Crenosoma vulpis	Dogs, foxes	Trachea, bronchi, bronchioles
Dictyocaulus arnfieldi	Horses, donkeys	Bronchi, bronchioles
D. filaria	Sheep, goats	Bronchi, bronchioles
D. viviparus	Cattle, buffalo	Bronchi, bronchioles
Filaroides hirthi	Dogs	Bronchi, bronchioles, alveoli
F. milksi	Dogs	Bronchi, bronchioles, alveoli
F. osleri	Dogs	Trachea, bronchi
Metastrongylus apri	Pigs	Bronchi, bronchioles
M. pudendotectus	Pigs	Bronchi, bronchioles
M. salmi	Pigs	Bronchi, bronchioles
Muellerius capillaris	Sheep, goats	Alveoli
Protostrongylus rufescens	Sheep, goats	Bronchioles

Life Cycle

Dictyocaulus species have **a direct life cycle**. Adults live in the bronchi, where eggs a re deposited, some of which hatch in the airways. Eggs a nd/or larvae are coughed up, s wallowed, and p assed in the faeces. They then d e-velop into **infective third-stage larvae** in moist, cool soil. **Ingested larvae** penetrate the intestinal mucosa and migrate through lymphatics to mesenteric lymph nodes, where they develop into **fourth-stage larvae**. These reach the lungs through lymphatics and pulmonary arteries. They enter the pulmonary alveoli, and u ltimately bronchioles and bronchi, w here they reach sexual maturity.

Clinical Signs

Clinical signs with **Dictyocaulus** sp. in **cattle, s heep,** and **goats** may be hardly noticeable, or so severe that death results. **Severe infection is mostly limited to young animals.** The presence of a few lungworms causes only a hacking (dry) cough. However, heavy infestation may result in laboured res-piration, anorexia, diarrhoea, and stunted growth. Sometimes, death may follow pulmonary consolidation caused by secondary bacterial infection of occluded bronchioles and alveoli. Infection with *D. arnfieldi* is usually mild.

Lesions

As larvae break through the capillaries and alveolar walls, they cause haemorrhage and necrosis. They also stimulate an inflammatory cellular in-filtration mainly c omposed of e osinophils, w hich fills t he alveoli, a lveolar septae, and terminal bronchioles. Some larvae, and later adults and eggs, die and may be surrounded by a g ranulomatous reaction, with multinucleated **giant cells.** When the number of the larvae is large, this initial phase of infec-tion can cause grossly visible foci of consolidation throughout the lungs. Heavy infestation is u sually associated w ith **extensive pulmonary oedema a nd interstitial emphysema,** b elieved to r esult f rom a h yperimmune response. With maturation to adults in bronchioles and bronchi, alveolar lesions begin to resolve whereas lesions in the bronchi become prominent. While the larvae induce lesions throughout the lungs, lesions associated with the adults tend to concentrate in t he d orso-caudal lung. **The bronchial epithelium becomes hyperplastic, and eosinophils and lymphocytes infiltrate the wall and peribronchial tissues.** Eosinophils and mucus plug the bronchial lumens, which when occluded lead to atelectasis or consolidation of the related alveoli. The adults, feeding on mucus and cellular debris, deposit ova. These are coughed up as embryonating eggs or hatched larvae. Or, they may lodge in alveoli, initiating a foreign body r eaction.

Aelurostrongylus

Aelurostrongylus abstrusus is a common **lungworm of cats (Table 51),** and has **indirect life cycle**. The adult parasites live in terminal bronchioles and alveolar ducts. Larvae are passed in the faeces, and must be ingested by various snails or slugs for further development. These, in turn, are ingested by transport hosts, which include rodents, frogs, lizards, and birds, in which the larvae remain infective. **Cats become infected by eating the intermediate or transport hosts.**

Larvae released in the gastrointestinal tract reach the lung through the bloodstream to ultimately lie in the bronchial tree. Eggs, which hatch to larvae, form **small, nodular collections** within alveoli. These tend to be located at the periphery of the lung and can be seen grossly as 1-10 mm pale projections. **Microscopically,** the lesions consist of alveoli packed with eggs and larvae, disrupted alveolar septa, and an infiltration of eosinophils, lymphocytes, macrophages, and multinucleated giant cells. The adult worms initiate a mild peribronchiolar inflammation containing eosinophils and mononuclear cells. **Aelurostrongylus** is believed to be the chief cause of medial hyperplasia and hypertrophy of the smooth muscle of pulmonary arteries, which is so often encountered in cats.

Angiostrongylus

Several species of genus **Angiostrongylus** infect the lung and pulmonary arteries. The adults of *Angiostrongylus vasorum* live in the **pulmonary arteries and right ventricle of dogs and foxes (Table 51)**, and stimulate a **proliferative endarteritis** similar to that produced by *Dirofilaria immitis*.

Eggs go up the pulmonary capillaries, where they lodge and hatch. Released larvae penetrate into the alveolar spaces, are coughed up, swallowed, and passed in the faeces. They may then be ingested by snails and slugs, which serve as intermediate hosts. In the lungs, eggs and larvae damage capillaries and small arterioles, causing thrombosis and occlusion. This is accompanied by a **granulomatous reaction** surrounding the parasites. Severe infections may lead to pulmonary hypertension, as well as right heart hypertrophy and failure.

Capillaria

Capillaria species affect a wide variety of animals (Table 54). They live in many different tissues, including the small intestine, urinary bladder, skin, and liver. *Capillaria aerophila* localizes in the trachea and bronchi of **dogs,** foxes, various wild animals, and sometimes **cats. Its life cycle is direct** The infective larvae develop in operculated eggs. Larvae released in the intestine eventually reach the respiratory tract, where the adults develop and cause **mild tracheitis** and **bronchitis.**

Crenosoma

Crenosoma species a re common p arasites of t he t rachea, bronchi, and bronchioles of **wild carnivores**. The best studied is *Crenosoma vulpis*, a parasite of **foxes** and sometimes **dogs (Table 51)**. Its life cycle requires a snail, which after being ingested, r eleases larvae w hich finally r each the l ung through lymphatics. The parasites cause bronchitis, bronchiolitis, and tracheitis, characterized by an infiltration of **eosinophils**. Focal areas of alveolar consolidation may also develop.

Filaroides

Several species of the genus **Filaroides** parasitize the **respiratory tract of dogs and cats (Table 51)**. *Filaroides osleri* affects the **trachea and bronchi of dogs**. It l ives in the mucosa, w here i t produces **n odules** about 1 c m in diameter. **The life cycle is direct**. Mature worms deposit eggs which contain larvae. Larvae leave the nodules through small pores, a nd are passed in the faeces. **Pups** usually acquire the i nfection from their dam. The **nodules are composed mainly of parasites**, which are surrounded by a connective tissue capsule containg a few inflammatory cells. Dead worms stimulate a stronger reaction. The presence of nodules may cause a chronic cough, but it does not affect the overall health of the dog. Although *F. osleri* occurs throughout the world, **it is not common**.

F. hirthi and *F. milksi* also have direct life cycles, and live in the **alveoli and small bronchioles of dogs**. Reaction may be minimal, or granulomatous, with t he presence of eosinophils that cause s mall nodules s imilar to t hose induced by **Muellerius**.

Metastrongylus

Three species of the genus **Metastrongylus** parasitize the **bronchi and bronchioles of pigs**, namely, *Metastrongylus apri*, *M. pudendotectus*, and *M. salmi* **(Table 51)**. **The life cycle is indirect**. Eggs laid in the bronchial tree are coughed up, swallowed, and passed in the faeces. Eggs, or larvae that hatch in the s oil, must b e ingested b y an e arthworm, in w hich further d evelopment occurs. **Pigs get infected when they ingest infected earthworms**, or larvae that earthworms r eleased when t hey died. L arvae penetrate t he intestinal mucosa and migrate to mesenteric lymph nodes, where they undergo a moult. They then go to the lungs.

Lesions are similar to those produced by **Dictyocaulus** sp. in ruminants, but are n ot as severe. Usually, l esions are n ot grossly v isible, and c linical signs are more related to poor performance rather than respiratory signs. I n addition to alveolitis and bronchitis, **lungs** of affected pigs may **contain grossly visible granulomas** stimulated by dead parasites and their eggs.

Muellerius

Muellerius capillaris is a common lungworm of **sheep** and **goats** (Table 51). However, infestation rarely causes clinical disease. **The life cycle is indirect** and similar to **Protostrongylus**. The first-stage larvae are passed in the faeces, and a snail or slug is required for further development. After ingestion of the snail by sheep or goats, the fourth-stage larvae reach the lung through the lymphatics. The larvae enter alveoli, mature to adults, and deposit e ggs. The eggs then hatch to first-stage larvae, and eventually move up the bronchial tree. **The adults, eggs, and newly hatched larvae all live in the alveoli, where they stimulate an inflammatory reaction leading to grossly visible nodules.** Most of the parasites are located immediately beneath the pleura.

The inflammatory response varies with the age of the lesion and previous exposure. Early lesions are characterized by an infiltration of lymphocytes in the alveolar septae and some alveolar haemorrhage. Later, and also in previously exposed animals, the infiltrate contains numerous eosinophils, macrophages, and often multinucleated giant c ells. These d istend the septae and fill the alveoli surrounding the parasites. Alveolar walls also become fibrotic. The lesions may progress to **an inflammatory nodule or granuloma with a core of parasites**. The necrotic material is surrounded by macrophages and g iant cells, w hich in t urn are s urrounded by f ibrous connective t issue. Bronchioles contain mucus and inflammatory cells, and their lining may be hyperplastic. However, bronchiolitis is not a usual feature.

Protostrongylus

Protostrongylus rufescens is a nematode which parasitizes small bronchioles of **sheep, goats,** and **deer** (Table 51). It has **an indirect life cycle**. The eggs hatch in the lungs and are then passed as larvae in the faeces. Further development requires that they be ingested by a snail. After ingestion of the snail by the animal, larvae penetrate the intestinal mucosa, pass to mesenteric lymph nodes, moult, and then move on to the lungs. **The infection is not severe**, but the parasites stimulate an inflammatory response in the wall of the affected bronchiole, and cause consolidation of the related alveoli.

Diagnosis

Lungworm disease c an be s uspected from t he signs. **D iagnosis can be confirmed by identifying lungworm eggs or larvae in the faeces of the living animal.** However, demonstration of adult worms in the bronchi or bronchioles, and ova and larvae in the lung parenchyma at the postmortem examination, is usually necessary to establish the nature of a herd infection. Careful examination with the naked eye and with the help of a hand lens are advised, especially when searching for the smaller lungworms. Histopathological examination is recommended.

Renal Dioctophymosis

Also known as "**giant kidney worm infection**", the giant kidney worm *Dioctophyma renale* is a rare parasite of a wide variety of species that includes **dogs**, **cats**, foxes, **horses**, **cattle**, **pigs**, mink, and **humans**. In domestic animals it is **most common in the dog**. However, the dog is considered an abnormal host. Mink, which are the most commonly affected animals, are the normal final host.

The adult worms are the largest of all nematodes, and live in the pelvis of the kidney. However, they may also be encountered in the peritoneal cavity. Eggs laid by the adult worms pass in the urine and undergo development of one to several months in water. They are then ingested by the **intermediate host**, an annelid (e.g., earthworms, leeches). Here they hatch, undergo further development, and encyst. Frogs and fish may serve as paratenic hosts. Dogs and other susceptible species become infected by ingesting the intermediate, or paratenic, hosts. Larvae released in the intestinal tract penetrate the wall, and enter the peritoneal cavity. Afterwards, they penetrate the kidney to reside in the pelvis. This entire process requires a minimum of about three months, but may take several years.

Clinical Signs

Clinical signs may be absent. Compensatory hypertrophy of the unaffected kidney prevents renal failure. However, bilateral involvement leads to **death from uraemia**.

Lesions

In dogs, the **right kidney is more frequently affected than the left**. However, as dog is not a normal host, the parasite is usually found restricted to the peritoneal cavity, where it cannot complete its life cycle. The presence of worms in the renal **pelvis leads to slow destruction of the renal parenchyma**, ultimately producing a fluid-filled sac. In the peritoneal cavity, the worms and their eggs stimulate a **chronic peritonitis with adhesions**.

Diagnosis

Diagnosis can be made by finding **eggs in the urine**.

Rhabditis Dermatitis

Also known as "**rhabditic dermatitis**" and "**Pelodera dermatitis**", dermatitis caused by the larvae of the nematode *Pelodera strongyloides* is rare and **occurs mostly in the dog**. The Family **Rhabditidae** contains many nematodes which live in moist decaying organic matter. **Usually these are not pathogenic**. Sometimes, however, some may cause dermatitis or other superficial lesions.

In dogs, cattle, and rarely in horses *Pelodera strongyloides* (*Rhabditis strongyloides*) can be found within localized areas of dermatitis. The dermatitis occurs especially on the ventral abdomen and limbs, and is characterized by erythema, pustules, and hyperkeratosis. The nematodes are unable to penetrate the intact skin, but can invade skin previously damaged from other causes. **Microscopically**, the nematodes are most prominent within hair follicles, but may also be found within the dermis. They do not penetrate beyond the skin.

Diagnosis is confirmed by finding live, motile *P. strongyloides* larvae in skin scrapings of affected areas. The adult parasites can be identified in tissue section by their rhabditiform oesophagus (anterior wide portion, narrow midsection, and terminal bulbous portion).

Spirocercosis

Infection with the spiruroid worm *Spirocerca lupi* (oesophageal worm) is worldwide in distribution, **and is also widely prevalent in India**. The adult worms are usually bright red. **They are found coiled in nodules in the wall of the oesophagus, aorta, stomach**, and other organs of the **dog, cat**, fox and wolf. The males are 30-54 mm long; the females 54-80 mm. **The eggs are thick-walled, and contain larvae when deposited.**

Life Cycle

The life cycle of this nematode is complex. The embryonated eggs are passed in the faeces and do not hatch until ingested by certain beetles. In these **intermediate hosts**, the larvae develop into the **infective (third) stage**, then encyst. When eaten by an abnormal host (paratenic host), such as a frog, snake, lizard, or any of the birds and mammals, the larvae burrow into the mesentery, where they remain in a viable state for some time. **When infected beetles are eaten by one of the final hosts (dog, cat**, fox, wolf), **the larvae penetrate the stomach wall.** Then, by following the course of the arteries and migrating through the adventitia and media, they reach the wall of the aorta and localize in the adventitia, usually in the upper thoracic portion. **The parasites reach the aorta 1-2 weeks after ingestion.** Here, they develop for about 90 days, and then migrate to the neighbouring oesophagus and burrow into its wall. In the oesophagus, they develop to adults in cyst nodules. Patent (open) infection is established 50-70 days later when the eggs reach the oeosphageal lumen through a small opening in the nodule. Only rarely, the adults localize in an abnormal location, such as wall of the stomach or lungs.

Clinical Signs

Clinical signs may be absent in mild infections. Or, there may be persistent **dysphagia** (difficulty in swallowing) and **vomiting** caused by oesophageal obstruction. Sudden death from haemorrhage from aortic lesions has been reported.

Lesions

The main features are produced by the adult worms as a result of their localization in the adventitia of the aorta and submucosa of the **oesophagus**. The worms become the focus of a **tumour-like nodule in the aortic wall**. This may initiate the **formation of aneurysm**, with possible rupture and fatal haemorrhage. **In microscopic sections** of the lesions of the **aorta**, worms may be found in areas of the adventitia and media. Here, the normal tissue is destroyed and replaced by leukocytes and debris. Sometimes the worms burrow into the media, with necrotic tracts leading to the intima. The intima undergoes marked proliferation. Mineralization and ossification may occur in the intima and media. **Finally, the worm leaves the aortic media or adventitia for the oesophagus**.

The **oesophgeal lesions** are most common near its terminus, usually a few centimeters from the cardia of the stomach. **Grossly**, one or several nodules are seen on the luminal surface (i.e., of lumen), raising the epithelium. **One or several worms may be embedded in each nodule**, and parts of the worms protrude from a small orifice. Cross section of one of the nodules reveals a thick fibrous wall, enclosing a cavity containing worms and yellowish pus. **Microscopically**, the worms form the centre for a mass of neutrophils. These are surrounded by a thick wall of connective tissue infiltrated with macrophages, lymphocyes, and plasma cells. Surprisingly, eosinophils are usually absent. In the worms, ova within the gravid uterus are ovoid and are embryonated before they are discharged through the genital pore.

Some affected dogs develop "**vertebral spondylosis**" or "**deformative ossifying spondylitis**" of the thoracic vertebrae. It is believed to be related to the migration and encystment of *Spirocerca lupi*.

Malignant neoplasms may develop within the wall of *Spirocerca lupi* granulomas. These are either **fibrosarcomas** or **osteosarcomas** which may metastasize to the lungs. **Their pathogenesis is not known**, but their close association with the parasite indicates it is the cause. **Hypertrophic pulmonary osteopathy** is a common finding in dog with large oesophageal malignancies.

Diagnosis

Infection with *Spirocerca lupi* in the living animal is confirmed by the identification of the **embryonated ova in the faeces**. Postmortem diagnosis is easily made by demonstration of characteristic lesions in the aorta, oesophagus, or ventral surface of thoracic vertebrae in association with the adult parasites.

Stephanofilariasis

Stephanofilariasis is **a nematode dermatitis of cattle caused by several** related filarial worms (see **Table 50**). The condition is worldwide in distribution. *Stephanofilaria assamensis* **occurs in Assam and other parts of India.** It causes chronic dermatitis in **Zebu cattle**, known as "**hump sore**". *S. zaheeri* is associated with dermatitis of the ears of **buffaloes in India**, referred to as "**earsore**". *S. stilesi* occurs in the skin lesions of **cattle** in United States. It causes dermatitis usually on the abdomen. *S. dedoesi* has been reported from Indonesia. It produces lesions on the sides of the neck, withers, dewlap, shoulders, and around the eyes. In Malaysia. *S. kaeli* causes "**filarial sores**" on the lower legs of **cattle**. In Japan, a species of **Stephanofilaria** produces dermatitis of the muzzle and teats of **cattle.**

Each has an indirect life cycle. Various species of flies ingest microfilariae as they feed on the lesions. Infective larvae develop in the fly after an interval of about 10 days, and are present in the proboscis.

Lesions

Studies on *S. assamensis* in **Zebu cattle** with "**hump sore**" have revealed that microfilariae live within eggs whose shells do not stain with H & E. **However, they can be seen with Gram's stain.**

The adult forms of *S. stilesi* are found either in the base of hair follicles, or in the dermis near the epidermis. In either site, the worms are surrounded by a zone of inflammation, containing eosinophils, lymphocytes, neutrophils, macrophages, and usually a layer of connective tissue. The microfilariae and adults are found in the dermal papillae. Hyperkeratosis and parakeratosis may be seen in the epidermis of parasitized areas. Crusts of exuded serum and detritus (tissue debris) may collect on the surface. Death of the parasites and sensitization of the host result in **severe dermatitis.**

Diagnosis

The parasites can be collected by deep scrapings of skin and identified by microscopic examination. Diagnosis can be established by the demonstration of adults and microfilariae in biopsy, or postmortem samples of affected skin.

Stephanuriasis

Also known as "**swine kidney worm infection**" and "**kidney worm disease**", stephanuriasis is a disease of **pigs** caused by the nematode *Stephanurus dentatus*. The swine kidney worm is 20-40 mm long, and is found mainly in the **perirenal fat and neighbouring tissues**. These worms form cystic cavities which communicate with lumen of the ureter and permit the **discharge of ova with the urine.**

Life Cycle

The larvae hatch in moist, shaded soil, and remain infective for some time unless exposed to direct sunlight and drying. The **infective larvae** may be ingested by the host, or penetrate the skin. **Earthworms** may serve as transport hosts. The larvae lose their sheaths to reach the fourth stage. This depends upon the route of entry. Orally ingested worms moult in the wall of the stomach, while those that penetrate the skin undergo this change in the abdominal muscles. The **fourth-stage larvae** soon migrate to the liver either through the portal veins when ingested, or after penetration of the skin through the lungs and systemic circulation. They remain in the liver for 2-3 months. Their movements stimulate severe tissue reaction. Eventually larvae come out of the liver into the peritoneal cavity and wander extensively. Most of them ultimately reach the **perirenal fat**. Here, the adults copulate and the female lays eggs in a cyst, which then empty into the ureter. **This life cycle requires about six months**.

Clinical Signs

Infected pigs are usually emaciated in spite of a good appetite, and **ascites** is common as a result of liver damage. **Death** may occur following secondary infection, extensive tissue destruction, or urinary obstruction.

Lesions

Both the larvae and the adults produce severe effects upon the host. Nodules and oedema in the host subcutis and mild enlargement of the superficial lymph nodes are produced by the passage of larvae. However, their most serious effect is upon the **liver**. These worms burrow into the liver, then stay here for a relatively long time, and move about aggressively. This eventually results in **extensive portal fibrosis**, which may obliterate many liver lobules. The fibrotic change is accompanied by intense tissue eosinophilia, foci of coagulative necrosis, and infiltration by other leukocytes.

A feature of this parasite is that it wanders extensively through the host's tissue producing widespread damage. Although most worms find their way to the vicinity of the ureters, many wander to other sites, where they stimulate a local purulent tissue reaction. *S. dentatus* has been found in the kidney, lumbar muscles, myocardium, lungs, pleural cavity, spleen, and even the spinal cord. Paralysis may result from destruction of the lumbar spinal cord by the migration of these worms.

Diagnosis

The diagnosis may be made **by demonstrating ova in the urine**, or by finding the worms at postmortem examination. In the liver, leukocytic infiltration and fibrosis are much more intense and extensive than the changes caused by other larvae in this organ (e.g., ascarids). This point is helpful in histological differentiation.

Strongyloidosis (Strongyloidiasis)

Several species of the genus **Strongyloides** (not to be confused with **Strongylus**) affect animals. The most important species include: *S. papillosus* of cattle, sheep, and goats; *S. westeri* of horses, pigs, and zebras; *S. ransomi* of pigs; *S. cati* and *S. tumefaciens* of cats; *S. fuelleborni* of monkeys; and *S. stercoralis* of humans, monkeys, foxes, dogs, and cats.

Life Cycle

Strongyloides are unusual parasites. They may occur either as parasites of the intestinal tract, or as free-living non-parasitic worms. **Only the female worm,** which reproduces parthenogenetically (i.e., from **unfertilized** eggs), **is parasitic.** The worms are 1-6 mm long, and live deep in the c rypts of the small intestine. Embryonated eggs may hatch in the lumen of the small intestine, or are passed in the faeces. They are **of three types:** diploid, haploid, and triploid. In the soil, **triploid eggs** give rise to infective third-stage larvae; **diploid eggs** hatch to free-living female adults; and **haploid eggs** hatch to free-living male adults. **Larvae infect the host by penetrating the skin.** They then enter into the venous circulation. However, infection through **ingestion** can also occur.

The larvae are then carried to the **lungs.** Here, they enter into the alveoli, are coughed up and swallowed, and ultimately reach the **intestine,** where they develop into adults. Transmammary and prenatal (i.e. before birth) infection may occur for some species of Strongyloides in the absence of intestinal parasites, a situation similar to that of some species of ascarids. Another feature of **Strongyloides** is that **hyperinfection** may occur, with completion of the reproductive cycle within the host. In this situation, the larvae hatch in the lower intestine, penetrate the intestinal wall, and cycle through the lungs. **This is most common in humans.**

Lesions

Upon entry, larvae cause minimal damage to the skin and lungs. However, in previously exposed (i.e., hypersensitive) animals, this migration may cause **allergic dermatitis** and **pneumonia,** although usually mild. The adult parasites lie deep in the crypts of the small intestine. When their number is small, **clinical signs and significant lesions may not occur.** However, the presence of a large number leads to diarrhoea and usually serious disease, which may **cause death.**

The mucosa of the **small intestine** is oedematous and infiltrated with neutrophils, lymphocytes, and eosinophils. Sometimes, epithelioid cells form small granulomas. Small erosions and haemorrhages may occur. The diarrhoea results from malabsorption. In severe infections, especially in hyperinfection, numerous migrating **filariform larvae** are present throughout the wall of the intestine and in many distant organs, including the liver, lungs, and brain. Often, bacteria brought along with the larvae cause **sepsis**. This is not common in domestic animals, but is not uncommon in humans and monkeys. *S. tumefaciens* infection of cats is associated with nodular (tumour-like) proliferative lesions in the colon.

Diagnosis

Diagnosis is made by demonstrating the **eggs or larvae in the faeces**. Histopathologically, the lesions are characteristic.

Thelaziasis

Thelazia ("eye worms"; family **Thelaziidae) live in the conjunctival sac and lachrymal duct of many domestic animals.** *Thelazia gulosa* and *T. skrjabini* are parasites of **cattle**, and are distributed worldwide. *T. lachrymalis* affects **horses** and is also distributed worldwide. *T. californiensis* occurs in the United States in **sheep, dogs,** deer, and rarely cats and humans. *T. callipaeda* occurs in Asia in **dogs.** *T. alfortensis* affects cattle in Europe. *T. rhodesii* has been reported from Asia, Africa, and Europe in **cattle, sheep, goats,** and **buffaloes**.

The **life cycle** of these spiruroid worms depends upon various species of flies (**Musca**) as intermediate hosts and vectors. The larvae move from the gut to develop first in the ovary of the fly, where they penetrate and develop in ovarian follicles. They spend their second and third stages in the ovary. Then, as **third-stage infective larvae**, they migrate to the mouth parts of the fly, ready to be transferred to the **conjunctivae of cattle**.

Their presence in the conjunctival sac causes excessive photophobia (intolerance to light) and lachrymation, if not removed. They are reported to cause blindness through production of corneal opacity. The **diagnosis** is made by finding and identifying the parasites in the conjunctiva.

Trichinosis

Trichinosis is also known as "trichiniasis" and "trichinelliasis". **Animals are rarely affected seriously by trichinosis.** However, they are the **source of infection for humans**, in whom the disease may be debilitating or fatal. In other words, **trichinosis is a parasitic disease of public health significance**. The causative agent is a tiny, slender nematode, *Trichinella spiralis* (family: **Trichinellidae**). It spends its adult life in the mucosa of the small intestine in a wide variety of species, including **humans**, domestic and wild **pigs**, rats, bears, **dogs**, and **cats**. The female is 3-4 mm long, and the male about half as long. The females are viviparous. The **larvae** they produce are **the main cause of symptoms and lesions** because they burrow through tissues and encyst in striated muscles.

Life Cycle

The life cycle of *Trichinella spiralis* is completed only when raw or undercooked meat containing encysted larvae are consumed by the host. **Pork products provide the main source of infection for humans**. The action of digective enzymes releases the infective larvae from the ingested muscle. Then, rapidly they undergo successive moults and mature into adults. After copulation the male dies, but the female burrows into the lamina propria of the intestinal villi, and deposits large numbers of larvae in the lymphatic spaces. Some larvae may escape into the intestinal lumen, but most of them are carried to the bloodstream and reach the skeletal and cardiac muscles. **The larvae invade the muscle bundles**, where they encyst (i.e., become enclosed in a cyst) and remain throughout the life of the host. Further development of the parasite occurs after ingestion of the infected muscle by another host.

Clinical Signs

Clinical signs of trichinosis are rarely observed in animals. They are varied and non-specific in humans. Even in humans, small numbers of trichina larvae do not provoke visible symptoms though they reach the muscles, but in large numbers they produce muscle pain, nausea, vomiting, diarrhoea, fever, oedema of the face, increased respiratory rate, and urticarial skin manifestations. When larvae invade the central nervous system, signs include disorientation, apathy, stupor, delirium, paralysis, and coma. The most important clinical laboratory evidence of the infection is in the blood cell count. Leukocytosis with **eosinophilia**, which in extreme cases may reach 90%, is characteristic. Although eosinophils fluctuate within wide limits, the eosinophilia may persist for months, **or even years**. Identification of adult trichinae in the stools, or demonstration of larvae in biopsy specimens of muscle, confirms the clinical diagnosis of trichinosis.

Lesions

Except for the mild catarrhal enteritis produced by the activities of the adults, the lesions of trichinosis in animals are confined to the skeletal, and to a much smaller extent, the cardiac muscles. Lesions are the result of invasion and encystment of the larvae. **In humans**, the muscles usually parasitized are the diaphragmatic, intercostal, mesenteric, laryngeal, lingual, and ocular. **The larvae penetrate the skeletal muscle bundles, usually near the tendinous portion, stimulating some inflammatory reaction.** The inflammation soon subsides as each larva becomes encysted in a muscle bundle. The sarcoplasm is replaced at the site of invasion by the encapsulated worm, and neighbouring parts of the muscle bundle may undergo some degenerative changes. The parasite damages the sarcolemma, the nuclei increase in size and number, and the sarcoplasm may become granular and lose its cross striations. Droplets of **fatty material** collect in the sarcolemma near the cyst containing the parasite.

After sometime, **calcium salts may be deposited**. They are first deposited in the thick hyaline capsule around the parasite (now dead or dying); and later, in the parasite itself. Fully calcified lesions appear as short chalk-coloured streaks in skeletal muscle, and are sometimes visible to the naked eye.

Diagnosis

Microscopic demonstration of the trichina larvae in the muscles of animals is sufficient to establish the nature of the parasite. However, this is not enough to prove that the larvae were the cause of any clinical symptoms. Although this is a somewhat academic problem in animals, **it is more important in humans**. Trichina larvae can be demonstrated by digestion of muscle.

A common meat inspection practice uses small pieces of fresh skeletal muscle (usually the diaphragm). These are compressed between two heavy glass plates and examined under the low magnification (trichinoscopy). Larvae are readily seen in these preparations, but in mild infection this method may not show any larvae. Routine tissue sections also reveal the **encysted larvae coiled within a hyaline membrane inside a muscle bundle**.

Trichuriasis

Trichuriasis is also known as "**whipworm infestation**". Whipworms include members of the family **Trichuridae** (genus: **Trichuris**). They were so named because one part of their body is thick and rest is thin (G. trich = hair, i.e., thin like hair + G. oura = tail, i.e., having a hair-tail), **resembling the shape of a whip**. There are several species of importance. *Trichuris ovis* is found in the caecum of **cattle, sheep, goats,** and many wild ruminants. *T. discolour* occurs in the caecum and colon of **cattle, sheep,** and **goats**. *T. suis* lives in the caecum of domestic and wild **pig** and wild boar. It is similar morphologically to *T. trichiura*, a whipworm of humans. *T. vulpis* infects **dogs** and foxes, whereas *T. serrata* infects **cats**. *T. globulosa* occurs in **sheep, goats, cattle, and camels**.

The parasites are oviparous. Infective eggs are ingested and hatch in the intestine. The released larvae penetrate the mucosa of the caecum and colon. After a period of about two weeks, the posterior portion of the larvae protrudes into the intestinal lumen, while the head remains embedded in the mucosa.

Light to moderate infections produce little visible effects. However, heavy parasitic loads may lead to **catarrhal, haemorrhagic, or necrotizing typhlitis** (inflammation of the caecum) and **colitis. Clinical and pathological findings are most common in pigs**. During periods of drought, whipworms increase and may be found in large numbers in the caecum and colon of **sheep**. Death may occur under these conditions.

Trichostrongylosis

The Superfamily **Trichostrongyloidea** contains several families. One of these is **Trichostrongylidae**, which in turn contains several genera that infect the gastrointestinal tract of a number of animal species. The most important genera are those which inhabit the abomasum of sheep and cattle, particularly members of the genera **Haemonchus** and **Ostertagia**. The important genera of **Trichostrongylidae** and its members are presented in **Table 52**. Other significant families of the superfamily **Trichostrongyloidea** are **Dictyocaulidae**, **Metastrongylidae** and **Filaroididae** which contain many important lungworms, discussed under "**pulmonary nematodiasis**".

Helminths of the Superfamily **Trichostrongyloidea** are small slender worms (**hair worms, scour worms**) in which the buccal cavity is absent or rudimentary, and usually toothless. **Their life cycles are direct**. The ova pass to the ground in the faeces of the host, hatch into filariform larvae, develop through larval stages in the soil, and produce infection in a new host **when they are ingested with fresh grass**. The larvae burrow between and beneath the epithelial cells of the abomasum, stomach, or small intestine, but usually remain above the basement membrane. Here, they undergo further development to adult worms. They do not migrate systemically. **The results of infection differ with the trichostrongyles.**

Table 52. Important genera and species of the Family Trichostrongylidae

Parasite	Location of adult	Host(s)
Genus: Cooperia		
C. curticei	Small intestine, abomasum (rare)	Sheep, goat, cattle (rare)
C. oncophora	Small intestine, abomasum (rare)	Cattle, sheep, horse (rare)
C. pectinata	Small intestine, abomasum (rare)	Cattle, sheep (rare)
C. punctata	Small intestine, abomasum (rare)	Cattle, sheep (rare)
C. spatulata	Small intestine, abomasum (rare)	Sheep, cattle
Genus: Haemonchus		
H. contortus	Abomasum	Sheep, goat, cattle, other ruminants
H. placei	Abomasum	Cattle
H. similis	Abomasum	Cattle, deer

Genus: Nematodirus

N. battus	Small intestine	Sheep, cattle, other ruminants
N. filicollis	Small intestine	Sheep, goat, cattle, deer
N. helvetianus	Small intestine	Cattle
N. spathiger	Small intestine	Sheep, cattle, other ruminants

Genus: Ostertagia

O. circumcincta	Abomasum	Sheep, goat
O. ostertagi	Abomasum	Sheep, goat, cattle, horse
O. trifurcata	Abomasum	Sheep, goat, cattle

Genus: Trichostrongylus

T. affinus	Small intestine	Rabbit, sheep, other ruminants
T. axei	Abomasum, stomach	Sheep, goat, cattle, pig, horse, donkey, humans
T. capricola	Small intestine	Sheep, goat
T. colubriformis	Abomasum, small intestine	Sheep, goat, cattle, pig, dog, humans
T. longispicularis	Small intestine	Sheep, cattle
T. retortaeformis	Small intestine, stomach (rare)	Rabbit, goat
T. vitrinus	Small intestine	Sheep, goat, pig, deer, dog, humans

Cooperiasis and Nematodiriasis

Cooperia and Nematodirus sp. are trichostrongyles which infect the upper small intestine of cattle, sheep, and other ruminants, including goats and deer. The important species are: *Cooperia pectinata*, *C. punctata*, and *C. oncophora* of cattle; *C. curticei* of sheep and goats; *Nematodirus filicollis* and *N. spathiger* of sheep, cattle, goats and other ruminants, including deer; *N. battus* of sheep; and *N. helvetianus* of cattle and sheep (Table 52).

Their life cycles are direct. The ingested larvae penetrate the intestinal mucosa, which can lead to extensive destruction. Clinically, affected animals develop diarrhoea, hypoproteinaemia, and wasting. Microscopically, the mucosa is atrophic with villous atrophy, and dilated glands contain the parasites. There may be erosions and an inflammatory infiltration of the lamina propria.

Haemonchosis

Haemonchosis is an important disease of sheep, goats, and cattle. *Haemonchus contortus* **parasitizes sheep and goats, and** *H. placei* **cattle (Table 52). These are extremely important parasites of the abomasum, and are widely prevalent in India.** They are commonly known as "**barber-pole worms**", "**twisted stomach worms**", or "**common stomach worms**". **They are the largest of the trichostrongyles,** the female w orms measuring u p to 30 mm in length. The common names are given from the appearance of the female worms, i n which the ovaries a re s pirally w rapped around the blood filled intestine. D evelopment of larvae requires a warm and m oist environment. Therefore, serious infections are seen mostly in **rainy season**. Larvae do not survive cold winters nor hot dry summers. However, the parasites have adapted to u nfavourable environmental c onditions t hrough a rrested l arval d evelopment (**hypobiosis**) within their hosts, which allows their continuation.

Life Cycle

The life cycle is direct. Infective third-stage larvae, after they are ingested, reach the abomasum. Here, they penetrate between epithelial cells' and moult to t he fourth-stage, w hen they a ttach to t he submucosa. S exual maturity i s reached in a bout two w eeks for *H*. *contortus* and a bout four w eeks for *H*. *placei*. **Both fourth-stage larvae and adults suck blood**. They attach to the mucosa with their lancets (buccal teeth). Not only do they deprive the host of large quantities of blood, **but they leave lacerations on the mucosa which predispose to gastritis.**

Clinical Signs

Anaemia and **hypoproteinaemia** (due to blood loss) are the main clinical signs of haemonchosis. In s evere infections w ith large n umbers o f w orms, **death may occur in the absence of clinical signs**. Usually, the disease continues over a long period with signs of weakness, loss of weight, and oedema of dependent parts, especially under the jaw and along the abdomen.

Lesions

Lesions depend o n the duration of i nfection. However, t hey are a lways characterized by **multifocal haemorrhages** on the mucosa of the **abomasum** with **attached and free parasites easily visible**. The abomasal contents a re reddish brown. Mucous membranes are pale and oedema may be widespread. **Hydropericardium, hydrothorax, and ascites may be present**. The body fat undergoes mucoid d egeneration, and b ecomes highly o edematous. Liver i s light brown and usually friable with areas of fatty change.

Ostertagiasis

Ostertagia sp. are important parasites of **cattle** and **sheep**. *O. ostertagi* is **the most important species in cattle**, and *O. circumcincta* the most important **in sheep and goats (Table 52)**. *Ostertagia* sp. resemble abomasal *Trichostrongylus* sp., but are much more important as pathogens, especially in **cattle**.

Life Cycle

The life cycle is direct. The parasites are more resistant to drying and cold temperatures than **Trichostrongylus** sp. After ingestion, the larvae penetrate the mucosa, where they undergo further development. Mature worms may remain partially embedded in the mucosa, or be found free

Clinical Signs

Diarrhoea occurs, which may be severe and wasting. Hypoproteinaemia may be present, as well as oedema of dependent parts.

Lesions

Grossly, the **abomasum** is thickened and covered with **multiple nodules**. This has given rise to the term "**morocco leather appearance**". The **nodules**, which may coalesce, contain larvae and often a projecting adult worm. **Micro-scopically**, the **nodules** result from dilation of glands along with marked epithelial hyperplasia and mucous metaplasia. A loss of parietal cells occurs, as well as achlorhydria (absence of hydrochloric acid) in the stomach. The lamina propria is infiltrated with eosinophils, neutrophils, lymphocytes, and plasma cells. Areas of mucosal necrosis are also present in severe infections.

Trichostrongylosis

Many species of the genus **Trichostrongylus** affect animals. The most important are: *Trichostrongylus axei*, which parasitizes the **abomasum of cattle, sheep, and goats**; *T. vitrinus*, and *T. capricola* of the **sheep** and **goat small intestine**; and *T. longispicularis* of the small intestine of **cattle, sheep, and goats**. These and other species and their usual location are presented in **Table 52**.

Life Cycle

The life cycle is direct. Following ingestion of **infective third-stage larvae**, they exsheath (remove sheath) and penetrate the abomasal or intestinal epithelium. In the case of horses, they penetrate deep into dilated gastric glands. The larvae go through two or more stages to become sexually mature in about 20 days. These adults remain partially embedded in the superficial mucosa. Larvae of **Trichostrongylus** sp. are much more resistant to drying and winter temperatures than are **Haemonchus** sp. Their development is, however, best during the warm moist season (rainy season). Like **Haemonchus** sp., larvae may remain in arrested development for their survival against adverse environmental conditions. However, they usually depend on persistence of adults for their perpetuation.

Clinical Signs

Trichostrongylus sp. are not as important pathogens as **Haemonchus** sp., **and their presence may not be associated with clinical disease**. Trichostrongylosis can, however, be characterized by **wasting, diarrhoea, and hypoproteinaemia**.

Lesions

Usually, **Trichostrongylus** sp. are found along with other nematodes, including **Ostertagia** sp., which are more important parasites. Lesions include **abomasitis, gastritis,** or **enteritis**. The mucosa of the abomasum or stomach is usually covered with a layer of mucus, and **microscopically** epithelial hyperplasia and mucous hyperplasia are present. This leads to a chlorhydria (absence of hydrochloric acid in the stomach). Small erosions may be present, and the lamina propria is infiltrated with eosinophils, neutrophils, lymphocytes, and plasma cells. When small intestine is parasitized, **villous atrophy** with an increased number of goblet cells is the main finding.

Diagnosis of Gastrointestinal Parasitism in Ruminants

Infection can usually be confirmed **by demonstrating eggs on faecal examination**. However, eggs of the different species, other than **Nematodirus**, cannot be differentiated and **cultures** must be made if one wants to determine the species present. Except in young animals, there is little correlation between faecal egg count and worm burden. Therefore, parasitic gastroenteritis should not be diagnosed on the basis of faecal egg count alone. A total worm count should be done whenever possible, and the results considered together with the clinical signs, age of the animal, and season of the year. The critical test in an outbreak of disease is the response to treatment.

Helminthic Diseases of Poultry

A great variety of helminths infect birds. However, in poultry, **helminths are not usually a major cause of disease or economic loss** because indoor rearing prevents contact with intermediate hosts, and because of the relatively short life span of broilers.

Trematodes (Flukes)

A large number of trematodes have been described in birds. **Most are of low pathogenicity**. Trematodes (flukes) are flat, leaf-like parasites ("**flat worms**") belonging to the Phylum **Platyhelminthes**, Class **Trematoda**. They differ from the cestodes (Class **Cestoda**) **in having a digestive system, and they do not form proglottids.** The life cycle of all trematodes parasitizing birds requires a **molluscan as an intermediate host.** Some species also use **a second intermediate host.** Since adult trematodes and larval metacercariae invade almost every cavity and tissue of birds, they may show up unexpectedly at postmortem examination.

Flukes are less host-specific than tapeworms. Therefore wild birds usually introduce infection in areas where domestic poultry are reared. Since many snails live in ponds and streams, **ducks and geese are the most commonly parasitized.** Of all the trematodes, **Prosthogonimus** sp., commonly known as the **oviduct fluke** may cause problems in chickens. *P. macrorchis* has caused economic losses to poultry producers **by drastically reducing egg production.** Sometimes it is enveloped within a hen's egg and is later discovered by a complaining customer.

Cestodes (Tapeworms)

A large number of cestodes (tapeworms) have been described in birds. **Most are of low pathogenicity.** Tapeworms are in the Class **Cestoda**, and flukes are in the Class **Trematoda.** Both belong to the Phylum **Platyhelminthes.** Cestodes utilize arthropod and other invertebrate **intermediate hosts.** Some of the more important tapeworms are listed in **Table 53.**

Table 53. Some important tapeworms of poultry

Tapeworm	Main final host	Intermediate host
Amoebotaenia cuneata	Chicken	Earthworms
Choanotaenia infundibulum	Chicken	Housefly, beetles
Davainea proglottina	Chicken	Slugs, snails
Hymenolepis cantaniana	Chicken	Beetles
Hymenolepis carioca	Chicken	Stable fly, dung beetles
Raillietina cesticillus	Chicken	Beetles
Raillietina echinobothrida	Chicken	Ants
Raillietina tetragona	Chicken	Ants

Chickens may be infected with tapeworms if they are reared on deep litter or in backyard flocks. These parasites are found usually in warmer seasons, when intermediate hosts are abundant. **Many species of tapeworms are now rare in intensive poultry farming because the birds do not come in contact with intermediate hosts.**

Tapeworms or cestodes are flattened, ribbon shaped, usually segmented worms. The term "**proglottid**" is used to describe these **individual "segments".** One to several gravid proglottids are shed daily from the posterior end of the worm. Each proglottid contains one or more sets of reproductive organs, which may become crowded with eggs as the maturing proglottid becomes a gravid proglottid.

Tapeworms are characterized by complete absence of a digestive tract and obtain their nourishment by absorption from the intestinal contents of the host. **Duodenum, jejunum, or ileum is the usual site for attachment.** Birds become infected by eating an **intermediate host**, and thus the larval stage of the tapeworm enters the intestine. This larval tapeworm is known as a "cysticercoid". The intermediate host may be an insect, earthworm, snail, slug, crustacean, or leech depending on the species of the tapeworm.

Pathogenicity

Some of the large tapeworms, *Raillietina cesticillus* and *Choanotaenia infundibulum*, may block completely the intestine of an infected bird. Different species vary considerably in pathogenicity. Of the various species, those which are of pathological importance include *Davainea proglottina, Raillietina tetragona* and *Raillietina echinobothrida*. *D. proglottina* is one of the more harmful species in young birds. The **clinical signs** of infection include **emaciation, dull plumage, breathing difficulties, leg weakness, paralysis, and death.** *R. tetragona* can cause weight loss and decreased egg production. *R. echinobothrida* is usually described as one of the most pathogenic tapeworms, since its presence has been associated with **nodular disease of chickens.** It produces **parasitic granulomas** about 1-6 mm in diameter at the sites of attachment. The condition is associated with catarrhal hyperplastic enteritis as well as lymphocytic, heterophilic, and eosinophilic infiltration.

Diagnosis

Distinctive characteristics of different species of tapeworms can be demonstrated by examining the scolex, the eggs, or individual proglottids of recently shed, live worms. Wet-mount preparations of the scolex examined under a coverslip with X 100 or higher magnification may reveal enough characteristics to make a species identification. Hook characteristics may require measurement with an ocular micrometer under higher magnification. Distinctive egg characteristics can be demonstrated by teasing apart a gravid proglottid under a coverslip. Wet preparations of mature or gravid proglottids under low magnification may reveal diagnostic characteristics such as the location, size, and shape of the cirrus pouch and the location of the genital pore and the gonads. If further details of the internal structures of the proglottid are required for identification, it may be necessary to kill, fix, stain, destain, dehydrate, and permanently mount the specimen.

Nematodes (Roundworms)

Nematodes constitute the most important group of helminthic parasites

of poultry. In both the number of species and the amount of damage done, they far exceed the trematodes and cestodes. The important nematodes of poultry are presented in **Table 54**.

Table 54. Some important nematodes of poultry

Nematode	Location	Intermediate host
Ascaridia galli	Small intestine	None
Capillaria anatis	Small intestine, caecum, cloaca	None
C. annulata	Oesophagus, crop	Earthworm
C. bursata	Small intestine	Earthworm
C. caudinflata	Small intestine	Earthworm
C. contorta	Mouth, oesophagus, crop	None or earthworm
C. obsignata	Small intestine, caecum	None
Heterakis gallinarum	Caecum	None
Syngamus trachea	Trachea	None
Trichostrongylus tenuis	Caecum	None

Avian nematodes usually have a broad host range. Therefore, nematodes found in wild birds may constitute a danger for commercially raised birds. **The nematodes are**, with very few exceptions, **sexually different**. The male can usually be differentiated from the female by the presence of two (rarely one) chitinous (horny) structures known as **"spicules"**, located in the posterior end of the body. **The spicules are considered as intromittent** (that which inserts) **organs for use during copulation**. They keep the vulva and vagina open and guide the sperm into the female. Eggs or larvae are discharged through the vulva.

Development

Nematodes of poultry have either **direct or an indirect type of development**. About one-half require no intermediate hosts, whereas the others depend on such **intermediate hosts** as insects, snails, and slugs for the early stage of development.

Nematodes normally pass through four developmental stages before reaching the **fifth or final stage**. Successive stages are preceded by shedding of the skin (**"moulting"**). In some nematodes, the loosened skin or cuticle is retained for a short time as a protective covering; in others it is shed at once.

Eggs deposited reach the outside in the droppings. Existence outside the body is necessary for eggs to become infective. The conditions existing within the definitive (final) host are usually unfavourable to the development of the eggs. Outside the host, in the required optimum moisture and temperature, eggs undergo development. Eggs of some nematodes require only a few days to complete embryonation; others require several weeks. **In case of nematodes with direct life cycle, the final host becomes infected by eating embryonated eggs containing the second-stage larvae,** or free larvae. In case of those **with indirect life cycle, the intermediate host** ingests the embryonated eggs or free larvae, and retains the larvae within the body tissues. **The final host becomes infected either by eating the infected intermediate host, or by injection of the larvae by a blood-feeding arthropod.**

Nematodes of the Digestive Tract

Ascaridia galli

Ascaridia are the largest nematodes of birds. The adults live in the lumen of the **small intestine, but the larval stages invade the mucosa.** *A. galli* occurs in **chickens,** turkey, duck, and goose. It is usually found in the lumen of the intestine, sometimes in the oesophagus, crop, gizzard, oviduct, and body cavity. *A. galli* are large worms. The male is 50-76 mm long; the female is 60-116 mm long. The eggs are oval-shaped, thick-shelled, and not embryonated at the time of deposition.

The life cycle of *A. galli* **is direct.** Infective eggs hatch either in the proventriculus or the duodenum. The **young larvae,** after hatching, live free in the lumen of the duodenum for the first 9 days, then **penetrate the mucosa and cause haemorrhage.** The young worms enter the lumen of the duodenum by the 17th or 18th day and remain there until maturity, at about 28-30 days after ingestion of embryonated eggs. Larvae may enter the tissues, and the large majority spend from 8th to the 17th day in the intestinal mucosa. A few of the larvae penetrate deep into the tissue. However, the majority have only a brief association with the intestinal mucosa during the "**tissue phase".** *A. galli* eggs are ingested by earthworms or grasshoppers, hatch, and are infective to chickens. However, no development of the larvae occurs.

Under optimun conditions of temperature and moisture, eggs in the droppings become infective in 10-12 days. Eggs are quite resistant to low temperatures.

Pathogenicity

A. galli infection causes **weight loss in the bird,** which correlates with increasing worm burden. **In severe infections, intestinal obstruction can occur.** Chickens infected with a large number of ascarids suffer from loss of blood, reduced blood sugar content, increased urates, shrunken thymus glands, **retarded growth, and greatly increased mortality.** However, there are no effects of infection on blood protein level, packed cell volume, or haemoglobin levels. *A. galli* can also have harmful effects through synergism (interaction) with other diseases such as coccidiosis and infectious bronchitis. *A.*

galli have also been shown to contain and **transmit avian reoviruses**.

Sometimes, *A. galli* is found in the hen's egg. It is believed that the worms migrate up the oviduct through the cloaca, and later get included in the egg. Infected eggs can be detected by candling.

Capillaria Infection

Capillaria sp., **though they are the smallest of the nematodes** (given in Table 54), **can be highly pathogenic** when present in large numbers. Different species parasitize different parts of the alimentary tract, and may have **direct or indirect life cycles**. Of all the Capillaria sp., the most common and pathogenic is *C. obsignata*. It is a hair-like worm, which has **a direct life cycle** and can be a problem in birds on litter.

Pathogenicity

Clinical signs include emaciation, diarrhoea, haemorrhagic enteritis, and death. A catarrhal exudate in the upper intestine, and some thickening of the wall, are the most severe gross pathological changes in heavy infections. **The most important effect of infection from a practical point of view is the less efficient utilization of the feed.**

Heterakis gallinarum

H. gallinarum occurs in **chicken**, turkey, duck, goose, pheasant, and quail. It is found in the lumen of the **caecum**. It is a small white worm. **The male is 7-13 mm long, and the female 10-15 mm in length. The eggs are thick-shelled, oval-shaped**, unsegmented when deposited, and similar in appearance to those of *A. galli*.

Life Cycle

The life cycle is direct. Eggs pass out in the faeces in an unsegmented state. In about two weeks, under favourable conditions of temperature and moisture, eggs reach the infective stage. When they are swallowed by a susceptible host, the embryos hatch in the upper part of the intestine. At the end of 24 hours, most of the young worms reach the **caeca**. The larvae are closely associated with and sometimes embedded in the caecal tissue. At postmortem, most of the adult worms are found in the tips or blind ends of the caeca. Earthworms may also ingest the eggs of the **caecal worms**, and may be the means of causing infection in poultry.

Pathogenicity

H.gallinarum is not pathogenic. **The importance of the caecal worm lies in its role in the transmission of histomoniasis (blackhead)**. It acts as a carrier of its causative organism *Histomonas meleagridis*. Histomoniasis can be produced in susceptible birds by feeding embryonated eggs of *H.*

gallinarum taken from histomoniasis-infected birds. This protozoan parasite is found incorporated in the worm egg. Its presence has been identified in the intestinal wall and in the reproductive systems of the male and female and in the developing eggs of the caecal worm.

The **caeca** of infected birds show **marked inflammation and thickening of the walls. In heavy infections, nodules form in the mucosa and submucosa,** as the response of already sensitized caeca to subsequent infection. **Hepatic granulomas** containing the worms have also been reported in chickens.

Nematodes of the Respiratory Tract

Syngamus trachea

S. trachea is the only nematode of importance in the respiratory tract. It occurs in **chicken,** turkey, goose, quail, and many other species. It is **found in the trachea, bronchi, and bronchioles,** and causes the condition of "**gapes**" (laboured breathing due to parasites). *S. trachea* is therefore commonly known as "**gapeworm**". It is sometimes called "**redworm**" because of its colour, or "**forked worm**" because the male and female are in permanent copulation so that they appear like the letter "**Y**". The male is 2-6 mm long, and female 5-20 mm in length. The eggs are oval-shaped and operculated.

Life Cycle

The life cycle may be **direct, or more commonly, indirect,** involving the **earthworms.** Infection can occur either directly from the feeding of embryonated eggs or **infective** larvae, or indirectly by ingestion of earthworms containing free or encysted larvae they had obtained by feeding on contaminated soil. The female gapeworm deposits eggs through the vulvar opening. The eggs reach the mouth cavity, are swallowed, and pass to the outside in the droppings. Within 8-14 days under optimum conditions of moisture and temperature, eggs embryonate, and soon thereafter hatch, with the larvae living free in the soil. The earthworms become infected with gapeworm larvae. **Within the earthworm,** the larvae penetrate the intestinal wall, enter the body cavity, and finally invade the body musculature. **Gapeworm larvae in the earthworm remain infective to young chickens for as long as 4 years.** Snails and slugs may also serve as transfer hosts of larvae. Snails are not true intermediate hosts, since they are not necessary for the transfer of gapeworms to birds.

Some **infective larvae** penetrate the wall of the crop and oesophagus, and then penetrate the **lungs** directly. However, the majority penetrate the duodenum and are carried to the lungs by the portal circulation through the liver and heart. Larvae break out of the capillaries of the lung into the interlobular connective tissue and migrate into the parabronchia and atria through air capillaries. Moulting and development to the adult stage can occur within 4 days of infection, and copulation by 6 days. Adults enter the trachea by 7 days, and males are firmly attached to the tracheal wall by 11 days. **About 2 weeks are required for the infective larvae to reach sexual maturity and for eggs to appear in the droppings**. Soil can remain infected for years. The disease is now usually seen in birds reared in outdoor pens, such as game birds and zoo birds.

Pathogenicity

S. trachea causes **"gapes" in chickens**. Disease is due to physical blockage of the airway by parasites. This causes **dyspnoea** (laboured breathing), **characterized by an outstretched neck with open mouth. Young birds are most seriously affected with gapeworms**. The rapidly growing worms soon obstruct the lumen of the trachea **and cause the birds to suffocate**. Turkey poults and baby chicks are most susceptible to infection. Turkey poults usually develop gapeworm signs earlier and begin to die sooner after infection, than young chickens.

Clinical Signs

Birds infected with gapeworms show signs of weakness and emaciation. They spend much of their time with **eyes closed and head drawn back against the body**. From time to time, they throw their heads forward and upward **and open the mouth wide to draw in air (gape)**. An infected bird may give its head a convulsive shake in an attempt to remove the obstruction from the trachea so that normal breathing is restored. Little or no food is taken by birds in the advanced stages of infection, and **death usually occurs**.

Lesions

Trachea shows extensive inflammation of the mucous membrane. Coughing is the result of irritation to the mucous lining. Lesions are usually found in the trachea of turkeys, but rarely in the trachea of young chickens. These lesions or **nodules** are produced as a result of an inflammatory reaction **at the site of attachment of the male worm, which remains permanently attached to the tracheal wall throughout the duration of its life**. The female worms detach and reattach from time to time to obtain a good supply of food. The net blood loss with *S. trachea* is minimal.

10

Arthropod Diseases

Parasitic Arthropods

The Phylum Arthropoda has five classes. Of these, only Insecta and Arachnida contain most of the parasitic species and the vectors of disease-producing viruses, protozoa, nematodes, rickettsia and spirochaetes. The Class Insecta contains six-legged insects, mosquitoes and flies, and Class Arachnida, ticks and mites.

Many species in both the Classes, Insecta and Arachnida, are parasites which bite animals or suck their blood. Horse flies, stable flies, tsetse flies, horn flies, gnats or black flies, sheep keds, midges, mosquitoes, kissing bugs, bees, wasps, hornets, biting and sucking lice and fleas come under this category. Many are merely annoying, or cause only temporary discomfort. However, their irritation can lead to traumatic dermatitis due to the animals rubbing, or biting the irritated skin. Others, such as fleas or lice, can be present in sufficient numbers to cause blood loss anaemia. These and several of the other superficial insects and arachnids may also incite hypersensitivity skin diseases.

Myiasis

Myiasis is the infestation of animal tissues by the larvae of flies. Clinical classification is based on the sites of invasion by these larvae.

1. **Cutaneous** : Larvae live in or under the skin. Example: cattle warble;

2. **Intestinal** : Larvae live in the stomach or intestines. Example: horse "bots";

3. **Atrial** : Larvae live in the oral, nasal, ocular, sinusal, vaginal, and urethral cavities. Example : *Oestrus ovis;*

4. **Wound-invading** : ("Screw-worm larvae"); and

5. **External** : (Blood-sucking larvae).

Some fly larvae occupy more than one of these sites during the course of development in the host. Many fly larvae are specific parasites of a certain host; others are non-specific. That is, they are deposited in or near diseased or wounded tissues in which they find a favourable environment.

Botflies

The genus **Gasterophilus** contains **five species** whose **larvae**, i.e., **bots** ("**bot**" is larva of a fly) are parasitic for **horses**. *Gasterophilus intestinalis* is a brown fly and **occurs mainly in the United States**. It deposits its eggs mostly on the hair of horse's fetlocks or forelegs. These eggs are ready to hatch in 5-10 days. However, hatching requires licking or rubbing by the horse. This action helps the **larvae** reach the animal's mouth, where they penetrate the mucosa of the tongue. The developing larvae remain in the tongue for 21-28 days. Then they migrate to the stomach, and with their mouth parts, attach to the cardiac portion of the mucosa. The bot larvae at this stage have a reddish colour. **Each larva causes** a small, umbilicated (having a central depression) **ulcer at the site of attachment.** Large numbers of bots obviously interfere with function in the affected part of the stomach. However, only occasionally do they produce general debility in the host. Usually, the host tolerates them well without visible effect. The larvae remain attached to the mucosa, living on blood and tissue, for 10-12 months. After this period, they loosen their hold and pass out with the faeces. The larvae pupate in soil for 3-5 weeks, and then emerge as adults.

G. haemorrhoidalis, the '**nose botfly**', is a small red-tailed fly. It also **occurs mainly in the United States**. It lays its eggs on hairs around the mouth, nose, and cheeks of **horses**. The larvae hatch from these eggs, then penetrate the skin of the face and wander into the mouth. The young red-coloured larvae eventually become attached at the cardia of the stomach. Here they have a similar effect to that of *G. intestinalis*, and remain for 10-12 months at this site before passing to the rectum. There, they again attach for a few days before passing out with the faeces. The rest of the life cycle is similar to that of *G. intestinalis*.

G. nasalis, the '**chin**' or '**throat**' **fly**, lays its eggs on hairs in the intermandibular region of **horses**. It also **occurs mainly in the United States**. The larvae migrate to attach to the mucosa of the pylorus and duodenum. Otherwise, their life cycle and effects upon the host are similar to those of *G. intestinalis*.

G. pecorum is a botfly whose female deposits eggs on the hoofs of **horses**. **It occurs mainly in Europe**. The eggs must be rubbed or licked by the horse before the larvae can emerge. The larvae penetrate the mucosa of the cheeks. The third-stage larvae attach to the stomach mucosa, and before leaving the host, attach to the rectal mucosa for a few days.

G. inermis is a botfly whose female deposits eggs on hairs around the mouth and cheeks of horses. It also occurs mainly in Europe. The larvae penetrate the skin, and leave tracks as they wander towards the mucosa. The third-stage larvae attach to the mucosa of rectum. Otherwise the life cycle is similar to that of *G. intestinalis*. The species which occurs in Asia is *G. nigricornis*.

Oestrus ovis is the botfly or **"head grub"** (grub = larva, bot) of **sheep.** It **deposits its larvae in the nose of sheep.** The larvae migrate into the nasal cavity and nasal sinuses, where they undergo further development. Their growth and development result in **serious damage to the tissue, and may cause death**. The larvae eventually drop to the ground, where they pupate and later emerge as adult flies.

Warbles, Heel Flies (Hypoderma)

The genus **Hypoderma**, which is in the same Family (**Oestridae**) to which *O. ovis* belongs, contains **two important species** : *Hypoderma bovis* and *H. lineatum*. These are the yellow and black **"warble" or heel flies of cattle,** which sometimes attack **horses,** and rarely **humans.** These flies produce 'warbles', hence the name **warble fly. A 'warble' is a swelling under the skin caused by the maggots of a warble fly or botfly.**

The female fly deposits eggs on the hair of the legs (hence the name '**heel flies**'), flanks, or dewlap of **cattle.** This produces irritation. The larvae hatch from these eggs and penetrate the skin, and begin to wander throughout the body. *H. lineatum* eventually reaches the wall of the oesophagus, whereas *H. bovis* reaches the epidermal tissues of the spinal cord. Here they reside for weeks and then they migrate to the subcutaneous tissue of the back, where they remain in **an encapsulated nodule (warble).** They gradually produce holes in the epidermis, through which the group of larvae eventually emerge. After reaching the ground, the larvae pupate and emerge as adult flies 40-50 days later. Heavy infestation leaves the skin with many holes which make the hide unfit for use. **Larvae may migrate to abnormal sites, such as brain, and cause death**. Mechanical rupture of a cyst containing larvae in the skin can also lead to **serious hypersensitivity reactions, including anaphylaxis.**

Screw-Worm Fly

The 'screw-worm' flies *Callitroga hominivorax* and *C. macellaria* are parasitic flies, which **are obligate parasites.** Their larvae develop only in wounds of animals and man leading to **myiasis. The pathogenic effects of this fly are produced by the larvae,** which feed upon living tissues and thus produce serious effects upon their host. **In humans,** harmful effects are produced by maggots invading the nasopharynx (naso-pharyngeal myiasis). **In animals,** the larvae attack any wound by which they can gain entrance. In

cluding e quine encephalomyelitis a nd canine d irofilariasis, are t ransmitted. **Mosquito bite hypersensitivity** has been recently described **in cats** characterized by alopecia, depigmentation, and swelling of the skin.

Acariasis

Within the Class **Arachnida**, the Order **Acarina** contains **ticks** and **mites**. Both of these are at times parasitic to animals. These and other ectoparasites, such as fleas and lice, are usually not associated with serious disease, **except when present in large numbers.** All these parasites **cause variable degrees of inflammation at the site of attachment or bite,** which results from mechanical irritation, **immediate hypersensitivity reactions** (localized anaphylaxis or Arthus-type reaction), **d elayed hypersensitivity reaction** (contact d ermatitis), or the introduction of secondary bacteria.

Ticks are particularly important as vectors of disease-producing agents. Except when present in large numbers or in particular sites, as in the ears, they do not produce any immediate or serious effect upon the host. An important exception is **tick paralysis.** It is a striking paralytic disease observed in **humans, sheep, dogs, cats,** and other species. **Twenty-two species of ticks have been associated with paralysis in various parts of the world.** Paralysis may disappear quickly when the offending ticks a re removed. **Young and small animals are more susceptible,** a nd require f ewer t icks t o induce p aralysis. **Death** occurs i n a nimals a nd h umans when the ticks a re n ot d etected a nd removed in time. The **paralysis** results from a **neuroparalytic toxin secreted by the tick.** However, its mode of action is not entirely clear, although it is believed to **interfere with the release of acetylcholine.**

The **tissue-burrowing habits of mites** cause them to produce more visible lesions in animals than do ticks. Common mites which are pathogenic for animals are listed in **Table 55.** These mites are described in groups according to the body system which they attack, that is, **pulmonary, intestinal,** and **urinary.**

Table 55. Important acarid (mite) animal parasites

Mite	Site	Disease	Hosts
Demodex folliculorum, D. phylloides, D. cati, D. canis, D. bovis, D. equi, D. ovis	Hair follicles, sebaceous glands	Demodectic mange	Humans, pig, dog, cat, cattle, horse, sheep
Sarcoptes scabiei var. *suis, bovis,* etc.	Epidermis, general	Scabies, sarcoptic mange	Dog, cat, cattle, sheep, pig, horse, humans
Notoedres cati	Epidermis, esp. ears, face, neck	Notoedric mange	Cat

Psoroptes ovis	Epidermis, general	Psoroptic mange, sheep scab	Sheep, cattle
Psoroptes equi	Epidermis, general	Psoroptic mange	Horse
Psoroptes cuniculi	Ears	Psoroptic mange	Rabbit, sheep, goat, horse
Chorioptes equi, C. bovis, C. ovis	Epidermis, legs, base of tail	Chorioptic mange	Horse, cattle, sheep
Otodectes cynotis	Ears	Otodectic mange	Dog, cat,
Psorergates ovis	Epidermal cysts, skin	Psorergatic mange	Sheep
Pneumonyssus caninum	Paranasal sinuses	Mite infection	Dog
Pneumonyssus simicola	Bronchioles, alveoli	Pulmonary acariasis	Monkeys
Linguatula serrata	Nasal and respiratory passages	Pentastomiasis or linguatuliasis	Dog, horse, goat, sheep, humans

Pulmonary Acariasis

This occurs in **monkeys** and is caused by the **lung mite** *Pneumonyssus simicola*. It is most common in **rhesus monkeys**. The presence of mites in the bronchi and bronchioles produces characteristic lesions. These include bronchiolitis, peribronchiolitis, and occasional bronchiectasis.

A related mite, *Pneumonyssus caninum*, is seen at times in the paranasal sinuses and upper respiratory tracts of **dogs**. The presence of these mites may result in **purulent sinusitis**.

Pentastomiasis (Linguatuliasis)

Organisms related to the mites and grouped in the Class **Pentastomida** include several genera which are parasitic in mammals. *Linguatula serrata* (*Pentastomum taenioides*) is a tongue-shaped, worm-like arthropod that inhibits the nasal and respiratory passages of the **dog, horse, goat, sheep, and human**. Eggs expelled from the nostrils are ingested by suitable intermediate hosts. These are **usually sheep or cattle**, but **pigs, horses**, and other species can be infected. The eggs hatch in the digestive tract, penetrate the intestinal wall, and localize in mesenteric lymph nodes or other tissues. There, the larvae grow to the infective stage. **Dogs become infected by eating tissues containing larvae**.

Cutaneous Acariasis (Mange, Scabies, Scab, Mite Infestation)

A **wide variety of mites parasitize the skin of animals**. Many of them produce serious lesions. In general, each species of mite has its specific host and will not flourish on any other. Collectively, **parasitism with mites is called "mange"**.

Demodectic Mange (Follicular Mange, Red Mange)

Mites of the genus **Demodex** are parasites of **hair follicles and sebaceous glands of most animals, including humans**. When they are present in large numbers they produce severe lesions in the skin. It is not clear what allows the mites to proliferate unchecked in some animals. **Demodex** species include *D. canis*, *D. cati*, *D. bovis*, *D. ovis*, *D. equi*, *D. phylloides* (pigs), and *D. folliculorum* (humans). **Demodex sp. are obligate parasites.** No stage of their cycle occurs outside the skin. Transmission is by direct contact. **Clinical disease is most common in dogs, cattle, and pigs.**

These mites burrow into the hair follicles of the skin. This produces **intense itching** accompanied by alopecia and scaling of the epidermis. Rubbing of the affected part promotes exudation of serum and scab formation on the denuded surface. The mites may burrow into sebaceous or sweat glands, or to the depths of hair follicles. This causes proliferation and then necrosis of the epithelium, and is followed by intense inflammation of the underlying dermis. This takes the form of **small abscesses, granulomas** with giant cells, and diffuse infiltration of lymphocytes. In some cases, the mites migrate even deeper and reach lymph nodes. **Secondary pyogenic infections can result in death.** Tissue sections reveal deep **folliculitis** (inflammation of hair follicles) and **dermatitis**, in which the parasites are easily demonstrated. **Deep scrapings of affected skin may also be examined microscopically for the mites.**

Sarcoptic Mange

This is caused by a specific mite, *Sarcoptes scabiei* (**sarcoptic mange mite**), which **affects many species**, including **cattle, sheep, dogs, pigs, horses, and humans**. Varieties of *S. scabiei*, such as *bovis* and *suis*, are found in each host species. They are morphologically indistinguishable. Each variety of mite has its definite host preference.

The sarcoptic mange mite burrows in the deeper parts of the stratum corneum, or the superficial layers of the stratum Malpighii of the skin, and rarely goes deeper. It completes its entire life cycle at this level. Even in this superficial position, the mites cause severe itching, hyperkeratosis, and acanthosis. This leads to **loss of hair or wool**. The intense pruritus causes rubbing of the skin, which in turn causes loss of epithelium and secondary infection of the dermis. **In dogs, pruritus is much more intense in sarcoptic than in demodectic mange.**

Notoedric Mange

This is mainly a disease of **cats** caused by *Notoedres cati*. It resembles sarcoptic mange. **Lesions** usually occur around the ears, face and neck, but may extend and become generalized.

Psoroptic Mange

Psoroptic mange occurs in several species of animals. However, it is **most important in sheep (sheep scab) and cattle**, where it is caused by *Psoroptes ovis*. Psoroptes species do not burrow into the epidermis, but **remain on the surface**.

Chorioptic Mange

This is caused by different species of **Chorioptes**. It is most common in **horses** (*C. equi*), **cattle**, (*C. bovis*), and **sheep** (*C. ovis*). In **horses**, the mites tend to localize on the legs. This leads to **foot mange** or **leg itch**.

Otodectic Mange

This is common in **dogs** and **cats**. It is caused by *Otodectes cynotis*, which lives in the **ear canal**. The mites live on the surface but produce intense itching. This leads to head-shaking and scratching. This usually results in **haematomas of the pinna**. It may also lead to **otitis media or interna**, and even **encephalitis**.

Psorergatic Mange

This is mainly a disease of **sheep** caused by *Psorergates ovis*. The mite lives on the skin surface and causes **pruritus** (severe itching) and **dermatitis**.

Ectoparasites of Poultry

Lice

Lice are common external parasites of birds. **Several species of biting (chewing) lice (order Mallophaga) may infect poultry**. More than 40 species have been reported from the chicken. Birds usually harbour several species at the same time. Lice move from one bird species to another if these hosts are in close contact (**cross contamination**). For example, pigeon lice are usually found on domestic fowl if pigeons nest above the fowl.

Lice vary in size from less than 1 mm to over 6 mm in length. They spend their entire life cycle on the host and **cause irritation by feeding on skin and feather**. Eggs are attached to the feathers, often in clusters, and require 4-7 days to hatch. The entire life cycle takes about three weeks for completion. **One pair of lice may produce 1,20,000 progeny within a few months.**

Menacanthus stramineus is probably the **commonest in chickens.** It is found on the skin, especially around the cloaca and on the breast and thighs. They lay eggs on the base of the feathers. Although lice usually eat feather products, *M. stramineus* may **consume blood by puncturing soft quills near the bases** and gnawing through the covering layers of the skin itself.

Severe lousiness in poultry may lead to **weight loss and low production.** Lice are not highly pathogenic to mature birds, but **lice-infected chicks may die.** Lousiness is usually associated with manifestations of poor health, such as internal parasitism, infectious disease, and malnutrition, as well as poor **sanitation.** Lice infestations tend to increase in **winter.**

Other species of the lice in chickens include *Lipeurus caponis* in the wing and tail feathers, *Cuclotogaster heterographus* on feathers of the head and *Goniocotes gallinae* on down feathers.

Lousiness (pediculosis) is **diagnosed** by finding the straw-coloured lice on skin, or feathers of birds.

Fleas

Several species of flea have been reported from poultry worldwide. Fleas breed away from the host and can keep infesting the environment for many months. However, *Echidnophaga gallinacea* is an unusual flea in that it remains attached to the host for days or weeks. **The irritation and blood loss caused can be severe.** The adult fleas are susceptible to treatment, but re-infestation can occur from the environment where the eggs and larvae develop.

Mites

Two species of non-burrowing mite can be serious ectoparasites due to their blood-sucking habits. These are *Dermanyssus gallinae* (**the red mite**) and *Ornithonyssus* (*Liponyssus*) *sylviarum* (**the northern fowl mite**). They are blood-suckers and can run rapidly on skin and feathers. *D. gallinae* is widely distributed throughout the world and infests chickens and other birds. **It feeds mainly at night,** hiding during the day in cracks and crevices in cages and buildings, where the eggs are laid. As a result, inspection of birds during the day may not reveal infestation. **Inspection during the night is usually necessary to find mites on the birds. Sparrows** may transmit this parasite because of the habit of lining their nests with chicken feathers. These mites may not only produce **anaemia,** thereby seriously **lowering production** and increasing feed consumption, but actually **kill birds,** particularly **chicks** or **laying hens. Dermanyssus** can transmit *Borrelia anserina,* the cause of **spirochaetosis.**

O. sylviarum may be common in caged layers. Unlike **D**. *gallinae*, this mite can easily be found on birds in the day as well as night, since it breeds continuously and **never leaves the host**. When birds are handled, mites quickly crawl over the examiner's hands and arms. Parting feathers reveals mites and their eggs. In heavy infestations, they cause **blackening of feathers** due to the excreta and dark egg masses. **These mites suck blood**. Of greater concern is the economic importance of this mite to **egg production** from infested caged layers.

Burrowing mites of the genus **Cnemidocoptes** may cause feather loss **(depluming itch mite,** *C. gallinae*), or excessive scaliness of the skin, leading to thickening and even deformation of the legs (**scaly leg mite,** *C. mutans*). Some affected birds with *C. gallinae* lose weight and show lowered production. **Diagnosis is confirmed by examining skin scrapings** cleared in 10% potassium or sodium hydroxide. Other mites which may cause problems include **some invasive species which may be found in airsacs** (*Cytodites nudis/nudus*) or in the loose subcutaneous connective tissue (*Laminiosioptes cysticola*).

C. nudis (*C. nudus*) may also be found in bronchi, lungs, airsacs and bone cavities of chickens. These mites are believed to be responsible for **emaciation, peritonitis, pneumonia, and obstruction of air passages, and are predisposing factors for tuberculosis.** *L. cysticola* does not appear to influence the health of the infested birds. These subcutaneous mites occur inside yellowish nodules, **which are often mistaken for tuberculous lesions**. The nodules appear to be caseo-calcareous deposits formed by the bird to enclose mites after they die in the tissues.

Ticks

The most important tick is the soft tick, *Argas persicus* (Family **Argasidae**). It is widely distributed in tropical and subtropical areas. The instars (the stage between two successive moults) feed blood for short periods at night. However, they spend most of their time away from the host, hidden in cracks and crevices. Apart from causing **anaemia, anorexia, weight loss and decreased egg production**, *Argas persicus* transmits *Borrelia anserina* (cause of **spirochaetosis**).

INDEX

Page numbers ending in the letter 't' refer to tables.

A

Aberrant hosts, 553
Acanthocephala, 523, 566
AcAP, 553
Acariasis, 602
Acholeplasma, 443, 446, 449
Actinobacillosis, 275
Actinobacillus, 275
Actinobacillus capsulatus, 275
Actinobacillus equuli, 275, 277
Actinobacillus lignieresii, 275, 276
Actinobacillus mallei, 314
Actinobacillus seminis, 275, 277
Actinobacillus suis, 275, 277
Actinomyces, 347
Actinomyces bovis, 347, 348
Actinomyces hordeovulneris, 348
Actinomyces israeli, 348
Actinomyces naeslundii, 348
Actinomyces pyogenes, 351
Actinomyces suis, 348
Actinomycosis, 347
    in cattle, 348
Adenitis equorum, 272
Adenoviridae, 194, 195t
Adhesins, 231
Aegyptianella, 426
Aelurostrongylus, 571
Aelurostrongylus abstrusus, 571
Aflatoxicosis, 396, 411
    acute, 399
    chronic, 400
Aflatoxin(s), 396, 410
African horse sickness, 136
African pig disease, 205
African swine fever, 205

African trypanosomiasis, 461, 467
Agranulocytosis, 146
Agriostomum vryburgi, 554
Airsac disease, 294
Akabane disease (of cattle), 36, 38
Akabane virus, 38
Alimentary lymphoma, 85
Alpha-herpes virus(es), 150, 152
Alpha toxin, 241, 243, 251, 258, 267
Alphavirus, 20
American leishmaniasis, 461
American trypanosomiasis, 461, **469**
Amoebiasis, 472
Amoebic abscesses, 472, 473
Amoebotaenia cuneata, 589t
Amyloid plaques, 217
Anaemia dermatitis syndrome, 144
Anaplasma, 426
Anaplasma centrale, 426
Anaplasma marginale, 426
Anaplasma ovis, 426
Anaplasmataceae, 426, 430
Anaplasmosis, 426
Ancylostoma braziliense, 553
Ancylostoma caninum, 552, 553
Ancylostomiasis, 551
Ancylostomidae, 551
Anergy, 368
Angara disease, 200, 210, 211
Angiostrongylus, 572
Angiostrongylus cantonensis, 557
Angiostrongylus vasorum, 572
Ankylosis, 452
Anthrax, 236
    zoonotic importance, 238
Anthropophilic (fungus), 378
Antigenic drift, 50
Antigenic shift, 50
Antigenic variation, 467, 528